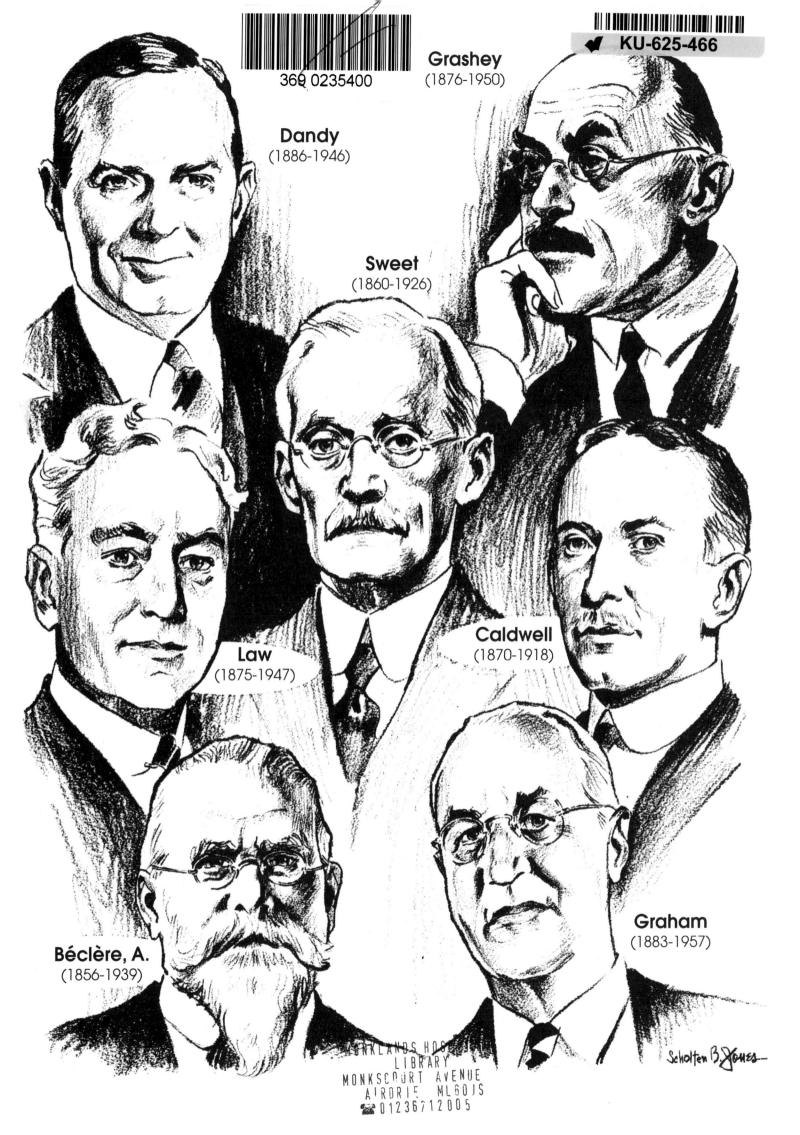

Dandy
(1886-1946)

Grashey
(1876-1950)

Sweet
(1860-1926)

Law
(1875-1947)

Caldwell
(1870-1918)

Béclère, A.
(1856-1939)

Graham
(1883-1957)

Scholten B. Jones

MERRILL'S ATLAS OF
RADIOGRAPHIC POSITIONING & PROCEDURES

THIRTEENTH EDITION | VOLUME THREE

MERRILL'S ATLAS OF
RADIOGRAPHIC POSITIONING & PROCEDURES

Bruce W. Long, MS, RT(R)(CV), FASRT, FAEIRS
Director and Associate Professor
Radiologic Imaging and Sciences Programs
Indiana University School of Medicine
Indianapolis, Indiana

Jeannean Hall Rollins, MRC, BSRT(R)(CV)
Associate Professor
Medical Imaging and Radiation Sciences Department
Arkansas State University
Jonesboro, Arkansas

Barbara J. Smith, MS, RT(R)(QM), FASRT, FAEIRS
Instructor, Radiologic Technology
Medical Imaging Department
Portland Community College
Portland, Oregon

ELSEVIER

ELSEVIER
MOSBY

3251 Riverport Lane
St. Louis, Missouri 63043

MERRILL'S ATLAS OF RADIOGRAPHIC POSITIONING
& PROCEDURES, THIRTEENTH EDITION

ISBN: 978-0-323-26342-9 (vol 1)
ISBN: 978-0-323-26343-6 (vol 2)
ISBN: 978-0-323-26344-3 (vol 3)
ISBN: 978-0-323-26341-2 (set)

Notices

Knowledge and best practice in this field are constantly changing. As new research and experience broaden our understanding, changes in research methods, professional practices, or medical treatment may become necessary.

Practitioners and researchers must always rely on their own experience and knowledge in evaluating and using any information, methods, compounds, or experiments described herein. In using such information or methods, they should be mindful of their own safety and the safety of others, including parties for whom they have a professional responsibility.

With respect to any drug or pharmaceutical products identified, readers are advised to check the most current information provided (i) on procedures featured or (ii) by the manufacturer of each product to be administered, to verify the recommended dose or formula, the method and duration of administration, and contraindications. It is the responsibility of practitioners, relying on their own experience and knowledge of their patients, to make diagnoses, to determine dosages and the best treatment for each individual patient, and to take all appropriate safety precautions.

To the fullest extent of the law, neither the Publisher nor the authors, contributors, or editors assume any liability for any injury and/or damage to persons or property as a matter of product liability, negligence, or otherwise, or from any use or operation of any methods, products, instructions, or ideas contained in the material herein.

The Publisher

Previous editions copyrighted 2012, 2007, 2003, 1999, 1995, 1991, 1986, 1982, 1975, 1967, 1959, 1949

International Standard Book Numbers:
978-0-323-26342-9 (vol 1)
978-0-323-26343-6 (vol 2)
978-0-323-26344-3 (vol 3)
978-0-323-26341-2 (set)

Executive Content Strategist: Sonya Seigafuse
Content Development Manager: Billie Sharp
Content Development Specialist: Betsy McCormac
Publishing Services Manager: Julie Eddy
Senior Project Manager: Richard Barber
Designer: Margaret Reid

Printed in the United States of America

Last digit is the print number: 9 8 7 6 5 4 3 2 1

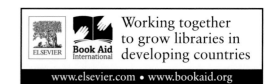

Working together
to grow libraries in
developing countries

www.elsevier.com • www.bookaid.org

PREVIOUS AUTHORS

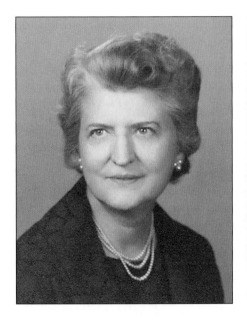

Vinita Merrill
1905-1977

Vinita Merrill was born in Oklahoma in 1905 and died in New York City in 1977. Vinita began compilation of Merrill's in 1936, while she worked as Technical Director and Chief Technologist in the Department of Radiology, and Instructor in the School of Radiography at the New York Hospital. In 1949, while employed as Director of the Educational Department of Picker X-ray Corporation, she wrote the first edition of the *Atlas of Roentgenographic Positions.* She completed three more editions from 1959 to 1975. Sixty-six years later, Vinita's work lives on in the thirteenth edition of *Merrill's Atlas of Radiographic Positioning & Procedures.*

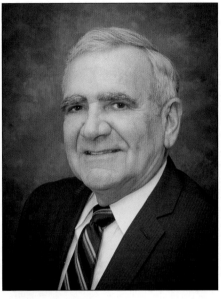

Philip W. Ballinger, PhD, RT(R), FASRT, FAEIRS, became the author of *Merrill's Atlas* in its fifth edition, which published in 1982. He served as author through the tenth edition, helping to launch successful careers for thousands of students who have learned radiographic positioning from *Merrill's.* Phil currently serves as Professor Emeritus in the Radiologic Sciences and Therapy, Division of the School of Health and Rehabilitation Sciences, at The Ohio State University. In 1995, he retired after a 25-year career as Radiography Program Director and, after ably guiding *Merrill's Atlas* through six editions, he retired as *Merrill's* author. Phil continues to be involved in professional activities, such as speaking engagements at state, national, and international meetings.

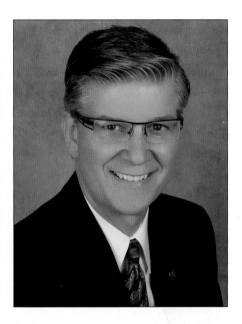

Eugene D. Frank, MA, RT(R), FASRT, FAEIRS, began working with Phil Ballinger on the eighth edition of *Merrill's Atlas* in 1995. He became the coauthor in its ninth and 50th-anniversary edition, published in 1999. He served as lead author for the eleventh and twelfth editions and mentored three coauthors. Gene retired from the Mayo Clinic/Foundation in Rochester, Minnesota, in 2001, after 31 years of employment. He was Associate Professor of Radiology in the College of Medicine and Director of the Radiography Program. He also served as Director of the Radiography Program at Riverland Community College, Austin, Minnesota, for 6 years before fully retiring in 2007. He is a Fellow of the ASRT and AEIRS. In addition to *Merrill's,* he is the coauthor of two radiography textbooks, *Quality Control in Diagnostic Imaging* and *Radiography Essentials for Limited Practice.* He now works in hospice through Christian Hospice Care and helps design and equip x-ray departments in underdeveloped countries.

THE MERRILL'S TEAM

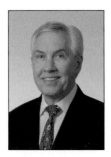

Bruce W. Long, MS, RT(R)(CV), FASRT, FAEIRS, is Director and Associate Professor of the Indiana University Radiologic and Imaging Sciences Programs, where he has taught for 29 years. A Life Member of the Indiana Society of Radiologic Technologists, he frequently presents at state and national professional meetings. His publication activities include 28 articles in national professional journals and two books, *Orthopaedic Radiography* and *Radiography Essentials for Limited Practice,* in addition to being coauthor of the *Atlas.* The thirteenth edition is Bruce's third on the Merrill's team and first as lead author.

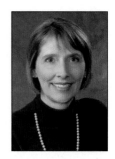

Barbara J. Smith, MS, RT(R)(QM), FASRT, FAEIRS, is an instructor in the Radiologic Technology program at Portland Community College, where she has taught for 30 years. The Oregon Society of Radiologic Technologists inducted her as a Life Member in 2003. She presents at state, regional, national, and international meetings, is a trustee with the ARRT, and is involved in professional activities at these levels. Her publication activities include articles, book reviews, and chapter contributions. As coauthor, her primary role on the Merrill's team is working with the contributing authors and editing Volume 3. The thirteenth edition is Barb's third on the Merrill's team.

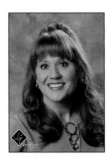

Jeannean Hall Rollins, MRC, BSRT(R) (CV), is an Associate Professor in the Medical Imaging and Radiation Sciences department at Arkansas State University, where she has taught for 22 years. She is involved in the imaging profession at local, state, and national levels. Her publication activities include articles, book reviews, and chapter contributions. Jeannean's first contribution to *Merrill's Atlas* was on the tenth edition as coauthor of the trauma radiography chapter. The thirteenth edition is Jeannean's third on the Merrill's team and first as a coauthor. Her previous role was writing the workbook, Mosby's Radiography Online, and the Instructor Resources that accompany *Merrill's Atlas.*

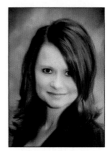

Tammy Curtis, PhD, RT(R)(CT)(CHES), is an associate professor at Northwestern State University, where she has taught for 14 years. She presents on state, regional, and national levels and is involved in professional activities on state level. Her publication activities include articles, book reviews, and book contributions. Previously, Tammy served on the advisory board and contributed the updated photo for Vinita Merrill, as well as other projects submitted to the *Atlas.* Her primary role on the Merrill's team is writing the workbook. The thirteenth edition is Tammy's first on the Merrill's team.

ADVISORY BOARD

This edition of *Merrill's Atlas* benefits from the expertise of a special advisory board. The following board members have provided professional input and advice and have helped the authors make decisions about Atlas content throughout the preparation of the thirteenth edition:

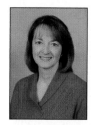

Andrea J. Cornuelle, MS, RT(R)
Professor, Radiologic Technology
Director, Health Science Program
Northern Kentucky University
Highland Heights, Kentucky

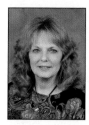

Patricia J. (Finocchiaro) Duffy, MPS, RT(R)(CT)
Clinical Education Coordinator/Assistant
   Professor
Medical Imaging Sciences Department
College of Health Professions
SUNY Upstate Medical University
Syracuse, New York

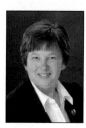

Lynn M. Foss, RT(R), ACR, DipEd, BHS
Instructor, Saint John School of Radiological
   Technology
Horizon Health Network
Saint John, New Brunswick, Canada

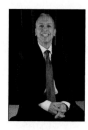

Joe A. Garza, MS, RT(R)
Associate Professor, Radiography Program
Lone Star College—Montgomery
Conroe, Texas

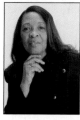

Parsha Y. Hobson, MPA, RT(R)
Associate Professor, Radiography
Passaic County Community College
Paterson, New Jersey

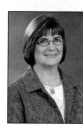

Robin J. Jones, MS, RT(R)
Associate Professor and Clinical Coordinator
Radiologic Sciences Program
Indiana University Northwest
Gary, Indiana

CHAPTER CONTENT EXPERTS

Valerie F. Andolina, RT(R)(M)
Senior Technologist
Elizabeth Wende Breast Care, LLC
Rochester, New York

Dennis Bowman, AS, RT(R)
Clinical Instructor
Community Hospital of the Monterey
  Peninsula
Monterey, California

Terri Bruckner, PhD, RT(R)(CV)
Instructor and Clinical Coordinator,
  Retired
Radiologic Sciences and Therapy
  Division
The Ohio State University
Columbus, Ohio

**Leila A. Bussman-Yeakel, MEd,
RT(R)(T)**
Director, Radiation Therapy Program
Mayo School of Health Sciences
Mayo Clinic College of Medicine
Rochester, Minnesota

Derek Carver, MEd, RT(R)(MR)
Clinical Instructor
Manager of Education and Training
Department of Radiology
Boston Children's Hospital
Boston, Massachusetts

Kim Chandler, MEdL, CNMT, PET
Program Director
Nuclear Medicine Technology Program
Mayo School of Health Sciences
Rochester, Minnesota

**Cheryl DuBose, EdD, RT(R)(MR)
(CT)(QM)**
Assistant Professor
Program Director, MRI Program
Department of Medical Imaging and
  Radiation Sciences
Arkansas State University
Jonesboro, Arkansas

**Angela M. Franceschi, MEd,
CCLS**
Certified Child Life Specialist
Department of Radiology
Boston Children's Hospital
Boston, Massachusetts

Joe A. Garza, MS, RT(R)
Professor, Radiologic Science
Lone Star College—Montgomery
Conroe, Texas

**Nancy Johnson, MEd, RT(R)(CV)
(CT)(QM)**
Faculty Diagnostic Medical Imaging
GateWay Community College
Phoenix, Arizona

**Sara A. Kaderlik, RT(R)(VI), RCIS,
CEPS**
Special Procedures Radiographer
St. Charles Medical Center
Bend, Oregon

Lois J. Layne, MSHA, RT(R)(CV)
Covenant Health
Centralized Privacy
Knoxville, Tennessee

**Cheryl Morgan-Duncan, MAS,
RT(R)(M)**
Radiographer Lab Coordinator/Adjunct
  Instructor
Passaic County Community College
Paterson, New Jersey

Susanna L. Ovel, RT(R), RDMS, RVT
Sonographer, Clinical Instructor
Sutter Medical Foundation
Sacramento, California

**Paula Pate-Schloder, MS, RT(R)
(CV)(CT)(VI)**
Associate Professor, Medical Imaging
  Department
Misericordia University
Dallas, Pennsylvania

**Bartram J. Pierce, BS, RT(R)(MR),
FASRT**
MRI Supervisor
Good Samaritan Regional Medical
  Center
Corvallis, Oregon

Jessica L. Saunders, RT(R)(M)
Technologist
Elizabeth Wende Breast Care, LLC
Rochester, New York

**Sandra Sellner-Wee, MS,
RT(R)(M)**
Program Director, Radiography
Riverland Community College
Austin, Minnesota

Raymond Thies, BS, RT(R)
Department of Radiology
Boston Children's Hospital
Boston, Massachusetts

Jerry G. Tyree, MS, RT(R)
Program Coordinator
Columbus State Community College
Columbus, Ohio

**Sharon R. Wartenbee, RT(R)(BD),
CBDT, FASRT**
Senior Diagnostic and Bone
  Densitometry Technologist
Avera Medical Group McGreevy
Sioux Falls, South Dakota

Kari J. Wetterlin, MA, RT(R)
Lead Technologist, General and
  Surgical Radiology
Mayo Clinic/Foundation
Rochester, Minnesota

Gayle K. Wright, BS, RT(R)(MR)(CT)
Instructor, Radiography Program
CT & MRI Program Coordinator
Medical Imaging Department
Portland Community College
Portland, Oregon

PREFACE

Welcome to the thirteenth edition of *Merrill's Atlas of Radiographic Positioning & Procedures*. This edition continues the tradition of excellence begun in 1949, when Vinita Merrill wrote the first edition of what has become a classic text. Over the past 66 years, *Merrill's Atlas* has provided a strong foundation in anatomy and positioning for thousands of students around the world who have gone on to successful careers as imaging technologists. *Merrill's Atlas* is also a mainstay for everyday reference in imaging departments all over the world. As the coauthors of the thirteenth edition, we are honored to follow in Vinita Merrill's footsteps.

Learning and Perfecting Positioning Skills

Merrill's Atlas has an established tradition of helping students learn and perfect their positioning skills. After covering preliminary steps in radiography, radiation protection, and terminology in introductory chapters, the first two volumes of *Merrill's* teach anatomy and positioning in separate chapters for each bone group or organ system. The student learns to position the patient properly so that the resulting radiograph provides the information the physician needs to correctly diagnose the patient's problem. The atlas presents this information for commonly requested projections, as well as for those less commonly requested, making it the only reference of its kind in the world.

The third volume of the atlas provides basic information about a variety of special imaging modalities, such as mobile and surgical imaging, pediatrics, geriatrics, computed tomography (CT), vascular radiology, magnetic resonance imaging (MRI), sonography, nuclear medicine technology, bone densitometry, and radiation therapy.

Merrill's Atlas is not only a comprehensive resource to help students learn, but also an indispensable reference as they move into the clinical environment and ultimately into practice as imaging professionals.

New to This Edition

Since the first edition of *Merrill's Atlas* in 1949, many changes have occurred. This new edition incorporates many significant changes designed not only to reflect the technologic progress and advancements in the profession, but also to meet the needs of today's radiography students. The major changes in this edition are highlighted as follows.

NEW PATIENT PHOTOGRAPHY

All patient positioning photographs have been replaced in Chapters 4 and 8. The new photographs show positioning detail to a greater extent and in some cases from a more realistic perspective. In addition, the equipment in these photos is the most modern available, and computed radiography plates are used. The use of electronic central ray angles enables a better understanding of where the central ray should enter the patient.

REVISED IMAGE EVALUATION CRITERIA

All image evaluation criteria have been revised and reorganized to improve the student's ability to learn what constitutes a quality image. In addition, the criteria are presented in a way that improves the ability to correct positioning errors.

WORKING WITH THE OBESE PATIENT

Many in the profession, especially students, requested that we include material on how to work with obese and morbidly obese patients. *Joe Garza*, of our advisory board, assisted in the creation of this new section. For this edition, new information and illustrations have been added related to equipment, transportation, communication, and technical considerations specific to this patient population. This was accomplished with input from a wide variety of educators and practitioners with expertise working with obese patients.

FULLY REVISED PEDIATRIC CHAPTER

The pediatric chapter has been completely reorganized, with new photos, images, and illustrations. Time-tested techniques and current technologies are covered. New material has been added addressing the needs of patients with autism spectrum disorders.

UPDATED GERIATRIC CHAPTER

To meet the need of imaging professionals to provide quality care for all elderly patients, material has been added, addressing elder abuse and Alzheimer's disease. Imaging aspects, in addition to patient care challenges, are included.

CONSOLIDATED CRANIAL CHAPTERS

The chapters on the skull, facial bones, and paranasal sinuses have been combined. This facilitates learning by placing the introductory and anatomy material closer to the positioning details for the facial bones and sinuses.

DIGITAL RADIOGRAPHY COLLIMATION

With the expanding use of digital radiography (DR) and the decline in the use of cassettes in Bucky mechanisms, concern was raised regarding the collimation sizes for the various projections. Because collimation is considered one of the critical aspects of obtaining an optimal image, especially with computed radiography

(CR) and DR, this edition contains the specific collimation sizes that students and radiographers should use when using manual collimation with DR in-room and DR mobile systems. The correct collimation size for projections is now included as a separate heading.

ENGLISH/METRIC IR SIZES

English and metric sizes for image receptors (IRs) continue to challenge radiographers and authors in the absence of a standardized national system. With film/screen technology, the trend was toward the use of metric measurements for most of the cassette sizes. However, with CR and DR, the trend has moved back toward English sizes. Most of the DR x-ray systems use English for collimator settings. Because of this trend, the IR sizes and collimation settings for all projections are stated in English, and the metric equivalents are provided in parentheses.

INTEGRATION OF CT AND MRI

In the past three editions, both CT and MRI images have been included in the anatomy and projection pages. This edition continues the practice of having students learn cross-section anatomy with regular anatomy.

NEW ILLUSTRATIONS

Many who use *Merrill's* in teaching and learning have stated that the line art is one of the most useful aspects in learning new projections. New illustrations have been added to this edition to enable the user to comprehend bone position, central ray (CR) direction, and body angulations.

DIGITAL RADIOGRAPHY UPDATED

Because of the rapid expansion and acceptance of CR and direct DR, either selected positioning considerations and modifications or special instructions are indicated where necessary. A special icon alerts the reader to digital notes. The icon is shown here:

COMPUTED RADIOGRAPHY

OBSOLETE PROJECTIONS DELETED

Projections identified as obsolete by the authors and the advisory board continue to be deleted. A summary is provided at the beginning of any chapter containing deleted projections so that the reader may refer to previous editions for information. Continued advances in CT, MRI, and ultrasound have prompted these deletions. The projections that have been removed appear on the Evolve site at evolve.elsevier.com.

NEW RADIOGRAPHS

Nearly every chapter contains updated, optimum radiographs, including many that demonstrate pathology. With the addition of updated radiographic images, the thirteenth edition has the most comprehensive collection of high-quality radiographs available to students and practitioners.

Learning Aids for the Student
POCKET GUIDE TO RADIOGRAPHY

The new edition of *Merrill's Pocket Guide to Radiography* complements the revision of *Merrill's Atlas*. Instructions for positioning the patient and the body part for all the essential projections are presented in a complete yet concise manner. Tabs are included to help the user locate the beginning of each section. Space is provided for the user to write in specifics of department techniques.

RADIOGRAPHIC ANATOMY, POSITIONING, AND PROCEDURES WORKBOOK

The new edition of this workbook features extensive review and self-assessment exercises that cover the first 29 chapters in *Merrill's Atlas* in one convenient volume. The features of the previous editions, including anatomy labeling exercises, positioning exercises, and self-tests, are still available. However, this edition features more image evaluations to give students additional opportunities to evaluate radiographs for proper positioning and more positioning questions to complement the workbook's strong anatomy review. The comprehensive multiple-choice tests at the end of each chapter help students assess their comprehension of the whole chapter. New exercises in this edition focus on improved understanding of essential projections and the need for appropriate collimated field sizes for digital imaging. Additionally, review and assessment exercises in this edition have been expanded for the chapters on pediatrics, geriatrics, vascular and interventional radiography, sectional anatomy, and computed tomography in Volume 3. Exercises in these chapters help students learn the theory and concepts of these special techniques with greater ease. Answers to the workbook questions are found on the Evolve website.

Teaching Aids for the Instructor
EVOLVE INSTRUCTOR ELECTRONIC RESOURCES

This comprehensive resource provides valuable tools, such as lesson plans, PowerPoint slides, and an electronic test bank for teaching an anatomy and positioning class. The test bank includes more than 1,500 questions, each coded by category and level of difficulty. Four exams are already compiled in the test bank to be used "as is" at the instructor's discretion. The instructor also has the option of building new tests as often as desired by pulling questions from the ExamView pool or using a combination of questions from the test bank and questions that the instructor adds.

Evolve may be used to publish the class syllabus, outlines, and lecture notes; set up "virtual office hours" and e-mail communication; share important dates and information through the online class Calendar; and encourage student participation through Chat Rooms and Discussion Boards. Evolve allows instructors to post exams and manage their grade books online. For more information, visit *www.evolve.elsevier.com* or contact an Elsevier sales representative.

MOSBY'S RADIOGRAPHY ONLINE

Mosby's Radiography Online: Merrill's Atlas of Radiographic Positioning & Procedures is a well-developed online course companion for the textbook and workbook. This online course includes animations with narrated interactive activities and exercises, in addition to multiple-choice assessments that can be tailored to meet the learning objectives of your program or course. The addition of this online course to your teaching resources offers greater learning opportunities while accommodating diverse learning styles and circumstances. This unique program promotes problem-based learning with the goal of developing critical thinking skills that will be needed in the clinical setting.

EVOLVE—ONLINE COURSE MANAGEMENT

Evolve is an interactive learning environment designed to work in coordination with

Merrill's Atlas. Instructors may use Evolve to provide an Internet-based course component that reinforces and expands on the concepts delivered in class.

We hope you will find this edition of *Merrill's Atlas of Radiographic Positioning &Procedures* the best ever. Input from generations of readers has helped to keep the atlas strong through 10 editions, and we welcome your comments and suggestions. We are constantly striving to build on Vinita Merrill's work, and we trust that she would be proud and pleased to know that the work she began 66 years ago is still so appreciated and valued by the imaging sciences community.

Bruce W. Long
Jeannean Hall Rollins
Barbara J. Smith
Tammy Curtis

ACKNOWLEDGMENTS

In preparing for the thirteenth edition, our advisory board continually provided professional expertise and aid in decision making on the revision of this edition. The advisory board members are listed on p. vii. We are most grateful for their input and contributions to this edition of the *Atlas.*

Scott Slinkard, a radiography student from the College of Nursing and Health Sciences in Cape Girardeau, Missouri, and a professional photographer, provided many of the new photographs seen throughout the *Atlas.*

Contributors

The group of radiography professionals listed below contributed to this edition of the *Atlas* and made many insightful suggestions. We are most appreciative of their willingness to lend their expertise.

Special recognition and appreciation to the imaging staff of St. Vincent Hospital, Carmel, Indiana, for sharing their extensive experience and expertise in imaging obese and morbidly obese patients, as a Bariatric Center of Excellence. We especially thank Carolyn McCutcheon, RT(R), director of Medical Imaging; Todd Judy, BS, RT(R), team leader of Medical Imaging; and Lindsay Black, BS, RT(R), clinical instructor. Thanks also to Mark

Adkins, MSEd, RT(R)(QM), Radiography Program director, for his assistance.

Special recognition and appreciation to the imaging professionals at NEA Baptist Hospital and St. Bernard's Medical Center in Jonesboro, Arkansas. The time, expertise, and efforts of Gena Morris, RT(R), RDMS, PACS administrator, and Loisey Wortham, RT(R), at NEA Baptist Hospital, and also to Mitzi Pierce, MSHS, RT(R)(M), radiology educator at St. Bernard's Medical Center, have been essential to this revision.

Suzie Crago, AS, RT(R)
Senior Staff Technologist
Riley Hospital for Children
Indianapolis, Indiana

Dan Ferlic, RT(R)
Ferlic Filters
White Bear Lake, Minnesota

Susan Herron, AS, RT(R)
Ezkenazi Health
Indianapolis, Indiana

Joy Menser, MSM, RT(R)(T)
Radiography Program Director
Owensboro Community & Technical
  College
Owensboro, Kentucky

Michael Mial
Student Radiographer
Indiana University Radiography Program
Indianapolis, Indiana
(Patient model for Chapter 8)

Kate Richmond, BS, RT(R)
Radiographer
Indianapolis, Indiana
(Patient model for Chapter 4)

Susan Robinson, MS, RT(R)
Associate Professor of Clinical
  Radiologic and Imaging Sciences
Clinical Instructor at Riley Hospital
  for Children
Indiana University School of Medicine
Indianapolis, Indiana

**Andrew Woodward MA,
RT(R)(CT)(QM)**
Assistant Professor and Clinical
  Coordinator
University of North Carolina at
  Chapel Hill
Chapel Hill, North Carolina

CONTENTS

VOLUME ONE

1 Preliminary Steps in Radiography, 1
2 Compensating Filters, 53
3 General Anatomy and Radiographic Positioning Terminology, 65

4 Upper Limb, 99
5 Shoulder Girdle, 173
6 Lower Limb, 225
7 Pelvis and Proximal Femora, 325
8 Vertebral Column, 363

9 Bony Thorax, 445
10 Thoracic Viscera, 477
Addendum A
Summary of Abbreviations, 521

VOLUME TWO

11 Long Bone Measurement, 1
12 Contrast Arthrography, 7
13 Trauma Radiography, 17
   Joe A. Garza
14 Mouth and Salivary Glands, 57
15 Anterior Part of Neck, 69

16 Abdomen, 81
17 Digestive System: Alimentary Canal, 95
18 Urinary System and Venipuncture, 181
19 Reproductive System, 237
20 Skull, Facial Bones, and Paranasal Sinuses, 255

21 Mammography, 369
   Valerie F. Andolina and Jessica L. Saunders
Addendum B
Summary of Abbreviations, 475

VOLUME THREE

22 Central Nervous System, 1
   Paula Pate-Schloder
23 Vascular, Cardiac, and Interventional Radiography, 19
   Sara A. Kaderlik and Lois J. Layne
24 Pediatric Imaging, 99
   Derek Carver, Angela Franceschi, and Raymond Thies
25 Geriatric Radiography, 161
   Sandra J. Sellner-Wee and Cheryl Morgan-Duncan

26 Mobile Radiography, 183
   Kari J. Wetterlin
27 Surgical Radiography, 213
   Kari J. Wetterlin
28 Sectional Anatomy for Radiographers, 251
   Terri Bruckner
29 Computed Tomography, 301
   Gayle K. Wright and Nancy M. Johnson
30 Magnetic Resonance Imaging, 341
   Bartram J. Pierce and Cheryl DuBose

31 Diagnostic Ultrasound, 369
   Susanna L. Ovel
32 Nuclear Medicine, 399
   Kim Chandler
33 Bone Densitometry, 441
   Sharon R. Wartenbee
34 Radiation Oncology, 479
   Leila A. Bussman-Yeakel

22
CENTRAL NERVOUS SYSTEM
PAULA PATE-SCHLODER

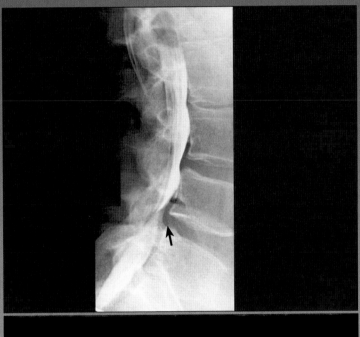

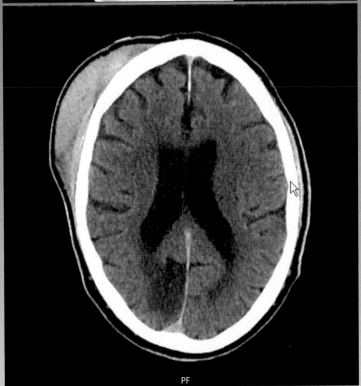

PF

OUTLINE

ANATOMY, 2
Brain, 2
Spinal Cord, 3
Meninges, 3
Ventricular System, 4
RADIOGRAPHY, 5
Plain Radiographic
    Examination, 5
Myelography, 6
Computed Tomography, 10
Magnetic Resonance Imaging, 12
Vascular and Interventional
    Procedures, 14
Other Neuroradiographic
    Procedures, 16
Definition of Terms, 18

For descriptive purposes, the central nervous system (CNS) is divided into two parts: (1) the *brain,** which occupies the cranial cavity, and (2) the *spinal cord,* which is suspended within the vertebral canal.

---

*Many italicized words are defined at the end of the chapter.

Brain

The brain is composed of an outer portion of gray matter called the *cortex* and an inner portion of *white matter.* The brain consists of the *cerebrum; cerebellum;* and *brain stem,* which is continuous with the spinal cord (Fig. 22-1). The brain stem consists of the *midbrain, pons,* and *medulla oblongata.*

The cerebrum is the largest part of the brain and is referred to as the *forebrain.* Its surface is convoluted by sulci and grooves that divide it into lobes and lobules. The stemlike portion that connects the cerebrum to the pons and cerebellum is termed the *midbrain.* The cerebellum, pons, and medulla oblongata make up the *hindbrain.*

A deep cleft, called the *longitudinal sulcus* (interhemispheric fissure), separates the cerebrum into *right* and *left hemispheres,* which are closely connected by bands of nerve fibers, or commissures. The largest commissure between the cerebral hemispheres is the *corpus callosum.* The corpus callosum is a midline structure inferior to the longitudinal sulcus. Each cerebral hemisphere contains a fluid-filled cavity called a *lateral ventricle.* At the diencephalon, or second portion of the brain, the thalami surround the *third ventricle.* Inferior to the diencephalon is the *pituitary gland,* the master endocrine gland of the body. The pituitary gland resides in the hypophyseal fossa of the sella turcica.

The cerebellum, the largest part of the hindbrain, is separated from the cerebrum by a deep transverse cleft. The hemispheres of the cerebellum are connected by a median constricted area called the *vermis.* The surface of the cerebellum contains numerous transverse sulci that account for its cauliflower-like appearance. The tissues between the curved sulci are called *folia.* The pons, which forms the upper part of the hindbrain, is the commissure or bridge between the cerebrum, cerebellum, and medulla oblongata. The medulla oblongata, which extends between the pons and spinal cord, forms the lower portion of the hindbrain. All the fiber tracts between the brain and spinal cord pass through the medulla.

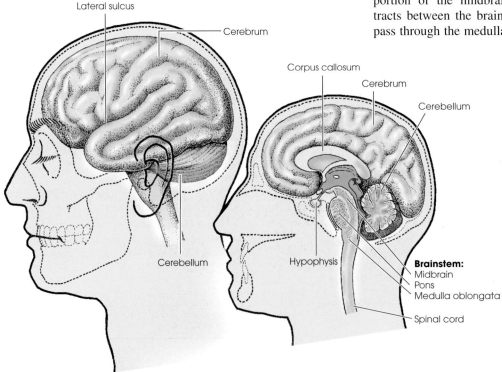

Fig. 22-1 Lateral surface and midsection of brain.

Spinal Cord

The *spinal cord* is a slender, elongated structure consisting of an inner, gray, cellular substance, which has an H shape on transverse section and an outer, white, fibrous substance (Figs. 22-2 and 22-3). The cord extends from the brain, where it is connected to the medulla oblongata at the level of the foramen magnum, to the approximate level of the space between the first and second lumbar vertebrae. The spinal cord ends in a pointed extremity called the *conus medullaris* (see Fig. 22-3). The *filum terminale* is a delicate fibrous strand that extends from the terminal tip and attaches the cord to the upper coccygeal segment.

In an adult, the spinal cord is 18 to 20 inches (46 to 50 cm) long and is connected to 31 pairs of spinal nerves. Each pair of spinal nerves arises from two roots at the sides of the spinal cord. The nerves are transmitted through the intervertebral and sacral foramina. Spinal nerves below the termination of the spinal cord extend inferiorly through the vertebral canal. These nerves resemble a horse's tail and are referred to as the *cauda equina*. The spinal cord and nerves work together to transmit and receive sensory, motor, and reflex messages to and from the brain.

Meninges

The brain and spinal cord are enclosed in three continuous protective membranes called *meninges*. The inner sheath, called the *pia mater* (Latin, meaning "tender mother"), is highly vascular and closely adherent to the underlying brain and cord structure.

The delicate central sheath is called the *arachnoid*. This membrane is separated from the pia mater by a comparatively wide space called the *subarachnoid space*, which is widened in certain areas. These areas of increased width are called *subarachnoid cisterns*. The widest area is the cisterna magna (cisterna cerebellomedullaris). This triangular cavity is situated in the lower posterior fossa between the base of the cerebellum and the dorsal surface of the medulla oblongata. The subarachnoid space is continuous with the ventricular system of the brain and communicates with it through the foramina of the fourth ventricle. The ventricles of the brain and the subarachnoid space contain *cerebrospinal fluid* (CSF). CSF is the tissue fluid of the brain and spinal cord; it surrounds and cushions the structures of the CNS.

The outermost sheath, called the *dura mater* (Latin, meaning "hard mother"), forms the strong fibrous covering of the brain and spinal cord. The dura is separated from the arachnoid by the *subdural space* and from the vertebral periosteum by the *epidural space*. These spaces do not communicate with the ventricular system. The dura mater is composed of two layers throughout its cranial portion. The outer layer lines the cranial bones, serving as periosteum to their inner surface. The inner layer protects the brain and supports the blood vessels. The inner layer also has four partitions that provide support and protection for the various parts of the brain. One of these partitions, the *falx cerebri*, runs through the interhemispheric fissure and provides support for the cerebral hemispheres. The *tentorium* is a tent-shaped fold of dura that separates the cerebrum and cerebellum. Changes in the normal positions of these structures often indicate pathology. The dura mater extends below the spinal cord (to the level of the second sacral segment) to enclose the spinal nerves, which are prolonged inferiorly from the cord to their respective exits. The lower portion of the dura mater is called the *dural sac*. The dural sac encloses the cauda equina.

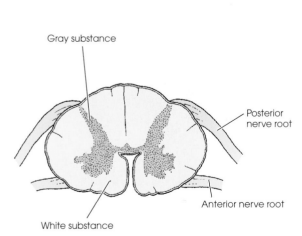

Gray substance

Posterior nerve root

Anterior nerve root

White substance

Fig. 22-2 Transverse section of spinal cord.

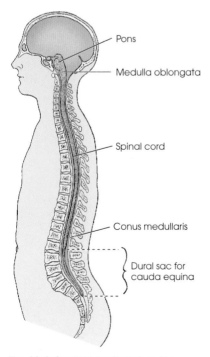

Pons

Medulla oblongata

Spinal cord

Conus medullaris

Dural sac for cauda equina

Fig. 22-3 Sagittal section showing spinal cord.

Ventricular System

The ventricular system of the brain consists of four irregular, fluid-containing cavities that communicate with one another through connecting channels (Figs. 22-4 through 22-6). The two upper cavities are an identical pair and are called the *right* and *left lateral ventricles*. They are situated, one on each side of the midsagittal plane, in the inferior medial part of the corresponding hemisphere of the cerebrum.

Each lateral ventricle consists of a central portion called the *body* of the cavity. The body is prolonged anteriorly, posteriorly, and inferiorly into hornlike portions that give the ventricle an approximate U shape. The prolonged portions are known as the *anterior, posterior,* and *inferior horns*. Each lateral ventricle is connected to the third ventricle by a channel called the *interventricular foramen* or foramen of Monro, through which it communicates directly with the third ventricle and indirectly with the opposite lateral ventricle.

The *third ventricle* is a slitlike cavity with a quadrilateral shape. It is situated in the midsagittal plane just inferior to the level of the bodies of the lateral ventricles. This cavity extends anteroinferiorly from the pineal gland, which produces a recess in its posterior wall, to the optic chiasm, which produces a recess in its anteroinferior wall.

The interventricular foramina, one from each lateral ventricle, open into the anterosuperior portion of the third ventricle. The cavity is continuous posteroinferiorly with the fourth ventricle by a passage known as the *cerebral aqueduct,* or aqueduct of Sylvius.

The *fourth ventricle* is diamond shaped and is located in the area of the hindbrain. The fourth ventricle is anterior to the cerebellum and posterior to the pons and the upper portion of the medulla oblongata. The distal, pointed end of the fourth ventricle is continuous with the central canal of the medulla oblongata. CSF exits the fourth ventricle into the subarachnoid space via the *median aperture* (foramen of Magendie) and the *lateral apertures* (foramen of Luschka).

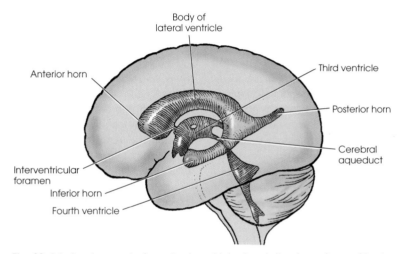

Fig. 22-4 Lateral aspect of cerebral ventricles in relation to surface of brain.

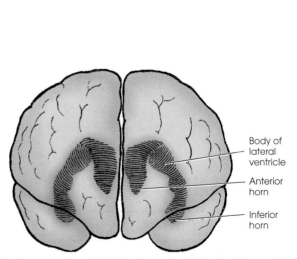

Fig. 22-5 Anterior aspect of lateral cerebral ventricles in relation to surface of brain.

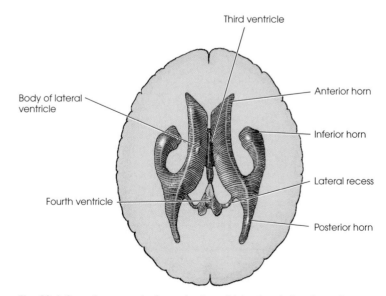

Fig. 22-6 Superior aspect of cerebral ventricles in relation to surface of brain.

Plain Radiographic Examination

Neuroradiologic assessment should begin with noninvasive imaging procedures. Radiographs of the cerebral and visceral cranium and the vertebral column may be obtained to show bony anatomy. In traumatized patients (see Chapter 8), radiographs are obtained to detect bone injury, subluxation, or dislocation of the vertebral column and to determine the extent and stability of the bone injury. Computed tomography is often employed first in a trauma setting due to its speed and ability to demonstrate both soft tissue and bony anatomy (see Chapter 29).

For a traumatized patient with possible CNS involvement, a cross-table lateral cervical spine radiograph may be obtained to rule out fracture or misalignment of the cervical spine. Approximately two thirds of significant pathologic conditions affecting the spine can be detected on this initial image. Care must be taken to show the entire cervical spine adequately including the C7-T1 articulation. Employing the Twining (swimmer's) method (see Chapter 8) may be necessary to show this anatomic region radiographically.

After the cross-table lateral radiograph has been checked and cleared by a physician, the following cervical spine projections should be obtained: anteroposterior (AP), bilateral AP oblique (trauma technique may be necessary), and AP to show the dens. A vertebral arch, or pillar image, of the cervical spine may provide additional information about the posterior portions of the cervical vertebrae (see Chapter 8). An upright lateral cervical spine radiograph may also be requested to show alignment of the vertebrae better and to assess the normal lordotic curvature of the spine.

Radiographs of the spine should always be obtained before myelography. Routine images of the vertebral column are helpful in assessing narrowed disk spaces because of degeneration of the disk, osteoarthritis, postoperative changes in the spine, and other pathologies of the vertebral column. Because the contrast agents used in myelography may obscure some anomalies, noncontrast spinal images complement the myelographic examination and often provide additional information.

Routine skull images may be obtained when the possibility of a skull fracture exists. In trauma patients, a cross-table lateral or upright lateral skull radiograph may be obtained to show air-fluid levels in the sphenoid sinus. In many instances, these air-fluid levels may be the initial indication of a basilar skull fracture. A noncontrast head CT is indicated in head trauma patients who experience a loss of consciousness or other neurologic symptoms. In addition, skull images are helpful in diagnosing reactive bone formation and general alterations in the skull resulting from various pathologic conditions, including Paget disease, fibrous dysplasia, hemangiomas, and changes in the sella turcica.

Myelography

Myelography (Greek, *myelos,* "marrow; the spinal cord") is the general term applied to radiologic examination of the CNS structures situated within the vertebral canal. This examination is performed by introducing a nonionic, water-soluble contrast medium into the subarachnoid space by spinal puncture, most commonly at the L2-3 or L3-4 interspace or at the cisterna magna between C1 and the occipital bone. Injections into the subarachnoid space are termed *intrathecal injections.*

Most myelograms are performed on an outpatient basis, with patients recovering for approximately 4 to 8 hours after the procedure before being released to return home. In many parts of the United States, magnetic resonance imaging (MRI) (see Chapter 30) has largely replaced myelography. Myelography continues to be the preferred examination method for assessing disk disease in patients with contraindications to MRI, such as pacemakers or metallic posterior spinal fusion rods.

Myelography is employed to show extrinsic spinal cord compression caused by a herniated disk, bone fragments, or tumors and spinal cord swelling resulting from traumatic injury. These encroachments appear radiographically as a deformity in the subarachnoid space or an obstruction of the passage of the column of contrast medium within the subarachnoid space. Myelography is also useful in identifying narrowing of the subarachnoid space by evaluating the dynamic flow patterns of the CSF.

CONTRAST MEDIA

A non–water-soluble, iodinated ester (iophendylate [Pantopaque]) was introduced in 1942. Because the body could not absorb it, this lipid-based contrast medium required removal after the procedure. Frequently, some contrast remained in the canal and could be seen on noncontrast radiographs of patients who had the myelography procedure before the introduction of the newer medium. Iophendylate was used in myelography for many years but is no longer commercially available. The first water-soluble, nonionic, iodinated contrast agent, metrizamide, was introduced in the late 1970s. Thereafter, water-soluble contrast media quickly became the agents of choice. Nonionic, water-soluble contrast media provide good visualization of nerve roots (Fig. 22-7) and good enhancement for follow-up CT of the spine. In addition, the body readily absorbs these agents. Over the past 2 decades, nonionic, water-soluble agents, including iopamidol (Isovue) and iohexol (Omnipaque), have become the most commonly used agents for myelography. To reduce the chance of infection, single dose vials are recommended. Improvements in nonionic contrast agents have resulted in fewer side effects.

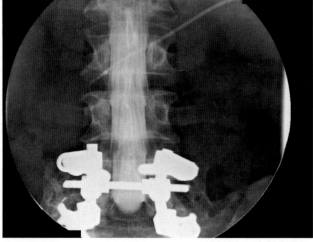

Fig. 22-7 Myelogram using nonionic, water-soluble contrast medium (iopamidol) on a postsurgical patient.

Technologists who perform myelography should be educated regarding the use of contrast media. Intrathecal administration of ionic contrast media may cause severe and fatal neurotoxic reactions. Because vials of ionic and nonionic agents may look similar, radiology departments are encouraged to store contrast media for myelography separately from other agents. Proper medication guidelines must be followed when administering intrathecal agents. Contrast vials should be checked three times, checked with the physician performing the examination, and kept until the procedure has been completed. All appropriate documentation should be completed.

PREPARATION OF EXAMINING ROOM

One of the radiographer's responsibilities is to prepare the examining room before arrival of the patient. The radiographic equipment should be checked. Because the procedure involves aseptic technique, the table and overhead equipment must be cleaned. The footboard should be attached to the table, and the padded shoulder supports should be placed and ready for adjustment to the patient's height. The image intensifier should be locked so that it cannot accidentally come in contact with the spinal needle, sterile field, or both (Fig. 22-8).

The spinal puncture and injection of contrast medium are performed in the radiology department utilizing sterile technique. The Centers for Disease Control and Prevention (CDC) require surgical masks be worn when placing a catheter or injecting material into the spinal canal or subdural space. Under fluoroscopic observation, placement of the 20-gauge to 22-gauge spinal needle in the subarachnoid space is verified, and the contrast medium is injected. The sterile tray and the nonsterile items required for this initial procedure should be ready for convenient placement.

EXAMINATION PROCEDURE

Premedication of the patient for myelography is rarely necessary. The patient should be well hydrated, however, because a nonionic, water-soluble contrast medium is used. To reduce apprehension and prevent alarm at unexpected maneuvers during the procedure, the radiographer should explain the details of myelography to the patient before the examination begins. The patient should be informed that the angulation of the examining table will change repeatedly and acutely. The patient should also be told why the head must be maintained in a fully extended position when the table is tilted to the Trendelenburg position. The radiographer must assure that the patient will be safe when the table is acutely angled and that everything possible will be done to avoid causing unnecessary discomfort. Most facilities require an informed consent form to be completed and signed by the patient and physician.

Scout images including a cross-table lateral lumbar spine prone (Fig. 22-9) are often requested. Some physicians prefer to have the patient placed on the table in the prone position for the spinal puncture. Many physicians have the patient adjusted in the lateral position, however, with the spine flexed to widen the interspinous spaces for easier introduction of the needle.

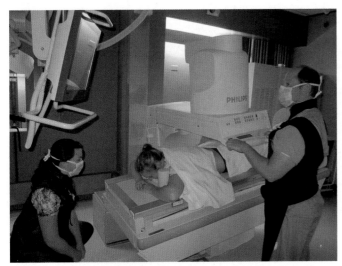

Fig. 22-8 Patient set up with shoulder supports and image intensifier in locked position.

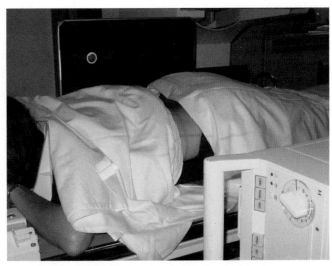

Fig. 22-9 Lateral scout projection of cross-table lumbar spine myelogram.

The physician may withdraw CSF for laboratory analysis. Approximately 9 to 12 mL of nonionic contrast medium is slowly injected. After completing the injection, the physician removes the spinal needle. Travel of the contrast medium column is observed and controlled fluoroscopically. Angulation of the table allows gravity to direct the contrast medium to the area of interest. Spot images are taken throughout the procedure. The radiographer obtains images at the level of any blockage or distortion in the outline of the contrast column. Conventional radiographic studies, with the central ray directed vertically or horizontally, may be performed as requested by the radiologist. The *conus projection* is used to show the *conus medullaris*. For this projection, the patient is placed in the AP position with the central ray centered to T12-L1. A 10- × 12-inch (24- × 30-cm) cassette is used. Cross-table lateral radiographs are obtained with grid-front cassettes or a stationary grid; they must be closely collimated (Figs. 22-10 through 22-14).

The position of the patient's head must be guarded as the contrast medium column nears the cervical area to prevent the medium from passing into the cerebral ventricles. Acute extension of the head compresses the cisterna magna and prevents further ascent of the contrast medium. Because the cisterna magna is situated posteriorly, neither forward nor lateral flexion of the head compresses the cisternal cavity.

After completion of the procedure, the patient must be monitored in an appropriate recovery area. Most physicians recommend that the patient's head and shoulders be elevated 30 to 45 degrees during recovery. Bed rest for several hours is recommended, and fluids are encouraged. The puncture site must be examined before the patient is released from the recovery area.

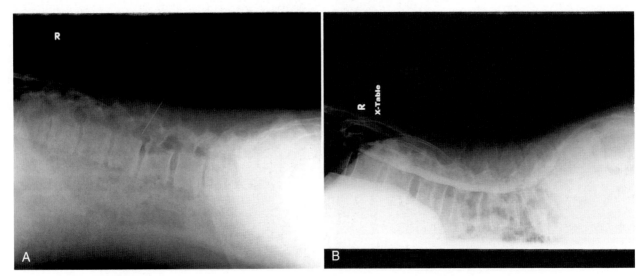

Fig. 22-10 A, Lumbar myelogram. Cross-table lateral showing needle tip in subarachnoid space. **B,** Lumbar myelogram. Cross-table lateral showing contrast enhancement.

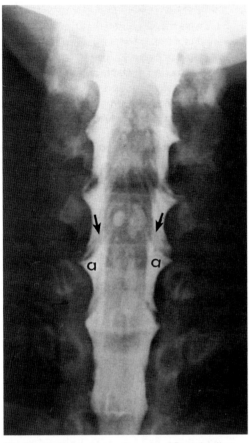

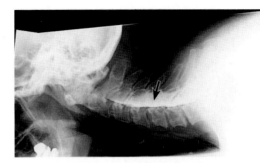

Fig. 22-12 Myelogram. Prone cross-table lateral projection showing dentate ligament and posterior nerve roots (*arrow*).

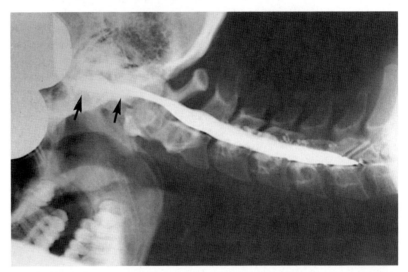

Fig. 22-11 Cervical myelogram. AP projection showing symmetric nerve roots (*arrows*) and axillary pouches (*a*) on both sides and spinal cord.

Fig. 22-13 Myelogram. Prone, cross-table lateral projection showing contrast medium passing through foramen magnum and lying against lower clivus (*arrows*).

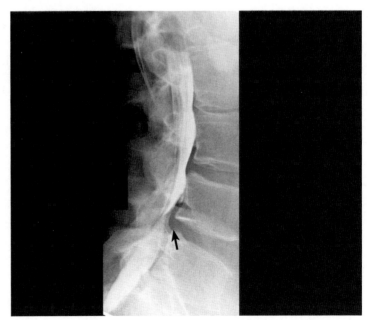

Fig. 22-14 Myelogram. Lateral projection showing subarachnoid space narrowing (*arrow*).

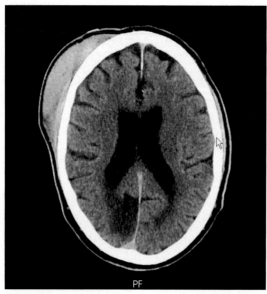

Fig. 22-15 Postinfusion (C1) CT scan of brain showing scalp hematoma in the right frontal region and old infarct in right occipital lobe.

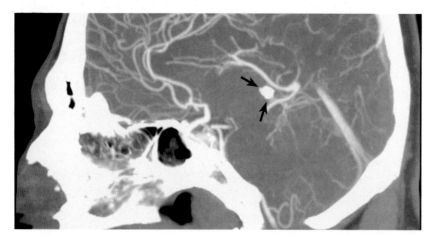

Fig. 22-16 CT angiography of the brain showing aneurysm (*arrows*), later confirmed by vascular imaging.

Computed Tomography

CT is a rapid, noninvasive imaging technique that was first introduced for clinical use in the early 1970s. It produces sectional images of the brain called *slices*. CT imaging of the head and spine expanded rapidly because of improvements in computer technology and the ability of this imaging modality to show abnormalities with a precision never before possible. Digital image processing techniques in CT allow for changes in the density and contrast of an image, called *windowing*. The use of different windows allows for visualization of soft tissue and bony structures, which makes it an essential tool in the diagnosis of traumatic brain injury. (See Chapter 29 for more detail.)

CT examination of the brain is commonly performed in an axial orientation with the gantry placed at an angle of 20 to 25 degrees to the orbitomeatal line, which allows the lowest slice to provide an image of the upper cervical/foramen magnum and the roof of the orbit. Normally, 12 to 14 slices are obtained, depending on the size of the patient's head and the thickness of the CT image slices. Imaging continues superiorly until the entire head has been examined. A slice thickness of 8 to 10 mm is often used; most institutions use 3- to 5-mm slices through the area of the posterior fossa. Coronal images may also be obtained and are helpful in evaluating abnormalities of the pituitary gland and sella turcica and facial bones and sinuses. The computer may be used to reconstruct and display the images in a variety of imaging planes.

CT scans of the brain are often obtained before and after intravenous (IV) injection of a nonionic, water-soluble contrast agent. These are often referred to as *pre-infusion* (C−) and *postinfusion* (C+) scans (Fig. 22-15). Common indications for scans with and without contrast agents include suspected primary neoplasms; suspected metastatic disease; suspected arteriovenous malformation (AVM); demyelinating disease, such as multiple sclerosis; seizure disorders; and bilateral, isodense hematomas. Common indications for CT of the brain without an IV infusion of contrast material include assessment of dementia, craniocerebral trauma, hydrocephalus, and acute infarcts. In addition, CT is often used for postevacuation follow-up examinations of hematomas.

CT of the brain is particularly useful in showing the size, location, and configuration of mass lesions and surrounding edema. CT is also helpful in assessing cerebral ventricle or cortical sulcus enlargement. Shifting of midline structures resulting from the encroachment of a mass lesion, cerebral edema, or a hematoma can be visualized without contrast media. CT of the head is also the imaging modality of choice in evaluating hematomas, suspected aneurysms (Fig. 22-16), ischemic or hemorrhagic strokes, and acute infarcts within the brain. CT of the brain is the initial diagnostic procedure performed to assess craniocerebral trauma because it provides an accurate diagnosis of acute intracranial injuries, such as brain contusions and subarachnoid hemorrhage. Bone windows are used for fracture evaluation of trauma patients (Fig. 22-17).

CT of the spine is helpful in diagnosing vertebral column hemangiomas and lumbar spinal stenosis. CT of the cervical spine is performed frequently after trauma to rule out fractures of the axis and atlas and to show the lower cervical and upper thoracic vertebrae better. This examination can clearly show the size, number, and location of fracture fragments in the cervical, thoracic, and lumbar spine. The information gained from the CT scans can greatly assist the surgeon in distinguishing neural compression by soft tissue from compression by bone (Fig. 22-18). Postoperatively, CT is used to assess the outcome of the surgical procedure. Multiplanar reconstructions are often performed (Fig. 22-19).

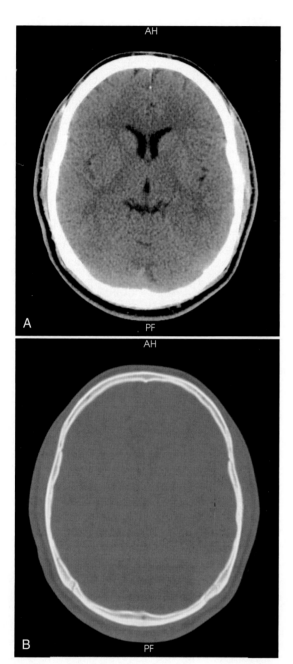

Fig. 22-17 A, Normal CT scan of brain using brain windows. **B,** Normal CT scan of brain using bone windows for fracture evaluation.

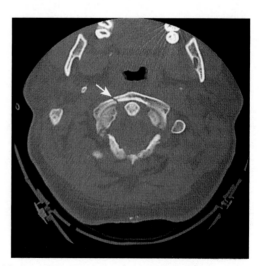

Fig. 22-18 Axial CT image of cervical spine showing fracture of anterior arch of C1 (*arrow*).

Computed tomography myelography (CTM) involves CT examination of the vertebral column after the *intrathecal* injection of a water-soluble contrast agent. The examination may be performed at any level of the vertebral column. At the present time, most conventional myelograms are followed by CTM. Multiple thin sections (1.5 to 3 mm) are obtained with the gantry tilted to permit imaging parallel to the plane of the intervertebral disk. Because CT has the ability to distinguish among relatively small differences in contrast, the contrast agent may be visualized 4 hours after the conventional myelogram. CTM shows the size, shape, and position of the spinal cord and nerve roots (Fig. 22-20). CTM is extremely useful in examining patients with compressive injuries or in determining the extent of dural tears resulting in extravasation of the CSF. (CT is discussed further in Chapter 29.)

Magnetic Resonance Imaging

MRI was approved for clinical use in the early 1980s and quickly became the modality of choice for evaluating many anomalies of the brain and spinal cord. MRI is a noninvasive procedure that provides excellent anatomic detail of the brain, spinal cord, intervertebral disks, and CSF within the subarachnoid space. In contrast to conventional myelography, MRI of the spinal cord and subarachnoid space does not require intrathecal injection of a contrast agent. (MRI is discussed in Chapter 30.)

Because magnetic resonance images are created primarily by the response of loosely bound hydrogen atoms to the magnetic field, this modality is basically "blind" to bone, in contrast to other conventional radiologic imaging modalities. MRI allows clear visualization of areas of the CNS normally obscured by bone, such as the vertebral column and structures in the base of the skull. The exact relationship between soft tissue structures and surrounding bony structures can be seen. This makes MRI the preferred modality in evaluating the middle cranial fossa and posterior fossa of the brain. When these structures are imaged with CT, they are often obscured by artifacts. MRI is also the preferred modality for evaluating the spinal cord because it allows direct visualization of the cord, nerve roots, and surrounding CSF. In addition, MRI may be performed in various planes (sagittal, axial, and coronal) after acquisition to aid in the diagnosis and treatment of neurologic disorders. Various imaging protocols, including T1-weighted and T2-weighted images, may be obtained to assist in the diagnosis, with a head coil used for the brain and cervical spine images and a body coil used in combination with a surface coil for the remainder of the spine. Paramagnetic IV contrast agents, such as gadolinium, are used to enhance tumor visualization (Fig. 22-21).

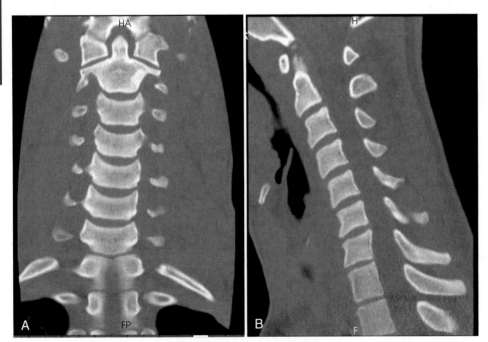

Fig. 22-19 CT coronal and sagittal reconstructions of cervical spine.

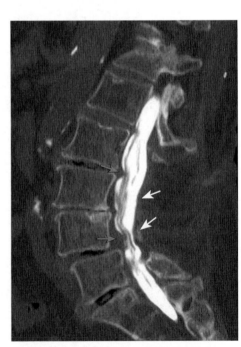

Fig. 22-20 CT myelogram of lumbar spine showing subarachnoid space narrowing (*red arrows*) and cauda equina (*white arrows*).

MRI is helpful in assessing demyelinating disease, such as multiple sclerosis, spinal cord compression, paraspinal masses, postradiation therapy changes in spinal cord tumors, metastatic disease, herniated disks, and congenital anomalies of the vertebral column (Fig. 22-22). In the brain, MRI is excellent for evaluating middle and posterior fossa abnormalities, acoustic neuromas, pituitary tumors, primary and metastatic neoplasms, hydrocephalus, AVMs, and brain atrophy.

Contraindications to MRI are primarily related to the use of a magnetic field. MRI should not be used in patients with pacemakers, ferromagnetic aneurysm clips, or metallic spinal fusion rods. In addition, MRI is of little value in assessing osseous bone abnormalities of the skull, intracerebral hematomas, and subarachnoid hemorrhage. CT provides better visualization of these pathologies.

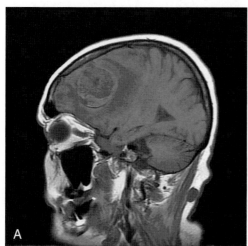

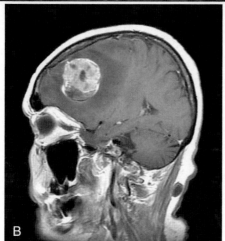

Fig. 22-21 A, Sagittal MRI section through brain showing frontal lobe mass without contrast agent. **B,** After gadolinium injection.

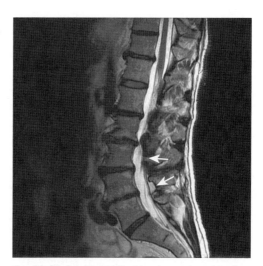

Fig. 22-22 Sagittal MRI of lumbar spine showing distal spinal cord and cauda equina (*arrows*).

Vascular and Interventional Procedures

Vascular and interventional procedures generally are performed after noninvasive evaluation techniques when it is necessary to obtain information about the vascular system or to perform an interventional technique. *Angiography* may be used to assess vascular supply to tumors; show the relationship between a mass lesion and intracerebral vessels; or illustrate anomalies of a vessel, such as an aneurysm or a vascular occlusion. An angiographic procedure is performed in a specialized imaging suite under sterile conditions. (Cardiovascular and interventional radiology of the cerebral circulation is discussed in more detail in Chapter 23.)

Cardiovascular and interventional imaging equipment requires multiplanar imaging and digital subtraction capabilities. Angiographic x-ray tubes should have a minimum focal spot size of 1.3 mm for routine imaging and a magnification focal spot size of 0.3 mm. The procedure requires the introduction of a catheter into the vascular system under fluoroscopic guidance. The image intensifier must be designed to move around the patient so that various tube angles may be obtained without moving the patient. The catheter is most commonly placed in the femoral artery; however, access may be gained using other arteries or veins, depending on the patient's clinical history and the area of interest. After the catheter is placed in the appropriate vessel, a nonionic water-soluble contrast agent is injected into the vessels, and rapid-sequence images are obtained for evaluation.

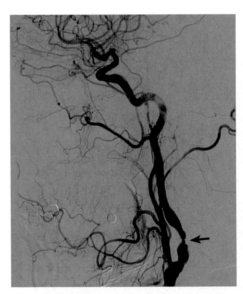

Fig. 22-23 Digital subtraction angiography showing stenosis of internal carotid artery at bifurcation (*arrow*).

Angiography is helpful in assessing vascular abnormalities within the CNS, such as arteriosclerosis (Fig. 22-23), AVMs, aneurysms, subarachnoid hemorrhage, transient ischemic attacks, certain intracerebral hematomas, and cerebral venous thrombosis. Cerebral angiography provides a presurgical road map (Figs. 22-24 and 22-25) and is performed in combination with interventional techniques to assess the placement of devices before and after the procedures.

Interventional radiology involves the placement of various coils, medications, filters, stents, or other devices to treat a particular problem or provide therapy. One type of interventional technique involves the introduction of small spheres, coils, or other materials into vessels to occlude blood flow. Embolization techniques are often performed to treat AVMs and aneurysms and to decrease blood supply to various vascular tumors. Other interventional techniques are used to open occluded vessels by the injection of specialized thrombolytic medications or by the inflation of small balloons within the vessel, as in the case of percutaneous angioplasty. In addition, therapeutic devices such as filters, stents, and shunts may be placed in the vascular and interventional area, eliminating the need for a more invasive surgical procedure.

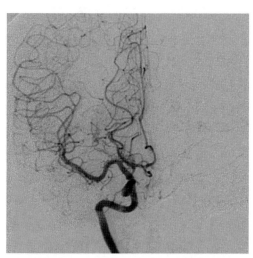

Fig. 22-24 Digital subtraction angiography showing anterior and middle cerebral arteries.

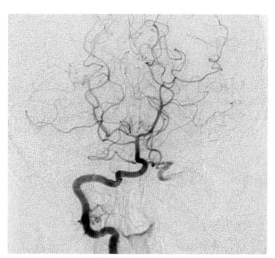

Fig. 22-25 Digital subtraction angiography showing vertebrobasilar circulation.

VERTEBROPLASTY AND KYPHOPLASTY

Vertebroplasty and kyphoplasty are interventional radiology procedures used to treat spinal compression fractures and other pathologies of the vertebral bodies that do not respond to conservative treatment. Vertebral fractures are common, especially in older patients with a history of osteoporosis. Estimates indicate that osteoporosis causes more than 700,000 vertebral fractures per year in the United States. About half of these fractures occur silently without any pain. Some fractures are extremely painful, however, and severely limit the patient's quality of life. Vertebroplasty and kyphoplasty are used in cases of severe pain that does not improve over many weeks of treatment.

Percutaneous vertebroplasty is defined as the injection of a radiopaque bone cement (e.g., polymethyl methacrylate) into a painful compression fracture under fluoroscopic guidance. This procedure is typically performed in the special procedures suite or the operating room with the patient sedated but awake. A specialized trocar needle is advanced into the fractured vertebral body under fluoroscopy (Fig. 22-26). Intraosseous venography using nonionic contrast media is performed to confirm needle placement. When the physician is satisfied with the needle placement, the cement is injected (Fig. 22-27). The cement stabilizes fracture fragments and leads to reduction in pain. Postprocedural imaging includes AP and lateral projections of the spine to confirm cement position (Fig. 22-28). A CT scan may also be performed.

Percutaneous kyphoplasty differs from vertebroplasty in that a balloon catheter is used to expand the compressed vertebral body to near its original height before injection of the bone cement. Inflation of the balloon creates a pocket for the placement of the cement. Kyphoplasty can help restore the spine to a more normal curvature and reduce hunchback deformities.

The success of these procedures is measured by reduction of pain reported by the patient. With proper patient selection and technique, success rates of 80% to 90% have been reported. Vertebroplasty and kyphoplasty have risks of serious complications, however. The most common complication is leakage of the cement before it hardens. Pulmonary embolism and death, although rare, have been reported. Patients should be encouraged to discuss risks, benefits, and alternatives with their physicians. Technologists who perform these procedures need to be properly educated and ensure that informed consent has been documented.

Other Neuroradiographic Procedures

PROVOCATIVE DISKOGRAPHY

Diskography is a procedure performed under fluoroscopic guidance to determine the source of a patient's chronic back pain. The examination is performed with a small quantity of water-soluble, nonionic iodinated media injected into the center of the disk. Diskography is used in the investigation of internal disk lesions, such as rupture of the nucleus pulposus, which cannot be shown by other imaging procedures (Fig. 22-29). Patients are given only a local anesthetic so that they remain fully conscious and able to inform the physician about pain when the needles are inserted and the injection is made. Attempts are made to replicate the patient's chronic pain during the injection. Spinal fusion is often recommended based on a positive provocation of pain. The need for this procedure should be carefully evaluated because there is controversy regarding the sensitivity and specificity of the examination. Some authors suggest diskography may increase the chance of later disk disruption. MRI and CTM have largely replaced diskography. (More information on diskography is presented in Chapter 29 of the seventh edition of this atlas.)

INTERVENTIONAL PAIN MANAGEMENT

Image-guided interventional pain management is becoming a common treatment for chronic back pain that does not respond to conservative treatment. Pretreatment assessment of the patient's pain and a thorough history are necessary. Fluoroscopy, CT, and ultrasonography are often used to confirm needle placement. Interventional pain management physicians perform a variety of injections using corticosteroids and local anesthetics to reduce

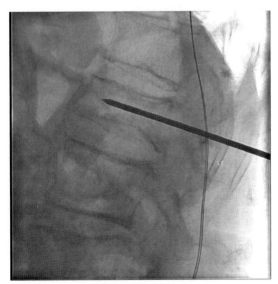

Fig. 22-26 Lateral projection of compressed vertebral body with bone needle in place.

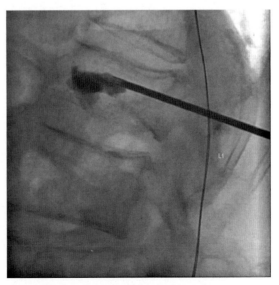

Fig. 22-27 Bone cement injected during vertebroplasty under image guidance.

inflammation and improve symptoms. Procedures can be performed at all levels of the spine. Various needle types can be used, but needles with a stylet are commonly used to prevent tissue from being trapped in the lumen. Size and tip configuration are determined by the physician. C-arm fluoroscopy is commonly used to determine needle placement. Contrast medium is sometimes used. Posteroanterior (PA) and lateral projections are needed to confirm needle depth. The tip of the needle and an identifiable bony landmark must be included in the images. The precise nature of the injections is thought to improve patient outcomes compared with blind injections. The success of the treatment is based on the patient's self-report of pain reduction.

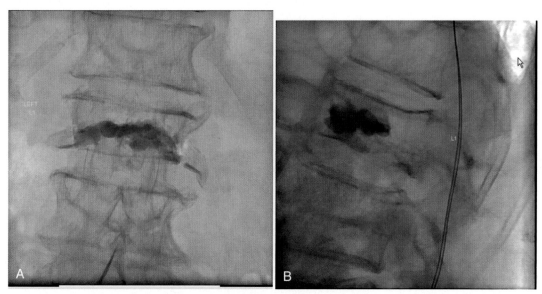

Fig. 22-28 A and **B,** AP and lateral projections show bone cement in L1.

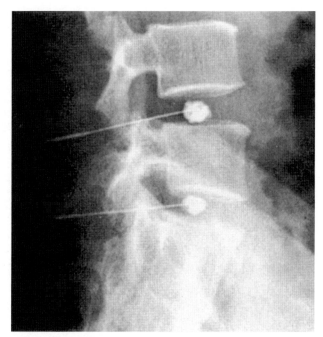

Fig. 22-29 Lumbar diskogram showing normal nucleus pulposus of round contour type.

Definition of Terms

angiography Radiographic examination of blood vessels after injection of contrast medium.

arachnoid Thin delicate membrane surrounding the brain and spinal cord.

brain Portion of the central nervous system contained within the cranium.

cauda equina Collection of nerves located in the spinal canal inferior to the spinal cord.

cerebellum Part of the brain located in the posterior cranial fossa behind the brain stem.

cerebral aqueduct Opening between the third and fourth ventricles.

cerebrospinal fluid Fluid that flows through and protects the ventricles, subarachnoid space, brain, and spinal cord.

cerebrum Largest uppermost portion of the brain.

conus medullaris Inferiormost portion of the spinal cord.

cortex Outer surface layer of the brain.

dura mater Tough outer layer of the meninges, which lines the cranial cavity and spinal canal.

epidural space Outside or above the dura mater.

falx cerebri Fold of dura mater that separates the cerebral hemispheres.

filum terminale Threadlike structure that extends from the distal end of the spinal cord.

gadolinium IV contrast medium used in MRI.

hindbrain Portion of the brain within the posterior fossa; it includes the pons, medulla oblongata, and cerebellum.

interventional radiology Branch of radiology that uses catheters to perform therapeutic procedures.

intrathecal injection Injection into the subarachnoid space of the spinal canal.

kyphoplasty Interventional radiology procedure used to treat vertebral body compression fractures using a specialized balloon and bone cement.

pons Oval-shaped area of the brain anterior to the medulla oblongata.

slices Sectional images of the body produced with either CT or MRI.

spinal cord Extension of the medulla oblongata that runs through the spinal canal to the upper lumbar vertebrae.

stereotactic surgery Radiographic procedure performed during neurosurgery to guide needle placement into the brain.

tentorium Layer of dura that separates the cerebrum and cerebellum.

vermis Wormlike structure that connects the two cerebellar hemispheres.

vertebroplasty Interventional radiology procedure used to treat vertebral body compression fractures by stabilizing bone fragments with cement.

Selected bibliography

Boyajian SS: Interventional pain management: an overview for primary care physicians, *J Am Osteopath Assoc* 105(9 Suppl 4):S1, 2005.

Brown DB et al: Treatment of chronic symptomatic vertebral compression fractures with percutaneous vertebroplasty, *AJR Am J Roentgenol* 182:319, 2004.

Carragee EJ et al: A gold standard evaluation of the discogenic pain diagnosis as determined by provocative discography, *Spine* 31:18, 2006.

Centers for Disease Control and Prevention: *Safe injection practices to prevent transmission of infections to patients.* Retrieved from http://www.cdc.gov/injectionsafety/ip07, 2007.

Furlow B: Pain management imaging, *Radiol Technol* 80:447, 2009.

Kelly LL, Petersen CM: *Sectional anatomy for imaging professionals*, ed 2, St Louis, 2007, Mosby.

Landers MH: Indications for spinal injections in the chronic pain patient, *Pain Med* V9:S1, 2008.

Linger L: Percutaneous polymethacrylate vertebroplasty, *Radiol Technol* 76:109, 2004.

Martin JB et al: Vertebroplasty: clinical experience and follow-up results, *Bone* 25:11, 1999.

Ortiz AO: Vertebral body reconstruction: review and update on vertebroplasty and kyphoplasty, *Appl Radiol* 37:10-24, 2008.

Seeram E: *Computed tomography physical principles, clinical applications and quality control*, ed 3, Philadelphia, 2009, Saunders.

Spivak JM: *Vertebroplasty and kyphoplasty: percutaneous injection procedures for vertebral fractures,* Available at: http://www.spine-health.com. Accessed May 2004.

Wheeler AH: *Therapeutic injections for pain management,* Available at: http://emedicine.medscape.com. Accessed September 2009.

Zoarski GH et al: Percutaneous vertebroplasty for osteoporotic compression fractures: quantitative prospective evaluation of long-term outcomes, *J Vasc Interv Radiol* 13:139, 2002.

23

VASCULAR, CARDIAC, AND INTERVENTIONAL RADIOGRAPHY

SARA A. KADERLIK
LOIS J. LAYNE

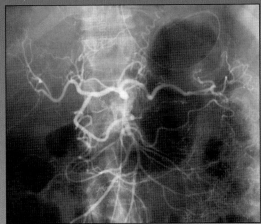

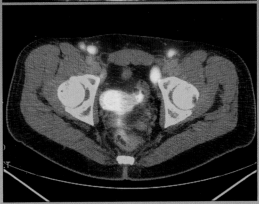

OUTLINE

Historical Development, 20
ANATOMY, 22
Circulatory System, 22
Blood-Vascular System, 23
Lymphatic System, 26
ANGIOGRAPHY, 28
Definitions and Indications, 28
Angiographic Studies, 29
Digital Subtraction
    Angiographic
    Procedures, 30
Angiographic Supplies and
    Equipment, 35
Patient Care, 38
Preparation of Examining
    Room, 39
Radiation Protection, 39
Angiography Team, 39
Angiography in the Future, 39
AORTOGRAPHY, 40
Thoracic Aortography, 40
Abdominal Aortography, 41
Pulmonary Arteriography, 42
Visceral Arteriography, 42
Peripheral Angiography, 46
CEREBRAL ANGIOGRAPHY, 49
Cerebral Anatomy, 49
Aortic Arch Angiogram
    (for Cranial Vessels), 55

Anterior Circulation, 56
Posterior Circulation, 58
Venography, 60
Visceral Venography, 61
INTERVENTIONAL RADIOLOGY, 62
Percutaneous Transluminal
    Angioplasty and Stenting, 62
Abdominal Aortic Aneurysm
    Endografts, 65
Transcatheter Embolization, 66
Inferior Vena Cava Filter
    Placement, 68
Transjugular Intrahepatic
    Portosystemic Shunt, 72
Other Procedures, 72
Interventional Radiology: Present and
    Future 74
CARDIAC CATHETERIZATION, 75
Specialized Equipment, 78
Patient Positioning for Cardiac
    Catheterization, 81
Catheterization Methods and
    Techniques, 81
Catheterization Studies and
    Procedures, 82
Postcatheterization Care, 95
Cardiac Catheterization Trends, 95

Historical Development

In January 1896, just 10 weeks after the announcement of Roentgen's discovery of x-rays, Haschek and Lindenthal announced that they had produced a radiograph showing the blood vessels of an amputated hand using Teichman's mixture, a thick emulsion of chalk, as the contrast agent. This work heralded the beginning of angiography. The advancement of angiography was hindered, however, by the lack of suitable contrast media and low-risk techniques to deliver the media to the desired location. By the 1920s, researchers were using sodium iodide as a contrast medium to produce lower limb studies comparable in quality to studies seen in modern angiography.

The first human cardiac catheterization was reported in 1929 by Forssman, a 25-year-old surgical resident who placed a catheter into his own heart and then walked to the radiology department where a chest radiograph was produced to document his medical achievement. Catheterization of the heart soon became a valuable tool used primarily for diagnostic purposes. Through the 1940s, the basic catheterization study remained relatively uncomplicated and easy for physicians to perform; however, the risk to the patient was significant.

Until the 1950s, contrast media were most commonly injected through a needle that punctured the vessel or through a ureteral catheter that passed into the body through a surgically exposed peripheral vessel. In 1952, shortly after the development of a flexible thin-walled catheter,

Seldinger announced a *percutaneous** method of catheter introduction. The Seldinger technique eliminated the surgical risk, which exposed the vessel and tissues (see Fig. 23-16). Selective coronary *angiography* was first reported by Sones in 1959, when he inadvertently injected contrast media into the right coronary artery of a patient who was undergoing routine aortography. In 1962, Ricketts and Abrams described the first percutaneous method for selective coronary angiography. This method was further perfected in the late 1960s with the introduction of preformed catheters designed to engage the ostium of the right and left coronary arteries.

Pioneers in the field overcame equipment obstacles. It has been said the "Fathers of Interventional Radiology and Cardiology" were Charles Dotter and Andreas Gruntzig, respectively. Dotter performed the first successful dilation of a superficial femoral artery in 1964 using coaxial catheters. Percutaneous transluminal angioplasty (PTA) was described in *Circulation* in November, 1964 with co-author Dr. Melvin Judkins. In 1966, Dotter fabricated a reinforced balloon dilating catheter, but it was not used on patients. Dr. Werner Portsman (Berlin, Germany) introduced *"Korsett Balloon Kather"* an 8 French outer Teflon catheter with four longitudinal slits in 1973. A latex balloon catheter was inflated inside the longitudinal slits. In September 1977, Dr. Andreas Gruntzig used successfully

*Almost all italicized words on the succeeding pages are defined at the end of the chapter.

used a balloon PTA to treat a left anterior descending coronary artery stenosis. Gruntzig and Hopff introduced the double-lumen, balloon-tipped catheter. One lumen allows the passage of a guidewire and fluids through the catheter. The other lumen communicates with a balloon at the distal end of the catheter. When inflated, the balloon expands to a size much larger than the catheter. Double-lumen, angioplasty balloon catheters are available in sizes ranging from 3 to 9 French, with attached balloons varying in length and expanding to diameters of 2 to 20 mm or more (see Figs. 23-60 and 23-61). Transluminal angioplasty can be performed in virtually any vessel that can be reached percutaneously with a catheter (see Figs. 23-62 and 23-63). In 1978, Molnar and Stockum described the use of balloon angioplasty for dilation of strictures within the biliary system. Balloon angioplasty is also conducted in venous structures, ureters, and the gastrointestinal tract.

The 1980s saw the development of expandable metallic stents. Andrew Cragg, Charles Dotter, Cesare Gianturco, Dierk Mass, Julio Palmaz, and Hans Wallsten were the first stent pioneers. These stents were composed primarily of a stainless steel alloy or thermal memory stents made of nitinol (alloy of nickel and titanium) and were self or balloon expandable. Three stents available for use in 1985 were the Gianturco Z, Palmaz, and Wallstent. Dotter continued advancement of cardiovascular procedures by first using Streptokinase for selective thrombolysis. In the 1980s, Urokinase was used for this widely performed procedure. Continued growth of thrombolysis was due to the advancement of fibrinolytic agents *(recombinant tissue plasminogen activators)*.

Therapeutic vascular occlusion procedures began in 1931 with an open surgical embolization of a carotid cavernous fistula. Dr. Shoji Ishimore used Gelfoam pieces through a polyethylene tube into an exposed carotid artery. Embolization became popular during the 1980s and 1990s with advancement of embolization agents, such as gelatin sponges (Gelfoam), polyvinyl alcohol (Ivalon), liquid and rapidly solidifying polymers including cyanoacrylate glue, coils, and detachable balloons.

Early angiograms consisted of single radiographs or the visualization of vessels by fluoroscopy. Because the advantage of *serial imaging* was recognized, cassette changers, roll film changers, cut film changers, and cine and serial spot-filming/digital devices were developed. Until the early 1990s, most angiograms recorded flowing contrast media in a series of images that required *rapid film changers* or cinefluorography devices; however, presently digital subtraction angiography (DSA) systems are used almost exclusively. Although some institutions may still have rapid film changers, most often the filming technique is by DSA. The newer imaging equipment has much better image quality and can produce images at a rate of 30 frames per second. In addition, digital imaging is cost-effective because images are stored electronically, reducing the need for expensive film and film storage. Digital images can be archived and retrieved in seconds from within the institution or any network connection. DSA imaging provides the interventionalist with a variety of tools for image manipulation analysis and measurement.

The resolution possible with early digital equipment was a drawback to the use of digital imaging in the cardiovascular laboratory. Larger matrix size, the obvious solution to this problem, allowed for acceptable resolution but also created another problem: how to acquire and store large volumes of digital information. In the late 1970s and early 1980s, the high-speed parallel transfer disk was introduced to solve the acquisition and short-term storage problem. This new disk acquired and stored an entire coronary angiogram and made real-time digital playback during the procedure possible. Permanent storage of the digital images remained a problem, however. Floppy disk and computer tape storage were inadequate solutions because they required significant time and supplies. Long-term storage of large amounts of digital images has benefited from advances in computer technology, which provide high-speed, large-capacity methods of storage, capable of acquiring large amounts of data (terabytes) with very high resolution. A problem incumbent with digital imaging was the incompatibility of the storage media from one system to the other. Today, networking, security, redundancy, and image integrity are issues for laboratories equipped with digital technology.

The 1960s and 1970s brought tremendous advances in radiologic and cardiovascular medicine and technology. Radiographic imaging and recording equipment, physiologic monitoring equipment, and cardiovascular pharmaceuticals and supplies became increasingly reliable. The uses of computers in the cardiovascular interventional laboratories have facilitated the development of this rapidly growing subspecialty of the cardiovascular medical and surgical sciences. These advances and trends have enabled angiography to evolve from a simple diagnostic investigation to its current state as a sophisticated diagnostic study and interventional procedure.

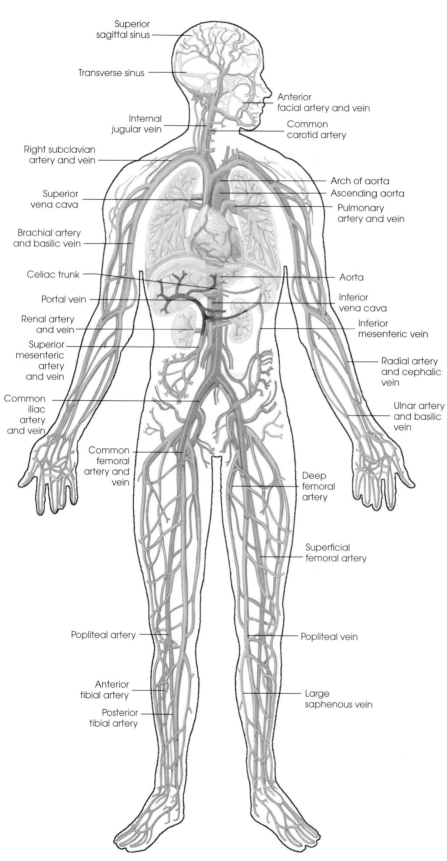

Superior
sagittal sinus

Transverse sinus

Internal
jugular vein

Right subclavian
artery and vein

Superior
vena cava

Brachial artery
and basilic vein

Celiac trunk

Portal vein

Renal artery
and vein

Superior
mesenteric
artery
and vein

Common
iliac
artery
and vein

Common
femoral
artery and
vein

Popliteal artery

Anterior
tibial artery

Posterior
tibial artery

Anterior
facial artery and vein

Common
carotid artery

Arch of aorta
Ascending aorta

Pulmonary
artery and vein

Aorta

Inferior
vena cava

Inferior
mesenteric vein

Radial artery
and cephalic
vein

Ulnar artery
and basilic
vein

Deep
femoral
artery

Superficial
femoral artery

Popliteal vein

Large
saphenous vein

Fig. 23-1 Major arteries and veins: *red*, arterial; *blue*, venous; *purple*, portal.

Circulatory System

The *circulatory system* has two complex systems of intimately associated vessels. Through these vessels, fluid is transported throughout the body in a continuous, unidirectional flow. The major portion of the circulatory system transports blood and is called the *blood-vascular system* (Fig. 23-1). The minor portion, called the *lymphatic system,* collects fluid from the tissue spaces. This fluid is filtered throughout the lymphatic system, which conveys it back to the blood-vascular system. The fluid conveyed by the lymphatic system is called *lymph.* Together, the blood-vascular and lymphatic systems carry oxygen and nutritive material to the tissues. They also collect and transport carbon dioxide (CO_2) and other waste products of metabolism from the tissues to the organs of excretion: the skin, lungs, liver, and kidneys.

Blood-Vascular System

The blood-vascular system consists of the *heart, arteries, capillaries,* and *veins.* The *heart* serves as a pumping mechanism to keep the blood in constant circulation throughout the vast system of blood vessels. *Arteries* convey the blood *away* from the heart. *Veins* convey the blood *back* toward the heart.

Two circuits of blood vessels branch out of the heart (Fig. 23-2). The first circuit is the arterial circuit or the *systemic circulation,* which carries oxygenated blood to the organs and tissues. Every organ has its own vascular circuit that arises from the trunk artery and leads back to the trunk vein for return to the heart. The systemic arteries branch out, treelike, from the aorta to all parts of the body. The arteries are usually named according to their location. The systemic veins usually lie parallel to their respective arteries and are given the same names.

The second circuit is the *pulmonary circulation,* which takes blood to the lungs for CO_2 exchange and for the reoxygenation of the blood, which is carried back to the arterial systemic circulation. The pulmonary trunk arises from the right ventricle of the heart, passes superiorly and posteriorly for a distance of about 2 inches (5 cm), and then divides into two branches, the right and left pulmonary arteries. These vessels enter the root of the respective lung and, following the course of the bronchi, divide and subdivide to form a dense network of capillaries surrounding the alveoli of the lungs. Through the thin walls of the capillaries, the blood discharges CO_2 and absorbs oxygen from the air contained in the alveoli. The oxygenated blood passes onward through the pulmonary veins for return to the heart. In the pulmonary circulation, the deoxygenated blood is transported by the pulmonary arteries, and the oxygenated blood is transported by the pulmonary veins.

Two main trunk vessels arise from the heart. The first is the aorta for the systemic circulation: the arteries progressively diminish in size as they divide and subdivide along their course, finally ending in minute branches called *arterioles.* The arterioles divide to form the capillary vessels, and the branching process is then reversed: the *capillaries* unite to form *venules,* the beginning branches of the veins, which unite and reunite to form larger and larger vessels as they approach the heart. These venous structures empty into the right atrium, then into the right ventricle, and then into the second main trunk that arises from the heart—the pulmonary trunk, or the pulmonary circulation. The process of oxygen exchange is carried out in small venous structures and then in larger and larger pulmonary veins. The pulmonary veins join to form four large veins (two from each lung), which empty into the left atrium, then into the left ventricle, and then into the aorta, which starts the circulation again throughout the body.

The pathway of venous drainage from the abdominal viscera to the liver is called the *portal system.* In contrast to the systemic and pulmonary circuits, which begin and end at the heart, the portal system begins in the capillaries of the abdominal viscera and ends in the capillaries and sinusoids of the liver. The blood is filtered and then exits the liver via the hepatic venous system, which empties into the inferior vena cava just proximal to the right atrium.

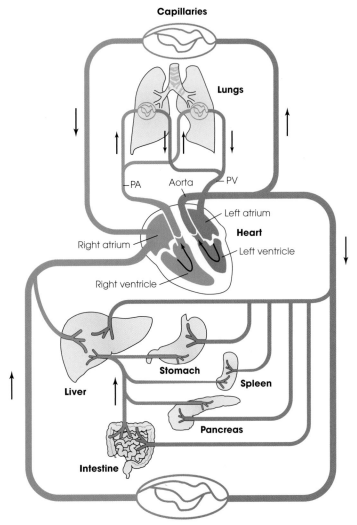

Fig. 23-2 Pulmonary, systemic, and portal circulation: oxygenated (*red*), deoxygenated (*blue*), and nutrient-rich (*purple*) blood.

The systemic veins are arranged in a superficial set and in a deep set with which the superficial veins communicate; both sets converge at a common trunk vein. The systemic veins end in two large vessels opening into the heart: the *superior vena cava* leads from the portion of the body above the diaphragm, and the *inferior vena cava* leads from below the level of the diaphragm.

The capillaries connect the arterioles and venules to form networks that pervade most organs and all other tissues supplied with blood. The capillary vessels have exceedingly thin walls through which the essential functions of the blood-vascular system take place: the blood constituents are filtered out, and the waste products of cell activity are absorbed. The exchange takes place through the medium of tissue fluid, which is derived from the blood plasma and is drained off by the lymphatic system for return to the blood-vascular system. The tissue fluid undergoes modification in the lymphatic system. As soon as this tissue fluid enters the lymphatic capillaries, it is called *lymph.*

The *heart* is the central organ of the blood-vascular system and functions solely as a pump to keep the blood in circulation. It is shaped like a cone and measures approximately 4¾ inches (12 cm) in length, 3½ inches (9 cm) in width, and 2½ inches (6 cm) in depth. The heart is situated obliquely in the central mediastinum, largely to the left of the midsagittal plane. The base of the heart is directed superiorly, posteriorly, and to the right. The apex of the heart rests on the diaphragm against the anterior chest wall and is directed anteriorly, inferiorly, and to the left.

The muscular wall of the heart is called the *myocardium.* Because of the force required to drive blood through the extensive systemic vessels, the myocardium is about three times as thick on the left side (the arterial side) as on the right (the venous side). The membrane that lines the interior of the heart is called the *endocardium.* The heart is enclosed in the double-walled *pericardial sac.* The exterior wall of this sac is fibrous. The thin, closely adherent membrane that covers the heart is referred to as the *epicardium* or, because it also serves as the serous inner wall of the pericardial sac, the *visceral pericardium.* The narrow, fluid-containing space between the two walls of the sac is called the *pericardial cavity.*

The heart is divided by septa into right and left halves, with each half subdivided by a constriction into two cavities, or chambers. The two upper chambers are called *atria,* and each atrium consists of a principal cavity and a lesser cavity called the *auricle.* The two lower chambers of the heart are called *ventricles.* The opening between the right atrium and right ventricle is controlled by the right atrioventricular (tricuspid) valve, and the opening between the left atrium and left ventricle is controlled by the left atrioventricular (mitral or bicuspid) valve.

The atria and ventricles separately contract (systole) in pumping blood and relax or dilate (diastole) in receiving blood. The atria precede the ventricles in contraction; while the atria are in systole, the ventricles are in diastole. One phase of contraction (referred to as the heartbeat) and one phase of dilation are called the *cardiac cycle.* In the average adult, one cardiac cycle lasts 0.8 second. The heart rate, or number of pulsations per minute, varies, however, with size, age, and gender. Heart rate is faster in small persons, young individuals, and females. The heart rate is also increased with exercise, food, and emotional disturbances.

The atria function as receiving chambers. The superior and inferior venae cavae empty into the right atrium (Fig. 23-3); the two right and left pulmonary veins empty into the left atrium. The ventricles function as distributing chambers. The right side of the heart handles the venous, or deoxygenated, blood, and the left side handles the arterial, or oxygenated, blood. The left ventricle pumps oxygenated blood through the aortic valve into the aorta and the systemic circulation. The three major portions of the aorta are the ascending aorta, the aortic arch, and the descending aorta. The right ventricle pumps deoxygenated blood through the pulmonary valve into the pulmonary trunk and the pulmonary circulation.

Blood is supplied to the myocardium by the right and left coronary arteries. These vessels arise in the aortic sinus immediately superior to the aortic valve (Fig. 23-4). Most of the cardiac veins drain into the coronary sinus on the posterior aspect of the heart, and this sinus drains into the right atrium (Fig. 23-5).

The ascending aorta arises from the superior portion of the left ventricle and passes superiorly and to the right for a short distance. It then arches posteriorly and to the left and descends along the left side of the vertebral column to the level of L4, where it divides into the right and left common iliac arteries. The common iliac arteries pass to the level of the lumbosacral junction, where each ends by dividing into the internal iliac, or hypogastric, artery and the external iliac artery. The internal iliac artery passes into the pelvis. The external iliac artery passes to a point about midway between the anterior superior iliac spine and pubic symphysis and then enters the upper thigh to become the common femoral artery.

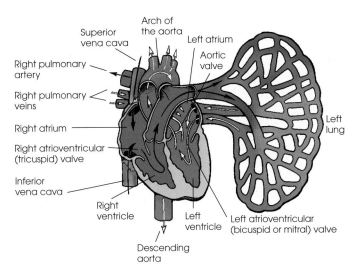

Fig. 23-3 Heart and great vessels: deoxygenated blood flow (*black arrows*); oxygenated blood flow (*white arrows*).

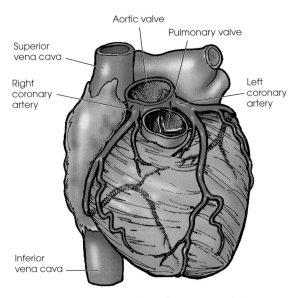

Fig. 23-4 Anterior view of coronary arteries.

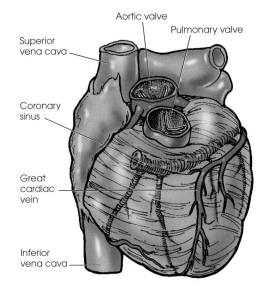

Fig. 23-5 Anterior view of coronary veins.

The velocity of blood circulation varies with the rate and intensity of the heartbeat. Velocity also varies in the different portions of the circulatory system based on distance from the heart. The speed of blood flow is highest in the large arteries arising at or near the heart because these vessels receive the full force of each wave of blood pumped out of the heart. The arterial walls expand with the pressure from each wave. The walls then rhythmically recoil, gradually diminishing the pressure of the advancing wave from point to point, until the flow of blood is normally reduced to a steady, nonpulsating stream through the capillaries and veins. The beat, or contraction and expansion of an artery, may be felt with the fingers at several points and is called the *pulse.*

Complete circulation of the blood through the systemic and pulmonary circuits, from a given point and back again, requires about 23 seconds and an average of 27 heartbeats. In certain contrast examinations of the cardiovascular system, tests are conducted to determine the circulation time from the point of contrast media injection to the site of interest.

Lymphatic System

The lymphatic system consists of an elaborate arrangement of closed vessels that collect fluid from the tissue spaces and transport it to the blood-vascular system. Almost all lymphatic vessels are arranged in two sets: (1) a superficial set that lies immediately under the skin and accompanies the superficial veins and (2) a deep set that accompanies the deep blood vessels and with which the superficial lymphatics communicate (Fig. 23-6). The lymphatic system lacks a pumping mechanism such as the heart of the blood-vascular system. The lymphatic vessels are richly supplied with valves to prevent backflow, and the movement of the lymph through the system is believed to be maintained largely by extrinsic pressure from the surrounding organs and muscles.

The lymphatic system begins in complex networks of thin-walled, absorbent capillaries situated in the various organs and tissues. The capillaries unite to form larger vessels, which form networks and unite to become still larger vessels as they approach the terminal collecting trunks. The terminal trunks communicate with the blood-vascular system.

The lymphatic vessels are small in caliber and have delicate, transparent walls. Along their course the collecting vessels pass through one or more nodular structures called *lymph nodes.* The nodes occur singly but are usually arranged in chains or groups of 2 to 20. The nodes are situated so that they form strategically placed centers toward which the conducting vessels converge. The nodes vary from the size of a pinhead to the size of an almond or larger. They may be spherical, oval, or kidney shaped. Each node has a hilum through which the arteries enter and veins and efferent lymph vessels emerge; the afferent lymph vessels do not enter at the hilum. In addition to the lymphatic capillaries, blood vessels, and supporting structures, each lymph node contains masses, or follicles, of lymphocytes that are arranged around its circumference and from which cords of cells extend through the medullary portion of the node.

Numerous conducting channels, here called *afferent lymph vessels,* enter the node opposite the hilum and break into wide capillaries that surround the lymph follicles and form a canal known as the *peripheral* or *marginal lymph sinus.* The network of capillaries continues into the medullary portion of the node, widens to form medullary sinuses, and then collects into several *efferent lymph vessels* that leave the node at the hilum. The conducting vessels may pass through several nodes along their course, each time undergoing the process of widening into sinuses. Lymphocytes—a variety of white blood cells formed in the lymph nodes—are added to the lymph while it is in the nodes. It is thought that most of the lymph is absorbed by the venous system from these nodes, and only a small portion of the lymph is passed on through the conducting vessels.

The absorption and interchange of tissue fluids and cells occur through the thin walls of the capillaries. The lymph passes from the beginning capillaries through the conducting vessels, which eventually empty their contents into terminal lymph trunks for conveyance to the blood-vascular system. The main terminal trunk of the lymphatic system is called the *thoracic duct.* The lower, dilated portion of the duct is known as the *cisterna chyli.* The thoracic duct receives lymphatic drainage from all parts of the body below the diaphragm and from the left half of the body above the diaphragm. The thoracic duct extends from the level of L2 to the base of the neck, where it ends by opening into the venous system at the junction of the left subclavian and internal jugular veins.

Three terminal collecting trunks—the right jugular, the subclavian, and the bronchomediastinal trunks—receive the lymphatic drainage from the right half of the body above the diaphragm. These vessels open into the right subclavian vein separately or occasionally after uniting to form a common trunk called the *right lymphatic duct.*

Lymphography is seldom performed in current practice because of the superior imaging capabilities of newer modalities such as magnetic resonance imaging (MRI) and computed tomography (CT) (Fig. 23-7). At present, it is primarily used to assess the clinical extent of lymphomas or to stage radiation treatment. Lymphography may also be indicated in patients who have clinical evidence of obstruction or other impairment of the lymphatic system. A more detailed description of lymphography is provided in previous editions of this text.

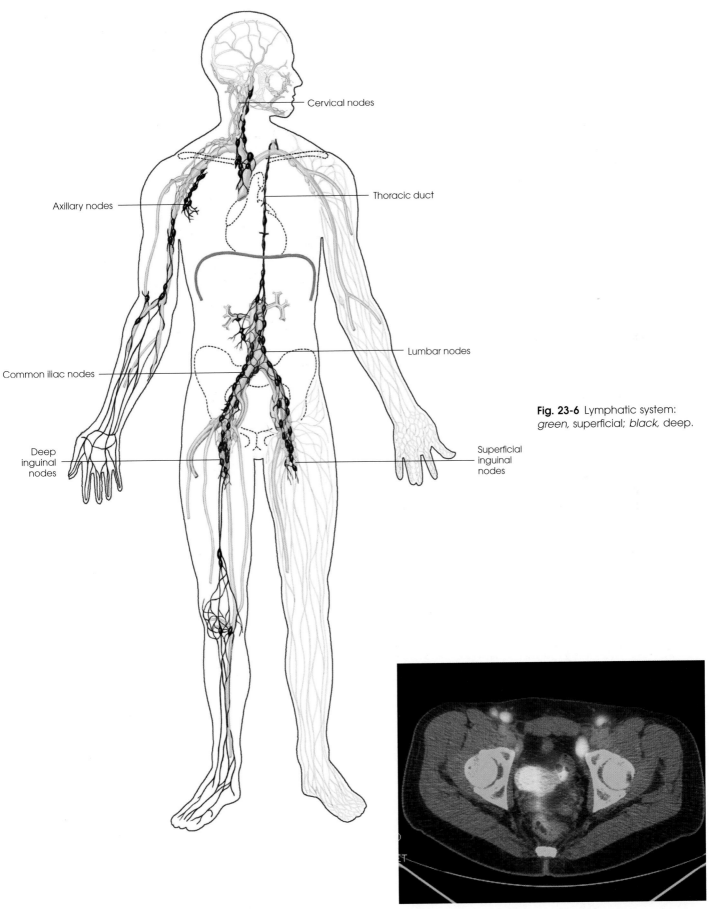

Cervical nodes

Thoracic duct

Axillary nodes

Lumbar nodes

Common iliac nodes

Fig. 23-6 Lymphatic system: *green,* superficial; *black,* deep.

Deep inguinal nodes

Superficial inguinal nodes

Fig. 23-7 Axial PET/CT of lymph nodes with lymphoma.

Definitions and Indications

Blood vessels are not normally visible on conventional radiography because no natural contrast exists between them and other soft tissues of the body. These vessels must be filled with a radiopaque contrast media to delineate them for radiography. *Angiography* is a general term that describes the radiologic examination of vascular structures within the body after the introduction of an iodinated contrast media or gas.

The visceral and peripheral angiography procedures identified in this chapter can be categorized generally as either *arteriography* or *venography.* Examinations are more precisely named for the specific blood vessel opacified and the method of injection.

Angiography is primarily used to identify the anatomy or pathologic process of blood vessels. Chronic cramping leg pain after physical exertion, a condition known as *claudication,* may prompt a physician to order an arteriogram of the lower limbs to determine whether atherosclerosis is diminishing the blood supply to the leg muscles. A *stenosis* or *occlusion* is commonly caused by *atherosclerosis* and is an indication for an arteriogram. Cerebral angiography is performed to detect and verify the existence and exact position of an intracranial vascular lesion such as an *aneurysm.* Although most angiographic examinations are performed to investigate anatomic variances, some evaluate the motion of the part. Other vascular examinations evaluate suspected tumors by opacifying the organ of concern; after a diagnosis is made, these lesions may be amendable to some type of intervention. Interventional radiology assists in the diagnosis of lesions and then is used to treat these lesions through an endovascular approach.

Angiographic Studies
CONTRAST MEDIA

Opaque contrast media containing organic iodine solutions are used in angiographic studies. Although usually tolerated, the injection of iodinated contrast media may cause undesirable consequences. The contrast medium is subsequently filtered out of the bloodstream by the kidneys. It causes physiologic cardiovascular side effects, including peripheral vasodilation, blood pressure decrease, and cardiotoxicity. It may also produce nausea and an uncomfortable burning sensation in about 1 of 10 patients. Most significantly, the injection of iodinated contrast media may invoke allergic reactions. These reactions may be minor (hives or slight difficulty in breathing) and require minimal treatment, or they may be severe and require immediate medical intervention. Severe reactions are characterized by a state of shock in which the patient exhibits shallow breathing and a high pulse rate and may lose consciousness. Historically, 1 of every 14,000 patients has a severe allergic reaction. The administration of contrast media is one of the significant risks in angiography.

At the kilovolt (peak) (kVp) used in angiography, iodine is slightly more radiopaque, atom for atom, than lead. The iodine is incorporated into water-soluble molecules formed as tri-iodinated benzene rings. Nonionic contrast media are used almost exclusively.

These forms have three iodine atoms on each particle in solution (a 3:1 ratio) because they do not dissociate and are only two to three times as osmolar as plasma. Studies indicate that these properties of nonionic contrast media result in decreased nephrotoxicity to the kidneys. Nonionic contrast media also cause fewer physiologic cardiovascular side effects, less intense sensations, and fewer allergic reactions.

Another form of contrast medium is a dimer, in which the two benzene rings are bonded together as the anion. Ionic contrast media with a dimer result in six iodine atoms for every two particles in solution, which yields the same 3:1 ratio as nonionic contrast media. The ionic dimer has advantages over the ionic monomeric molecule, primarily by reducing osmolality, but it lacks some of the properties of the nonionic molecule. Nonionic contrast media can also be found as a dimer, which yields a ratio of 6:1 because it does not dissociate into two particles, producing an osmolality similar to blood.

All forms of iodinated contrast media are available in various iodine concentrations. The agents of higher concentration are more opaque. Typically, 30% iodine concentrations are used for cerebral and limb arteriography, whereas 35% concentrations are used for visceral angiography. Peripheral venography may be performed with 30% or lower concentrations. Ionic agents of higher concentration and nonionic agents are more viscous and produce greater resistance in the catheter during injection.

Patients with a predisposition to allergic reaction may be pretreated with a regimen of antihistamines and steroids to help prevent anaphylactic reactions to contrast media. Patients who have a history of severe reaction to iodinated contrast media or with compromised renal function may undergo procedures in which CO_2 is used as a contrast agent. CO_2 is less radiopaque than blood and appears as a negative or void in angiographic imaging. CO_2 is approved for use only below the diaphragm because the possibility of emboli is too great near the brain. CO_2 imaging is possible only in the DSA environment because it requires a narrow contrast window and the ability to stack or combine multiple images to provide a single image free of bubbles or fragmented vascular opacification. Specific kVp values should be employed to display the CO_2 optimally in contrast to the rest of the body.

INJECTION TECHNIQUES

Selective injection through a catheter involves placing the catheter within a vessel so that the vessel and its major branches are opacified. In a selective injection, the catheter tip is positioned into the orifice of a specific artery so that only that specific vessel is injected. This technique has the advantage of more densely opacifying the vessel and limiting the superimposition of other vessels.

A contrast medium may be injected by hand with a syringe, but ideally it should be injected with an automatic injector. The major advantage of automatic injectors is that a specific quantity of contrast media can be injected during a predetermined period. Another advantage to automatic injectors is the ability to operate these remotely from a shielded control room. This reduces radiation exposure to physician and staff while still allowing visualization of images and patient. Automatic injectors have controls to set the injection rate, injection volume, and maximum pressure. Another useful feature is a control to set a time interval during which the injector gradually achieves the set injection rate, which is the linear rise. This may prevent a catheter from being dislodged by whiplash.

Because the opacifying contrast media are often carried away from the area of interest by blood flow, the injection and demonstration of opacified vessels usually occur simultaneously. The injector is often electronically connected to the rapid imaging equipment to coordinate the timing between the injector and the onset of imaging.

Digital Subtraction Angiographic Procedures

A DSA study begins with catheter placement performed in the same manner as for conventional angiography. Injection techniques vary, but typically similar rates and volumes are used as in cut film. An automatic pressure injector is used to ensure consistency of injection and to facilitate computer control of injection timing and image acquisition.

The intravascular catheter is positioned using conventional fluoroscopic apparatus and technique, and a suitable imaging position is selected. At this point, an image that does not have a large dynamic range should be established; no part of the image should be significantly brighter than the rest of the image. This image can be accomplished by proper positioning, but it often requires the use of compensating filters. The filters can be bags of saline or thin pieces of metal inserted in the imaging field to reduce the intensity of bright regions. Metal filters are often part of the collimator, and water or saline bags are placed directly on or adjacent to the patient. Most newer imaging systems have built-in compensating filters.

If compensating filters are not properly placed, image quality is reduced significantly. Automatic controls in the system adjust the exposure factors so that the brightest part of the image is at that level. An unusually bright spot satisfies the automatic controls and causes the rest of the image to lie at significantly reduced levels, where the camera performance is worse. An alternative to proper filter placement is to adjust the automatic sensing region, similar to automatic exposure control (AEC) for conventional radiography, to exclude the bright region. This solution is less desirable than the use of compensating filters, and it is not always effective for some positions of the bright spot on the image. Proper positioning and technique are essential for high-quality imaging.

As the imaging sequence begins, an image that will be used as a subtraction mask (without contrast media) is acquired, digitized, and stored in the digital memory. This mask image and those that follow are produced when the x-ray tube is energized and x-rays are produced, usually 1 to 30 exposures per second at 65 to 95 kVp and between 5 mAs and 1000 mAs. The radiation dose received by the patient for each image can be adjusted during installation. The dose may be reduced or the same as that used for a conventional radiograph. Images can be acquired at variable rates, from 1 image every 2 to 3 seconds up to 30 images per second.

The *acquisition rate* can also be varied during a run. Most commonly, images are acquired at a faster rate during the passage of iodine contrast media through the arteries and then at a reduced rate in the venous phase, during which the blood flow is much slower. This procedure minimizes the radiation exposure to the patient but provides a sufficient number of images to show the clinical information. Each of these digitized images is electronically *subtracted* from the mask, and the subtraction image is amplified (contrast enhanced) and displayed in real time so that the subtraction images appear essentially instantaneously during the imaging procedure. The images are simultaneously stored on a *digital disk*.

Some DSA equipment allows the table or the image intensifier (II) or flat panel detector system to be moved during acquisition. The movement is permitted to "follow" the flow of iodine contrast material as it passes through the arteries. Sometimes called the "bolus chase" or "DSA stepping" method, this technique is particularly useful for evaluating the arteries in the pelvis and lower limb. Previously, several separate imaging sequences would be performed with the II or flat panel positioned in a different location for each sequence, but this method required an injection of iodine contrast material for each sequence. The bolus chase method requires only one injection of iodine, and the imaging sequence follows (or "chases") the iodine as it flows down the limb. The imaging sequence may be preceded or followed by a duplicate sequence without iodine injection to enable subtraction. Occasionally, this method may need to be repeated because the contrast media in one leg may flow faster than in the other.

Misregistration, a major problem in DSA, occurs when the mask and the images displaying the vessels filled with contrast media do not exactly coincide. Misregistration is sometimes caused by voluntary movements of the patient, but it is also caused by involuntary movements such as bowel peristalsis or heart contractions. Preparing the patient by describing the sensations associated with injection of contrast media and the importance of holding still can help eliminate voluntary movements. It is also important to have the patient suspend respiration during the procedure.

During the imaging procedure, the subtraction images appear on the display monitor (Fig. 23-8). Often a preliminary diagnosis can be made at this point or as the images are reviewed immediately after each exposure sequence. A formal reading session occurs after the patient study has been completed; the final diagnosis is made at that time.

Some *postprocessing* is performed after each exposure sequence to improve visualization of the anatomy of interest or to correct misregistration. More involved postprocessing, including quantitative analysis, is performed after the patient study has been completed. The processed images are available on the computer monitor for review by the radiologist. Because the images are digital, it is possible to store them in a *picture archive and communication system (PACS).* PACS allows images to be archived in digital format on various computer devices, including magnetic tape and optical disk. The images also can be transmitted via a computer network throughout the hospital or to remote locations for consultation with an expert or the referring physician. As an alternative to digital storage and reading, hard-copy images may be produced using a *laser printer* or *multiformat camera,* with several images appearing on each radiograph.

Fluoroscopy, cine, and DSA systems consist essentially of a flat panel digital detector containing the output phosphor similar to that of an image intensification system. In DSA, the fluoroscopic image is digitized into serial images that are stored by a computer. The computer subtracts an early image, the mask image (before contrast media enter the vessel), from a later image (after the vessel opacifies) and displays the difference, or subtraction image, on the fluoroscopy monitor.

Imaging systems may be used either singly or in combination at right angles to obtain simultaneous frontal and lateral images of the vascular system under investigation with one injection of contrast media. This arrangement of units is called a *biplane* imaging system (Fig. 23-9). When two image receptors operate together for simultaneous biplane imaging, exposures in both planes cannot be made at the same moment because scatter radiation would fog the opposite plane image. Yet biplane imagers must cycle exactly together so that synchronization can be electronically controlled. It is necessary to alternate the exposures in the two planes. The x-ray tubes in a biplane system must

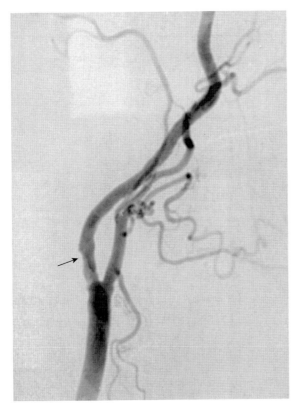

Fig. 23-8 DSA image of common carotid artery showing stenosis *(arrow)* of internal carotid artery.

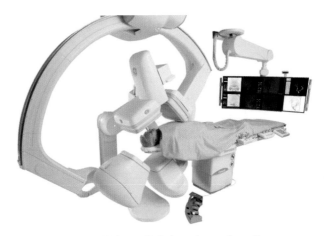

Fig. 23-9 Modern biplane digital angiography suite.

(Courtesy GE Medical.)

fire alternately to prevent exposure of the opposite II. In addition, the II that is not being exposed is "blanked" or is powered off for an instant so as not to receive any input from the opposite exposure. The difference in the alternating exposures is about 3 msec.

Rapid serial radiographic imaging requires large focal-spot x-ray tubes capable of withstanding a high heat load. Magnification studies require fractional focus tubes with focal spot sizes of 0.1 to 0.3 mm. X-ray tubes may have to be specialized to satisfy these extreme demands.

Rapid serial imaging also necessitates radiographic generators with high-power output. Because short exposure times are needed to compensate for all patient motion, the generators must be capable of producing high-milliampere output. The combination of high kilowatt–rated generators and rare earth film-screen technology significantly aids in decreasing the radiation dose to the patient while producing radiographs of improved quality, with the added advantage of prolonging the life of the high-powered generators and x-ray tubes.

A comprehensive angiography suite contains a great amount of equipment other than radiologic devices. Monitoring systems record patient electrocardiogram (ECG) data, blood pressure readings, and pulse oximetry. Emergency equipment includes resuscitation equipment (e.g., a defibrillator for the heart) and anesthesia apparatus. The cardiovascular and interventional technologist (CIT) must be familiar with the use of each piece of equipment (Fig. 23-10).

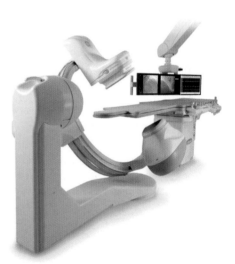

Fig. 23-10 Modern single-plane digital angiography suite.

(Courtesy GE Medical.)

MAGNIFICATION

Magnification occurs intentionally and unintentionally in angiographic imaging sequences. DSA imaging allows different magnification levels by employing different focusing filters inside the image intensifier. Varying the distance of the image receptor can increase this type of magnification. Intentional use of magnification can result in a significant increase in resolution of fine vessel recorded detail. Fractional focal spot tubes of 0.3 mm or less are necessary for direct radiographic magnification techniques. The selection of a fractional focal spot necessitates the use of low milliamperage. Short exposure time (1 to 200 msec) is necessary because the size and load capacity of the smaller focal spot.

The formula for manual magnification is as follows:

$$M = \frac{SID}{SOD} \; or \; \frac{SID}{SID - OID}$$

The SID is the *source-to-image-receptor distance,* the SOD is the *source-to-object distance,* and the OID is the *object-to-image-receptor distance.* For a 2 : 1 magnification study using SID of 40 inches (101 cm), the focal spot and the image receptor are positioned 20 inches (50 cm) from the area of interest. A 3 : 1 magnification study using a 40-inch (101-cm) SID is accomplished by placing the focal spot 13 inches (33 cm) from the area of interest and the image receptor 27 inches (68 cm) from the area of interest.

Unintentional magnification occurs when the area of interest cannot be placed in direct contact with the image receptor. This is particularly a problem in the biplane imaging sequence, in which the need to center the area of interest in the first plane may create some unavoidable distance of the body part to the image receptor in the second plane. Even in single-plane imaging, vascular structures are separated from the image receptor by some distance. The magnification that occurs as a result of these circumstances is frequently 20% to 25%. A 25% magnification occurs when a vessel within the body is 8 inches (20 cm) from the image receptor—OID of 8 inches (20 cm)—and SID is 40 inches (101 cm).

Angiographic images do not represent vessels at their actual size, and this must be taken into account when direct measurements are made from angiographic images. Increasing SID while maintaining OID can reduce unintentional magnification. Increasing SID may not be an option, however, if the increase in technical factors would exceed tube output capacity or exposure time maximum. When any measurement is necessary, the DSA post-processing quantitative analysis programs require the angiographer to calibrate the system by measuring an object in the imaging field of known value. Some systems calibrate by using the known position of the table, the II or detector, and x-ray tube and the tube angulation.

THREE-DIMENSIONAL INTRAARTERIAL ANGIOGRAPHY

The latest diagnostic tool is three-dimensional angiography. To acquire a three-dimensional model of a vascular structure, a C-arm is rotated around the region of interest (ROI) at speeds up to 60 degrees per second. The C-arm makes a preliminary sweep while mask images are acquired. Images are acquired at 7.5 to 30 frames per second. The C-arm returns to its initial position, and a second sweep is initiated. Just before the second sweep, a contrast medium is injected to opacify the vascular anatomy. The second sweep matches mask images from the first sweep, producing a rotational subtracted DSA sequence. The DSA sequence is sent to a three-dimensional rendering computer where a three-dimensional model is constructed. This model provides an image that can be manipulated and analyzed. It has proved to be a valuable tool for interventional approaches and for evaluation before surgery. Various methods of vessel analysis are available with three-dimensional models. Aneurysm volume calculation, interior wall analysis, bone fusion, and device display all are possible (Figs. 23-11 and 23-12).

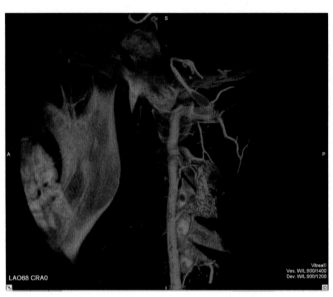

Fig. 23-11 Three-dimensional angiography provides for reconstruction of the vessels and the skeletal anatomy.

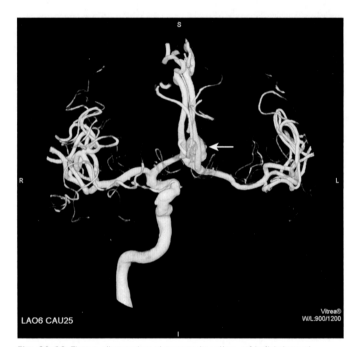

Fig. 23-12 Three-dimensional reconstruction of left internal carotid artery. Note the anterior communicating artery aneurysm (*arrow*).

Angiographic Supplies and Equipment

NEEDLES

Vascular access needles are necessary when performing percutaneous procedures. Needle size is based on the external diameter of the needle and is assigned a gauge size. To allow for appropriate guidewire matching, the internal diameter of the needle must be known. Vascular access needles come in different types, sizes, and lengths. The most commonly used access needle for adult cardiovascular procedures is an 18-gauge needle that is 2.75 inches (7 cm) long. This particular needle is compatible with a 0.035-inch guidewire, which is the most frequently used guidewire in cardiovascular procedures. Appropriate needle size is predicated on the type or size of guidewire needed, the size of the patient, and the targeted entry vessel. To decrease the chances of vascular complications, the smallest gauge needle that meets the above-mentioned criteria is used for vascular access. Access needles for pediatric patients come in smaller gauge sizes with shorter lengths (Fig. 23-13).

GUIDEWIRES

Guidewires are used in angiography and other special procedures as a platform over which the catheter is to be advanced. To decrease the possibilities of complications, the guidewire should be advanced into the vasculature ahead of the catheter. After the guidewire is positioned in the area of interest, the position of the guidewire is fixed, and the catheter is advanced until it meets the tip of the guidewire. Similar to needles, guidewires come in various sizes, shapes, and lengths, and care must be taken to match the proper guidewire to the selected access needle and catheter.

Most guidewires are constructed of stainless steel, with a core or mandrel encased circumferentially within a tightly wound spiral outer core of spring wire. The mandrel gives the guidewire its stiffness and body. The length of the mandrel within the wire determines the flexibility of the wire. The shorter the mandrel, the more flexible the wire, and the more likely it is to traverse tortuous anatomy. A safety ribbon is built into the tip of the guidewire to prevent wire dislodgment in case the wire fractures. Many stainless steel guidewires are coated with polytef (Teflon) to provide lubricity and to decrease the friction between the catheter and wire. Similarly, the Teflon coating is thought to help decrease the thrombogenicity of the guidewire.

More recently, plastic alloy guidewires consisting of a hydrophilic plastic polymer coating have been introduced. These new wires provide a smooth outer coating, with a pliable tip, and exhibit a high degree of torque or maneuverability (Fig. 23-14).

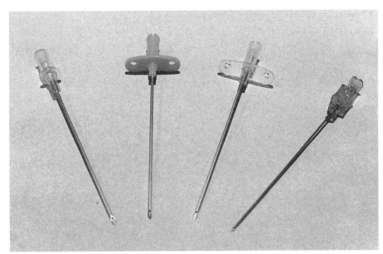

Fig. 23-13 Various needles used during catheterization.

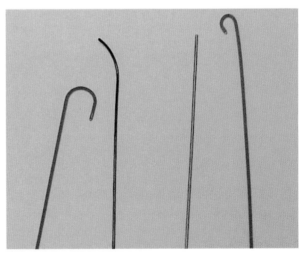

Fig. 23-14 A guidewire allows the user a high degree of torque and maneuverability. Various lengths and shaped tips are available.

INTRODUCER SHEATHS

Introducer sheaths are frequently used in angiographic procedures when multiple catheters are used. When the sheath has been placed, controlled access of the vasculature is ensured while reducing vessel trauma by limiting numerous catheter passages through the vessel wall.

Introducer sheaths are short catheters consisting of a slotted, rubberized backbleed valve and a sidearm extension port. The backbleed valve prevents the loss of blood volume during catheter exchanges or guidewire manipulations. The sidearm extension port may be used to infuse medications, monitor blood pressure, or inject contrast media to visualize the vessel or adjacent vessels.

Similar to vascular catheters, introducer sheaths come in various sizes and lengths. Typically, most introducer sheaths range in length from 4 to 35 inches (10 to 90 cm). Catheters are measured by their outside diameters and expressed in units of French size (Fr), and introducer sheaths are named according to the French size catheter they can accommodate. To accomplish this, the outer diameters of introducer sheaths are 1.5 to 2 Fr sizes larger than the catheter they can accept. A 5-Fr introducer has an outer diameter of nearly 7 Fr and accepts a 5-Fr catheter (Fig. 23-15).

CATHETERIZATION

Catheterization for filling vessels with contrast media is preferred to needle injection of the media. The advantages of catheterization are as follows:
1. The risk of *extravasation* is reduced.
2. Most body parts can be reached for selective injection.
3. The patient can be positioned as needed.
4. The catheter can be safely left in the body while radiographs are being examined.

The femoral, axillary, brachial, and radial arteries are the most commonly punctured vessels. The transfemoral site is preferred because it is associated with the fewest risks.

The most widely used catheterization method is the Seldinger technique.[1] Seldinger described the method as puncture of both walls of the vessel (the anterior and posterior walls). The modified Seldinger technique allows for puncture of the anterior wall only and has become the preferred method. The steps of the technique are described in Fig. 23-16. The procedure is performed under sterile conditions. The catheterization site is suitably cleaned

---

[1]Seldinger SI: Percutaneous selective angiography of the aorta: preliminary report, *Acta Radiol (Stockh)* 45:15, 1956.

and surgically draped. The patient is given local anesthesia at the catheterization site. With this percutaneous technique, the arteriotomy or venotomy is no larger than the catheter itself, so hemorrhage is minimized. Patients can usually resume normal activity within 24 hours after the examination. In some diagnostic angiographic studies, the procedure can be performed in the early morning, and the patient may be discharged later that same day. Most often, an uncomplicated interventional procedure may be performed, and the patient recovers in an ambulatory care area and is discharged home usually within 24 hours. The risk of infection is less than in surgical procedures because the vessel and tissues are not exposed.

After a catheter is introduced into the blood-vascular system, it can be maneuvered by pushing, pulling, and turning the part of the catheter still outside the patient so that the part of the catheter inside the patient travels to a specific location. A wire is sometimes positioned inside the catheter to help manipulate and guide the catheter to the desired location. When the wire is removed from the catheter, the catheter is infused with sterile solution, most commonly heparinized saline, to help prevent clot formation. Infusing the catheter and assisting the physician in the catheterization process may be the responsibility of the CIT.

When the examination is complete, the catheter is removed. Pressure is applied to the site until complete hemostasis is achieved, but blood flow through the vessel is maintained. The patient is placed on complete bed rest and observed for the development of bleeding or *hematoma.* Newer closure devices, which close the vessel percutaneously, can also be used to close the puncture site.

When peripheral artery sites are unavailable, a catheter may sometimes be introduced into the aorta using the translumbar aortic approach. For this technique, the patient is positioned prone, and a special catheter introducer system is inserted percutaneously through the posterolateral aspect of the back and directed superiorly so that the catheter enters the aorta around the T11-12 level.

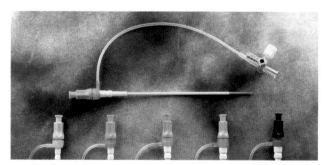

Fig. 23-15 Various types of introducer sheaths used during catheterization.

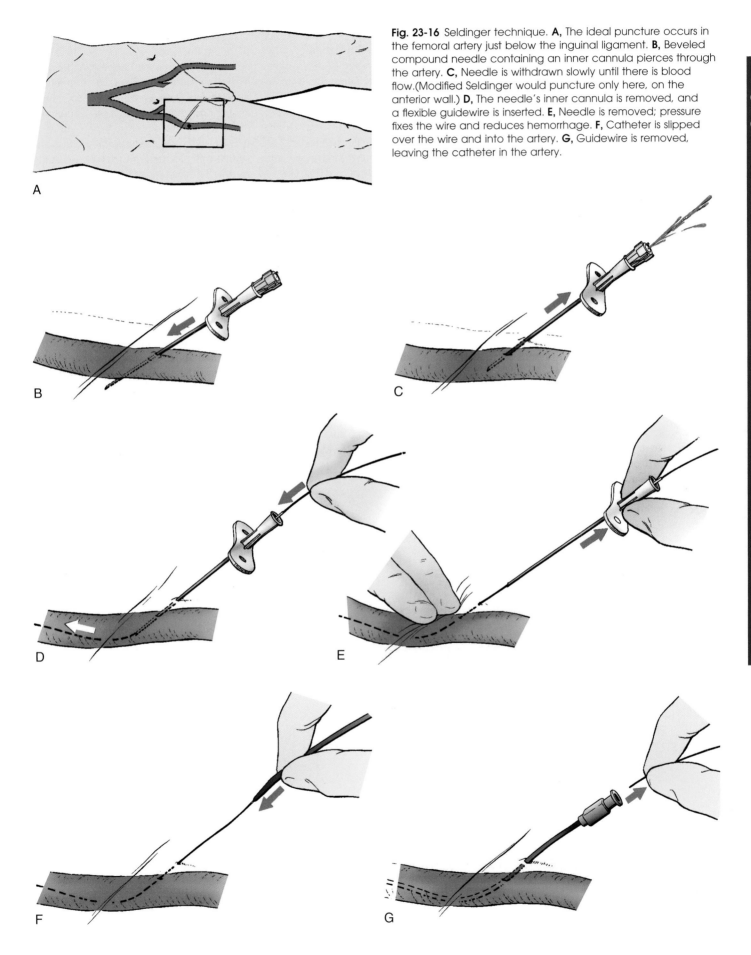

Fig. 23-16 Seldinger technique. **A,** The ideal puncture occurs in the femoral artery just below the inguinal ligament. **B,** Beveled compound needle containing an inner cannula pierces through the artery. **C,** Needle is withdrawn slowly until there is blood flow.(Modified Seldinger would puncture only here, on the anterior wall.) **D,** The needle's inner cannula is removed, and a flexible guidewire is inserted. **E,** Needle is removed; pressure fixes the wire and reduces hemorrhage. **F,** Catheter is slipped over the wire and into the artery. **G,** Guidewire is removed, leaving the catheter in the artery.

Catheters are produced in various forms, each with a particular advantage in shape, maneuverability or torque, and maximum injection rate (Fig. 23-17). Angiographic catheters are made of pliable plastic that allows them to straighten for insertion over the guide-wire, also called a *wire guide*. They normally resume their original shape after the guidewire is withdrawn. It usually requires manipulation from the angiographer to resume its original shape, however. Catheters with a predetermined design or shape are maneuvered into the origins of vessels for selective injections. They may have only an end hole, or they may have multiple side holes. Some catheters have multiple side holes to facilitate high injection rates but are used only in large vascular structures for flush injections. A pigtail catheter is a special multiple-side hole catheter that allows higher volumes of contrast media to be injected with less whiplash effect, causing less damage to the vessel being injected.

Common angiographic catheters range in size from 4 Fr (0.05 inch) to 7 Fr (0.09 inch), although smaller or larger sizes may be used. Most angiographic catheters have inner lumens that allow them to be inserted over guidewires ranging from 0.032 to 0.038 inch in diameter.

Patient Care

Before the initiation of an angiographic procedure, it is appropriate to explain the process and the potential complications to the patient. Written consent is obtained after an explanation. Potential complications include a vasovagal reaction; stroke; heart attack; death; infection; bleeding at the puncture site; nerve, blood vessel, or tissue damage; and an allergic reaction to the contrast media. Bleeding at the puncture site is usually easily controlled with pressure to the site. Blood vessel and tissue damage may require a surgical procedure. A vasovagal reaction is characterized by sweating and nausea caused by a decrease in blood pressure. The patient's legs should be elevated, and intravenous (IV) fluids may be administered to help restore blood pressure. Minor allergic reactions to iodinated contrast media, such as hives and congestion, are usually controlled with medications and may not require treatment. Severe allergic reactions may result in shock, which is characterized by shallow breathing, high pulse rate, and possibly loss of consciousness. Angiography is performed only if the benefits of the examination outweigh the risks.

Patients are usually restricted to clear liquid intake and routine medications before undergoing angiography. Adequate hydration from liquid intake may minimize kidney damage caused by iodinated contrast media. Solid food intake is restricted to reduce the risk of aspiration related to nausea. Contraindications to angiography are determined by physicians and include previous severe allergic reaction to iodinated contrast media, severely impaired renal function, impaired blood clotting factors, and inability to undergo a surgical procedure or general anesthesia.

Because the risks of general anesthesia are greater than the risks associated with most angiographic procedures, conscious sedation may be used for the procedure. Thoughtful communication from the CIT and physician calms and reassures the patient. The CIT or physician should warn the patient about the sensations caused by the contrast media and the noise produced by the imaging equipment. This information also reduces the patient's anxiety and helps ensure a good radiographic series with no patient motion.

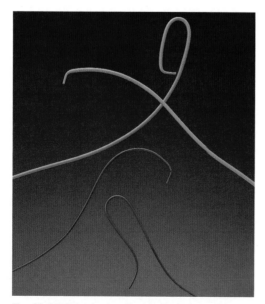

Fig. 23-17 Selected catheter shapes used for angiography.

(Courtesy Cook, Inc., Bloomington, IN.)

Preparation of Examining Room

The angiography suite and every item in it should be scrupulously clean. The room should be fully prepared, with every item needed or likely to be needed on hand before the patient is admitted. Cleanliness and advance preparation are of vital importance in procedures that must be carried out under aseptic conditions. The CIT should observe the following guidelines in preparing the room:

- Check the angiographic equipment and all working parts of the equipment, and adjust the controls for the exposure technique to be employed.
- Have restraining bands available for application in combative patients.
- Adapt immobilization of the head (by suitable strapping) to the type of equipment employed.
- Ensure patient information is entered correctly on acquisition equipment.

The sterile and nonsterile items required for introduction of the contrast media vary according to the method of injection. The supplies specified by the interventionalist for each procedure should be listed in the angiographic procedure book. Sterile trays or packs, set up to specifications, can usually be obtained from the central sterile supply room. Otherwise, it is the responsibility of a qualified member of the interventional team to prepare them. Extra sterile supplies should always be on hand in case of a complication. Preparation of the room includes having life-support and emergency equipment immediately available.

Radiation Protection

As in all radiographic examinations, the patient is protected by filtration totaling not less than 2.5 mm of aluminum, by sharp restriction of the beam of radiation to the area being examined, and by avoidance of repeat exposures. In angiography, each repeated exposure necessitates repeated injection of the contrast material. For this reason, only skilled and specifically educated CITs should be assigned to participate in these examinations. Gonadal shielding should be available and used when it would not interfere with the examination.

Angiography suites should be designed to allow observation of the patient at all times and provide adequate protection to the physician and radiology personnel. These goals are usually accomplished with leaded glass observation windows.

Angiography Team

The angiography team consists of the physician (usually an interventional radiologist), the CIT, and other specialists, such as an anesthetist or a nurse. The CIT assists in performing procedures that require sterile technique. Other duties may include operating monitoring devices, emergency equipment, and radiographic equipment. Instruction in patient care techniques and sterile procedure is included in the basic preparation of the CIT.

Angiography in the Future

Visceral and peripheral angiography is a dynamic area that challenges angiographers to keep abreast of new techniques and equipment. New diagnostic modalities that reduce or eliminate irradiation may be developed and may replace many current angiographic procedures. Some diagnostic information can be obtained only through conventional angiographic methods, however. Consequently, angiography will continue to be used to examine vasculature and, through therapeutic procedures, to provide beneficial treatment. Noninvasive imaging techniques, such as ultrasound, magnetic resonance angiography, and CT angiography, are being used more often. These less invasive procedures may eliminate some diagnostic angiographic procedures, but at the present time, therapeutic procedures continue.

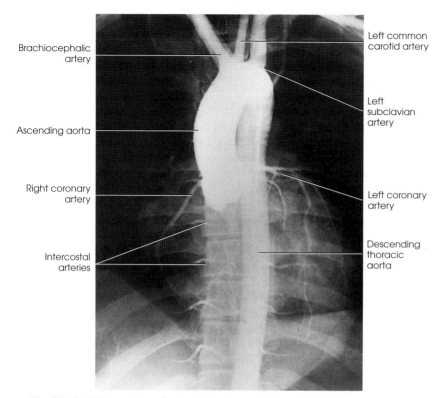

Brachiocephalic artery

Ascending aorta

Right coronary artery

Intercostal arteries

Left common carotid artery

Left subclavian artery

Left coronary artery

Descending thoracic aorta

Fig. 23-18 AP thoracic aorta that also shows right and left coronary arteries.

Visualization of the aorta is achieved by placing a multihole catheter into the aorta at the desired level, using the modified Seldinger technique. *Aortography* is usually performed with the patient in the supine position for simultaneous frontal and lateral imaging, with the central ray perpendicular to the imaging system. For introduction of a translumbar aortic catheter, the patient must be in the prone position.

Thoracic Aortography

Thoracic aortography may be performed to rule out an aortic aneurysm or to evaluate congenital or postsurgical conditions. The examination is also used in patients with *aortic dissection*. Biplane imaging is recommended so that anteroposterior (AP) or posteroanterior (PA) and lateral projections can be obtained with one injection of contrast media. The CIT observes the following guidelines:

- For lateral projections, move the patient's arms superiorly so that they do not appear in the image.
- For best results, increase lateral SID, usually to 60 inches (152 cm), so that magnification is reduced.
- If biplane equipment is unavailable, use a single-plane, 45-degree right posterior oblique (RPO) or left anterior oblique (LAO) body position, which often produces an adequate study of the aorta.
- For all projections, direct the perpendicular central ray to the center of the chest at the level of T7. The entire thoracic aorta should be visualized, including the proximal brachiocephalic, carotid, and subclavian vessels. The contrast media are injected at rates ranging from 23 to 35 mL/sec for a total volume of 50 to 70 mL.
- Make the exposure at the end of suspended inspiration (Fig. 23-18).

Abdominal Aortography

Abdominal aortography may be performed to evaluate abdominal aortic aneurysm (AAA), occlusion, or atherosclerotic disease. Simultaneous AP and lateral projections are recommended. The CIT observes the following guidelines:

- For the lateral projection, move the patient's arms superiorly so that they are out of the image field.
- Usually, collimate the field in the AP aspect of the lateral projection.
- Direct the perpendicular central ray at the level of L2 so that the aorta is visualized from the diaphragm to the aortic bifurcation. The AP projection shows best the renal artery origins, the aortic bifurcation, and the course and general condition of all abdominal visceral branches. The lateral projection best shows the origins of the celiac and superior mesenteric arteries because these vessels arise from the anterior abdominal aorta.
- Make the exposure at the end of suspended expiration (Figs. 23-19 and 23-20).

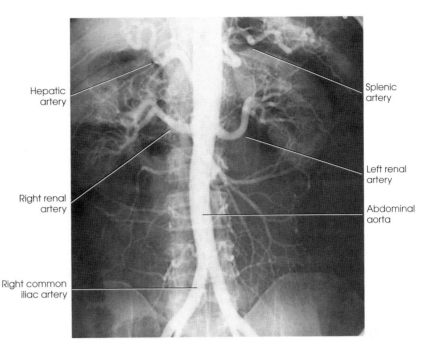

Fig. 23-19 AP abdominal aorta.

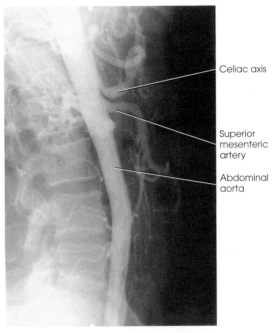

Fig. 23-20 Lateral abdominal aorta.

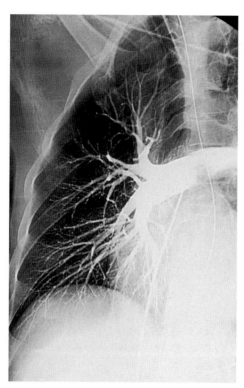

Fig. 23-21 Right pulmonary artery.

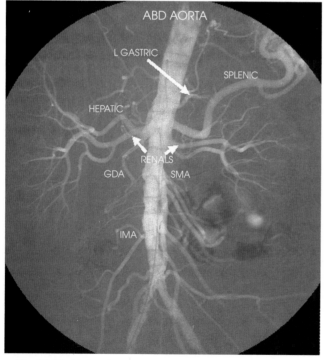

Fig. 23-22 Abdominal aortogram showing visceral arteries.

Pulmonary Arteriography

Under fluoroscopic control, a catheter is passed from a peripheral vein through the vena cava and right side of the heart and into the pulmonary arteries. This technique is usually employed for a selective injection, and the examination is primarily performed for the evaluation of pulmonary embolic disease (Fig. 23-21). Pulmonary angiography has widely been replaced with pulmonary CT angiography because it provides superior imaging.

Visceral Arteriography

Abdominal visceral arteriographic studies (Fig. 23-22) are usually performed to visualize tumor vascularity or to rule out atherosclerotic disease, thrombosis, occlusion, and bleeding. An appropriately shaped catheter is introduced, usually from a transfemoral artery puncture, and advanced into the orifice of the desired artery. The CIT observes the following steps:

- Perform all selective studies initially with the patient in the supine position for single-plane frontal images.
- Direct the central ray perpendicular to the image receptor.
- If necessary, use oblique projections to improve visualization or avoid superimposition of vessels.
- For all abdominal visceral studies, obtain angiograms during suspended expiration.

Selective abdominal visceral arteriograms are described in the following sections.

CELIAC ARTERIOGRAM

The celiac artery normally arises from the aorta at the level of T12 and carries blood to the stomach and proximal duodenum, liver, spleen, and pancreas. The CIT follows these steps:

• For the angiographic examination, center the patient to the image receptor.
• Direct the central ray to L1 (Fig. 23-23).

HEPATIC ARTERIOGRAM

The common hepatic artery branches from the right side of the celiac artery and supplies circulation to the liver, stomach and proximal duodenum, and pancreas. The CIT does the following:

• Position the patient so that the upper and right margins of the liver are at the respective margins of the image receptor (Fig. 23-24).

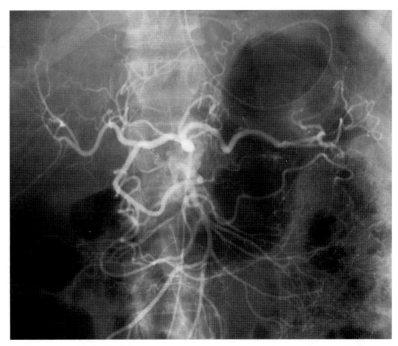

Fig. 23-23 Superselective celiac artery injection.

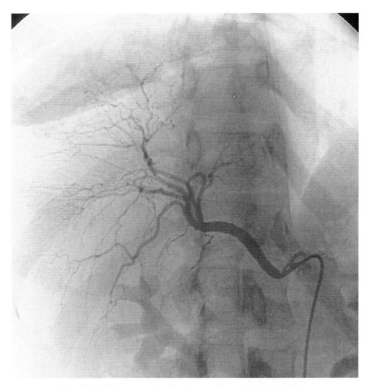

Fig. 23-24 Superselective hepatic artery injection.

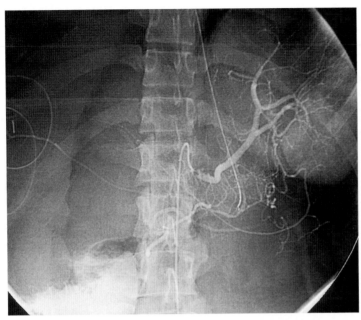

Fig. 23-25 Superselective splenic artery injection.

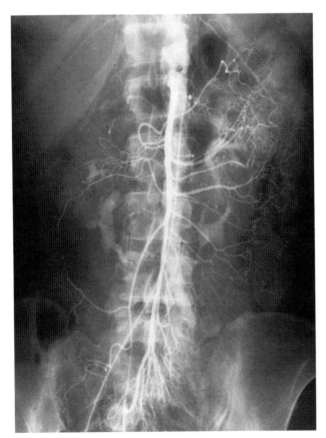

Fig. 23-26 Selective SMA injection.

SPLENIC ARTERIOGRAM

The splenic artery branches from the left side of the celiac artery and supplies blood to the spleen and pancreas. The steps are as follows:

- Position the patient to place the left and upper margins of the spleen at the respective margins of the image receptor (Fig. 23-25).
- Injection of the splenic artery can show the portal venous system on the late venous images.
- To show the portal vein, center the patient to the image receptor.

SUPERIOR MESENTERIC ARTERIOGRAM

The superior mesenteric artery (SMA) supplies blood to the small intestine and the ascending and transverse colon. It arises at about the level of L1 and descends to L5-S1. The CIT follows these steps:

- To show the SMA, center the patient to the midline of the image receptor.
- Direct the central ray to the level of L3 (Fig. 23-26).
- When attempting to visualize bleeding sites, extend the exposure duration to 60 seconds or as requested by the radiologist.

INFERIOR MESENTERIC ARTERIOGRAM

The inferior mesenteric artery (IMA) supplies blood to the splenic flexure, descending colon, and rectosigmoid area. It arises from the left side of the aorta at about the level of L3 and descends into the pelvis. The CIT does the following:

- To visualize the IMA best, use a 15-degree right anterior oblique (RAO) or left posterior oblique (LPO) position that places the descending colon and rectum at the left and inferior margins of the image (Fig. 23-27). The imaging is the same as that for the SMA.

RENAL ARTERIOGRAM

The renal arteries arise from the right and left side of the aorta between L1 and L2 and supply blood to the respective kidney. The CIT observes the following steps:

- A renal flush aortogram may be accomplished by injecting 25 mL/sec for a 40-mL total volume of contrast media through a multiple–side hole catheter positioned in the aorta at the level of the renal arteries. A representative selective injection is 8 mL/sec for a 12-mL total volume.

- For a right renal arteriogram, position the patient so that the central ray enters at the level of L2 midway between the center of the spine and the patient's right side.

- For a selective left renal arteriogram, position the patient so that the central ray usually enters at the level of L1 midway between the center of the spine and the patient's left side (Fig. 23-28).

OTHER ABDOMINAL ARTERIOGRAMS

Other arteries branching from the aorta may be selectively studied to show anatomy and possible pathology. The positioning for these procedures depends on the area to be studied and the surrounding structures (these may include spinal, lumbar, adrenal, and phrenic).

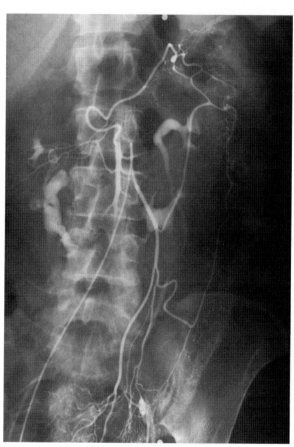

Fig. 23-27 Selective IMA injection.

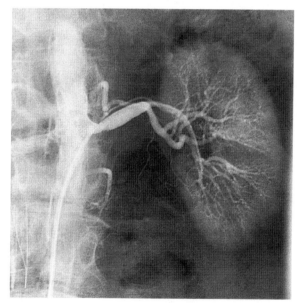

Fig. 23-28 Selective left renal artery injection in early arterial phase.

Peripheral Angiography
UPPER LIMB ARTERIOGRAMS

Upper limb arteriography is most often performed to evaluate traumatic injury, atherosclerotic disease, or other vascular lesions. Arteriograms are usually obtained using the modified Seldinger technique to introduce a catheter, most often at a femoral artery site for selective injection into the subclavian or axillary artery. The contrast media may also be injected at a more distal site through a catheter. The area to be radiographed may be a hand or another selected part of the arm or the entire upper extremity and thorax.

The recommended projection is a true AP projection with the arm extended and the hand supinated. Hand arteriograms may be obtained in the supine or prone arm position (Figs. 23-29 and 23-30). The injection varies from 3 to 4 mL/sec through a catheter positioned distally to 10 mL/sec through a proximally positioned catheter. Images are obtained by using a bolus chase technique or by performing serial runs over each segment of the extremity.

UPPER LIMB VENOGRAMS

Upper limb venography is most often performed to look for thrombosis or occlusions. The contrast medium is injected through a needle, IV line, or catheter into a superficial vein at the elbow or wrist. Radiographs should cover the vasculature from the wrist or elbow to the superior vena cava (Fig. 23-31).

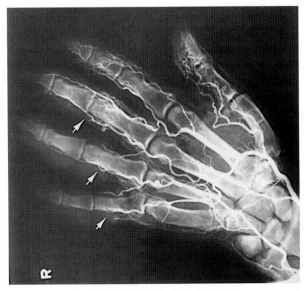

Fig. 23-29 Right hand arteriogram (2:1 magnification) showing severe arterial occlusive disease (*arrows*) affecting digits after cold temperature injury.

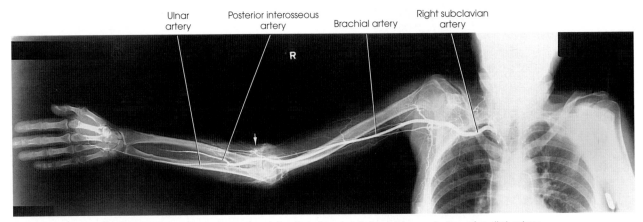

Ulnar artery   Posterior interosseous artery   Brachial artery   Right subclavian artery

Fig. 23-30 Right subclavian artery injection showing iatrogenic occlusion of radial artery (*arrow*).

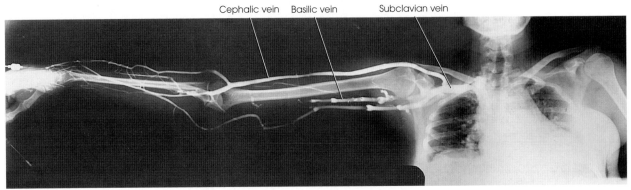

Cephalic vein   Basilic vein   Subclavian vein

Fig. 23-31 Normal right upper limb venogram.

LOWER LIMB ARTERIOGRAMS

Aortofemoral arteriography is usually performed to determine whether atherosclerotic disease is the cause of *claudication*. A catheter is usually introduced into a femoral artery using the modified Seldinger technique. The catheter tip is positioned superior to the aortic bifurcation so that bilateral arteriograms are obtained simultaneously. When only one leg is to be examined, the catheter tip is placed below the bifurcation, or the contrast medium is injected through a catheter or sheath placed in the femoral artery on the side of interest. The CIT observes the following guidelines:

- For a bilateral examination, place the patient in the supine position for single-plane AP projections and center the patient to the midline of the image receptor to include the area from the renal arteries to the ankles (Fig. 23-32).
- For either patient position, internally rotate the legs 30 degrees.
- Subtracted or unsubtracted bolus chase selections can be used to follow the contrast media down the legs or single-station DSA.
- Make exposures of the opacified lower abdominal aorta and aortic bifurcation with the patient in suspended expiration.

Examinations of a specific area of the leg such as the popliteal fossa or foot are occasionally performed. For these procedures, the preferred injection site is usually the femoral artery. AP, lateral, or both projections may be obtained with the patient centered to the designated area.

LOWER LIMB VENOGRAMS

Lower limb venography is usually performed to visualize thrombosis of the deep veins of the leg. Ultrasound of the legs is the first-line diagnostic tool to diagnose deep vein thrombosis. Venograms are usually obtained with contrast media injected through a sheath or catheter placed directly into the popliteal vein with the patient prone (Fig. 23-33).

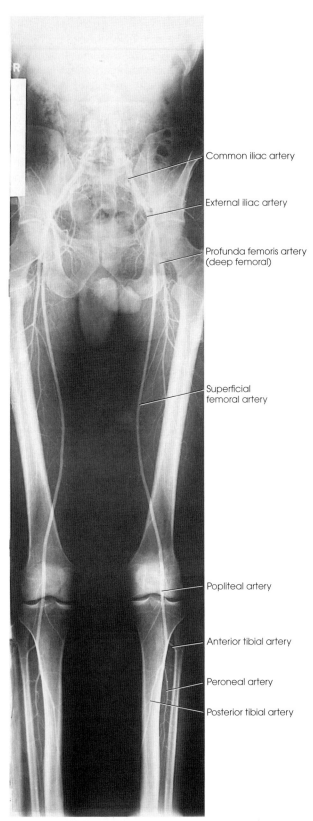

Common iliac artery

External iliac artery

Profunda femoris artery (deep femoral)

Superficial femoral artery

Popliteal artery

Anterior tibial artery

Peroneal artery

Posterior tibial artery

Fig. 23-32 Normal abdominal aortogram and bilateral femoral arteriogram in late arterial phase.

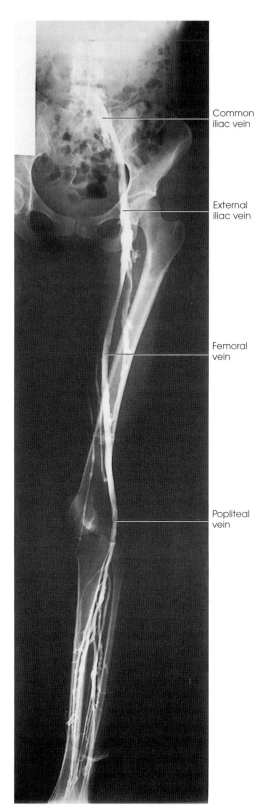

Common iliac vein

External iliac vein

Femoral vein

Popliteal vein

Fig. 23-33 Normal left lower limb venogram.

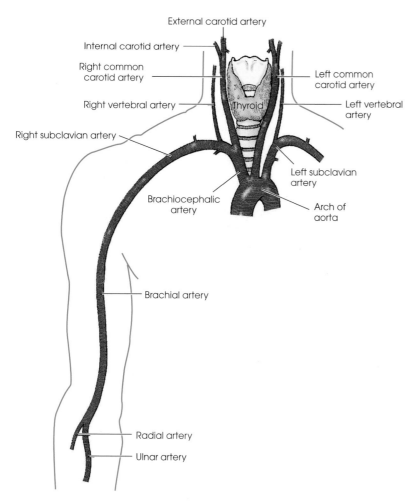

External carotid artery

Internal carotid artery

Right common carotid artery

Left common carotid artery

Right vertebral artery

Left vertebral artery

Thyroid

Right subclavian artery

Left subclavian artery

Brachiocephalic artery

Arch of aorta

Brachial artery

Radial artery

Ulnar artery

Fig. 23-34 Major arteries of upper chest, neck, and arm.

Cerebral Anatomy

Cerebral angiography is the radiologic and angiographic examination of the blood vessels of the brain. The procedure was introduced by Egas Moniz[1] in 1927. It is performed to investigate intracranial vascular lesions such as aneurysms, arteriovenous malformations (AVMs), tumors, and atherosclerotic or stenotic lesions.

The brain is supplied by four trunk vessels or great vessels (Fig. 23-34): the right and left common carotid arteries, which supply the anterior circulation, and the right and left vertebral arteries, which supply the posterior circulation. These paired arteries branch from the arch of the aorta and ascend through the neck.

---

[1]Egas Moniz AC: L'encéphalographie artérielle, son importance dans la localisation des tumeurs cérébrales, *Rev Neurol* 2:72, 1927.

Cerebral Anatomy

49

The first branch of the aortic arch is the *innominate artery* or the *brachiocephalic artery*. It bifurcates into the right common carotid and the right subclavian artery. The second branch of the aortic arch is the left common carotid, followed by the left subclavian artery. Each of the vessels originates directly from the aortic arch. Both vertebral arteries most commonly take their origins from the subclavian arteries. Although this branching pattern is common in most patients, there can be some *anomalous* origins of these great vessels. Each common carotid artery passes superiorly and laterally alongside the trachea and larynx to the level of C4 and then divides into internal and external carotid arteries. The external carotid artery contributes blood supply to the extracranial and extraaxial circulation. There can be some collateral circulation into the internal carotid circulation in some situations. The internal carotid artery enters the cranium through the carotid foramen of the temporal bone and bifurcates into the anterior and middle cerebral arteries (Fig. 23-35). These vessels branch and rebranch to supply the anterior circulation of the respective hemisphere of the brain.

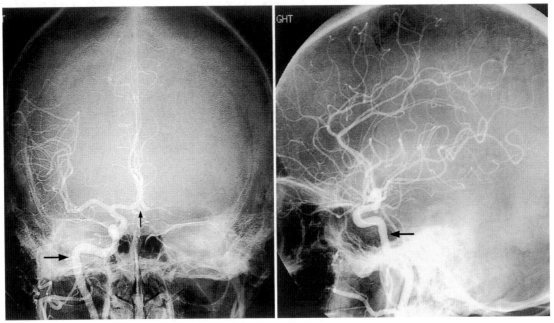

Fig. 23-35 Right common carotid artery injection showing right internal carotid artery (*arrows*) and anterior cerebral blood circulation, including reflux across anterior communicating artery (*small arrow*).

The vertebral arteries ascend through the cervical transverse foramina and pass medially to enter the cranium through the foramen magnum. The vertebral arteries unite to form the basilar artery, which, after a short superior course along the posterior surface of the dorsum sellae, bifurcates into the right and left posterior cerebral arteries. The blood supply to the posterior fossa (cerebellum) originates from the vertebral and basilar arteries (Fig. 23-36).

The anterior and posterior cerebral arteries are connected by communicating arteries at the level of the midbrain to form the *circle of Willis*. The anterior communicating artery forms an anastomosis between the anterior cerebral arteries, which communicate between the right and left hemispheres. The right and left posterior communicating arteries each form an anastomosis between the internal carotid artery and the posterior cerebral artery connecting the anterior and posterior circulation. A chart detailing intracerebral circulation is provided in Figs. 23-37 and 23-38.

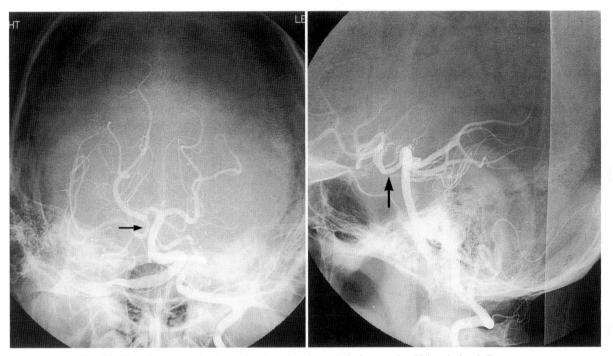

Fig. 23-36 Left vertebral artery injection showing posterior cerebral blood circulation, including reflux into posterior communicating artery (*arrows*).

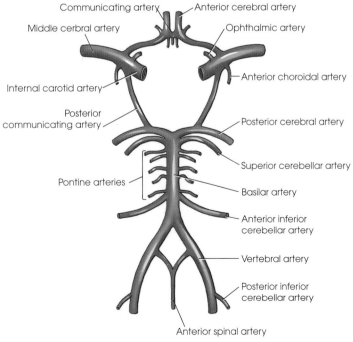

Fig. 23-37 Circle of Willis.

51

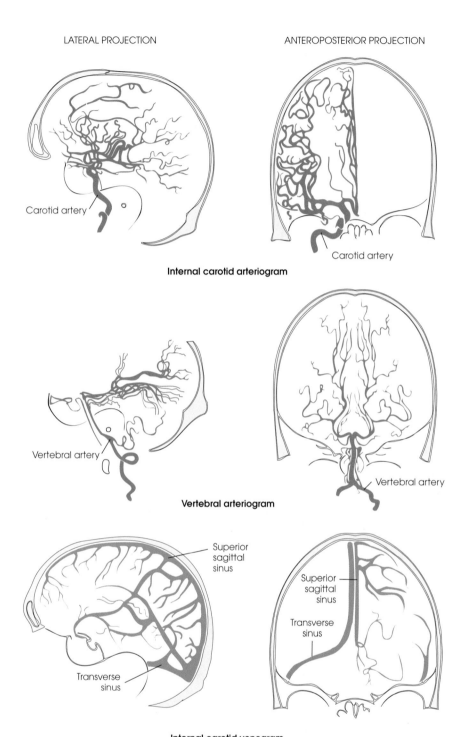

LATERAL PROJECTION

ANTEROPOSTERIOR PROJECTION

Carotid artery

Carotid artery

Internal carotid arteriogram

Vertebral artery

Vertebral artery

Vertebral arteriogram

Superior sagittal sinus

Superior sagittal sinus

Transverse sinus

Transverse sinus

Internal carotid venogram

Fig. 23-38 Diagram of intracranial circulation: arterial and venous phase.

(From Bean BC: A chart of the intracerebral circulation, ed 2, *Med Radiogr Photogr* 34:25, 1958; courtesy Dr. Berton C. Bean and Eastman Kodak Co.)

Technique

Cerebral angiography should be performed only in facilities equipped to produce studies of high technical quality with minimal risk to the patient. The ability to obtain rapid-sequence biplane images with automatic injection represents the minimum standard. This equipment is available in all major medical centers and in most large hospitals (see Fig. 23-9).

Cerebral angiography is most commonly performed from a transfemoral approach; however, a brachial or axillary artery approach can be employed. Selective catheterization techniques also allow the internal and external carotid circulation to be studied separately, which is useful in delineating the blood supply of some forms of cerebral tumors and vascular malformations.

The final position of the catheter depends on the information sought from the angiographic study. When atherosclerotic disease of the extracranial carotid, subclavian, and vertebral arteries is being evaluated, injection of the aortic arch with imaging of the extracranial portion of these vessels is an appropriate way to begin.

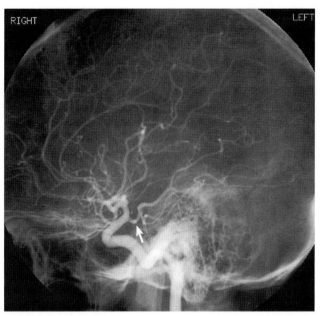

Fig. 23-39 Right internal carotid injection, lateral projection, shows arterial phase of circulation. Note posterior communicating artery (*arrow*).

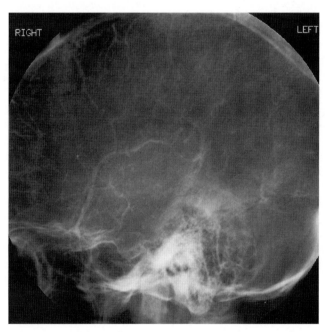

Fig. 23-40 Right internal carotid injection, lateral projection, shows capillary phase of carotid circulation.

CIRCULATION TIME AND IMAGING PROGRAM

Egas Moniz[1] stated that the transit time of the cerebral circulation is only 3 seconds for the blood to circulate from the internal carotid artery to the jugular vein, with the circulation time being slightly prolonged by the injected contrast solution. Greitz,[2] who measured the cerebral circulation time as "the time between the points of maximum concentration (of contrast media) in the carotid siphon and in the parietal veins," found a normal mean value of 4.13 seconds. This time is a highly important factor in cerebral angiography.

Certain pathologic conditions significantly alter the cerebral circulation time. AVMs shorten the transit time; arterial vasospasm may cause a considerable delay.

A standard radiographic program should include a radiograph taken before the arrival of contrast material to serve as a subtraction mask and rapid-sequence images at $1\frac{1}{2}$ to 3 images per second in the AP and lateral projections during the early, or arterial, phase (first $1\frac{1}{2}$ to $2\frac{1}{2}$ seconds) of the arteriogram (Fig. 23-39). After the arterial phase, imaging may be slowed to one image per second for the capillary, or parenchymal, phase (Fig. 23-40) and maintained at one image per second or every other second for the venous phase (Fig. 23-41) of the angiogram. The entire program should cover 7 to 10 seconds, depending on the preference of the angiographer. The imaging program must be tailored to show the suspected pathologic condition.

Injection rates and volumes through the catheter are coupled with the imaging program, usually by automatic means. Injections at rates of 5 to 9 mL/sec for 1 to 2 seconds are most often employed in the cerebral vessels, with variations dependent on vessel size and the patient's circulatory status.

[1]Egas Moniz AC: *L'angiographie cérébrale,* Paris, 1934, Masson & Cie.
[2]Greitz T: A radiologic study of the brain circulation by rapid serial angiography of the carotid artery, *Acta Radiol* 46(Suppl 140):1, 1956.

Technique

53

EQUIPMENT

Rapid-sequence biplane imaging with DSA electronically coupled with an automatic injector is employed almost universally in cerebral angiography. Collimating to the area of the head and neck is essential for improving image quality in a nonmagnified study. The standard tube collimator may be used for this purpose.

POSITION OF HEAD

The centering and angulation of the central ray required to show the anterior circulation differ from those required to show the posterior circulation. The same head position is used for the basic AP and lateral projections of both regions. The following steps are observed:

- For the initial right-angle studies, center the head to the AP and lateral image receptors.
- Adjust the patient's head to place its midsagittal plane exactly perpendicular to the headrest and consequently exactly parallel with the laterally placed image receptor.
- Place the infraorbitomeatal line (IOML) perpendicular to the horizontal plane when positioning is done manually.
- Angle the central ray for caudally inclined AP and AP oblique projections from the vertically placed IOML, or adjust the central ray so that it is parallel to the floor of the anterior fossa, as indicated by a line extending from the supraorbital margin to a point ¾ inch (1.9 cm) superior to the external acoustic meatus (EAM).

In this chapter, head positioning is presented as if the image receptors were fixed in the horizontal and vertical planes; this necessitates the use of facial landmarks for precise positioning of the head in relation to the central ray to achieve certain projections. In some angiography suites, fluoroscopy can be used to determine the final position of the head and the angulation of the central ray required to achieve the desired image.

Frontal projections are described in this section as AP projections, but equivalent PA projections also exist. Many angiographic imaging systems place the image receptor above the tabletop and the x-ray tube below. Because patients usually lie supine for cerebral angiography, the central ray, coming from below, enters the posterior cranium and exits the anterior cranium on its course to the image receptor. The position of the central ray results in PA projections equivalent to the AP projections described.

The literature on cerebral angiography contains numerous position variations concerning the degree of central ray angulation, the base from which the central ray should be angled or the line that it should parallel, and the degree of part rotation for oblique studies. This chapter discusses the most frequently employed images and reasonably standard specifications for obtaining them.

The number of radiographs required for satisfactory delineation of a lesion depends on the nature and location of the lesion. Oblique projections or variations in central ray angulation are used to separate the vessels that overlap in the basic positions and to evaluate any existing abnormality.

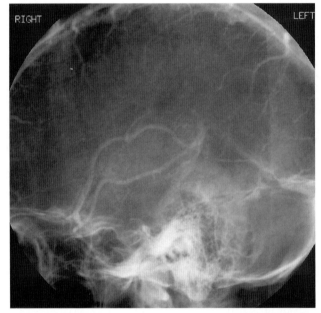

Fig. 23-41 Right internal carotid injection, lateral projection, shows venous phase of circulation.

Aortic Arch Angiogram (for Cranial Vessels)

An aortic arch angiogram is most commonly obtained to visualize atherosclerotic or occlusive disease of the extracranial or common carotid, vertebral, and subclavian arteries. A multiple–side hole catheter is positioned in the ascending thoracic aorta so that the subsequent injection fills all of the vessels simultaneously.

SIMULTANEOUS BIPLANE OBLIQUE PROJECTIONS

For best results, simultaneous biplane oblique projections are produced so that superimposition of vessels is minimized (Fig. 23-42). The CIT observes the following steps:

- Place the image receptor in a 35-degree RPO position. This position opens the aortic arch and the origins of the great vessels for the AP oblique projection, which frees the carotid and vertebral arteries from superimposition.
- Raise the patient's chin to superimpose the inferior margin of the mandible onto the occiput so that as much of the neck as possible is exposed in the frontal image.
- Move the patient's shoulders inferiorly so that they are removed as much as possible from the lateral image.
- Position the lateral image receptor similarly to the AP projection to get another image of the origins of the great vessels.
- For the AP and lateral projection, direct the central ray perpendicular to the center of the image receptor to enter the patient at a level $1\frac{1}{4}$ inch (3 cm) superior to the sternal angle.

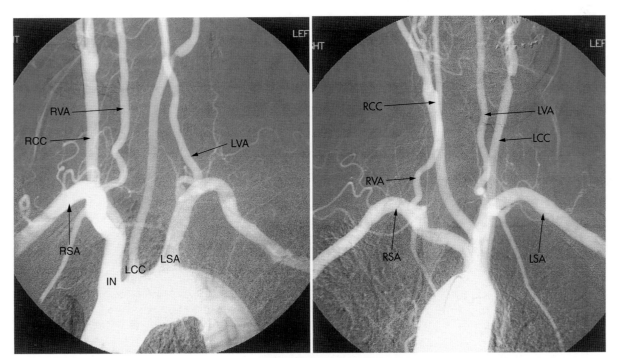

Fig. 23-42 Digital subtracted images of thoracic aortogram showing the origins of the great vessels. RVA: right vertebral artery, RCC: right common carotid, LVA: left vertebral artery, LSA: left subclavian artery, IN: innominate, RSA: right subclavian artery.

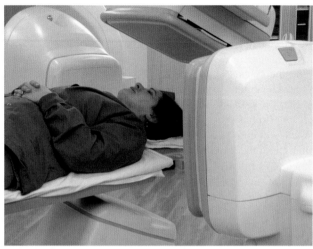

Fig. 23-43 Cerebral angiogram: lateral projection as part of a biplane setup.

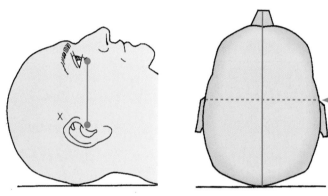

Fig. 23-44 Lateral projection.

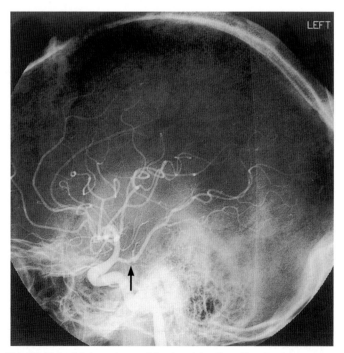

Fig. 23-45 Left internal carotid artery injection. Cerebral angiogram: lateral projection showing anterior circulation. Note posterior communicating artery (*arrow*).

Anterior Circulation
LATERAL PROJECTION

The CIT observes the following steps:
- Center the patient's head to the vertically placed image receptor.
- Extend the patient's head enough to place the IOML perpendicular to the horizontal.
- Adjust the patient's head to place the midsagittal plane vertical and parallel with the plane of the image receptor.
- Adapt immobilization to the type of equipment being employed.
- Perform lateral projections of the anterior, or carotid, circulation with the central ray directed horizontally to a point slightly cranial to the auricle and midway between the forehead and the occiput. This centering allows for patient variation (Figs. 23-43 through 23-45).

NOTE: See Fig. 23-38 for assistance in identifying the cerebral vessels in the image.

ANTEROPOSTERIOR AXIAL PROJECTION (SUPRAORBITAL)

The CIT observes the following steps:

- Adjust the patient's head so that the midsagittal plane is centered over and perpendicular to the midline of the grid and so that it is extended enough to place the IOML vertically.
- Immobilize the patient's head.
- Keep in mind that achieving the goal in this angiogram requires superimposition of the supraorbital margins on the superior margin of the petrous ridges so that the vessels are projected above the floor of the anterior cranial fossa.
- To obtain this result in most patients, direct the central ray 20 degrees caudally for the AP axial projection or 20 degrees cephalad for the PA axial projection along a line passing ¾ inch (1.9 cm) superior to and parallel with a line extending from the supraorbital margin to a point ¾ inch (1.9 cm) superior to the EAM; the latter line coincides with the floor of the anterior fossa (Figs. 23-46 through 23-48).

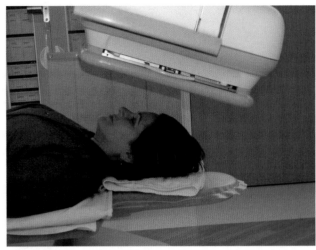

Fig. 23-46 Carotid angiogram: PA axial (supraorbital) projection.

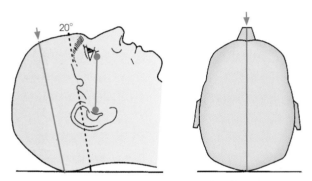

Fig. 23-47 AP axial (supraorbital).

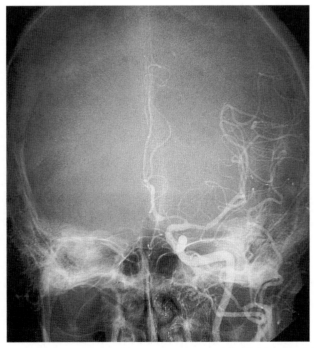

Fig. 23-48 Left common carotid artery injection showing AP axial (supraorbital) projection. Arterial phase of circulation.

ANTEROPOSTERIOR AXIAL OBLIQUE PROJECTION (TRANSORBITAL)

The oblique transorbital projection shows the internal carotid bifurcation and the anterior communicating and middle cerebral arteries within the orbital shadow. The steps are as follows:

- From the position for the basic AP transorbital projection, rotate the patient's head approximately 30 degrees away from the injected side, or angle the central ray 30 degrees toward the injected side.
- Angle the central ray 20 degrees cephalad and center it to the mid-orbit of the uppermost side (Figs. 23-49 and 23-50).

Posterior Circulation
LATERAL PROJECTION

The CIT observes the following steps:
- Center the patient's head to the vertically placed image receptor.
- Extend the patient's head enough to place the IOML perpendicular to the horizontal plane, and adjust the head to place the midsagittal plane vertically and parallel with the plane of the image receptor.

- Rigidly immobilize the patient's head.
- Perform lateral projections of the posterior, or vertebral, circulation with the central ray directed horizontally to the mastoid process at a point about ⅜ inch (1 cm) superior to and ¾ inch (1.9 cm) posterior to the EAM.
- Restrict the exposure field to the middle and posterior fossae for lateral studies of the posterior circulation (Figs. 23-51 and 23-52). Inclusion of the entire skull

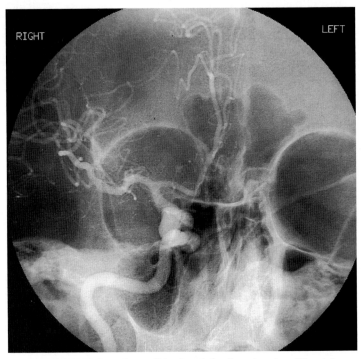

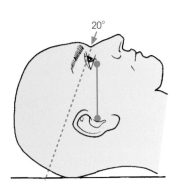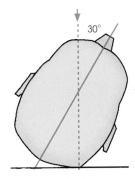

Fig. 23-49 AP axial oblique (transorbital) projection.

Fig. 23-50 Right internal carotid artery injection showing AP axial oblique (transorbital) projection.

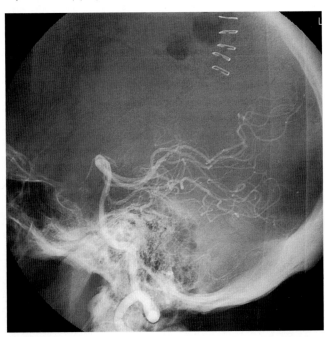

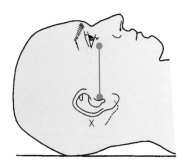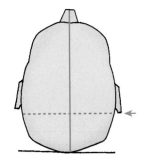

Fig. 23-51 Lateral projection for posterior circulation.

Fig. 23-52 Right vertebral artery injection showing lateral projection of vertebrobasilar system.

is neither necessary nor, from the standpoint of optimal technique, desirable.

ANTEROPOSTERIOR AXIAL PROJECTION

The following steps are observed:
- Adjust the patient's head so that the midsagittal plane is centered over and perpendicular to the midline of the grid, and extend the head enough so that the IOML is vertical.
- Immobilize the patient's head.

Direct the central ray to the region approximately $1\frac{1}{2}$ inches (3.8 cm) superior to the glabella at an angle of 30 to 35 degrees caudad. The central ray exits at the level of the EAM. For this projection, the supraorbital margins are positioned approximately $\frac{3}{4}$ inch (1.9 cm) below the superior margins of the petrous ridges (Figs. 23-53 and 23-54).

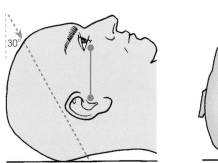

Fig. 23-53 AP axial projection for posterior circulation.

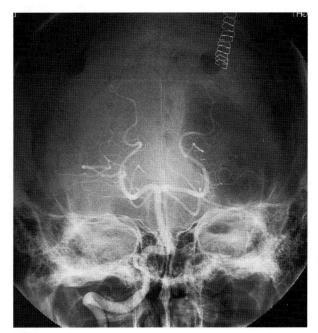

Fig. 23-54 Right vertebral artery injection showing AP axial projection of vertebrobasilar system.

Venography

Venous blood in veins flows proximally toward the heart. Injection into a central venous structure may not opacify the peripheral veins that *anastomose* to it. The position of peripheral veins can be indirectly documented, however, by the filling defect from unopacified blood in the opacified central vein. The CIT observes the following guidelines:

- Place the patient in the supine position for either a single-plane AP or PA projection or biplane projections. Move the patient's arms out of the field of view.
- Obtain lateral projections at increased SID, if possible, to reduce magnification.
- Remember that collimation to the long axis of the vena cava improves image quality but may prevent visualization of peripheral or *collateral veins.*

SUPERIOR VENACAVOGRAM

Venography of the superior vena cava is performed primarily to rule out the existence of thrombus or the occlusion of the superior vena cava. The contrast media may be injected through a needle or an angiographic catheter introduced into a vein in an antecubital fossa, although superior opacification results from injection through a catheter positioned in the axillary or subclavian vein. Radiographs should include the opacified subclavian vein, brachiocephalic vein, superior vena cava, and right atrium (Fig. 23-55).

INFERIOR VENACAVOGRAM

Venography of the inferior vena cava is performed primarily to identify the location of the renal veins for placement of an inferior vena cava filter. The contrast media are injected through a multiple–side hole catheter inserted through the femoral vein and positioned in the common iliac vein or the inferior aspect of the inferior vena cava (Fig. 23-56).

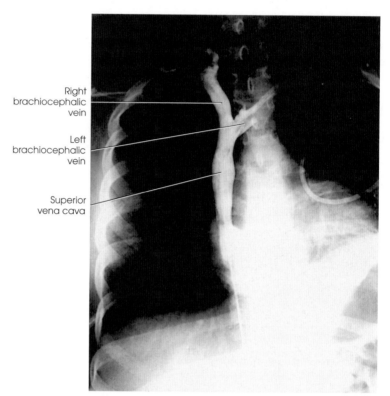

Fig. 23-55 AP superior vena cava.

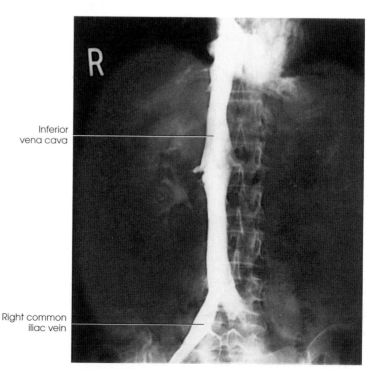

Fig. 23-56 AP inferior vena cava.

Visceral Venography

The visceral veins are often visualized by extending the imaging program of the corresponding visceral artery injection. The veins that drain the small bowel are normally visualized by extending the imaging program of a superior mesenteric arteriogram. Portal venography (Fig. 23-57) can be performed by injecting the portal vein directly from a percutaneous approach, but it is usually accomplished by late-phase imaging of a splenic artery injection or SMA injection.

HEPATIC VENOGRAM

Hepatic venography is usually performed to rule out stenosis or thrombosis of the hepatic veins. These veins are also catheterized to obtain pressure measurements from the interior of the liver. The hepatic veins carry blood from the liver to the inferior vena cava. (The portal vein carries nutrient-rich blood from the viscera to the liver.) The hepatic veins are most easily catheterized from a jugular vein or an upper limb vein approach, but a femoral vein approach may also be used. The CIT follows these steps:

- Place the patient in the supine position for AP or PA projections that include the liver tissue and the extreme upper inferior vena cava (Fig. 23-58).
- Make exposures at the end of suspended expiration.

RENAL VENOGRAM

Renal venography is usually performed to rule out thrombosis of the renal vein. The renal vein is also catheterized for blood sampling, usually to measure the production of renin, an enzyme produced by the kidney when it lacks adequate blood supply. The renal vein is most easily catheterized from a femoral vein approach. The following steps are observed:

- Place the patient in the supine position for a single-plane AP or PA projection.
- Center the selected kidney to the image receptor, and collimate the field to include the kidney and area of the inferior vena cava (Fig. 23-59).
- Make exposures at the end of suspended expiration.

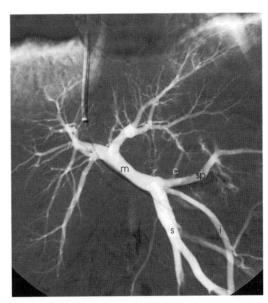

Fig. 23-57 Portal venogram. *c,* Coronary varices; *i,* inferior mesenteric vein; *m,* main portal vein; *s,* superior mesenteric vein; *sp,* splenic vein.

Hepatic veins

Inferior vena cava

Renal veins

Fig. 23-58 Hepatic vein visualization from reflux from inferior vena cava injection. (Note reflux into bilateral renal veins.)

Left renal veins

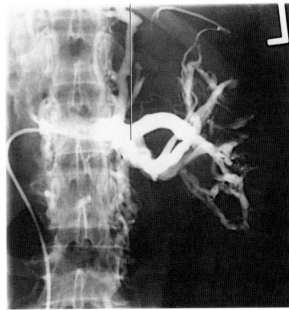

Fig. 23-59 Selective left renal venogram. AP projection.

Interventional radiology has a therapeutic rather than diagnostic purpose in that it intervenes in, or interferes with, the course of a disease process or other medical condition. Since the conception of this form of radiology in the early 1960s, its realm has become so vast and sophisticated that publishers of periodicals struggle to keep abreast of this rapidly advancing specialty.

Interventional radiology allows the angiographer to assume an important role in the management and treatment of disease in many patients. Interventional radiologic procedures reduce hospital stays in many patients and help some patients avoid surgery, with consequent reductions in medical costs.

Every interventional radiologic procedure must include two integral processes.

The first is the interventional or medical side of the procedure, in which a highly skilled radiologist uses wires, catheters, and special medical devices (e.g., occluding coils, stents) to improve the patient's status or condition. The second process involves the use of fluoroscopy and radiography to guide and document the progress of the steps taken during the first process. A CIT must receive special education in the angiographic and interventional suite. This skilled CIT has an important role in assisting the angiographer in the interventional procedures.

The more frequently performed interventional procedures are described in this section. Resources containing more detailed information are cited in the selected bibliography at the end of the chapter.

Percutaneous Transluminal Angioplasty and Stenting

Percutaneous transluminal angioplasty (PTA) is a therapeutic radiologic procedure designed to dilate or reopen stenotic or occluded areas within a vessel using a catheter introduced by the Seldinger technique. In 1964, Dotter and Judkins[1] first described PTA using a coaxial catheter method. First, a guidewire is passed through the narrowed area of a vessel. A smaller catheter then is passed over the guidewire through the stenosis to begin the dilation process. Finally, a larger catheter is passed over the smaller catheter to cause further dilation. This method is referred to as the "Dotter method." Although this method can achieve dilation of stenosis, it has the significant disadvantage of creating an arteriotomy as large as the dilating catheters, and it is seldom used as a first-line therapy.

[1]Dotter CT, Judkins MP: Transluminal treatment of arteriosclerotic obstruction: description of a new technique and preliminary report of its application, *Circulation* 30:654, 1964.

In 1974, Gruntzig and Hopff[1] introduced the double-lumen, balloon-tipped catheter. One lumen allows the passage of a guidewire and fluids through the catheter. The other lumen communicates with a balloon at the distal end of the catheter. When inflated, the balloon expands to a size much larger than the catheter. Double-lumen, angioplasty balloon catheters are available in sizes ranging from 3 to 9 Fr, with attached balloons varying in length and expanding to diameters of 2 to 20 mm or more (Fig. 23-60).

[1]Gruntzig A, Hopff H: Perkutane rekanalisation chronischer arterieller Verschlusse mit einem neuen dilatationskatheter; modifikation der Dotter-Technik, *Deutsch Med Wochenschr* 99:2502, 1974.

Fig. 23-61 illustrates the process of *balloon angioplasty*. The stenosis is initially identified on a previously obtained angiogram. The balloon diameter used for a procedure is often the measured diameter of the normal artery adjacent to the stenosis. The angioplasty procedure is often performed at the same time and through the same catheterization site as the initial diagnostic examination.

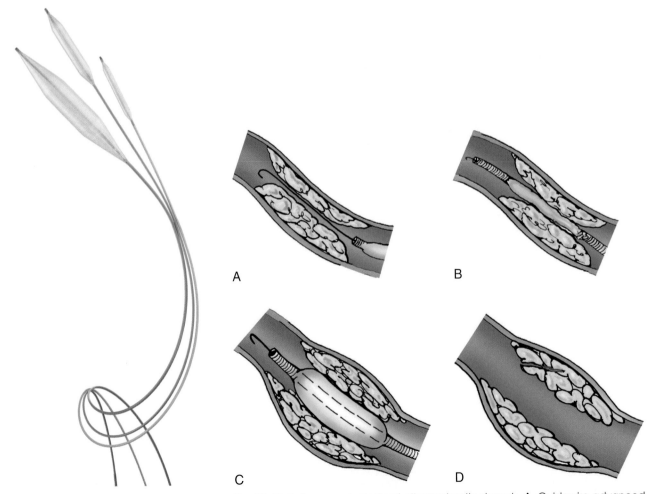

Fig. 23-60 Balloon angioplasty catheters with varied diameters and lengths.

Fig. 23-61 Balloon angioplasty of atherosclerotic stenosis. **A,** Guidewire advanced through stenosis. **B,** Balloon across stenosis. **C,** Balloon inflated. **D,** Postangioplasty stenotic area.

After the guidewire is positioned across the stenosis, the angiographic catheter is removed over the wire. The angioplasty balloon catheter is introduced and directed through the stenosis over the guidewire. The balloon is usually inflated with a diluted contrast media mixture for 15 to 45 seconds, depending on the degree of stenosis and the vessel being treated. The balloon is deflated and repositioned or withdrawn from the lesion. Contrast media can be injected through the angioplasty catheter for a repeat angiogram to determine whether or not the procedure was successful. The success of the angioplasty procedure may also be determined by comparing transcatheter blood pressure measurements from a location distal and a location proximal to the lesion site. Nearly equal pressures indicate a reopened stenosis.

Transluminal angioplasty can be performed in virtually any vessel that can be reached percutaneously with a catheter (Figs. 23-62 and 23-63). In 1978, Molnar

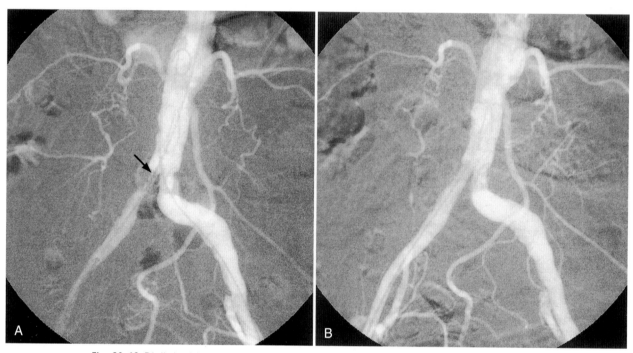

Fig. 23-62 Digital subtracted images of the abdominal aortogram and bilateral iliac arteries. **A,** High-grade stenosis of right common iliac artery (*arrow*). **B,** Abdominal aortogram and bilateral iliac arteries, postangioplasty, showing widely patent iliac system.

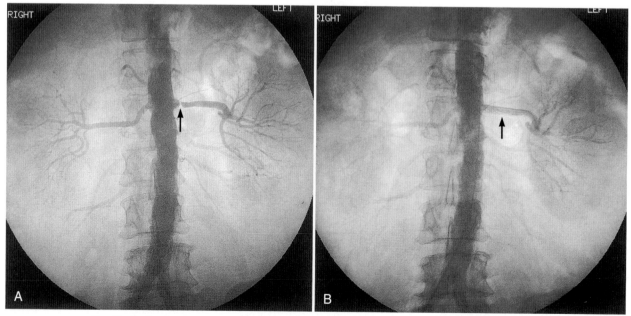

Fig. 23-63 Abdominal aortogram before and after angioplasty of the left renal artery. **A,** High-grade stenosis of left renal artery (*arrow*). **B,** Postangioplasty and stent placement within left renal artery (*arrow*).

and Stockum[1] described the use of balloon angioplasty for dilation of strictures within the biliary system. Balloon angioplasty is also conducted in venous structures, ureters, and the gastrointestinal tract.

Balloon angioplasty has been used successfully to manage various diseases that cause arterial narrowing. The most common form of arterial stenosis treated by transluminal angioplasty is caused by atherosclerosis. Dotter and Judkins[2] speculated that this atheromatous material was soft and inelastic and could be compressed against the artery wall. The success of coaxial and balloon method angioplasty was initially attributed to enlargement of the arterial lumen because of compression of the atherosclerotic plaque. Later research showed, however, that the plaque does not compress. If plaque surrounds the inner diameter of the artery, the plaque cracks at its thinnest portion as the arterial lumen is expanded. Continued expansion cracks the inner layer of the arterial wall, the *intima,* then stretches and tears the middle layer, the *media,* and finally stretches the outer layer, the *adventitia.* The arterial lumen is increased by permanently enlarging the artery's outer diameter. Restenosis, when it occurs, is usually caused by deposits of new plaque, not arterial wall collapse.

A final possibility for percutaneous treatment of vessel stenoses is the placement of vascular stents. A vascular *stent* is composed of a metal material, stainless steel or nitinol, and can be covered or uncovered with a biologic material that is introduced through a catheter system and positioned across a stenosis to keep the narrowed area spread apart. These devices remain in the vessel permanently (Figs. 23-64 and 23-65).

The success of PTA in the management of atherosclerosis has made it a significant alternative to surgical procedures in the treatment of this disease. PTA is not indicated in all cases, however. Long segments of occlusion may be best treated by surgery. PTA has a lower risk than surgery but is not totally risk-free. Generally, patients must be able to tolerate the surgical procedure that may be required to repair vessel damage that can be caused by PTA. Unsuccessful transluminal angioplasty procedures rarely prevent or complicate necessary subsequent surgery. In selected cases, the procedure is effective and almost painless and can be repeated as often as necessary with no apparent increase in risk to the patient. The recovery time is often no longer than the time required to stabilize the arteriotomy site, usually a matter of hours, and general anesthesia is normally not required. The hospital stay and the cost to the patient are reduced.

Abdominal Aortic Aneurysm Endografts

An interventional therapy started in the late 1990s treats AAAs with a transcatheter approach and stenting. AAAs historically have been treated with an open repair of the aneurysm by a vascular surgeon. This approach has risks associated with abdominal surgery and a long hospital stay for recovery of the incision. The stent graft or endograft is a nitinol-covered stent that comes in pieces or one intact device depending on the manufacturer (Fig. 23-66). A cutdown approach to bilateral femoral arteries is done, and sheaths and

---

[1]Molnar W, Stockum AE: Transhepatic dilatation of choledochoenterostomy strictures, *Radiology* 129:59, 1978.

[2]Dotter CT, Judkins MP: Transluminal treatment of arteriosclerotic obstruction: description of a new technique and preliminary report of its application, *Circulation* 30:654, 1964.

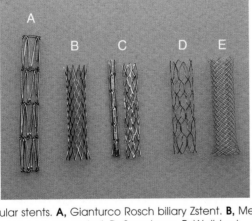

Fig. 23-64 Intravascular stents. **A,** Gianturco Rosch biliary Zstent. **B,** Memotherm. **C,** Palmez; unexpanded and expanded. **D,** Symphony. **E,** Wallstent.

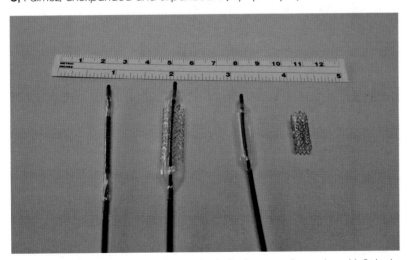

Fig. 23-65 Stent and balloon for angioplasty shown collapsed and inflated.

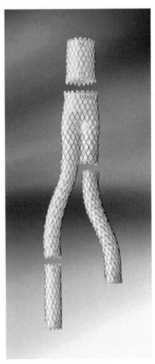

Fig. 23-66 Stent graft or endograft used to repair aneurysm in the aorta and iliac region.

delivery catheters are advanced to deliver the device. A large amount of planning is done before a patient can undergo this approach to treating AAA. Patients preferably should have an AAA that is infrarenal or occurring below the renal arteries. The stent is a covered device and would occlude the renal arteries. Some newer devices are designed to treat aneurysms that extend to involve the renal artery takeoffs.

Preliminary abdominal and iliac arteriograms may be obtained using a calibrated catheter that the radiologist or vascular surgeon can use for measuring (Fig. 23-67). CT is the preferred imaging modality and is used as the primary source for measurements. This procedure is done either in the catheterization laboratory or in the operating room depending on the hospital. If done in the operating room, a portable C-arm is needed with DSA capability. Some hospitals are building hybrid surgical suites that have a C-arm built in to the room like a standard angiography suite.

Although most PTA procedures are conducted in the angiography suite, angioplasty involving the arteries of the heart is generally performed in a more specialized laboratory. *Percutaneous transluminal coronary angioplasty (PTCA)* is performed in the cardiac catheterization laboratory because of the possibility of potentially serious cardiac complications. PTCA is discussed later in this chapter.

Transcatheter Embolization

Transcatheter embolization was first described by Brooks[1,2] in 1930. He described vessel occlusion for closure of arteriovenous fistula. Transcatheter embolization involves the therapeutic introduction of various substances to occlude or drastically reduce blood flow within a vessel (Box 23-1). The three main

[1]Brooks B: The treatment of traumatic arteriovenous fistula, *South Med J* 23:100, 1930.
[2]Brooks B: Discussion. In Nolan L, Taylor AS: Pulsating exophthalmos, *Trans South Surg Assoc* 43:176, 1931.

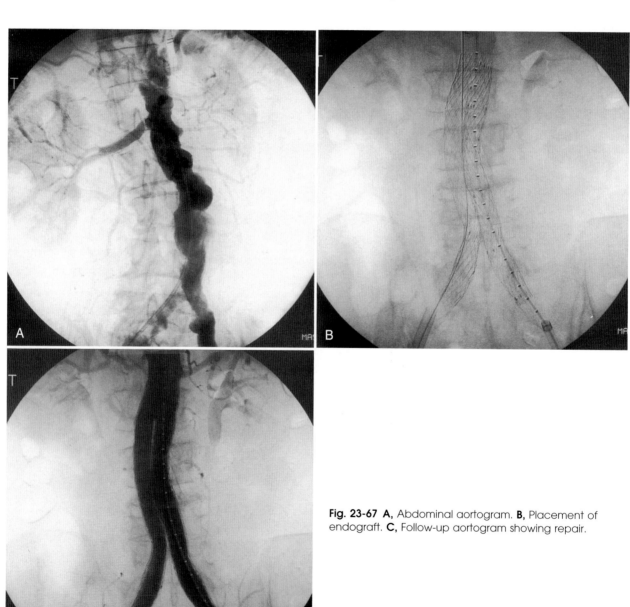

Fig. 23-67 A, Abdominal aortogram. **B,** Placement of endograft. **C,** Follow-up aortogram showing repair.

purposes for embolization are (1) to stop active bleeding sites, (2) to control blood flow to diseased or malformed vessels (e.g., tumors or AVMs), and (3) to stop or reduce blood flow to a particular area of the body before surgery.

The patient's condition and the situation must be considered when choosing an embolic agent. The interventionalist usually identifies the appropriate agent to be used. Embolic agents must be administered with care to ensure that they flow to the predetermined vessel or target. Embolization is a permanent treatment; the effects on the lesion are irreversible.

Many embolic agents are available (Box 23-2), and the choice of agent depends on whether the occlusion is to be temporary or permanent (Table 23-1).

Temporary agents such as Gelfoam* or Avitene may be used as a means to reduce the pressure head of blood to a specific site. These temporary agents reduce flow into a bleeding site so that hemostasis may be achieved. Temporary agents can also be used to prevent inadvertent embolization of normal vessels.

*Gelfoam is the trademark for a sterile, absorbable, water-insoluble, gelatin-base sponge.

BOX 23-1

Lesions amendable to embolization

Aneurysm
Pseudoaneurysm
Hemorrhage
Neoplasms
  Malignant
  Benign
Arteriovenous malformations
Arteriovenous fistula
Infertility (varicocele)
Impotence owing to venous leakage
Redistribution of blood flow

BOX 23-2

Embolic agents

Particulate agents
Polyvinyl alcohol
Embosphere
Avitene
Gelfoam

Metal coils
Gianturco coils
Metal coils
Detachable coils
  Platinum
  Coated

Vascular occluder plug
Liquid agents (occluding, sclerosing)
  Ethanol
  Thrombin
  Hypertonic glucose
  Sodium tetradecyl sulfate
  Ethibloc
  EVAL
  Onyx
Detachable balloons
  Latex—Debrun
  Silicone—Heishima
Liquid adhesives
  N-butyl 2-cyanoacrylate
Autologous material

TABLE 23-1

Particulate agent sizes

Agent	Size
Gelfoam powder	40-60 μ
Gelfoam sponges	Pledgets-torpedoes
Avitene	100-150 μ
Polyvinyl alcohol	100-1200 μ
Embosphere	100-1200 μ

Vasoconstricting drugs can be used to reduce blood flow temporarily. Vasoconstrictors such as vasopressin (Pitressin) drastically constrict vessels, resulting in hemostasis.

When permanent occlusion is desired, as in trauma to the pelvis that causes hemorrhage or when vascular tumors are supplied by large vessels, stainless steel coils may be used. This coil (Fig. 23-68), which functions to produce thrombogenesis, is simply a looped segment of guidewire with Dacron fibers attached to it. The coil is initially straight and is easily introduced into a catheter that has been placed into the desired vessel. The coil is then pushed out of the catheter tip with a guidewire. The coil assumes its looping shape immediately as it enters the bloodstream. It is important that the catheter tip be specifically placed in the vessel so that the coil springs precisely into the desired area. Numerous coils can be placed as needed to occlude the vessel. A new generation of coils promises to deliver more effective closure of vascular structures by using various coatings on the outside of the coil. One such coil uses a coating that initiates a foreign body/scarring response. Another type of coil is coated with an expansile gel that swells in the presence of blood, occluding the vessel. Tissue grows inside and around the gel to provide healing. Newer occlusion technology is a vascular plug which is a single occlusion device mounted on a delivery catheter. The new device is a three lobe design that reduces occlusion time. The device is placed at the ostium of a vessel and deployed once in position.

Fig. 23-69 shows a hypervascular uterine fibroid that was causing significant symptoms. Embolization of this uterine fibroid was successfully accomplished with total occlusion of the lesion.

Transcatheter embolization has also been used in the cerebral vasculature of the brain. Vascular lesions within the cerebral vasculature, such as aneurysms, AVMs, and tumors, can be managed using multiple embolic agents, PVA, or tissue adhesive. Very small catheters (2 or 3 Fr) are passed through a larger catheter, a coaxial system that is positioned in the cerebral vessels. The smaller catheter is manipulated into the appropriate cerebral vessel, and lesions such as an aneurysm and the embolic material are delivered through it until the appropriate embolization is achieved (Fig. 23-70).

Inferior Vena Cava Filter Placement

The idea of interrupting the pathway of an embolus is not a new one. Surgical interruption of the common femoral vein was first described in 1784, and surgical interruption of the inferior vena cava was described in 1868. These procedures and the partial surgical interruption procedures that evolved from them had a high rate of complications, not only owing to the surgical process but also owing to inadequate venous drainage from the lower limbs. Catheterization technology led to the development of detachable balloons for occluding the inferior vena cava, but that procedure also resulted in complications because of inadequate venous flow from the lower limbs.

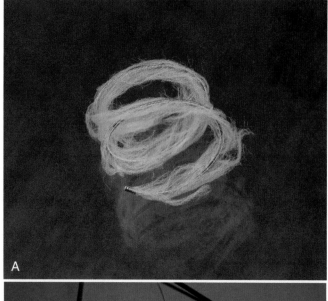

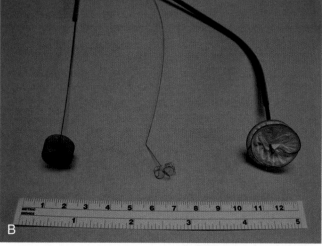

Fig. 23-68 A, Fibered Gianturco stainless steel occluding coil (magnified). **B,** Vascular plug for large vessel embolization, Guglielmi detachable neuroembolization coil used in aneurysm coiling or other high-risk small vessel embolization and Helex septal occluder used for repair of patent foramen ovale/atrial septal defects in pediatric and adult patients.

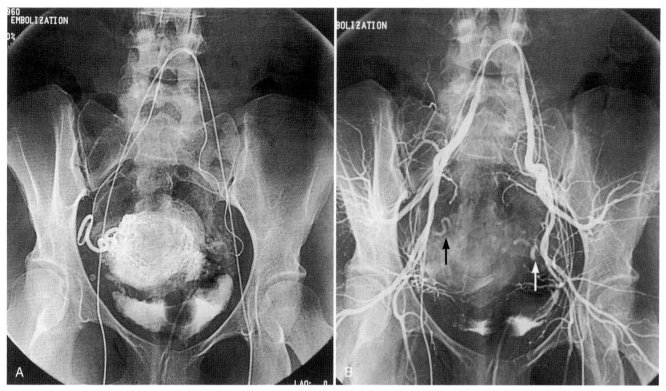

Fig. 23-69 Hypervascular uterine fibroid. **A,** Bilateral uterine artery injections using coaxial microcatheters, showing hypervascular uterine fibroid. **B,** Bilateral iliac artery injections, postembolization, showing total occlusion of both uterine arteries (*arrows*).

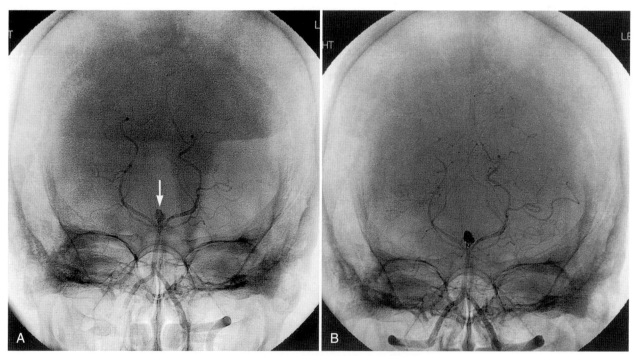

Fig. 23-70 Left vertebral artery injection. **A,** Basilar tip aneurysm (*arrow*). **B,** Left vertebral artery injection postembolization with the use of Guglielmi detachable coils (GDCs).

Pulmonary angiography primarily evaluates embolic disease of the lungs. CT angiography has been shown to be just as accurate as pulmonary angiography, however. A pulmonary embolus is a blood clot that forms as a thrombus and usually develops in the deep veins of the leg. When such a thrombus becomes dislodged and migrates, it is called an *embolus*. An embolus originating in the leg may migrate through the inferior vena cava and right side of the heart and finally lodge in the pulmonary arteries. A filter can be percutaneously placed in the inferior vena cava to trap such an embolus.

Lower limb vein thrombosis is not an indication for inferior vena cava filter placement. Normally, blood-thinning medications are administered to treat deep vein thrombosis. When anticoagulant therapy is contraindicated because of bleeding or the risk of hemorrhage, filter placement may be indicated. Filter placement itself has associated risks, including thrombosis of the vein through which the filter is introduced and thrombosis of the vena cava. These risks normally are not life threatening, however. Inferior vena cava filter placement is not a treatment for deep vein thrombosis of the leg but a therapy intended to reduce the chance of pulmonary embolism.

The first true filter designed to trap emboli while maintaining vena cava patency was introduced in 1967 by Mobin-Uddin. It consisted of six metal struts joined at one end to form a conical shape that was covered by a perforated plastic canopy. The plastic canopy proved to be too occlusive, which is the reason that the Mobin-Uddin filter is no longer in use. Because of this filter's striking resemblance to an open umbrella, vena cava filters of all types for many years were referred to as "umbrella filters."

Inferior vena cava filters are available in various shapes. All of these filters are initially compacted inside an introducer catheter delivery system and assume their functional shape as they are released (Fig. 23-71). The introducers are passed through sheaths ranging in size from 6 to 15 Fr.

Most filters are designed as a conical shape to trap clots in the central lumen. They are also designed to be placed in vena cavae ranging up to 20 to 30 mm in diameter. Each filter has its own mechanism of clot trapping. Fig. 23-71 shows the most currently available permanent inferior vena cava filters. These filters would be employed as a temporary means to prevent new pulmonary embolus. While patients are in an acute high-risk state, these temporary filters may help prevent pulmonary embolus. Regardless of whether the filter is permanent or temporary, the purpose is to prevent

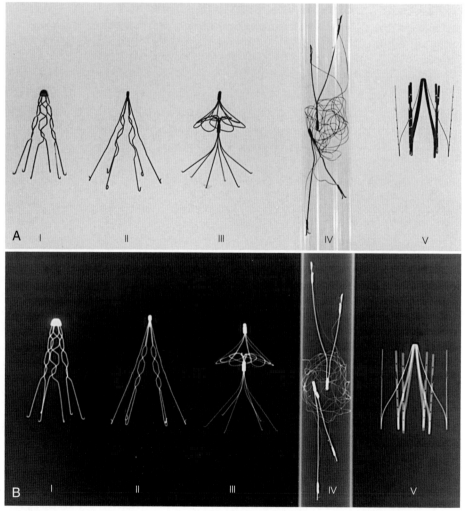

Fig. 23-71 Vena cava filters: *I,* Kimray-Greenfield; *II,* Titanium Greenfield; *III,* Simon Nitinol; *IV,* Gianturco-Roehm Bird's Nest; *V,* Vena Tech. **A,** Photographic image. **B,** Radiographic image.

and trap new onset of pulmonary embolus. These filters do treat preexisting clots, however.

Several filters are designed for temporary placement. They have hooks on the top and the bottom that allow them to be grasped by a catheter snare device and be removed percutaneously. Another temporary filter remains attached to its introducer catheter, which is used to retrieve it. Some temporary filters must be removed within approximately 10 days, or they become permanently attached to the vena cava endothelium. Various filter designs are in use in countries other than the United States. Development of inferior vena cava filters continues, and new designs are likely to become available.

The filters are percutaneously inserted through a femoral, jugular, or antecubital vein, usually for placement in the inferior vena cava just inferior to the renal veins. Placement inferior to the renal veins is important to prevent renal vein thrombosis, which can occur if the vena cava is occluded superior to the level of the renal veins by a large thrombus in a filter. An inferior vena cavogram is performed using the modified Seldinger technique, usually from the femoral vein approach. The inferior vena cavogram defines the anatomy, including the level of the renal veins, determines the diameter of the vena cava, and rules out the presence of a thrombus (Fig. 23-72). Filter insertion from the jugular or antecubital approach may be indicated if a thrombus is present in the inferior vena cava.

The diameter of the vena cava may influence the choice of filter because each filter has a maximum diameter. The filter insertion site is dilated to accommodate the filter introducer. The filter remains sheathed until it reaches the desired level and is released from its introducer by the angiographer. The introducing system is then removed, and external compression is applied to the venotomy site until hemostasis is achieved. A postplacement image is obtained to document the location of the filter (Fig. 23-73).

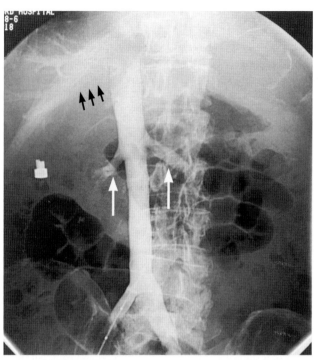

Fig. 23-72 Inferior vena cavogram. Note reflux into renal veins (*large arrows*) and hepatic veins (*small arrows*).

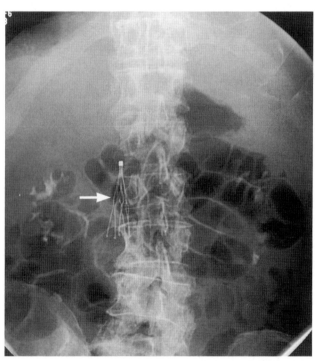

Fig. 23-73 Postplacement image showing Greenfield filter in place (*arrow*).

Transjugular Intrahepatic Portosystemic Shunt

The *portal circulation* consists of blood from the digestive organs, which drains into the liver. The portal system consists of the splenic vein, the superior mesenteric vein, and the inferior mesenteric vein. The blood passes through the liver tissue and is returned to the inferior vena cava via the hepatic veins. Disease processes can increase the resistance of blood flow through the liver, elevating the blood pressure of the portal circulation—a condition known as *portal hypertension.* It may cause the blood to flow through collateral veins. Venous *varices* are the result and can be life threatening if they bleed. The creation of a portosystemic shunt can decrease portal hypertension and the associated variceal bleeding by allowing the portal venous circulation to bypass its normal course through the liver. The percutaneous intervention for creating an artificial low-pressure pathway between the portal and hepatic veins is called a *trans-jugular intrahepatic portosystemic shunt (TIPS).*

Portography and hepatic venography are usually performed before a TIPS procedure to delineate anatomy and confirm *patency* of these vessels. Ultrasonography may be used for this purpose. Transcatheter blood pressure measurements may also confirm the existence of a pressure gradient between the portal and hepatic veins.

The most common approach for a TIPS procedure is from a right internal jugular venous puncture site to the middle or right hepatic vein. A hepatic venogram may be obtained using contrast material or CO_2 or both. A special long needle is passed into the hepatic vein and advanced through the liver tissue into the portal vein. The needle is exchanged for an angioplasty balloon catheter, and the tract through the liver tissue is dilated. An angiographic catheter may be passed through the tract and advanced into the splenic vein for a splenoportal venogram. An intravascular stent is positioned across the tract to maintain its patency (Figs. 23-74 and 23-75). The tract and stent may be enlarged further with an angioplasty balloon catheter until the desired reduction in pressure gradient between the portal and hepatic veins is achieved. The sheath is removed from the internal jugular vein, and external pressure is applied until hemostasis at the venotomy occurs.

Other Procedures

When an angiogram shows thrombosis, the procedure may be continued for thrombolytic therapy. Blood clot–dissolving medications can be infused through an angiographic catheter positioned against the thrombus. Special infusion catheters that have side holes may be manipulated directly into the clot. Periodic repeat *angiograms* evaluate the progress of *lysis* (dissolution). The catheter may have to be advanced under fluoroscopic control to keep it against or in the clot as lysis progresses.

Catheters can also be used to remove foreign bodies, such as catheter fragments or broken guidewires, percutaneously from the vasculature. Various snares can be used for this purpose. A snare catheter introduced using the Seldinger technique is manipulated under fluoroscopic control to grasp the foreign body. The snare and foreign body are then withdrawn as a unit.

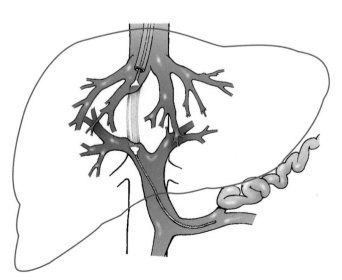

Fig. 23-74 Intravascular stent placement in a TIPS procedure.

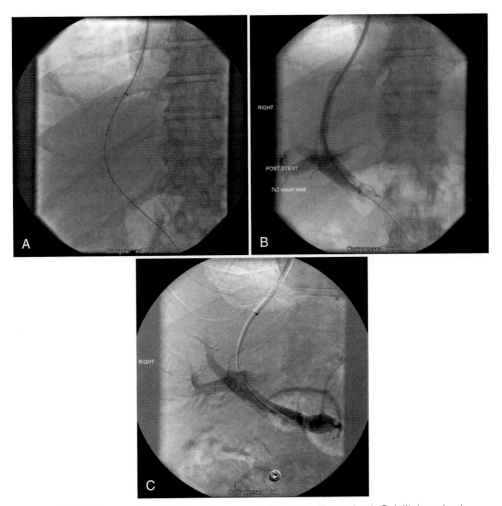

Fig. 23-75 TIPS procedure. **A,** Stent placement. **B,** Stent with contrast. **C,** Initial contrast agent injection.

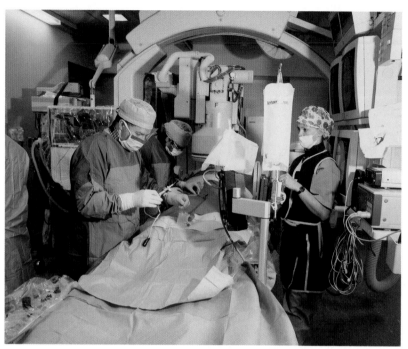

Fig. 23-76 The CIT plays an active role on the interventional team by assisting the interventionalist (*left*) or by circulating within the angiography suite (*right*).

Interventional Radiology: Present and Future

Interventional procedures bring therapeutic capabilities into the hands of the interventional radiologist. Procedures are done for diagnosis and treatment of multiple lesions. The treatment procedures can be performed at the same time as the diagnostic procedure. New equipment is continually becoming available to improve techniques and broaden the scope of percutaneous intervention. Although use of the catheter for angiographic diagnosis may wane, its ability to provide therapy percutaneously ensures a future for angiography. These procedures are highly technical, and a team approach is crucial. The cardiovascular and interventional technologist plays an active role on this interventional team (Fig. 23-76).[1] Along with the interventional technologist, the other members of the team include the nurse, support personnel, and the interventionalist. Although these procedures are performed in an angiography suite, this subspecialty of radiology can be considered less invasive surgery. The field can also be called *surgical angiography* and *surgical neuroangiography*. This field of interventional radiology has a bright future as more sophisticated equipment is developed.

[1]Scanlon PJ et al: ACC/AHA guidelines for coronary angiography: a report of the American College of Cardiology/American Heart Association Task Force on Practice Guidelines (Committee on Coronary Angiography), *J Am Coll Cardiol* 33:1758, 1999.

Cardiac catheterization is a comprehensive term used to describe a minor surgical procedure involving the introduction of specialized catheters into the heart and surrounding vasculature for the purpose of diagnostic evaluation and therapy (intervention) associated with various cardiovascular-related disorders in children and adults. Cardiac catheterization is classified as either a diagnostic or an interventional procedure. The primary purpose of diagnostic procedures is to collect data necessary to evaluate the patient's condition. Cardiac interventional procedures involve the application of therapeutic measures through catheter-based systems or other mechanical means to treat disorders of the vascular and conduction systems within the heart.

GENERAL INDICATIONS

Cardiac catheterization is performed to identify the anatomic and physiologic condition of the heart. The data gathered during catheterization provide the physi-

cian with information to develop management strategies for patients who have cardiovascular disorders. *Coronary angiography* is currently the most definitive procedure for visualizing the coronary anatomy. The anatomic information gained from this procedure may include the presence and extent of obstructive coronary artery disease, thrombus formation, coronary artery collateral flow, coronary anomalies, aneurysms, and spasm. Coronary artery size can also be determined.

Coronary artery disease is the most common disorder necessitating catheterization of the adult heart. This disease is caused primarily by the accumulation of fatty intracoronary *atheromatous* plaque, which leads to *stenosis* and *occlusion* of the coronary arteries. Coronary artery disease is symptomatically characterized by chest pain (angina pectoris) or a heart attack (myocardial infarction [MI]). Treatment of coronary artery disease includes medical and surgical interventions.

Diagnostic cardiac catheterization of an adult patient with coronary artery disease is conducted to assess the appropriateness and feasibility of various therapeutic options. Cardiac catheterization is performed before open-heart surgery to provide *hemodynamic* and *angiographic* data to document the presence and severity of disease. In selected circumstances, postoperative catheterization is performed to assess the results of surgery. An interventional procedure (e.g., PTCA, intracoronary stent, or atherectomy) may be indicated for the relief of arteriosclerotic coronary artery stenosis.

Diagnostic studies of the adult heart also aid in evaluating a patient who has confusing or obscure symptoms (e.g., chest pain of undetermined cause). These studies are also used to assess diseases of the heart not requiring surgical intervention, such as certain cardiomyopathies.

TABLE 23-2
Indications for cardiac catheterization

Indications	Procedures
1. Suspected or known coronary artery disease	
a. New-onset angina	LV, COR
b. Unstable angina	LV, COR
c. Evaluation before a major surgical procedure	LV, COR
d. Silent ischemia	LV, COR, ERGO
e. Positive ETT	LV, COR, ERGO
f. Atypical chest pain or coronary artery spasm	LV, COR, ERGO
2. Myocardial infarction	
a. Unstable angina postinfarction	LV, COR
b. Failed thrombolysis	LV, COR, RH
c. Shock	LV, COR, RH
d. Mechanical complications (ventricular septal defect)	LV, COR, RH (rupture of wall or papillary muscle)
3. Sudden cardiovascular death	LV, COR, R + L
4. Valvular heart disease	LV, COR, R + L, AO
5. Congenital heart disease (before anticipated corrective surgery)	LV, COR, R + L, AO
6. Aortic dissection	AO, COR
7. Pericardial constriction or tamponade	LV, COR, R + L
8. Cardiomyopathy	LV, COR, R + L, BX
9. Initial and follow-up assessment for heart transplant	LV, COR, R + L, BX

AO, Aortography; *BX,* endomyocardial biopsy; *COR,* coronary angiography; *ERGO,* ergonovine provocation of coronary spasm; *ETT,* exercise tolerance test; *LV,* left ventriculography; *R + L,* right and left heart hemodynamics; *RH,* right heart oxygen saturations and hemodynamics (e.g., placement of Swan-Ganz catheter).
From Kern MJ: *The cardiac catheterization handbook,* ed 4, St Louis, 2003, Mosby.

In children, diagnostic heart catheterization is employed to evaluate congenital and valvular disease, disorders of the cardiac conduction system, and selected cardiomyopathies. Interventional techniques are also performed in children, primarily to alleviate symptoms associated with certain congenital heart defects.

The indications for cardiac catheterization as established by a special task force to the American College of Cardiology and the American Heart Association (ACC/AHA) are summarized in Table 23-2. Commonly performed procedures based on diagnosis are also presented. The ACC/AHA[1] has classified the indications and appropriateness for coronary angiography by placing the previously discussed disease categories into three classifications, as follows:

Class 1: Conditions for which there is general agreement that coronary angiography is justified

[1]Scanlon PJ et al: ACC/AHA guidelines for coronary angiography: a report of the American College of Cardiology/American Heart Association Task Force on Practice Guidelines (Committee on Coronary Angiography), *J Am Coll Cardiol* 33:1758, 1999.

Class 2: Conditions for which coronary angiography is frequently performed, but for which a divergence of opinion exists with respect to its justification in terms of value and appropriateness

Class 3: Conditions for which coronary angiography ordinarily is not justified

Other procedures that may be performed concurrently with coronary angiography are listed in Table 23-3. Some of these procedures are discussed later in the text.

TABLE 23-3

Procedures that may accompany coronary angiography

Procedures	Comment
1. Central venous access (femoral, internal jugular, subclavian)	Used as IV access for emergency medications or fluids, temporary pacemaker (pacemaker not mandatory for coronary angiography)
2. Hemodynamic assessment	
a. Left heart pressures (aorta, left ventricle)	Routine for all studies
b. Right and left heart combined pressures	Not routine for coronary artery disease; mandatory for valvular heart disease; routine for CHF, right ventricular dysfunction, pericardial diseases, cardiomyopathy, intracardiac shunts, congenital abnormalities
3. Left ventricular angiography	Routine for all studies; may be excluded with high-risk patients, left main coronary or aortic stenosis, severe CHF
4. Internal mammary selective angiography	Not routine unless used as coronary bypass conduit
5. Pharmacologic studies	
a. Ergonovine	Routine for coronary vasospasm
b. IC/IV/sublingual nitroglycerin	Optionally routine for all studies
6. Aortography	Routine for aortic insufficiency, aortic dissection, aortic aneurysm, with or without aortic stenosis; routine to locate bypass grafts not visualized by selective angiography
7. Digital subtraction angiography	Not routine for coronary angiography; excellent for peripheral vascular disease
8. Cardiac pacing and electrophysiologic studies	Arrhythmia evaluation
9. Interventional and special techniques	Intracoronary flow-pressure for lesion assessment Coronary angioplasty (PTCA) Myocardial biopsy Transseptal or direct left ventricular puncture Balloon catheter valvuloplasty Conduction tract catheter ablation
10. Arterial closure devices	Available for patients with conditions prone to puncture site bleeding

CHF, Congestive heart failure.
From Kern MJ: *The cardiac catheterization handbook,* ed 4, St Louis, 2003, Mosby.

CONTRAINDICATIONS, COMPLICATIONS, AND ASSOCIATED RISKS

Cardiac catheterization has associated inherent risk factors. Many physicians agree, however, that the only absolute contraindications to this procedure are the refusal of the procedure by a mentally competent person and the lack of adequate equipment or catheterization facilities.

There are few contraindications for cardiac catheterization when the appropriateness of the procedure is based on the benefit-risk ratio. Relative contraindications according to the guidelines of the ACC/AHA[1] include the following:

- Active gastrointestinal bleeding
- Acute or chronic renal failure
- Recent stroke
- Fever from infection or the presence of an active infection
- Severe electrolyte imbalance
- Severe anemia
- Short life expectancy because of other illness
- Digitalis intoxication
- Patient refusal of therapeutic treatment such as PTCA or bypass surgery
- Severe uncontrolled hypertension
- Coagulopathy and bleeding disorders
- Acute pulmonary edema
- Uncontrolled ventricular arrhythmias
- Aortic valve endocarditis
- Previous anaphylactic reaction to contrast media

Some of these conditions may be temporary, or they may be treated and reversed before cardiac catheterization is attempted. Cardiac catheterization may proceed if any of the above-listed conditions exist in a patient who is deemed to be unstable from a suspected cardiac cause.

As with any invasive procedure, complications can be expected during cardiac catheterization. The Society for Cardiac Angiography and Interventions (SCA&I) reviewed the catheterizations in more than 300,000 patients from three different time periods and found the major complication rate for the entire group was less than 2%. The risks associated with cardiac catheterization have decreased since the early days of the procedure. As the severity of the patient's disease increases, however, so do the risks associated with the procedure.

The risks of cardiac catheterization vary according to the type of procedure and the status of the patient undergoing the procedure. Significantly influencing the outcome of the procedure is the stability of the patient's condition before the procedure. Patients presenting with left main coronary stenosis have a greater than twofold higher risk of complications from coronary angiography than patients who have no left main coronary stenosis. The SCA&I database identified the main predictors of major complications after cardiac catheterization and determined that the following increased the risk of complications[1]:

- Moribund patient (patient with poor response to life-threatening condition)
- Cardiogenic shock
- Acute MI (within 24 hours)
- Renal insufficiency
- Cardiomyopathy

Risk variables of less significance include the anatomy to be studied, type of catheter and approach used, history of drug allergy, presence of basic cardiovascular disease or noncardiac disease such as asthma or diabetes, hemodynamic status, and age or other patient characteristics. The expected benefits of cardiac catheterization must be weighed against the associated risks when determining whether to perform the procedure.

---

[1]Laskey W et al: Multivariable model for prediction of risk of significant complication during diagnostic cardiac catheterization: the Registry Committee of the Society for Cardiac Angiography and Interventions, *Cathet Cardiovasc Diagn* 30:185, 1993.

---

[1]Scanlon PJ et al: ACC/AHA guidelines for coronary angiography: a report of the American College of Cardiology/American Heart Association Task Force on Practice Guidelines (Committee on Coronary Angiography), *J Am Coll Cardiol* 33:1758, 1999.

Specialized Equipment

Cardiac catheterization has developed into a highly complex, sophisticated procedure requiring specialized equipment and supplies. In contrast to earlier radiographic examinations of the intracardiac structures, modern cardiac catheterization requires more than a simple fluoroscope and a recording modality such as that used in overhead radiography.

Equipment and supplies required for cardiac catheterization can be categorized into three groups: (1) angiographic supplies and equipment, (2) imaging, and (3) ancillary equipment and supplies. Examples of equipment typically contained in each group are described next.

ANGIOGRAPHIC SUPPLIES AND EQUIPMENT

Cardiovascular equipment consists of supplies and equipment needed to perform the procedure. In addition to the equipment mentioned previously for angiographic procedures, there are variations in catheter design to accommodate the coronary arteries. The guidewires used also have several variations in length, stiffness, and coatings depending on the tortuosity of the aorta and iliac arteries leading to the heart. Because of the complexity and types of procedures performed in a cardiac catheterization laboratory, only a few of the main component items are discussed.

Catheters

The catheters used for left heart cardiac catheterization are similar to the angiographic catheters previously described except that cardiac catheters are preformed for the cardiac vasculature (Fig. 23-77). Specialized catheters are used for right heart catheterization procedures. In contrast to angiographic catheters, the main purpose of which is to serve as a conduit for contrast media, right heart catheters are typically flow-directed catheters that use an inflated balloon on the tip of the catheter to ease passage through the various chambers of the heart. Various types of flow-directed catheters are capable of performing more tasks than the standard angiographic catheter. Depending on the type of procedure to be performed, the physician decides which catheter to use.

The catheter (or catheters) placed in a patient's vasculature can function as a fluid-filled column for hemodynamic data or as a conduit for contrast media, thrombolytic agents, and mechanical devices. Blood samples can be drawn directly from selected cardiac chambers for the purpose of oximetry or other laboratory analysis. To perform these and other tasks, three or four valves *(stopcocks)* are combined to form a *manifold,* which is attached to the proximal end of the catheter (Fig. 23-78). Using a manifold allows such functions as drawing blood samples, administering medications, and recording blood pressures without disconnecting from the catheter.

Contrast media

Injection of contrast media is essential for angiographic visualization of the cardiac anatomy. Several iodinated radiographic contrast media are approved for intravascular, intracardiac, and intracoronary use in adults and children. Transient (temporary) ECG changes during and immediately after the injection of contrast media are common.

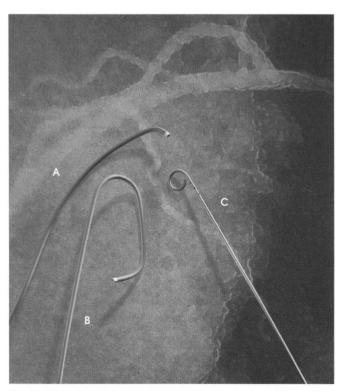

Fig. 23-77 Catheters used during cardiac catheterization. **A,** Judkins right. **B,** Judkins left. **C,** Pigtail.

(Courtesy Cordis Corp., Miami, FL.)

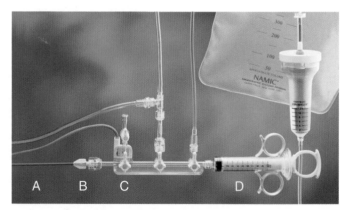

Fig. 23-78 Disposable three-valve Compensator Morse manifold, with a Selector catheter (**A**), rotating adapter (**B**), pressure transducer (**C**), and angiographic control syringe (**D**).

(Courtesy SCHNEIDER/NAMIC, Glens Falls, NY.)

Pressure injector

The pressure injector for the administration of radiographic contrast media (Fig. 23-79) as previously discussed in the section on injection techniques is also used during cardiac catheterization. In the catheterization laboratory, the pressure injector is used to inject a large amount (25 to 50 mL) of contrast material into either the right or the left ventricle (the main pumping chambers of the heart), the aortic root, or the pulmonary vessels. Because the coronary arteries are of small caliber and of low flow rate, administration of contrast media into these structures generally does not require a high-pressure injector. Instead, most physicians opt for manual injection using an angiographic control syringe (see Fig. 23-99). At some facilities, power injectors with a 4-Fr catheter system are used so that the least amount of contrast media is used, and the possibility of introducing air into a coronary artery is reduced.

IMAGING

The imaging equipment found in the cardiac catheterization laboratory is essentially the same as the equipment found in the vascular angiography suite. The catheterization laboratory requires a system capable of producing fluoroscopic images with the greatest amount of recorded detail available. Maximum resolution from the optical system is crucial because of the small size of the cardiac anatomy, which must be imaged while in motion. The imaging used for cardiac studies is typically 15 to 30 frames per second compared with 2 to 6 frames per second used for peripheral imaging. The motion of the heart beating requires this increased frame rate to visualize these small arteries properly. The imaging equipment neces-sary to produce high-resolution imaging is described in detail in the previous section on digital subtraction angiographic procedures.

Physiologic equipment

The physiologic monitor is essential to cardiac catheterization procedures. It is used to monitor and record vital patient functions, including electrical activity (ECG)* within the heart and blood pressure (hemodynamic) within the various intracardiac chambers (Fig. 23-80). The patient's ECG and hemodynamic pressures are continuously displayed throughout the various types of procedures. (Selective samplings of ECG and hemodynamic pressures are recorded for permanent documentation.)

---

*Interpretation of ECG is beyond the scope of this chapter.

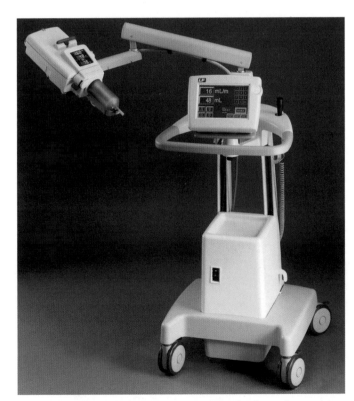

Fig. 23-79 The Angiomat (ILLUMENA) high-pressure injector for radiographic contrast media.

(Courtesy Liebel-Flarsheim, a product of Mallinckrodt, Inc., Cincinnati, OH.)

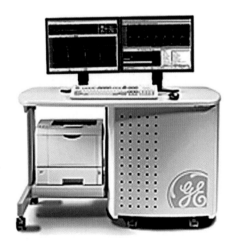

Fig. 23-80 Computer-based physiologic monitor used to monitor patient ECG and hemodynamic pressures during cardiac catheterization.

(Courtesy GE Medical Systems.)

For the collection of hemodynamic data during catheterization, the physiologic recorder (receiving information in electrical form) must be connected to the catheter (carrying information as physical fluid pressure). Devices called *pressure transducers* are interfaced between the manifold and the physiologic recorder to convert fluid (blood) pressure into an electrical signal.

For a standard cardiac catheterization procedure, four channels of the physiologic recorder are usually prepared: two for ECG recordings and two for pressure recordings. A physiologic recorder can have as many as 32 *channels,* however. A channel, or module, is an electrical component of the physiologic recorder that is capable of measuring an individual parameter, such as a specific type of ECG or intravascular pressure. The number of channels required for a particular catheterization increases as the amount of detailed information required increases. Increasingly, these monitoring systems are pro-duced with detailed procedural databases for the collection and maintenance of patient clinical data and the concurrent generation of a procedural report at the time of catheterization.

OTHER EQUIPMENT

Because of the nature of the patient's condition, the inherent risks of cardiac catheterization, and the types of procedures performed, each catheterization room should have the following equipment available:

- A fully equipped emergency cart. The cart typically contains emergency medications, cardiopulmonary resuscitation equipment, intubation equipment, and other related supplies.
- Oxygen and suction.
- Whole-blood oximeters used to determine the oxygen saturation of the blood samples obtained during adult and pediatric catheterizations (Fig. 23-81).
- Defibrillator, used to treat life-threatening arrhythmias. Ideally, the defibrillator would also have external pacemaking capabilities. Some laboratories have two defibrillators available in case one fails.
- Temporary pacemaker to treat potential asystole or symptomatic bradycardia.
- Pulse oximeter to monitor and assess level of oxygenation noninvasively during sedation.
- Noninvasive blood pressure cuff.
- Equipment to perform cardiac output studies.
- Intraaortic balloon pump console and catheters to treat cardiogenic shock.
- Activated clotting time machine to measure levels of heparinization during interventional procedures.

In addition to the basic coronary angiogram and left and right heart studies, many effective tools are available to diagnose and treat coronary artery disease (Table 23-4).

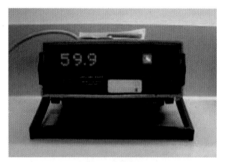

Fig. 23-81 Oximeter used to measure oxygen saturation in blood.

TABLE 23-4

Tools for diagnosis and treatment of coronary artery disease

Equipment	Use	Diagnostic or therapeutic
Pressure wire	Measures blood flow across lesion to determine severity of stenosis	Diagnostic
IVUS	Internal vessel visualization of stenosis, plaque, stent position	Diagnostic
OCT (optical coherence tomography)	Laser light to image the inside of the vessel wall	Diagnostic
Rotablator	Rotational atherectomy of intraluminal plaque or calcium	Therapeutic
Rheolytic thrombectomy	High-velocity saline spray for thrombectomy	Therapeutic
The Crosser	Study device to cross CTOs	Therapeutic

CTOs, Chronic total occlusions.

Patient Positioning for Cardiac Catheterization

Procedures such as selective coronary arteriography and certain pediatric catheterizations require imaging equipment to be positioned to reduce the superimposition created by the cardiac vasculature. Moving the patient during catheterization is undesirable, particularly when catheters have been carefully positioned to show specific anatomic structures or to record certain data.

In most catheterization laboratories, the image intensifier or flat panel detector and fluoroscopic tube are mechanically suspended in a C-arm configuration to allow for equipment rotation around the patient and to provide cranial or caudal angulation. In this configuration, the detector is above the plane of the table, and the fluoroscopic tube is beneath the table. During catheterization procedures, the patient is placed on the examination table in a supine position. For optimal images, the imaging equipment should be rotated around the patient. In some interventional procedures, biplane C-arms are advantageous because they allow simultaneous imaging of cardiac structures in two different planes (Fig. 23-82).

Adult and pediatric coronary anatomy has normal and pathologic variations. Projections for each type of catheterization procedure cannot be specified. Instead, each patient's anatomy must be fluoroscopically evaluated to ascertain the optimal degree of rotation and cranial or caudal angulation necessary to visualize each structure of interest.

Catheterization Methods and Techniques

Different cardiac catheterizations require various combinations of methods and techniques to allow for precise data acquisition and the application of therapeutic interventions. Some methods and techniques common to most cardiac catheterizations are discussed in the following sections.

PRECATHETERIZATION CARE

Before the catheterization is performed, the procedure is explained, and informed consent is obtained. Testing before catheterization normally includes the following:

- Patient history
- Physical examination
- Chest x-ray examination
- Blood work
- ECG
- Echocardiogram
- Exercise stress test
- Nuclear medicine cardiac perfusion studies

Various medications are frequently administered for sedation and control of nausea. Patients brought to the catheterization laboratory typically are not allowed anything to eat or drink for 4 to 6 hours before the procedure or after midnight. During all catheterizations, a protocol (or detailed record) of the procedure is maintained. The record includes hemodynamic data, fluoroscopy time, medications administered, supplies used, and other pertinent information.

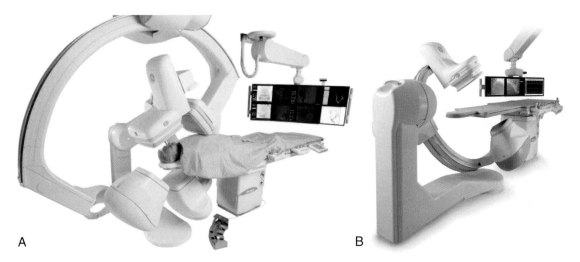

Fig. 23-82 A, Biplane radiology equipment used in the cardiac catheterization laboratory. **B,** Modern single-plane digital catheterization with "smart handle" technology.

(Courtesy GE Medical Systems.)

CATHETER INTRODUCTION

After the patient has been transported to the catheterization laboratory, ECG, noninvasive blood pressure monitoring, and *pulse oximetry* are initiated. The appropriate site for catheter introduction must be prepared using aseptic technique to minimize the risk of subsequent infection. The area of the body to be entered is shaved, and an antiseptic solution is applied. Numerous sites can be used for catheter introduction. The specific sites vary according to the age and body habitus of the patient, the preference of the physician, and the procedure attempted. The most frequent site used for catheterization is the femoral area. The radial, brachial, axillary, jugular (neck), and subclavian (chest) areas may also be chosen.

For catheterization of the femoral artery or vein, the percutaneous approach is employed (see the modified Seldinger technique, which is described and illustrated in Fig. 23-16). If the percutaneous approach cannot be used, a cutdown technique is employed. This technique requires that a small incision be made in the skin to allow for direct visualization of the artery or vein that the physician wants to catheterize. The skin is aseptically prepared and infiltrated with local anesthetic, and the vessel or vessels are bluntly dissected and exposed. After an opening is created in the desired vessel (arteriotomy or venotomy), the catheter is introduced and advanced toward the heart. Cutdown procedures are frequently performed in the right antecubital fossa to access the basilic vein or brachial artery.

PHYSIOLOGIC EQUIPMENT

The acquisition of certain data is essential, regardless of the type of catheterization performed. Physiologic data typically collected include hemodynamic parameters, ECG, and oximetry readings. For the collection of hemodynamic data during catheterization, the physiologic recorder (receiving information in electrical form) must be connected to the catheter (carrying information as physical fluid pressure). Devices called *pressure transducers* are interfaced between the manifold and the physiologic recorder to convert fluid (blood) pressure into an electrical signal.

Hemodynamic parameters include blood pressure and cardiac output. The monitoring and recording of intracardiac (within the heart) and extracardiac (outside the heart) vascular pressures require the use of the physiologic-transducer system described previously in this chapter. Cardiac output, an important indicator of the overall ability of the heart to pump blood, can be measured in the catheterization laboratory. Several methods are used to obtain estimates of cardiac output. ECG is continuously monitored during catheterization and can be simultaneously recorded with intracardiac or extracardiac pressures. Blood samples are obtained from the various chambers of the heart to determine oxygen saturation levels and the presence of any intracardiac shunts.

Catheterization Studies and Procedures

The primary purpose of the diagnostic cardiac catheterization is data collection, whereas the primary purpose of the interventional procedure is therapy. The following sections briefly describe commonly performed diagnostic and interventional heart catheterizations.

BASIC DIAGNOSTIC STUDIES OF THE VASCULAR SYSTEM

Adults

Catheterization of the left side of the heart is a widely performed basic diagnostic cardiac study. The catheter may be introduced through the radial, brachial, or femoral artery and advanced over a guidewire to the ascending aorta. When in the ascending aorta, the guidewire is removed, and the catheter is aspirated and flushed to prevent migration of any air bubbles. Aortic root angiography may be performed to document the competence of the aortic valve. A normal aortic valve prevents backward flow of contrast media into the left ventricle during injection, whereas an insufficient valve does not (Fig. 23-83). Arterial oximetry and blood pressure measurements within the aorta are taken using the manifold system. After these measurements have been taken, the catheter is passed through the aortic valve into the left ventricle.

Blood pressure measurements are taken in the left ventricle. Angiography of the left ventricle is performed in nearly all catheterization studies of the left side of the heart (Fig. 23-84). Left ventriculography provides information about valvular competence, interventricular septal integrity, and the efficiency of the pumping action of the left ventricle (ejection fraction). Mitral regurgitation is another example of valvular incompetence, and angiographically it is seen as the backward flow of contrast media from the left ventricle into the left atrium or pulmonary veins (Fig. 23-85). Computer *planimetry* software calculates how well the ventricle

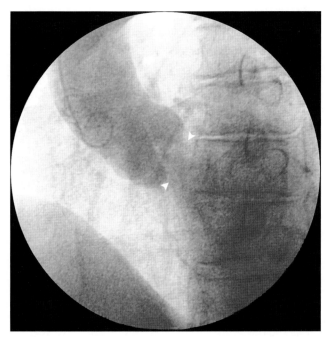

Fig. 23-83 Aortic root injection showing aortic insufficiency with contrast agent flowing back into left ventricle (*arrowheads*).

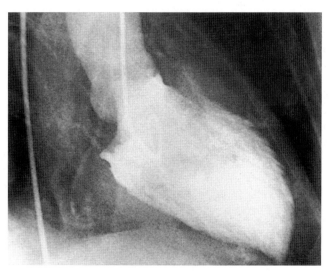

Fig. 23-84 Normal left ventriculogram during diastole.

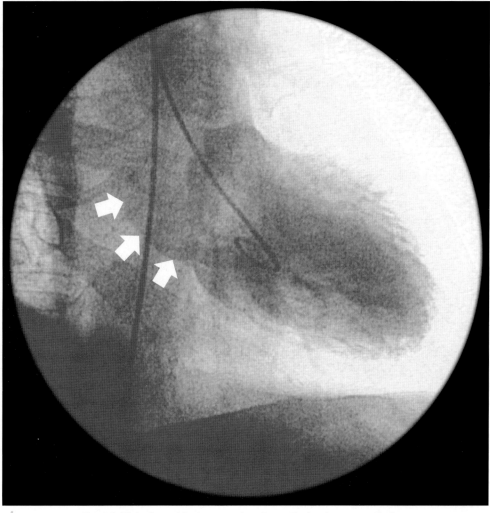

Fig. 23-85 Left ventriculogram showing mitral valve regurgitation.

functions (Fig. 23-86). After left ventriculography, the presence of aortic valve stenosis is determined as the blood pressure measurements are repeated while the catheter is withdrawn across the aortic valve. Normal flow of blood through the aortic valve allows the systolic pressure in the left ventricle to match the systolic pressure in the aorta. When the systolic blood pressure in the left ventricle is greater than the systolic blood pressure in the aorta, aortic stenosis is present.

Selective angiography of the right coronary artery and left coronary artery is performed, with different projections used for each coronary artery to prevent superimposition with overlapping structures. Coronary angiography allows the extent of

intracoronary stenosis to be evaluated (Figs. 23-87 and 23-88).

Because of the complexity of the anatomy involved, the variations in patient body habitus, and the presence of anomalies, a comprehensive guide for angiographic projections is difficult to establish. Projections commonly used during coronary angiography are listed in Table 23-5. The physician determines the projections that best show the artery of interest. Coronary arteriograms are obtained in nearly all catheterizations of the left side of the heart.

Catheterization of the right side of the heart is another commonly performed procedure. During right heart catheterization, a catheter is inserted into a vein in the

groin, antecubital fossa, internal jugular, or subclavian, and it is advanced to the vena cava, into the right atrium, across the tricuspid valve, to the right ventricle, and through the pulmonary valve to the pulmonary artery, until it is wedged distally in the pulmonary artery. Pressure measurements and oximetry are performed in each of the heart chambers as the catheter is advanced. The pressure measurements are used to determine the presence of disorders such as valvular heart disease, congestive heart failure, pulmonary hypertension, and certain cardiomyopathies. The oximetry data are used to determine the presence of an intracardiac shunt. Cineangiography is performed as appropriate.

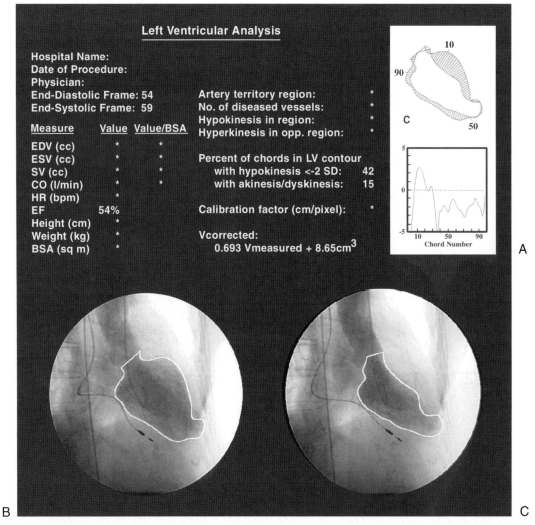

Fig. 23-86 Computerized planimetry for evaluation of left ventricular ejection fraction. **A,** Diastolic phase of contraction of the heart. **B,** Systolic phase of contraction of the heart. **C,** Digital representation of when the diastolic and systolic phases of contraction are superimposed.

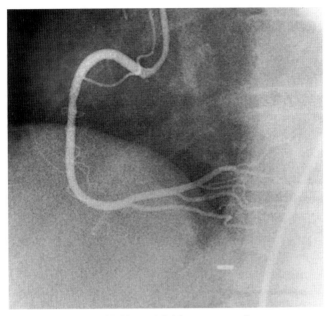

Fig. 23-87 Normal right coronary artery.

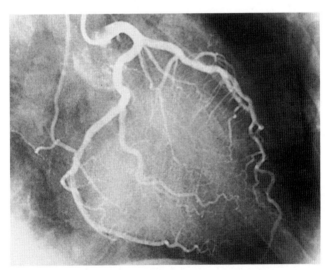

Fig. 23-88 Normal left coronary artery.

TABLE 23-5

Common angiographic angles for specific coronary arteries

Coronary artery	Vessel segment	Projections
Left coronary artery	Left main	PA or RAO 5-15 degrees
	Left anterior descending	LAO 30-40 degrees, cranial 20-40 degrees
		RAO 5-15 degrees, cranial 15-45 degrees
		RAO 20-40 degrees, caudal 15-30 degrees
		RAO 30-50 degrees
		Lateral
	Circumflex	RAO 20-40 degrees, caudal 15-30 degrees
		LAO 40-55 degrees, caudal 15-30 degrees
		LAO 40-60 degrees
Right coronary artery	Middle right	LAO 20-40 degrees
		RAO 20-40 degrees
	Posterior descending	LAO 5-30 degrees, cranial 15-30 degrees

Exercise hemodynamics are often required in the evaluation of valvular heart disease when symptoms of fatigue and dyspnea are present. In such cases, simultaneous catheterization and pressure measurements of the right and left heart are performed at rest and during peak exercise. Exercise often consists of pedaling a stationary bicycle ergometer that is placed on top of the examination table. During simultaneous catheterization, a catheter is placed in a vein (femoral or basilic) and an artery (femoral or brachial).

Children

A primary indication for diagnostic catheterization studies in children is the evaluation and documentation of specific anatomy, hemodynamic data, and selected aspects of cardiac function associated with congenital heart defects. Methods and techniques used for catheterization of the heart in a child vary depending on age, heart size, type and extent of defect, and other coincident pathophysiologic conditions.

Pediatric cardiac catheters are often introduced percutaneously into the femoral vein and, in older children, sometimes into the femoral artery. In very young patients, it may be possible to pass a catheter from the right atrium to the left atrium (allowing access to the left side of the heart) through either a patent foramen ovale or a preexisting atrial septal defect. If the atrial septum is intact, temporary access to the left atrium may be obtained using a transseptal catheter system. With the transseptal catheter system, a long introducer and needle are used to puncture the right atrial septum of the heart to gain access to the left atrium if access cannot be attained as previously described.

ADVANCED DIAGNOSTIC STUDIES OF THE VASCULAR SYSTEM IN ADULTS AND CHILDREN

An example of an advanced diagnostic study of the vascular system is endomyocardial biopsy, which is performed to provide a tissue sample for direct pathologic evaluation of cardiac muscle. A special biopsy catheter with a bioptome tip (Fig. 23-89) is advanced under fluoroscopic control from either the jugular or the femoral vein to the right ventricle (Fig. 23-90). After the bioptome is advanced into the ventricle, the jaws of the device are opened, and the catheter is advanced to the ventricular septum. After the bioptome is in contact with the septum, its jaws are closed, and a gentle tugging motion is applied to retrieve the tissue sample. Several biopsy specimens are acquired in this manner. The specimens are immediately fixed in either glutaraldehyde or buffered formalin before being sent for pathologic evaluation. Endomyocardial biopsy is frequently used to monitor cardiac transplantation patients for early signs of tissue rejection and to differentiate between various types of cardiomyopathies.

ADVANCED DIAGNOSTIC STUDIES OF THE CONDUCTION SYSTEM IN ADULTS AND CHILDREN

Electrophysiology studies involve the collection of sophisticated data to facilitate detailed mapping of the electrical conduction system within the heart. The procedures involve the placement of numerous multipolar catheters within the heart (Fig. 23-91). Electrophysiology studies are used to analyze the conduction system, induce and evaluate arrhythmias, and determine the effects of therapeutic measures in treating arrhythmias.

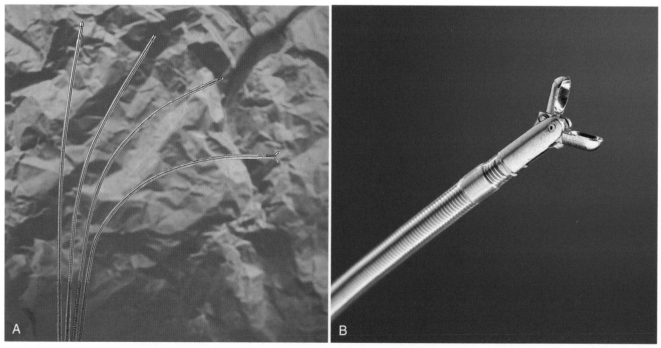

Fig. 23-89 A, Standard biopsy catheters. **B,** Bioptome catheter tip used for myocardial biopsy. The jaws on the tip close and take a "bite" from the inside of the heart muscle.

(Courtesy Cordis Corp., Miami, FL.)

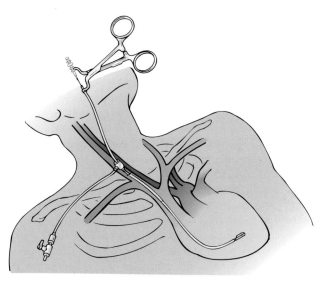

Fig. 23-90 Bioptome tip in the right ventricular apex points toward the ventricular septum.

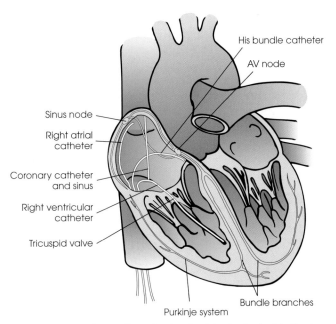

His bundle catheter

AV node

Sinus node

Right atrial
catheter

Coronary catheter
and sinus

Right ventricular
catheter

Tricuspid valve

Bundle branches

Purkinje system

Fig. 23-91 Catheter positions for routine electrophysiologic study. Multipolar catheters are positioned in the high right atrium near the sinus node, in the area of the atrioventricular apex, and in the coronary sinus.

Electrode catheters are introduced into the femoral vein, internal jugular vein, or subclavian vein. Because several catheters are used, multiple access sites are needed. It is common to have three introducer sheaths placed within the same vein. The catheters consist of several insulated wires, each of which is attached to an electrode on the catheter tip that serves as an interface with the intracardiac surface. The arrangements of the electrodes on the catheter allow its dual function of recording the electrical signals of the heart (intracardiac electrograms) and pacing the heart. The pacemaker function is performed to introduce premature electrical impulses to determine possible arrhythmias. After the precise defect is characterized, an appropriate course of therapy can be undertaken. Cardiac ablation, pacemaker, and internal cardiac defibrillator are the most common treatments for arrhythmias. In some cases, surgical intervention is required.

INTERVENTIONAL PROCEDURES OF THE VASCULAR SYSTEM
Adults

Interventional cardiac catheterization techniques requiring special-purpose catheters have expanded significantly since the late 1970s. PTCA is a technique that employs balloon dilation of a coronary artery stenosis to increase blood flow to the heart muscle. Gruentzig performed the first successful PTCA in 1977.

During PTCA, a specially designed guiding catheter is placed into the orifice of the stenotic coronary artery as determined by coronary angiography (Fig. 23-92). A steerable guidewire is inserted into the balloon catheter and advanced within the guiding catheter (Fig. 23-93). The guidewire is advanced across the stenotic area; it serves as a support platform so that the balloon catheter can be advanced and centered across the stenosis. Controlled and precise inflation of the balloon fractures and compresses the fatty deposits into the muscular wall of the artery. This compression, in conjunction with the stretching of the external vessel diameter, is necessary for successful angioplasty. The balloon is deflated to allow rapid reperfusion of blood to the heart muscle. The inflation procedure, followed by arteriography, may be repeated several times until a satisfactory degree of patency is observed (Fig. 23-94). The limiting factor of PTCA is restenosis, which occurs in approximately 30% to 50% of patients who undergo the procedure.

Restenosis of the coronary artery after revascularization is the major factor in failed long-term outcomes. Drug-coated or drug-eluting stents are now routinely used for the treatment of coronary artery disease. The goal is to reduce or inhibit restenosis that occurs after a revascularization procedure. Drugs are chemically bound or coated on a stent. The drug is released in small amounts over time to inhibit restenosis. The various drugs reduce restenosis by limiting the proliferation of smooth muscle cells or reducing the rate at which this occurs. The prevention of restenosis after revascularization remains to be proven.

Bare metal stents are used along with or independently of drug-eluting stents. Patient age, cost, and disease are the determining factors. The procedure is similar to PTCA and is performed in the same manner except that a metallic stent is mounted on the PTCA balloon (Fig. 23-95). For optimal stent deployment, the stent is centered across the entire length of the stenosis. Deployment of the stent is achieved with the inflation and deflation of the PTCA balloon. After the stent is deployed, the angioplasty balloon is removed, and a high-pressure balloon is advanced within the stent. Inflation of the high-pressure balloon is performed to embed the metallic struts of the stent in the walls of the artery. Restenosis rates are lower in patients receiving intracoronary stents than in patients who undergo conventional angioplasty. PTCA and stent

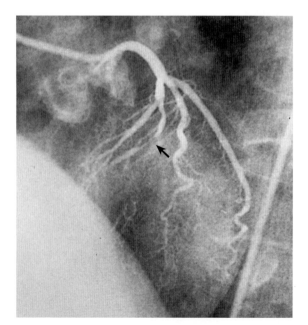

Fig. 23-92 Stenotic coronary artery before PTCA. *Arrow* indicates the stenotic area, estimated at 95%, with minimum blood flow distal to the lesion.

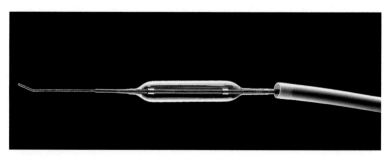

Fig. 23-93 Catheter system for PTCA. The three sections of the system are the outer guiding catheter (*right*), central balloon catheter (*middle*), and internal steerable guidewire (*left*).

(Courtesy Cordis Corp., Miami, FL.)

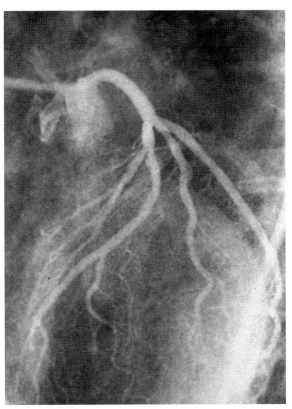

Fig. 23-94 Coronary arteriogram after PTCA in the same patient as in Fig. 23-92. Blood flow is estimated to be 100%.

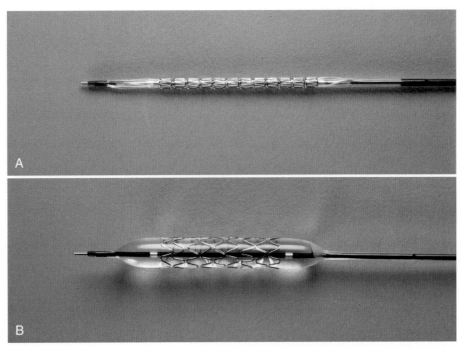

Fig. 23-95 Balloon expandable intracoronary stent. **A,** Before stent balloon inflation. **B,** After stent balloon inflation.

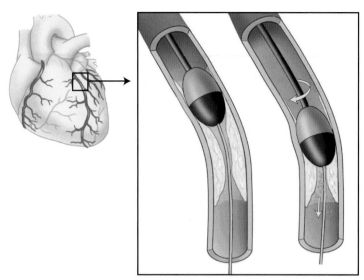

Fig. 23-96 Coronary atherectomy device.

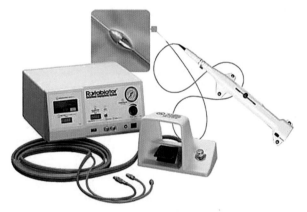

Fig. 23-97 Rotablator rotational atherectomy catheter with advancer unit. *Insert* shows football-shaped burr.

(Courtesy Boston Scientific.)

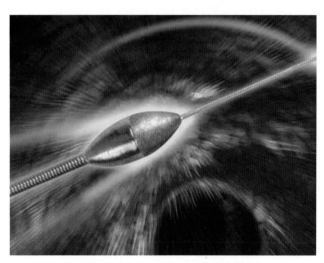

Fig. 23-98 Atherectomy catheter burr.

(Courtesy Boston Scientific.)

interventions constitute the bulk of the coronary interventions being performed at the present time. Of major concern are dissection at the proximal and distal ends of the stent and complete apposition of the stent against the vessel wall (see Fig. 23-101).

Atherectomy devices have also been used in the treatment of coronary artery disease. In contrast to PTCA balloons, atherectomy devices remove the fatty deposit or thrombus material from within the artery (Fig. 23-96).

A device called Rotablator has been indicated in the use of atherosclerotic coronary artery disease. Commonly referred to as percutaneous transluminal coronary rotational atherectomy (PTCRA), this procedure can be used in conjunction with PTCA or stenting. The tip of the catheter (1.25 to 2.5 mm in diameter) resembles a football and is embedded with microscopic diamond particles on the front half and is rotated on a special torque guidewire between 160,000 rpm and 200,000 rpm (Figs. 23-97 and 23-98).

Standard angioplasty catheter positioning techniques are used to position a guidewire distal to the targeted lesion. A rotational atherectomy burr size is selected and advanced over the special torque guidewire just proximal to the lesion. At this point, the burr is activated, and the plaque is pulverized and reduced to the size of a blood cell. The pulverized plaque is removed by the reticuloendothelial system. After an adequate amount of plaque is cleared, standard PTCA or stenting techniques are employed to maintain artery patency (Fig. 23-99). PTCRA has proven to be beneficial in the treatment of highly calcified lesions and in-stent restenosis compared with PTCA alone.

Although coronary angiography remains the gold standard for the diagnosis of coronary artery disease, *intravascular ultrasound* (IVUS) offers further diagnostic and interventional information that cannot be appreciated by angiography alone. IVUS allows a full 360-degree circumference visualization of the vessel wall, permits information regarding vascular pathology and longitudinal and volumetric measurements, and facilitates guidance of catheter-based interventions. The intervention-associated potential of IVUS is the ability to optimize the type and size of device (i.e., PTCA or stent vs. Rotablator, atherectomy) being used and to determine proper apposition of the stent after deployment against the artery wall.

Components consist of the ultrasound unit, recording device (usually stored on the hard drive and available for recording onto a CD-ROM, or digital imaging and communications in medicine [DICOM] system), printer, transducer, pullback device, and catheter (Fig. 23-100). The intravascular catheters in use today

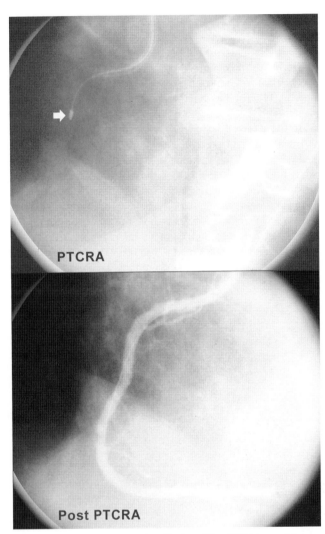

Fig. 23-99 PTCRA. *Arrow* points to burr of catheter. After PTCRA, a widely patent right coronary artery is shown.

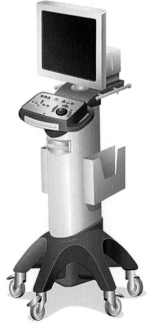

Fig. 23-100 IVUS unit. Shown here are the keyboard and monitor.

(Courtesy Volcano.)

employ 20- to 40-MHz silicon piezoelectric crystals and range in size from 5 Fr on the proximal end of the catheter to 2.9 Fr at the distal end. During the procedure, the IVUS catheter is advanced over the guidewire that was previously placed within the artery being imaged. The IVUS catheter is advanced distal to the targeted lesion, at which time the transducer and recording device are turned on. Slowly, the catheter is withdrawn using the pullback device to maintain a consistent withdrawal of the catheter and to help ascertain the length of the targeted lesion. Documentation of IVUS catheter position can be obtained with angiography. The images are stored on the hard drive of the IVUS system and can be retrieved later or saved to a DV-R; this allows the cardiologist to review, take measurements, and print images later (Figs. 23-101 and 23-102).

At present, IVUS remains an integral part of coronary interventions being performed. With advances in stent designs, brachytherapy, local drug delivery, and future technologies, IVUS will remain a vital source for information in improving the outcomes of percutaneous coronary interventions. IVUS equipment combines an imaging transducer with an interventional device, permitting guidance during the interventional procedure. The clinical use of IVUS imaging and other improved computerized image enhancements should allow for more precise data collection and more tailored methods of determining the interventional method to use in treating coronary artery disease.

The newest diagnostic tool available to visualize intravascular structures is optical coherence tomography (OCT). This technology uses infrared laser light to identify plaque rupture, stent apposition, dissection, and vessel size. This diagnostic tool creates extremely high resolution images with improved visualization of calcified plaques. The image is obtained while injecting contrast into the vessel of interest, thereby displacing the blood. The only limitation to using this intraprocedure is if a patient has impaired renal function (Fig. 23-103, *A* and *B*).

Because of the risks associated with mechanical interventions of the vascular system, open-heart surgical facilities must be immediately available. Coronary occlusion is a major complication requiring emergency surgery in patients undergoing catheter-based mechanical interventions.

Interventional pharmacologic procedures in adults consist of the therapeutic administration of medications that may be given before the patient reaches the cardiac catheterization laboratory. A thrombolytic agent can be used in the early hours of an acute MI in an effort to modify its course. Estimates indicate that thrombotic coronary artery occlusion is present in 75% to 85% of patients with acute MI. If reperfusion of the ischemic myocardium is effective, scarring is reduced. Reperfusion in the early stages of MI offers greater potential for heart muscle salvage. ST segment elevation MI is determined from a 12-lead ECG performed in the field or in the emergency department. These patients are the most critical and typically have a complete or almost complete blockage of a coronary artery. Rapid reperfusion to the heart muscle must be performed to minimize damage.

Children

Many congenital cardiac defects in children are amenable to interventional procedures performed in the catheterization laboratory. As with PTCA procedures, cardiovascular surgical support services must be readily available.

When successful, certain pediatric interventional procedures negate the need for surgical correction of defects. Some procedures are performed for palliative

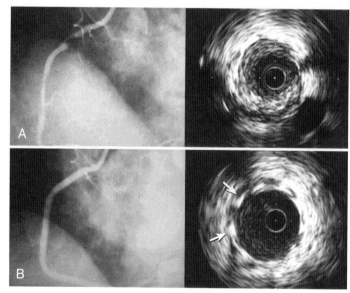

Fig. 23-101 IVUS images shown on the right correlated with angiography images on the left. *Arrows* in **B** show the echogenicity of the stent struts during IVUS.

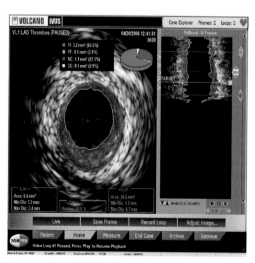

Fig. 23-102 IVUS artery images.

purposes, however, to allow the child to grow to a size and weight at which subsequent open-heart surgery is feasible.

One technique, *balloon septostomy*, may be used to enlarge a patent foramen ovale or preexisting *atrial septal defect*. Enlargement of the opening enhances the mixing of right and left atrial blood, thereby improving the level of systemic arterial oxygenation. Transposition of the great arteries is a condition for which atrial septostomy is performed.

Balloon septostomy requires a catheter similar to the type used in PTCA. The balloon is passed through the atrial septal opening into the left atrium, inflated with contrast media, and snapped back through the septal orifice. This maneuver causes the septum to tear. Often the technique must be repeated until the septal opening is sufficiently enlarged to allow the desired level of blood mixing as documented by oximetry, intracardiac pressures, and angiography.

If the atrial septum does not contain a preexisting opening, an artificial defect can be created. A transseptal system approach is employed, and a special catheter containing an internal folding knife-like blade is advanced into the left atrium (Fig. 23-104). After the catheter is inside the left atrium, the blade is advanced out of its protective outer housing and pulled back to the right atrium, creating an incision in the septal wall. This technique may be repeated. A balloon septostomy is performed to widen the new opening, and the condition of the patient is monitored by oximetry, blood pressures, and angiography.

A patent ductus arteriosus is sometimes evident in a newborn. In utero, the pulmonary artery shunts blood flow into the aorta through the ductus arteriosus, which normally closes after birth. Patent ductus arteriosus occurs when this channel fails to close spontaneously. In some instances, closure can be induced with medication. If this measure is unsuccessful, and the residual shunt is deemed significant, surgical closure (ligation) of the vessel is appropriate.

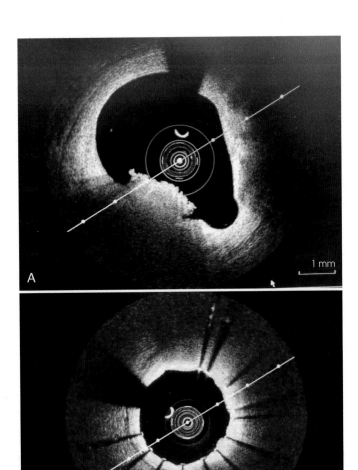

Fig. 23-103 A, OCT demonstrating plaque burden inside a coronary artery. **B,** OCT of coronary artery post stent deployment.

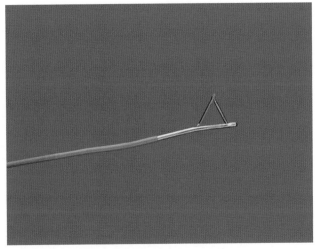

Fig. 23-104 Blade on catheter tip used to incise septal walls in pediatric interventional procedures.

For some patients, occlusion of a patent ductus arteriosus can be accomplished in the catheterization laboratory. A catheter containing an occlusion device, such as an umbrella, is advanced to the ductus. After the position of the lesion is confirmed by angiography, the occluder is released. Subsequent clotting and fibrous infiltration permanently stop the flow and subsequent mixing of blood.

INTERVENTIONAL PROCEDURES OF THE CONDUCTION SYSTEM IN ADULTS AND CHILDREN

Permanent implantation of an antiarrhythmic device is a manipulative procedure that is being performed in cardiac catheterization laboratories (Fig. 23-105). Antiarrhythmic devices include pacemakers for patients with bradyarrhythmias or disease of the electrical conduction system of the heart and implantable cardioverter defibrillators (ICDs) for patients with lethal ventricular tachyarrhythmias originating from the bottom of the heart.

Pacemaker implantation can be performed successfully under local anesthesia in selected adult and pediatric patients. ICD implantation requires conscious sedation or general anesthesia because of the type of testing required at the time of implantation. Insertion of either a pacemaker or an ICD involves puncturing the subclavian or cephalic vein and introducing leads (electrically insulated wires with distal electrodes). The leads are manipulated so that their tips are in direct contact with the right ventricular or right atrial endocardium, or both. The leads are tested for stimulation and sensing properties to ascertain proper functioning before they are attached to the pulse generator. During ICD implantation, defibrillation threshold testing is performed to determine the amount of energy required to defibrillate a patient from ventricular tachycardia or fibrillation. After testing is completed, the proximal end of the lead is attached to a battery (pacemaker or ICD) and implanted in a subcutaneous or subpectoral pocket created in the thorax (Fig. 23-106). Current pacemakers have longevity of 5 to 10 years, and ICDs have longevity of 6 to 8 years.

Another interventional procedure performed in the cardiac catheterization laboratory to treat disorders of the conduction system is radiofrequency (RF) ablation. Several different arrhythmias previously treated with ICD implantation or drug therapy can now be treated with RF ablation. The procedure is normally performed at the time of the diagnostic electrophysiology study if an underlying mechanism or arrhythmogenic focus is identified.

RF ablation is achieved by delivering a low-voltage, high-frequency alternating current directly to the endocardial tissue through a specially designed ablation catheter. The current desiccates the underlying abnormal myocardial conduction tissue and creates a small, discrete burn lesion. Localized RF lesions create areas of tissue necrosis and scar, subsequently destroying the arrhythmogenic focus. Several RF lesions may be necessary to eliminate the abnormal conduction circuit.

Follow-up electrophysiologic testing is performed to document the resolution of the arrhythmia. RF ablation of the atrioventricular node and pacemaker insertion are quickly becoming the preferred treatment for chronic atrial fibrillation with rapid, irregular responses. The atrioventricular junction is destroyed intentionally; consequently, the rapid, irregular electrical impulses from the atrium are not conducted into the ventricle. A pacemaker is implanted, and a more consistent, regular heart rate is achieved.

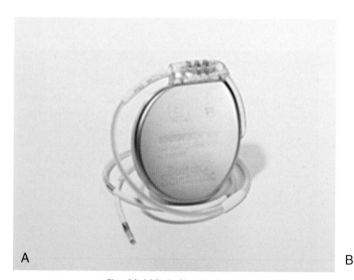
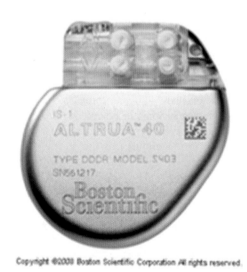

Fig. 23-105 A, Single-chamber ICD. **B,** Dual chamber pacemaker.

(Used with permission of Boston Scientific Corporation. Boston Scientific Corporation 2013 or its Affiliates. All rights reserved.)

Postcatheterization Care

When the catheterization procedure is completed, all catheters are removed. If a cutdown approach was used, the arteriotomy or venotomy is repaired as appropriate. If a percutaneous approach was used, multiple techniques can be employed to obtain hemostasis. Manual pressure is placed on the puncture site until bleeding is controlled. Devices used to close the arteriotomy include collagen seal, suture-mediated devices, or a metal clip. These are deployed under the skin against the artery wall. Wound sites are cleaned and dressed to minimize the risk of infection.

The physician prescribes postcatheterization medications. The puncture site must be observed for hemorrhage or hematoma, and the status of the distal pulse is recorded on the protocol record before the patient leaves the catheterization laboratory. Vital signs should be monitored regularly after the catheterization. The ingestion of fluids should be encouraged, and pain medication may be indicated.

Cardiac catheterization may also be performed on an outpatient or same-day treatment basis. The patient is monitored for 4 to 8 hours in a recovery area and then allowed to go home. Instructions for home care recovery procedures are usually given to the patient or a family member before the patient leaves the recovery area.

Cardiac Catheterization Trends

CATHETER-BASED THERAPIES

Many procedures previously performed only by cardiothoracic surgeons are presently being done in the catheterization laboratory. These are percutaneous procedures done by specially trained cardiologists and include placement of a device percutaneously to close patent foramen ovales and atrioseptal defects. New trials are also being done to develop percutaneous valve replacements.

MAGNETIC RESONANCE IMAGING

Techniques and methods for cardiac catheterization continue to be developed and refined. Angiographic imaging and recording devices are becoming even more sophisticated and yielding ever greater resolution and detail. MRI (see Chapter 30) of the cardiovascular system is now a well-recognized investigational technique. Magnetic resonance coronary arteriography is now able to assess anomalous coronary artery anatomy reliably and to identify the presence of calcification in the coronary arteries and bypass grafts.

ELECTRON BEAM COMPUTED TOMOGRAPHY

An area receiving much recognition more recently in the study of coronary artery disease is the use of electron beam tomography (EBT) imaging. Many manufacturers are working on similar imaging equipment by using ultrafast CT scanning coupled with software reconstruction algorithms to accomplish the goal of noninvasive coronary angiography (see Chapter 29). EBT can detect heart disease at its earliest and most treatable stages by measuring the amount of coronary calcium. The coronary calcium score provides a good indication of the amount of artery blockage.

The patient lies on a table similar to that used for a conventional CT scan. The significant difference between a conventional CT scanner and EBT is the exposure time. Exposure time for EBT is approximately 100 msec. This typically results in about 30 to 40 scans and the ability to scan the entire heart in a single breath hold.

Another technique using EBT involves the injection of contrast media intravenously. The term *electron beam angiography* (EBA) refers to a simple, noninvasive technique that uses an IV injection of contrast media. EBA is effective for visualization of the heart, great vessels, carotid arteries, and peripheral vasculature. EBA shows the coronary arteries with a high degree of accuracy compared with conventional angiography.

Many experts believe that the greatest area for growth in the field of cardiac catheterization is in interventional procedures. Despite the use of such techniques as PTCA, intracoronary stenting, and atherectomy in coronary artery disease, restenosis continues to be prevalent and of major concern. Most of the research in interventional procedures is geared toward finding a technique to prevent or limit greatly restenosis after an intervention. Procedures classified as experimental or investigational in the late 1980s are now being performed regularly. Existing and new interventional procedures should continue to provide patients with viable, relatively low-risk, financially reasonable alternatives to open-heart surgery. Current trends indicate that the number and variety of outpatient cardiac catheterizations will continue to increase. The equipment used and procedures performed in the cardiac catheterization laboratories of the future are likely to be significantly different from those associated with existing facilities. Despite changes in cardiovascular technology and medical techniques, cardiac catheterization laboratories will continue to provide the essential patient care services necessary for the diagnosis and treatment of a vast number of cardiovascular-related diseases.

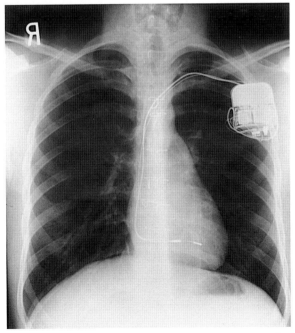

Fig. 23-106 Chest radiograph of a patient with a permanent pacemaker implanted. Note the pacemaker location in the superior and anterior chest wall, with the distal leads located in the right ventricle and right atrium of the heart.

Definition of Terms

afferent lymph vessel Vessel carrying lymph toward a lymph vessel.

anastomose Join.

aneurysm Sac formed by local enlargement of a weakened artery wall.

angina pectoris Severe form of chest pain and constriction near the heart; usually caused by a decrease in the blood supply to cardiac tissue; most often associated with stenosis of a coronary artery as a result of atherosclerotic accumulations or spasm. Pain generally lasts for a few minutes and is more likely to occur after stress, exercise, or other activity resulting in increased heart rate.

angiography Radiographic demonstration of blood vessels after the introduction of contrast media.

anomaly Variation from the normal pattern.

aortic dissection Tear in inner lining of the aortic wall that allows blood to enter and track along the muscular coat.

aortography Radiographic examination of the aorta.

arrhythmia Variation from normal heart rhythm.

arrhythmogenic Producing an arrhythmia.

arteriography Radiologic examination of arteries after injection of a radiopaque contrast medium.

arteriole Very small arterial vessel.

arteriosclerotic Indicative of a general pathologic condition characterized by thickening and hardening of arterial walls, leading to general loss of elasticity.

arteriotomy Surgical opening of an artery.

arteriovenous malformation Abnormal anastomosis or communication between an artery and a vein.

artery Large blood vessel carrying blood away from the heart.

atherectomy Excision of atherosclerotic plaque.

atheromatous Characteristic of degenerative change in the inner lining of arteries caused by the deposition of fatty tissue and subsequent thickening of arterial walls that occurs in atherosclerosis.

atherosclerosis Condition in which fibrous and fatty deposits on the luminal wall of an artery may cause obstruction of the vessel.

atrium One of the two upper chambers of the heart.

bifurcation Place where a structure divides into two branches.

biplane Two x-ray exposure planes 90 degrees from one another, usually frontal and lateral.

blood vascular system Vascular system comprising arteries, capillaries, and veins, which convey blood.

bradyarrhythmia Irregular heart rhythm in conjunction with bradycardia.

bradycardia Any heart rhythm with an average heart rate of less than 60 beats/min.

capillary Tiny blood vessel through which blood and tissue cells exchange substances.

cardiac output Amount of blood pumped from the heart per given unit of time; can be calculated by multiplying stroke volume (amount of blood in milliliters ejected from the left ventricle during each heartbeat) by heart rate (number of heartbeats per minute). A normal, resting adult with a stroke volume of 70 mL and a heart rate of 72 beats/min has a cardiac output of approximately 5 L/min.

cardiomyopathies Relatively serious group of heart diseases typically characterized by enlargement of the myocardial layer of the left ventricle and resulting in decreased cardiac output; hypertrophic cardiomyopathy is a condition often studied in the catheterization laboratory.

cardiovascular and interventional technologist Technologists specializing in angiographic and interventional procedures.

cerebral angiography Imaging of vascular system of the brain.

cineangiography High-speed, 35-mm motion picture film recording of a fluoroscopic image of structures containing radiographic contrast media.

cinefluorography Same as cineradiography; the production of a motion picture record of successive images on a fluoroscopic screen.

claudication Cramping of the leg muscles after physical exertion because of chronically inadequate blood supply.

coagulopathy Any disorder that affects the blood-clotting mechanism.

collateral Secondary or accessory.

diastole Relaxed phase of the atria or ventricles of the heart during which blood enters the chambers; in the cardiac cycle at which the heart is not contracting (at rest).

dyspnea Labored breathing.

efferent lymph vessel Vessel carrying lymph away from a node.

ejection fraction Measurements of ventricular contractility expressed as the percentage of blood pumped out of the left ventricle during contraction; can be estimated by evaluating the left ventriculogram; normal range is 57% to 73% (average 65%). A low ejection fraction indicates failure of the left ventricle to pump effectively.

embolus Foreign material, often thrombus, that detaches and moves freely in the bloodstream.

endocardium Interior lining of heart chambers.

epicardium Exterior layer of heart wall.

ergometer Device used to imitate the muscular, metabolic, and respiratory effects of exercise.

extravasation Escape of fluid from a vessel into the surrounding tissue.

fibrillation Involuntary, chaotic muscular contractions resulting from spontaneous activation of single muscle cells or muscle fibers.

French size Measurement of catheter sizes; 1 French = 0.33 mm; abbreviated Fr.

guidewire Tightly wound metallic wire over which angiographic catheters are placed.

hematoma Collection of extravasated blood in an organ or a tissue space.

hemodynamics Study of factors involved in circulation of blood. Hemodynamic data typically collected during heart catheterization are cardiac output and intracardiac pressures.

hemostasis Stopping of blood flow in a hemorrhage.

iatrogenic Caused by a therapeutic or diagnostic procedure.

innominate or brachiocephalic artery First major artery of the aortic arch supplying the cerebral circulation.

in-stent restenosis Renarrowing of an artery inside a previously placed stent.

intervention Therapeutic modality—mechanical or pharmacologic—used to modify the course of a disease process.

interventional Improving a condition; therapeutic.

interventricular septal integrity Continuity of the membranous partition that separates the right and left ventricles of the heart.

intracoronary stent Metallic device placed within a coronary artery across a region of stenosis.

introducer sheath Plastic tubing placed within the vasculature through which other catheters may be passed.

ischemic Indicative of a local decrease of blood supply to myocardial tissue associated with temporary obstruction of a coronary vessel, typically as a result of thrombus (blood clot).

lesion Injury or other damaging change to an organ or tissue.

lymph Body fluid circulated by the lymphatic vessels and filtered by the lymph nodes.

lymph vessels See *afferent* and *efferent lymph vessel.*

lymphadenography Radiographic study of the lymph nodes.

lymphangiography Radiographic study of the lymph vessels.

lymphography Radiographic evaluation of the lymphatic channels and lymph nodes.

mandrel Inner metallic core of a spiral wound guidewire.

meninges Three membranes that envelop the brain and spinal cord.

misregistration Occurs when the two images used to form a subtraction image are slightly displaced from one another.

myocardial infarction (MI) Acute ischemic episode resulting in myocardial damage and pain; commonly referred to as a heart attack.

myocardium Muscular heart wall.

neointimal hyperplasia Hyperproliferation of smooth muscle cells and extracellular matrix secondary to revascularization.

nephrotoxic Chemically damaging to the kidney cells.

nonocclusive Not completely closed or shut; allowing blood flow.

occlusion Obstruction or closure of a vessel, such as a coronary vessel, as a result of foreign material, thrombus, or spasm.

oximetry Measurement of oxygen saturation in blood.

oxygen saturation Amount of oxygen bound to hemoglobin in blood, expressed as a percentage.

patency State of being open or unobstructed.

patent foramen ovale Opening between the right atrium and left atrium that normally exists in fetal life to allow for the essential mixing of blood. The opening normally closes shortly after birth.

percutaneous Introduced through the skin.

percutaneous transluminal angioplasty (PTA) Surgical correction of a vessel from within the vessel using catheter technology.

percutaneous transluminal coronary angioplasty (PTCA) Manipulative interventional procedure involving the placement and inflation of a balloon catheter in the lumen of a stenosed coronary artery for the purpose of compressing and fracturing the diseased material, allowing subsequent increased distal blood flow to the myocardium.

percutaneous transluminal coronary rotational atherectomy (PTCRA) Manipulative interventional procedure involving a device called a Rotablator to remove atherosclerotic plaque from within the coronary artery using a high-speed rotational burr.

percutaneously Performed through the skin.

pericardium Fibrous sac that surrounds the heart.

planimetry Mechanical tracing to determine the volume of a structure.

pledget Small piece of material used as a dressing or plug.

portal circulation System of vessels carrying blood from the organs of digestion to the liver.

postprocessing Image processing operations performed when reviewing an imaging sequence.

pulmonary circulation System of vessels carrying blood from the heart to the lungs and back to the heart.

pulse Regular expansion and contraction of an artery that is produced by ejection of blood from the heart.

pulse oximetry Measurement of oxygen saturation in the blood via an optic sensor placed on an extremity.

reperfusion Reestablishment of blood flow to the heart muscle through a previously occluded artery.

restenosis Narrowing or constriction of a vessel, orifice, or other type of passageway after interventional correction of primary condition.

rotational burr atherectomy Ablation of atheroma through a percutaneous transcatheter approach using a high-speed rotational burr.

serial imaging Acquisition of images in rapid succession.

stenosis Narrowing or constriction of a vessel, an orifice, or another type of passageway.

stent Wire mesh or plastic conduit placed to maintain flow.

systemic circulation System of vessels carrying blood from the heart out to the body (except the lungs) and back to the heart.

systole Contraction phase of the atria or ventricles of the heart during which blood is ejected from the chambers; point in the cardiac cycle at which the heart is contracting (at work).

tachyarrhythmia Irregular heart rhythm in conjunction with tachycardia.

tachycardia Any heart rhythm having an average heart rate in excess of 100 beats/min.

targeted lesion Area of narrowing within an artery where a revascularization procedure is planned.

thrombogenesis Formation of a blood clot.

thrombolytic Capable of causing the breakup of a thrombus.

thrombosis Formation or existence of a blood clot.

thrombus Blood clot obstructing a blood vessel or cavity of the heart.

transducer Device used to convert one form of energy into another. Transducers used in cardiac catheterization convert fluid (blood) pressure into an electrical signal displayed on a physiologic monitor.

transposition of the great arteries Congenital heart defect requiring interventional therapy. In this defect, the aorta arises from the right side of the heart, and the pulmonary artery arises from the left side of the heart.

umbrella Prosthetic interventional device consisting of two opposing polyurethane disks connected by a central loop mounted on a spring-loaded assembly to provide opposing tension.

valvular competence Ability of the valve to prevent backward flow while not inhibiting forward flow.

varices Irregularly swollen veins.

vasoconstriction Temporary closure of a blood vessel using drug therapy.

vein Vessel that carries blood from the capillaries to the heart.

venography Radiologic study of veins after injection of radiopaque contrast media.

venotomy Surgical opening of a vein.

ventricle One of two larger pumping chambers of the heart.

venule Any of the small blood vessels that collect blood from the capillaries and join to become veins.

Selected bibliography

Ahn SS, Concepcion B: Current status of atherectomy for peripheral arterial occlusive disease, *World J Surg* 20:635, 1996.

Burke TH et al: Cardiovascular and interventional technologists: their growing role in the interventional suite, *J Vasc Interv Radiol* 8:720, 1997.

Caldwell DM et al: Embolotherapy: agents, clinical applications, and techniques, *Radio-Graphics* 14:623, 1994.

Colombo A et al: Intracoronary stenting without anticoagulation accomplished with intravascular ultrasound guidance, *Circulation* 91:1676, 1995.

Dorffner R et al: Treatment of abdominal aortic aneurysms with transfemoral placement of stent-grafts: complications and secondary radiologic intervention, *Radiology* 204:79, 1997.

Dyet JF: Endovascular stents in the arterial system—current status, *Clin Radiol* 52:83, 1997.

Eustace S et al: Magnetic resonance angiography in transjugular intrahepatic portosystemic stenting: comparison with contrast hepatic and portal venography, *Eur J Radiol* 19:43, 1994.

Fillmore DJ et al: Transjugular intrahepatic portosystemic shunt: midterm clinical and angiographic follow-up, *J Vasc Interv Radiol* 7:255, 1996.

Kandarpa K: Technical determinants of success in catheter-directed thrombolysis for peripheral arterial occlusions, *J Vasc Interv Radiol* 6(6 pt 2 Suppl):55S, 1995.

Kern MJ: *The cardiac catheterization handbook*, ed 4, St Louis, 2003, Mosby.

Kerns SR et al: Current status of carbon dioxide angiography, *Radiol Clin North Am* 33:15, 1995.

Laine C et al: Combined cardiac catheterization for uncomplicated ischemic heart disease in a Medicare population, *Am J Med* 105:373, 1998.

LeRoux PD, Winn HR: Current management of aneurysms, *Neurosurg Clin N Am* 9:421, 1998.

Nelson PK, Kricheff II: Cerebral angiography, *Neuroimaging Clin N Am* 6:1, 1996.

Norris TG: Principles of cardiac catheterization, *Radiol Technol* 72:109, 2000.

Pieters PC et al: Evaluation of the portal venous system: complementary roles of invasive and noninvasive imaging strategies, *RadioGraphics* 17:879, 1997.

Rees CR et al: Use of carbon dioxide as a contrast medium for transjugular intrahepatic portosystemic shunt procedures, *J Vasc Interv Radiol* 5:383, 1994.

Rogers CG Jr et al: Intrahepatic vascular shunting for portal hypertension: early experience with the transjugular intrahepatic porto-systemic shunt, *Am Surg* 60:114, 1994.

Scanlon PJ et al: ACC/AHA guidelines for coronary angiography: a report of the American College of Cardiology/American Heart Association Task Force on Practice Guidelines (Committee on Coronary Angiography), *J Am Coll Cardiol* 33:1756, 1999.

Seldinger SI: Percutaneous selective angiography of the aorta: preliminary report, *Acta Radiol (Stockh)* 45:15, 1956.

Vinuela F et al: Guglielmi detachable coil embolization of acute intracranial aneurysm: perioperative anatomical and clinical outcome in 403 patients, *J Neurosurg* 86:475, 1997.

Warner JJ et al: Recognizing complications of cardiac catheterization, *Emerg Med* 32:12, 2000.

24
PEDIATRIC IMAGING

DEREK CARVER
ANGELA FRANCESCHI
RAYMOND THIES

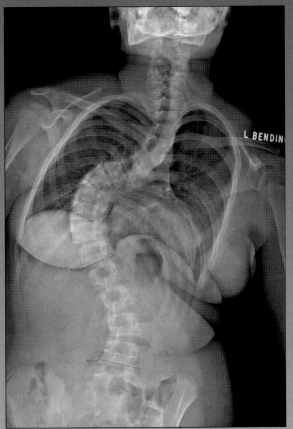

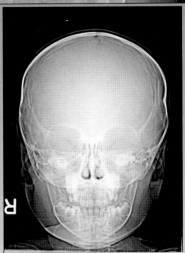

OUTLINE

Introduction to Pediatric
  Imaging, 100
Specific Pediatric
  Considerations, 101
Age-Based Development, 102
Patients with Special
  Needs, 105
Autism Spectrum Disorders, 105
Common Pediatric Positions and
  Projections, 112
Abdomen, Gastrointestinal, and
  Genitourinary Studies, 112
Chest, 118
Pelvis and Hips, 125
Limb Radiography, 127
Skull and Paranasal Sinuses, 132
Soft Tissue Neck, 137
Foreign Bodies, 139
Selected Pediatric Conditions and
  Syndromes, 141
Nonaccidental Trauma (Child
  Abuse), 143
Advances in Technology, 155

Introduction to Pediatric Imaging

Imaging children is one of the most fascinating and worthwhile specialties in radiography. To witness their cheerful resilience and the acceptance of immense challenges by the parents is a privilege. At the same time, pediatric imaging can be one of the most confounding experiences. Radiographers gain skills in multitasking such as quickly engaging and reassuring the child using an age-appropriate approach, then switching gears to gain the confidence of the parents, explaining and instructing them on immobilization techniques for the exam, all the while keeping in mind that other patients are waiting. It is important to be mindful of the various stressors parents may have endured before finding their way to the imaging room. In addition to the stress of a pending diagnosis, parents may have experienced an early and long commute, an unsettled child, a busy parking lot, and difficulty navigating their way through the institution. Do not personalize family moods. Your primary job is to actively listen, communicate, and understand the parents and their child. This is the primary path to achieving cooperation and quality diagnostic radiography. Children take their behavioral cues from facial expressions, intonations, and body postures; an ill-at-ease parent will convey that mood to the child, making the exam more difficult to perform. The sooner you can win the child's trust and turn his or her attention to the task at hand, the more successful the exam results will be and the family will leave praising your efforts. Part radiographer, psychologist, physicist, and caregiver, your job is always full of surprises and can be immensely satisfying. Whether you are an imaging professional looking for guidance on pediatric imaging or a student exploring career possibilities, this overview will give you a broad look at the specialty, details on how to conduct the most common pediatric exams including positioning and projections, and an understanding of the more prevalent pathologies and syndromes.

WAITING ROOM

Waiting and procedure rooms that are well equipped can reduce anxiety and act as a diversion for both the parents and children. Children are attracted to and amused by toys, thus leaving the parents free to check in, register, and ask pertinent questions. Gender-neutral toys or activities such as coloring with crayons located at a small age-appropriate table are most appropriate. (Children should be supervised to prevent them from putting the crayons in their mouths.) Books or magazines for older children are also good investments. The Child Life Department of the hospital can provide advice and make appropriate recommendations (Figs. 24-1 through 24-3).

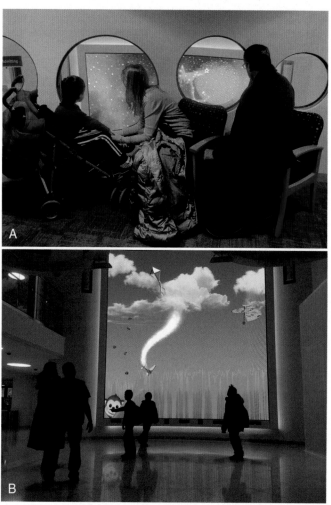

Fig. 24-1 A, Radiology outpatient and family viewing Interactive media wall. **B,** Interactive media wall from the first floor lobby.

Specific Pediatric Considerations

SAFETY

- Never leave your patient unattended.
- Keep items that could be swallowed out of reach.

COMMUNICATION

- Introduce yourself while making eye contact (if culturally appropriate) with patient and parents.
- Explain the radiography team role.
- Always speak to a child using language appropriate for the child's developmental level.
- Explain the exam.
- Take history (as required), and discuss pertinent medical information on a level the family can understand.
- Avoid medical jargon and unfamiliar terms. If a medical term cannot be avoided, explain in lay terms.

- Be mindful not to engage in conversations that are inappropriate in the presence of the patient.
- Before beginning the exam, ask if there are any questions or concerns.
- Use family teaching sheets when applicable. (These are web-based outlines of your hospital's procedures for the patient/family.)

RESPECT PATIENT/PARENT RIGHTS AND DIGNITY

- Listen to patient's/parent's questions and concerns.
- Some patients/parents speak English as a second language, which may impede their complete understanding of the exam and communication of exam results. To better serve the family and for medicolegal reasons, have an interpreter present.
- Be mindful of cultural preferences and taboos. Ask your interpreter, the family,

or seek out resources within your institution.
- Always knock before entering, and avoid entering an imaging room while an exam is in progress.

PROVIDE ADEQUATE CARE AND SERVICE TO THE PATIENT AND FAMILY

- Create a child-friendly environment.
- Use appropriately sized equipment.
- Remember, parents know their children best, so seek and make use of their advice.
- Utilize your child life specialist (CLS); they are invaluable for facilitating cooperation.
- If not contraindicated by the study, use a soft pad with a sheet on the exam table for patient comfort.
- Place the patient on the exam table when ready to proceed.

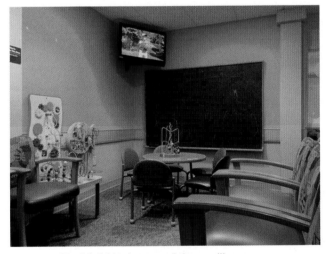

Fig. 24-2 Nuclear medicine waiting room.

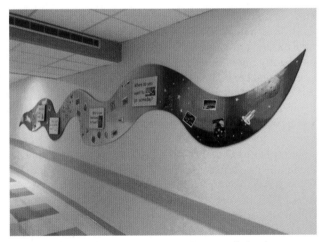

Fig. 24-3 Transition hallway from nuclear medicine to ultrasound.

Age-Based Development

The pediatric patient may not always fit neatly into the following developmental stages for a variety of reasons (e.g., pathology, developmental delays, parenting, chronic illness or prolonged hospital stay, or mood at the time of exam), but there are some universal approaches to interacting with children that will always apply (e.g., setting limits, making eye contact, and addressing their fears). Be observant, take your queues from the patient and family, and tailor your approach to them. Watch their eyes and body postures. Are the parents gripping things tightly? Do you need to set limits for their children? Is the child clinging to the parent's leg? Is the child tense? Listen to the child's choice of words.

With a team approach (gastrointestinal/genitourinary [GI/GU] exams, survey studies), pass on your experience in connecting with the family in a final strategy session before the team enters the exam room. Introductions should always be made in a slow and relaxed fashion so the family and patient understand them. Cultural norms are important, and although the family might make allowances for your ignorance, it is best to educate yourself on the norms and appropriate behavior in the family's country. Learn a few words or phrases in the languages most common to your patient's demographic. Cultural biases can also work in reverse; the family might make assumptions about you and how they treat you based on your sex or their socioeconomic status in their country of origin. Consulting your interpreter for advice is the first place to start.

PREMATURE INFANTS

Generally, bedside radiography and procedures in GI and GU using fluoroscopy encompass the majority of the contact radiographers will have with premature infants in the department. Elevate room temperature 10 to 15 minutes prior to the patient's arrival. When these babies are in radiology for a procedure, an intensive care unit (ICU) nursing team will accompany them. The nursing team will provide care for the patient, but you will need to explain the procedure and how the nursing team can help. Obtain the current status of the patient and any special requests from the nursing staff. As with any exam, suction and oxygen must always be available and the room well stocked. Leave the patient in the incubator/warmer until just before the procedure. Depending on the exam, you may be able to use a radiolucent cushion on the exam table for patient comfort. Discuss the patient immobilization plan (who will hold, how, what body part) with the nursing staff to ensure that you accommodate the patient's medical condition. Have warming lights available, wash hands, glove, and adhere to all isolation precautions.

NEONATE (0 TO 28 DAYS)

The neonatal period is a time of transition from the uterine environment to the outside world. During this first month the newborn is forming attachments with caregivers. They are sensitive to the way they are held, rocked, and positioned. They love to be swaddled, which gives them a sense of security and keeps them from being disturbed by their own startle reflex. Newborns startle easily when moved quickly or upon hearing a loud noise, and bright lights cause them to blink frequently or close their eyes. Understandably, the hospital environment creates particular stressors that can affect those at this very young age, which should be minimized whenever possible.

Because newborns are most secure and comfortable when swaddled, keep them in this position until just before you are ready for imaging. Decrease noise levels and bright lights whenever possible, maintain a warm room, and always use warming lights unless the nursing team directs otherwise. Speak soothingly and try to avoid sudden, quick movements. Let the caregivers know exactly what is expected during imaging and involve them in soothing and calming their infant. Pacifiers, oral sucrose (check with the nursing team), a personal blanket, and quiet singing can all help to sooth newborns, enabling them to feel safe and secure.

INFANT (28 DAYS TO 18 MONTHS)

During different periods of infancy, babies experience stranger and separation anxiety. When working with infants, involve the parents whenever possible; the comfort of seeing the parent's/caregiver's face, hearing that familiar voice, and feeling the caregiver's touch can be invaluable when calming the infant.

The radiographer and the CLS play important roles in establishing a relationship with the infant by talking and smiling; this will help put the parents at ease and demonstrate care and concern for their baby. The caregiver knows the infant best, so ask what soothes and comforts the baby when he or she is distressed. Personal objects such as a pacifier or a blanket can distract and soothe the infant during the exam. To ease the transition from the parent's arms to the exam table, it is advisable to decrease stimuli and eliminate loud noises. Keeping the baby swaddled or in their carrier until just prior to imaging minimizes transitions and reduces the baby's time on the exam table. The first rule of imaging infants is never leave the infant unattended; the radiographer or parent should always have a hand on the infant. The second rule is always cushion the exam table under the infant's skull. Be sure not to flex the head forward, which may cause respiratory difficulties.

TODDLER (18 MONTHS TO 3 YEARS)

Toddlers can be a challenge for both radiographers and staff. Toddlers are not abstract thinkers and are unable to understand the concept of "inside their body." They operate very much in the "here and now." They are seldom able to keep their bodies still, which can make imaging problematic, and they also have a short attention span and become overwhelmed quickly. Toddlers are fearful of medical experiences and often become unruly while they are being positioned for an exam. Unfamiliar exam positions and faces can escalate their movement.

In an effort to provide adequate care and minimize reactions, keep language brief and use concrete words. Because keeping their body still is most often an issue, efficiency is crucial. Be sure the room is organized before the patient and family enter. If the toddler has a toy or blanket, keep it within reach during the examination if possible. Distraction techniques can be extremely helpful in keeping the toddler calm. A screaming toddler can often be distracted and calmed by being allowed to blow bubbles or use a tablet computer with an age-appropriate application.

After the imaging has been completed, let children know they did a great job, that you are proud of them, and that they should be proud of themselves. Praise may be in the form of positive statements or a small reward like a sticker or balloon.

PRESCHOOLER (3 TO 5 YEARS)

New places, faces, and experiences can be overwhelming to preschoolers. Unfamiliar sights, sounds and faces can be quite intimidating and can leave the preschooler feeling frightened. In addition, preschoolers are establishing routines and greatly benefit from structure and knowing what to expect. For preschoolers, the medical environment is unpredictable, so often these patients need time to explore and familiarize themselves with the imaging room, even if it is brief. They also need to feel comfortable with the clinicians who will be working with them. Taking the time to establish rapport will be instrumental in making preschoolers feel comfortable, thus enhancing their coping ability (Fig. 24-4).

Additional steps include letting them know exactly what to expect and what you expect of them. For example, mention the loud sounds of the "camera," show the movement of the "camera," the coldness of a solution or cotton ball they may feel, and most important, assure them that you will let them know before you do anything. These simple courtesies facilitate trust and cooperation and help the child feel more comfortable. Some preschoolers may have difficulty understanding the exam through dialogue. Therefore, when speaking with them about imaging or "taking pictures," it may be helpful to model this process using a doll or stuffed animal.

Although preschoolers are developing independence and want to establish themselves as separate from their parents, they can become fearful if separated from them; utilizing parents can be instrumental to the success of the exam. If the parents are not able to remain with the child during imaging, be sure they can be first to pick up and comfort the child when the procedure is completed.

When working with patients of this age, use directive statements in an effort to facilitate cooperation; for example, "It's time to" or "You can help me by" are directive statements that will limit their response, leaving them more likely to comply. Open-ended questions that begin with "Do you want to (get on the table, get changed, etc.)" leave preschoolers feeling as if they have a choice when in reality getting on the table or having the exam is not a choice. Open-ended statements confuse preschoolers and can leave them feeling overwhelmed. Preschoolers are constantly seeking approval from others and respond well to positive affirmations. Praise and encouragement are beneficial for this age group, as they will create a positive experience and help to boost the preschooler's confidence for future medical appointments.

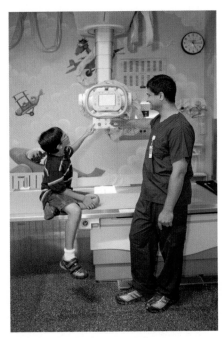

Fig. 24-4 The radiographer should make an introduction to the child and show the child how the collimator light is used.

SCHOOL AGE (6 TO 12 YEARS)

School-age children are becoming logical thinkers and have a fear of failure, so positive affirmations and reassurances are extremely beneficial. They are curious and full of questions; take the opportunity to connect using age-appropriate explanations. Break down the exam into steps, let them know exactly what to expect and what you expect of them, and, most important, let them know before you do anything. These simple courtesies will facilitate trust and cooperation and help the child feel more comfortable.

Avoid unfamiliar medical jargon, as this will only confuse school-age children and can decrease their ability to cope. School-agers are very literal, so it is crucial to avoid words that can be misconstrued like shoot, shot, or dye. School-age patients benefit from being given choices; this will give them a sense of control and entitlement, which inevitably enhances their coping abilities. However, be cautious to only give realistic choices; cajoling the child using open-ended questions could mislead the child.

It is important to make imperative or interrogative statements, such as "It's time to get changed; would you like the green gown or the blue one?" or "You need to get on the table; would you like me to help you or would you like your mom to help you?" These choices are direct and allow for a realistic choice. Coping and distraction techniques available to patients and staff like taking deep breaths, blowing bubbles, listening to music, watching a movie, or playing games with a tablet can be instrumental in helping children cope during exams.

ADOLESCENT (12 TO 18 YEARS)

When imaging adolescents, respect their need for privacy; a private area for changing, knocking before entering their exam room, and limiting the number of staff involved will help to alleviate stress. If you have clinicians (GI/GU, MR, CT) and radiographers of both sexes (and time permits), ask the patient if he or she would feel more comfortable with a male or female performing the exam. In many pediatric centers, girls who have reached the age of 10-12 years must be asked if there is any chance they might be pregnant. You may also ask if the girl has started menstruating. A truthful response is more probable if the parent is not present when these questions are asked. The patient's response will dictate whether further explanation is required. For example, you may need to add, "We ask these same questions of all girls because unborn babies are extremely sensitive to radiation exposure."

If it is necessary for adolescent patients to disclose their medical history, speak directly to them and their parents rather than just the parents. Radiographers have a tendency to ask the parents this information, and it is important to remember that adolescents most often know their body best. As adolescents, they don't always discuss things with their parents for reasons of embarrassment or shame. In addition, before beginning the exam, ask the adolescent patient if they would like to have a parent present during imaging. This gives adolescents a choice and also lets them know it is okay to ask parents to step out.

It is not uncommon for the adolescent patient to respond negatively to having an exam. In addition to being extremely modest, they see themselves as invincible and often do not believe that anything could possibly be wrong with them. Adolescents also fear "being different" and are afraid of something happening to their bodies that would alter their appearance or make them unlike their peers. Validating their feelings and letting them know you want to help will reassure them, such as by saying, "I understand the way you are feeling; lots of teenagers have this test done and they feel the same way" or "I am here to help you as best I can." Assisting adolescents with preparation, explaining the rationale for why the exam is taking place, and giving them tools for coping will facilitate cooperation and decrease fears. Deep breathing, listening to music, or having a conversation with a caregiver can help to put the patient at ease.

Patients with Special Needs

The radiographer should consider age and behavior when approaching children with physical and mental disabilities. School-age children with disabilities strive to achieve as much autonomy and independence as possible. They are sensitive to the fact that they are less independent than their peers. The radiographer should observe the following guidelines:

- Introduce yourself and identify the patients at their level (you may have to kneel down), then briefly explain the procedure to the child and parents. All children appreciate being given the opportunity to listen and respond. As with all patients, children want to be spoken to rather than talked about.
- If this approach proves ineffective, turn to the parents. Generally, the parents of these patients are present and can be very helpful. In strange environments, younger children may trust only one person—the parent. In that case, the medical team can gain cooperation from the child by communicating through the parent. Parents often know the best way to lift and transfer the child from the wheelchair or stretcher to the table. Children with physical disabilities often have a fear of falling and may want only a parent's assistance.
- Place the wheelchair or stretcher parallel to the imaging table, taking care to explain that you have locked the wheelchair or stretcher and will be getting help for the transfer. These children often know the way they should be lifted—*ask them*. They can tell you which areas to support and which actions they prefer to do themselves.

Finally, children with spastic contractions are often frustrated by their inability to control movements that are counterproductive to the exam. Gentle massage or a warm blanket should be used to help relax the muscles.

Communicating with a child who has a mental disability can be difficult, depending on the severity of the disability. Some patients react to verbal stimuli, whereas loud or abrupt noises may startle and agitate them. Ask the parent or caregiver if there is anything you should know about the child that would help achieve a quick and accurate exam. They will alert you to psychological, behavioral, or physical impairments that may not be obvious or referenced on the exam order.

AUTISM SPECTRUM DISORDERS*

Medical imaging of individuals with autism spectrum disorders can be difficult. In addition to difficulties with communication, there are also behavioral issues, medical issues, and environmental concerns that need to be considered. There are important steps that should be taken before the patient is brought into the examination room and, in some cases, before they come to the imaging facility.

According to the Centers for Disease Control and Prevention (CDC), autism spectrum disorders (ASDs) are a group of developmental disabilities that can cause significant social, communication, and behavioral challenges. People with ASDs handle information in their brain differently than other people. A spectrum means that autism can range from very mild to severe. There are some similar symptoms, such as problems with social interaction; however, there are differences in time of onset, severity, and the nature of the symptoms. One popular saying within the autism community is "If you know one person with autism, then, you know one person with autism." This makes creating treatment plans difficult for parents, caregivers, and physicians. What works well for one individual may not be effective for another. This also makes imaging individuals with ASDs challenging.

The prevalence of autism is on the rise; in 1998 the rate of Autism was 1 in 110, and by 2000 it had risen to 1 in 88. More recent studies have indicated that it may be as high as 1 in 35 for males and 1 in 50 for all children. It is five times more

---

*Written by Jerry Tyree.

common in males than females, and on average the diagnosis is earlier for those with more severe symptoms. Parents may notice the difference as early as 6 months, whereas high-functioning individuals, such as those with Asperger syndrome, are diagnosed at around 6 years of age.

Most patients with ASDs will be identified before scheduling imaging procedures. The CDC has several publications on the diagnosis for ASD; however, for facilitating imaging the following are commonly recognized signs of autism:

1. Difficulty with social interaction
2. Problems with verbal and nonverbal communication
3. Repetitive behaviors or narrow, obsessive interests

Special considerations for imaging

Once an ASD patient is identified, there are many things we can do to provide for a successful imaging experience for both radiographer and patient. Whether or not the patient is in the department, we should begin by asking more questions. Table 24-1 is an example of a patient questionnaire. It might be beneficial to schedule the exam at a time when the department is not busy. Loud noises or visual overstimulation can be distracting and in some cases can cause severe behaviors. This can be especially true during the adolescent years. Because these children are larger, aggressive or violent behavior can be dangerous for the patient or staff. It is wise to prepare for all possibilities. A good patient questionnaire can help gather resources and prepare the environment. You can use the questionnaire to eliminate noises when needed and adjust lighting.

TABLE 24-1

Autism patient questionnaire

Is your child sensitive to fluorescent lighting?
Is your child comfortable in a dimly lit room?
Is your child tactile defensive, or sensitive to touch?
    If yes, explain.
Is your child sensitive to loud noises?
    High frequencies?
    Low frequencies?
Is your child uncomfortable in cool or cold situations?
Is your child uncomfortable in warm or hot situations?
Do you have any calming objects you would like the child to have in the imaging suite?
Will your child find a video played during the procedure calming?

Try to give the patient with an ASD the first or last appointment of the day. People with an ASD find waiting around for an appointment extremely stressful. Waiting in busy hospital corridors will increase the stress levels of an already anxious child or adult. If possible, find a small side room the family can wait in. Alternatively, they may prefer to wait outside or in the car and a member of staff should be identified to collect them or call their cell phone when the radiographer is ready. If the appointment is likely to be delayed, the family may wish to leave the building completely and return at a later agreed time.

Temperature is often difficult to adjust, but patient dress can be modified if it is an issue. Many individuals with autism are sensitive to touch. They have difficulty habituating stimuli of any type. Some may wear socks inside out so they can't feel the seam on their toes. These are serious issues for individuals on the spectrum.

Sometimes we need to modify our positioning techniques for individuals who are tactile defensive, or sensitive to touch. A sensitivity to the "poking" often used to find anatomic landmarks can also be problematic. Some barbers have found that once you touch, you maintain the touch until you are finished with the haircut. One hand must remain on the head until the haircut is complete. We can use this same concept with imaging; once you begin to touch, don't remove your hand until you have all the information you need.

Videos can be a double-edged sword. Although a familiar video can be calming, if it varies in any small way from the one the child is used to, it can actually cause a severe reaction. This often happens with videos that are different depending on whether it is a VHS or a DVD version. It might be best if patients bring in videos of their own, especially if the procedure is expected to be long.

Personal space and body awareness

A crowded waiting room may be distressing for people with an ASD who may need their personal space. Similarly, close proximity to the radiographer could be uncomfortable for the patient.

Problems can also occur when trying to explain where pain is experienced. Those who have difficulty with body awareness may not be able to experience where different body parts are.

Touch

Individuals with ASDs may be hyposensitive to touch, or tactile defensive. They may find a light touch very painful. Some of these patients may prefer more deep pressure in touching, or you may not be able to touch them at all.

Patient responses

Do not be surprised if the patient does not make eye contact, especially if he or she is distressed. Lack of eye contact does not necessarily mean the patient is not listening to what you are saying. Allow the patient extra time to process what you have said. Do not assume that a nonverbal patient cannot understand what you are saying.

People with an ASD can have a high pain threshold. Even if the child does not appear to be in pain, he or she may, for example, have broken a bone. ASD patients may show an unusual response to pain that could include laughter, humming, singing, and removal of clothing. Agitation and behavior may be the only clues that the child or adult is in pain.

Communication

Use clear simple language with short sentences. People with an ASD tend to take everything literally. Thus, if you say, "It will only hurt for a minute," they will expect the pain to have gone within a minute.

Make your language concrete and avoid using idioms, irony, metaphors, and words with double meanings (e.g., "It's raining cats and dogs out there"). This could cause the patient to look outside for cats and dogs. Avoid using body language, gestures, or facial expressions without verbal instructions, as the patient may not understand these nonverbal messages.

Consider involving a caregiver to facilitate communication. Many individuals respond slowly, and patience is required.

Noise

Some departments use buzzers to indicate when it is a patient's turn to have an exam. They may also have music playing in a waiting room. Crying babies or children in the waiting room may also be quite noisy. For those with hypersensitive hearing, these types of noises can be magnified and become disturbing or even painful. Also with this heightened volume, surrounding sounds could become distorted. This could make it difficult for the person with an ASD to recognize sounds, such as a name being called. Individuals may respond by putting their fingers in their ears like the child at a racetrack, whereas others may "stim" (flap hands, flick fingers, rock, etc.). This kind of behavior is calming to the individual, so do not try and stop it unless absolutely essential. Individuals with ASDs often retreat when overstimulated.

Injections/needle sticks

If the patient needs an injection or blood test, divert their attention elsewhere. The use of pictures or a doll is a good idea to demonstrate what is going to happen. People with an ASD can be either under- or oversensitive to pain, so that some may feel the pain acutely and be very distressed whereas others may not appear to react at all.

It is advisable to assume that the patient will feel pain. Use a local anesthetic cream such as an eutectic mixture of local anesthetics (EMLA) to numb the site of injection. Sand timers and clocks can be used as distracters during procedures such as injections so that the person with autism can see a definite end.

Tips for radiographers

Relaxation techniques such as deep breathing, counting, singing favorite songs, talking about a favorite interest, or looking at favorite books/toys could also help during physical examination or treatments. Parents may be instructed to bring a favorite toy or video if a player is available in the procedure room.

Make sure directions are given step by step, verbally, visually, and by providing physical supports or prompts, as needed by the patient. Patients with autism spectrum disorders often have trouble interpreting facial expressions, body language, and tone of voice. Be as concrete and explicit as possible in your instructions and feedback to the patient. Demonstrating on others or toys to show what will happen during a physical examination can reassure an individual with an ASD.

Many children with autism fixate on routines. Most medical imaging will fall outside of their routines. Social stories can be used to make something unfamiliar seem more routine. A social story can be a written or visual guide describing various social interactions or situations. These stories can be a book, on flashcards, or the department can have them online so the family can share with the patient what it is like to go to the x-ray department. The caregiver can revisit or practice these social stories prior to the exam. Pictures of the parking garage, waiting room, imaging room, even the individual radiographer can be added. The more accurate these pictures are, the better they will work. It might even be helpful to take pictures from the perspective of the individual with the ASD. If the patient will be lying on an x-ray table, a picture taken up toward the tube or scanner might be appropriate. In this way, a social story can be used to make something the individual has never done before seem routine.

Parents of many children with ASDs create social stories for vacations, plane rides, trips to the amusement park, and so on. Parents and caregivers who use these social stories will vouch for their effectiveness. In addition to social stories, it may be helpful if you can allow the patient with autism and caregiver access to the facility before the exam. This allows a "dry run" of the procedure, which may reduce anxiety during the actual exam.

In summation, a combination of questionnaire, social stories, and the patient application of the aforementioned principles should greatly help when imaging individuals with ASDs. Preparation is key, but it need not be prohibitively time consuming. Creating a social story for every exam an imaging department does is ideal, but simplification is possible. Making social stories accessible online is desirable. Adding pictures and images, especially accurate ones of specific facilities, increases the comfort level of patients. These practices are also good for all patients, not just those with ASDs. Many advocates would say that better serving individuals with ASDs (or others with "different" abilities) has improved schools, social services, and the lives of all they touch. The same could be said of our imaging departments.

Radiation Protection

DOSE AND DIAGNOSTIC INFORMATION

The goal in administering radiation for a specific clinical indication is to ensure that the *diagnostic* information obtained will be of greater value than the potential risks associated with the radiation. To protect our patients, we should identify through scientific testing an acceptable level of quantum mottle for each exam, which will not compromise the diagnostic goal of the image. What we, as medical practitioners, are attempting to do is use the minimum radiation dose required to produce a *clinically diagnostic* image for a specific clinical indication; this is our primary goal as radiographers and radiologists. Radiographers should observe the following steps:

- Direct efforts toward proper centering and selection of exposure factors, and precise collimation, which all contribute to safe practice.
- Use strategic placement of gonadal and breast shielding, and employ effective immobilization techniques to reduce the need for repeat examinations.
- Instead of the anteroposterior (AP) projection, use the posteroanterior (PA) projection of the thorax and skull to reduce the amount of radiation reaching the breast tissue and lens of the eye, respectively.
- During radiography of the upper limbs, protect the upper torsos of all children.
- Pulsed fluoroscopy with "last image hold" also reduces patient dose and length of examination.

A cautionary note: The fact that digitally acquired images can be "postprocessed," thereby correcting some exposure errors, does not negate an important truth—images of proper density are achieved by proper positioning. The anatomy to be demonstrated must be in proper alignment with the photocell or ionization chamber.

Child versus adult

The possible long-term stochastic effects of a low linear energy transfer (LET) radiation dose on pediatric patients, if they exist, are much greater than the same dose to an adult because the child has a longer lifetime over which to express any long-term effects, and due to the child's smaller body volume, the potential exists to expose multiple organ systems to radiation for any given exam.

Shielding and dose reduction

A primary radiation shield should always be employed to protect gonadal, breast, and thyroid tissues when the exam protocol allows. Patients should always be shielded, including male breast tissue, unless the shielding will compromise the diagnostic area of interest for the exam (e.g., male or female lateral proximal femurs, female abdominal images, and male or female false profile lateral hips). Initial images for PA scoliosis and female pelvic exams should not be shielded (your clinical setting will have specific guidelines for shielding) (Fig. 24-5). Males can be shielded on the initial AP pelvic image provided the shield is positioned below the pubic symphysis (Fig. 24-6).

Discussing radiation risks and benefits with parents

Just as you have developed exam-based routines, you should have an example-based "script" for discussing the risk/benefit equation of radiation exposure. When parents have questions, listen carefully and hear their questions, fears (which may only be implied), point of reference for understanding radiation dose (usually CT), and educational level. Be aware that people in medical settings, especially when under stress, often hear only 50% of what is being said; additionally, they often give greater weight to negative information. Be knowledgeable and confident with your answers (body language, tone, interest, and clarity of presentation without technical jargon); a rambling or confusing presentation will do more harm than good. "In risk perception theory, perception equals reality. This means there may be no correlation between public perceptions of risk and scientific or technical information. Therefore, you must discuss the risk based on the perception."[1]

---

[1]Available at: www.imagewisely.org/Imaging-Professionals/Medical-Physicists/Articles/How-to-Understand-and-Communicate-Radiation-Risk. Accessed July 2013.

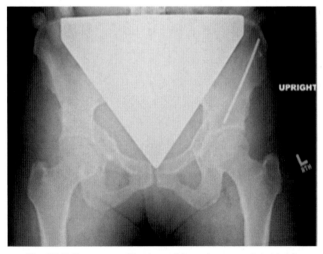

Fig. 24-5 Proper positioning of female gonadal shield.

Reframing the way parents and patients understand radiation risks (if they exist) and benefits should be your first goal. Human exposure to x-radiation is usually "understood" through the subjectivity of the lay press, the sensationalism of TV shows, and the half-truths of word of mouth. A wonderfully clear and effective, but often overlooked, approach to help place radiation exposure in perspective is to reference the dose the child will receive for any given exam to the background radiation we all receive daily. Background equivalent radiation time (BERT) equates a particular exam-based radiation dose to the equivalent amount of radiation dose received daily from our natural background (Table 24-2). The BERT method has several advantages: (1) the patient readily understands it; (2) it does not mention radiation risk, which is unknown; and (3) it educates the patient that he or she lives in a sea of natural background radiation.

The lay public's preoccupation with the perceived risks of x-radiation often overshadows the benefits of the diagnostic imaging exam. When a physician orders a radiation-based exam, it is with the confidence that the diagnostic information obtained will outweigh any potential risks (if there are any) of an image. Declining an exam based on perceived risks creates the real risk of a missed diagnosis.

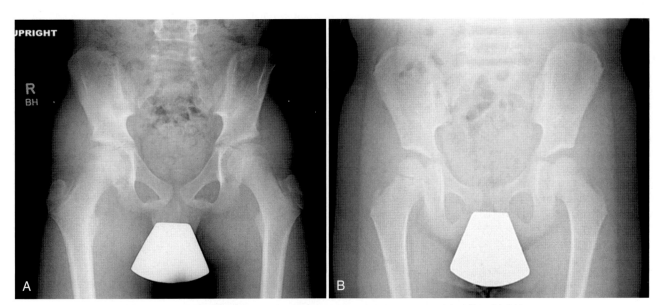

Fig. 24-6 Males can be shielded on the initial AP pelvic image provided the shield is positioned below the pubic symphysis. **A,** Shows correct shielding and positioning (femoral heads are centered), but collimation should be tighter and the patient should have been changed prior to imaging **B,** Incorrect shielding; shield covering part of symphysis and inferior rami.

TABLE 24-2

Comparison of pediatric exam dose to background radiation level

Exam	Natural background radiation equivalent* (time to receive equivalent background radiation)
Chest CT, high resolution (pulmonary embolism, angiogram)	730 days (6 mSv)
Abdominal CT	365 days (3 mSv)
Abdomen/pelvic radiograph	90 days (0.75 mSv)
Chest radiograph, two view	2.5 days (0.02 mSv)
Natural background radiation	1 day (0.008 mSv)

*Using an average background radiation level of 3 mSv/yr.
Data from http://www.imagewisely.org/Imaging-Professionals/Medical-Physicists/Articles/How-to-Understand-and Communicate-Radiation-Risk. Accessed July 2013.
Colang JE et al: Patient dose from CT: a literature review, *Radiol Technol* 79:17 2007.

Radiographers holding for exams

Effective use of immobilization techniques must always be attempted. Imaging pediatric patients may require the radiographer to hold the patient. Radiographers are encouraged to hold only as a last resort, but there are many challenging exams that would, even with the best of instruction, have a low chance of success using only parents to hold the patient. In deciding whether to hold for an exam, radiographers seek to balance the potential stochastic risks of radiation exposure to themselves (scatter) against the possibility of having to repeat a child's x-ray (primary beam) because of a parent's unsuccessful attempt at immobilization. If our ultimate goal is to reduce the dose to the patient and ourselves, where is the balance?

Evaluating the parents' ability to hold their child firmly enough to prevent movement and achieve correct positioning should begin when you introduce yourself. Is the parent/guardian attentive to what you say? Are they tentative first-time parents? Are they overindulgent and unable to set limits? Are they so concerned with radiation exposure that they have difficulty listening to instructions? Are they overwhelmed with parenting? Do they come with an attitude that will prevent them from listening? Does the patient's physical condition him or her a challenge to hold? An affirmative answer to any of these questions may suggest that a radiographer does the holding. Allowing a parent who is probably not capable to hold the patient in order to prevent a small, low linear energy transfer (LET), occupational dose (scatter) to the radiographer is not in the patient's best interest; the patient, now facing a repeat, receives twice the primary beam radiation dose and the radiographer will still end up having to hold. Before making the decision to hold, the radiographer should make every attempt at immobilization or to instruct the parent/caregiver clearly and slowly, using lay terms, while demonstrating the technique. After the parent has attempted to hold the child, the radiographer must decide whether to continue allowing the parent to hold the child or to step in himself or herself, thereby assuring that a diagnostic exam is achieved on the first try. The goal of any radiographic exam is to produce an image with a radiation dose as low as diagnostically achievable while providing good patient and family care. This is a lot to juggle even for the seasoned pediatric radiographer, and it takes a lot of experience to do it well.

Artifacts

The dynamic range of digital radiography has increased the universe (number and type) of artifacts visible on images. With film screen and digital images, the usual suspects are dirt, scratches, the presence of unwanted metallic or radiopaque objects on the patient, processing errors, and motion. The following is a partial list of artifacts unique to digital radiography:

- Soap or starches in patient gowns that appear as long slender irregular densities (Fig. 24-7).
- Silk-screening on t-shirts, and dirt on imaging plates.
- Textured or thick hair, cornrows, dreadlocks, ponytails, bobby pins, hair clips, or any object woven into the hair.
- Clothing seams, sweat pants eyelets, silkscreen designs, appliqué or embroidery, textured t-shirts, onesies, dry or wet diapers, and sanitary pads.
- Glitter, rhinestones, pearls, belly-button rings, or other piercings. You may encounter some resistance from parents concerning the removal of an infant's new ear piercing studs; assure the parent that the holes will not close during the time it takes to generate the exam images.

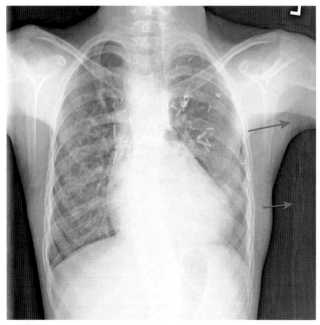

Fig. 24-7 Soap or starches in patient gowns appear as long slender irregular densities *(red arrows)*.

The ratio of artifact size and body volume is greater in pediatric patients than adults. In other words, given two images, one of an adult and one of an infant and both of the same anatomic area, and given two artifacts of the same size, shape, and density located in the same spot within those same anatomic areas, the likelihood of detecting the artifact in the infant's image would be greater due to the artifact's size relative to the anatomy. To reduce clothing artifacts, remove any piece of clothing covering the anatomy of interest. Paper shorts are radiolucent and can be used for pelvic and abdominal imaging. Years of experience support this approach; failure to remove clothing will result in repeat images. When there is a need to observe breathing patterns (chests), particularly on children who cannot hold their breath (those younger than 6 or 7 years old), clothes should be removed from the waist up so the radiographer can observe breathing. As noted earlier, it is well documented that patients in a hospital setting hear about 50% of what is said to them, so when the patients/parents enter the exam room after changing, ask them again if they have removed the requested pieces of clothing. Clear communication is paramount, followed closely by checking for compliance. Trust, but verify. Don't assume (Fig. 24-8).

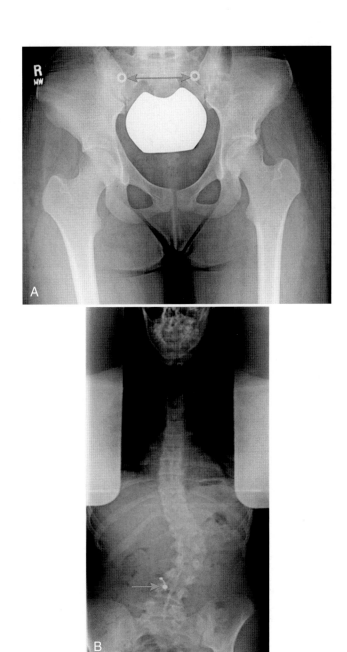

Fig. 24-8 A, Eyelets on sweatpants *(orange arrow).* **B,** Belly-button ring *(orange arrow).*

Common Pediatric Positions and Projections
ABDOMEN, GASTROINTESTINAL, AND GENITOURINARY STUDIES
Abdomen

Abdominal radiography in children is requested for different reasons than it is for adults. Consequently, the initial procedure or protocol differs significantly. In addition to supine and upright images, the assessment for acute abdomen conditions or the abdominal series in adult radiography usually includes images obtained in the left lateral decubitus position. Often the series is not considered complete without a PA projection of the chest. To keep radiation exposure to a minimum, the pediatric abdominal series need only include two images: the supine abdomen and an image to show air-fluid levels. The upright image is preferred over the lateral decubitus in patients younger than 2 or 3 years old because, from an immobilization and patient-comfort perspective, it is much easier to perform. The upright image can be obtained with a slight modification of the Pigg-O-Stat (Modern Way Immobilizers, Gainesboro, TN) (Fig. 24-9), whereas the lateral decubitus position requires significant modification of the Pigg-O-Stat. As mentioned for hip radiography, the diaper should be completely removed for all abdominal and pelvic imaging to avoid artifacts.

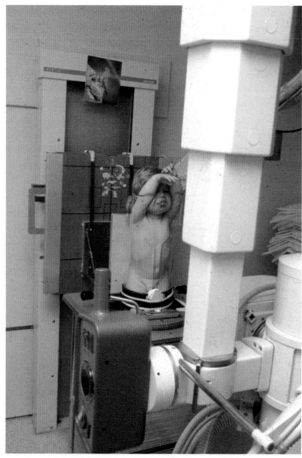

Fig. 24-9 The Pigg-O-Stat, modified with the seat raised to suit upright abdominal radiography. The sleeves and seat are cleaned, and the seat is covered with a cloth diaper or thick tissue before the patient is positioned. (Note the gonad shield placed anterior.)

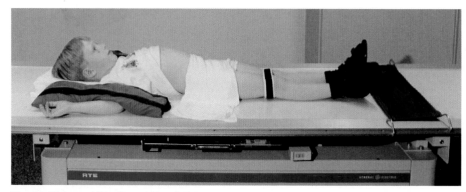

Fig. 24-10 Immobilization of the active child: sandbags over the arms, Velcro strips around the knees, and a Velcro band beside the patient's feet to be secured over the legs.

Positioning and immobilization

Young children can be immobilized for supine abdominal imaging with the same methods as those used for radiography of the hips and pelvis (Fig. 24-10), which provide basic immobilization of a patient for supine table radiography. All boys should be shielded using methods described for radiography of the hips and pelvis. The central ray should be located midway at the level of L2. The radiographer should observe the following guidelines for upright abdominal imaging:

- Effectively immobilize newborns and children up to 3 years old for the upright image using the Pigg-O-Stat.
- Raise the seat of the Pigg-O-Stat to avoid projecting artifacts from the bases of the sleeves over the lower abdomen (see Fig. 24-9).
- For the best results in an older child, have the child sit on a large box, trolley, or stool and spread the legs apart to prevent superimposition of the upper femora over the pelvis.

Lateral images of the abdomen are occasionally required in children, generally to localize something in the AP plane. Immobilization for lateral images is challenging; this difficulty, along with the fact that patient immobilization is the same as for lateral spine images, makes it worthy of mention here. Properly instructed, the parent can be helpful with obtaining this image. The radiographer should observe the following steps:

- Remember that the parent can do only one job.
- Ask the parent to stand on the opposite side of the table and hold the child's head and arms.
- Immobilize the rest of the child's body using available immobilization tools. These tools include large 45-degree sponges, sandbags (large and small), a "bookend," and a Velcro band.

- Accomplish immobilization by rolling the child on the side and placing a small sponge or sandbag between the knees.
- Snugly wrap the Velcro band over the hips; to prevent backward arching, place the "bookend" against the child's back with the 45-degree sponge and sandbag positioned anteriorly (Fig. 24-11).

Note that it is common for pediatric clinicians to request two projections of the abdomen. This should be supported by the clinical indications. A neonatal patient with necrotizing enterocolitis requires supine and left *lateral decubitus* images to rule out air-fluid levels indicative of bowel obstruction. However, the patient with an umbilical catheter needs supine and *lateral* images to verify the location and position of the catheter. *When in doubt, consult the radiologist.*

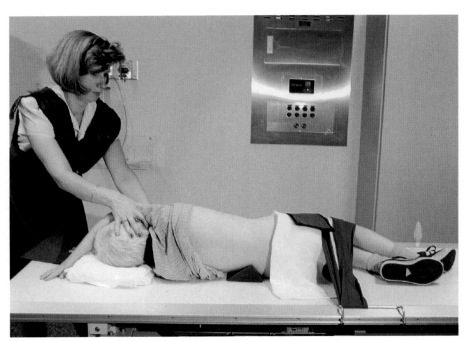

Fig. 24-11 The immobilization used for lateral abdominal imaging is also effective for lateral thoracic and lumbosacral spine images. A 45-degree sponge and sandbag are used anteriorly.

Pathology

Intussusception. Intussusception is the invagination or telescoping of the bowel into itself; the majority of cases (90%) are ileocolic (Fig. 24-12). Idiopathic intussusception is most common and is the most common cause of small intestinal obstruction in the infant-toddler age group, reaching a peak incidence between 2 months and 3 years of age. The majority of cases (60%) occur in males. Intussusception can present with an abrupt onset of abdominal pain that becomes more frequent. There can be bouts of diarrhea, vomiting, and lethargy. Blood and blood clots in stool with the consistency and color of currant jelly are highly suggestive of intussusception. No matter how high the clinical index of suspicion is for intussusception, an abdominal image is always indicated; in some patients this supine image may be negative. Bowel perforation and degree of obstruction are ruled out with a horizontal-beam image, whereas a prone or left-side-down decubitus is more likely to demonstrate a soft tissue mass than the supine position. The combination of diminished colonic stool and bowel gas, especially when accompanied by a visible soft tissue mass, indicates a high likelihood of intussusception. An abdominal physical exam by an experienced surgeon is a useful precaution before proceeding to reduction.

Although there are significant procedural variations among radiologists for the reduction of intussusceptions, many pediatric radiology departments use the pneumatic enema under fluoroscopic guidance as the treatment of choice because of its ease of use, a reduced risk for peritonitis in the event of a perforation (as compared with hydrostatic), reduced time of procedure, and reduced radiation dose. The pneumatic filling of a large portion of the small bowel is usually necessary to confirm reduction. Contraindications to radiologic reduction are intestinal perforation, frank peritonitis, and hypervolemic shock.

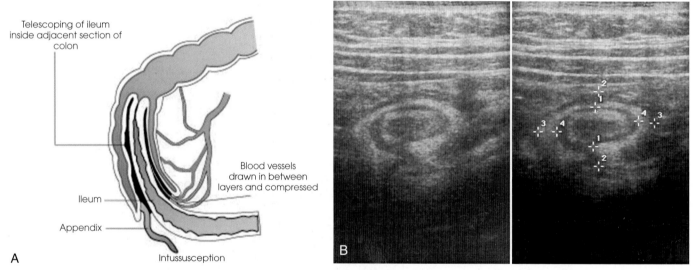

Fig. 24-12 A, Intussusception. **B,** Ultrasound image illustrates doughnut-shaped lesion marked for measurement.

(**A** from Van Meter K: Gould's pathophysiology for the health professions, ed 5, St. Louis, 2014, Elsevier. **B** from Eisenberg RL, Johnson NM: Comprehensive radiographic pathology, ed 5, St. Louis, 2010, Mosby/Elsevier.)

Telescoping of ileum inside adjacent section of colon

Blood vessels drawn in between layers and compressed

Ileum

Appendix

Intussusception

Pneumoperitoneum Intraperitoneal air/gas is most commonly the result of perforation of hollow viscera (stomach or intestines) or can be caused by surgical complications, such as abdominal drainage tubes, percutaneous gastronomy tubes, or insufflation of CO_2 or air during liver and renal biopsies or during laparoscopy (Fig. 24-13, *A*). These causes may have the same radiologic appearances but different clinical significance. Patients normally have pneumoperitoneum following abdominal surgery, which clears more rapidly in children than in adults. Studies have demonstrated clearing of free air in most postoperative children within 24 hours.

Diagnosis of pneumoperitoneum is most easily made with a cross-table horizontal beam projection, which is also indicated to rule out free air or intestinal obstruction, or when small amounts of free air are suspected, the decubitus position is recommended (Fig. 24-13, *B*). A properly positioned abdominal image, upright, cross-table, or decubitus will include both pubic symphysis and the bases of both diaphragms. In the upright image, free air is easily demonstrated under the diaphragms, displacing the liver on the right, and stomach, liver, and spleen on the left. A child who is younger than 1 year or unable to stand can be examined in the left decubitus position, which allows the liver to fall away from the wall of the peritoneal cavity revealing lucency between the abdominal wall and liver.

The gridded, tabletop, decubitus view is most successfully achieved when the patient's back is parallel and in contact with the imaging IR. Arms are on either side of the head and above the shoulders with elbows bent one on either side of the head. The patient's pelvis is perpendicular to the table with knees bent and legs stacked one atop the other. The person holding will immobilize the patient's arms and head as one unit (left hand) and hold the lower torso just below the buttocks (right hand). A gonadal shield should be used on males, but make sure to keep it below the pubic symphysis.

The horizontal beam image may be useful in distinguishing a pneumoperitoneum caused by bowel perforation (air fluid levels present) and a dissecting pneumomediastinum presenting with air in the peritoneal space and no fluid levels (this difference is not always present). Pneumomediastinum is usually suspected when there is a history of assisted ventilation or chest trauma and is best visualized in PA and lateral views of the chest.

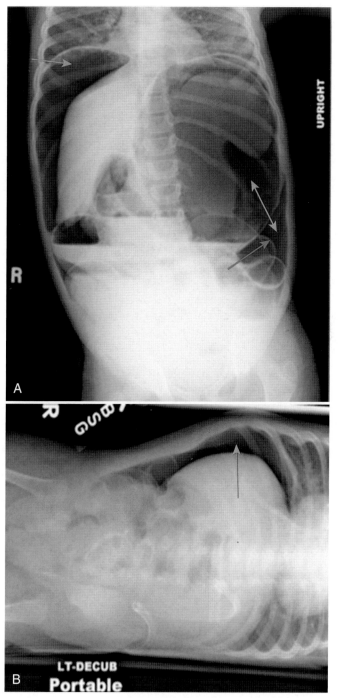

Fig. 24-13 A, Pneumoperitoneum resulting from a fundoplication procedure *(orange arrows)*. Rigler's sign (air on both sides of bowel wall) is present at *blue arrow*. **B,** Pneumoperitoneum seen *(orange arrow)* as a complication from percutaneous gastronomy tube procedure.

Gastrointestinal and genitourinary studies

As with any radiology procedure-based modality, a team approach to the care of the patient and family is essential. There are many procedures unique to pediatrics that fall under the headings gastrointestinal and genitourinary (GI/GU). Although it is beyond the scope of this chapter to delve into the specifics of each of these exams, many of which are complex, we will briefly discuss some of the most common procedures and indications. Common to each of these procedures is the use of a contrast medium, which enhances the visualization of soft tissue. These media can be either water-soluble iodine based or non-water-soluble barium sulfate based. The water-soluble contrast media are used for intravenous (IV) injection and non-IV excretory urography studies, for post-surgical assessments where leakage might occur, and for suspected perforations. They are characterized as being either nonionic (fewer side effects) with low osmolality (low-osmolality contrast agents [LOCAs]) or ionic (increased side effects) with high osmolality (high-osmolality contrast agents [HOCAs]). The choice of which LOCA to use is based on the concentration of iodine desired within the blood plasma and urine, the cost, and safety. Dosage is based on patient weight for IV injections; after injection of a bolus at a moderate rate, contrast excretion begins almost immediately and peaks at 10 to 20 minutes. Studies have shown that the adoption of a LOCA offers a definite improvement in patient experience and safety as compared to that of a HOCA. The American College of Radiology (ACR) has specific criteria for the use of LOCAs that include questions about previous history of contrast reactions, asthma, allergies (especially to shellfish), and cardiac issues. Adverse reactions can be life threatening. When administering a contrast agent, the trained radiographer should have a nurse present and doctor available.

Barium sulfate-based contrast agents are not water soluble and are for oral or rectal administration to rule out malrotation, investigation of esophageal problems, swallow studies, or to rule out Hirschsprung disease. The patient should be advised to drink plenty of liquids after the study, as the body does not break down barium. Barium is contraindicated for suspected perforations, instances of lower bowel obstructions, or attempted reduction of meconium ileus or meconium plug.

Radiation protection

When performing exams using conventional fluoroscopic units, it is good practice to cover most of the tabletop with large mats of lead rubber (the equivalent of 0.5 mm of lead is recommended) (Figs. 24-14 and 24-15). Operators and patients can be effectively protected by positioning the mats so that only the areas being examined are exposed.

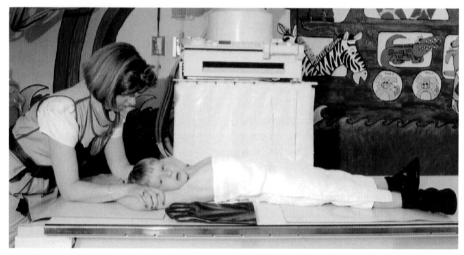

Fig. 24-14 Another modification of the "bunny" technique. The arms are left free and are raised above the head to prevent superimposition over the esophagus. In this example, tape is used to secure the blanket; however, Velcro strips are easier to use if a parent is not available to assist. (Note lead under patient when tube is under the table.)

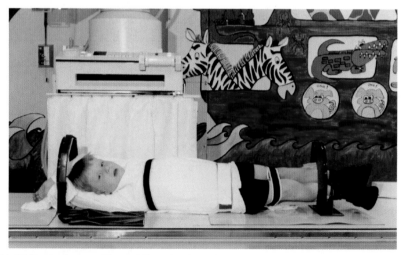

Fig. 24-15 The octagonal immobilizer (or, for this child, a "rocket ship") permits the child to be immobilized in a variety of positions. (Note lead under patient when tube is under the table.)

Vesicoureteral reflux

For infants and small children experiencing first-time febrile urinary tract infections, the goal after antibiotic treatment is to rule out the possibility of reflux, existing renal scarring, and structural or functional abnormalities of the urinary tract that may predispose the patient to reflux and infection, particularly to anomalies that may require prompt surgical treatment. This is accomplished with an ultrasound (US) and, if indicated, a voiding cystourethrogram (VCUG). Patient assessment may begin with a noninvasive US to assess the upper urinary tracts and kidneys. If the US is negative, the decision to proceed with the VCUG is made after a thorough discussion between the parents, attending urologist, and pediatrician. Some radiologists feel that a VCUG for a first-time nonfebrile urinary tract infection (UTI) with a negative ultrasound is not indicated. The VCUG is an invasive procedure in which a Foley catheter (5-8 French) is inserted into the urethra, advanced into the bladder, and then taped to the inside of the leg in a female or to the shaft of the penis in a male. An iodinated contrast agent designed for the lower urinary tract is instilled into the bladder by gravity. The volume used is based on the patient's age. Bilateral, oblique, pulsed fluoroscopy captures are made to check for reflux (Fig. 24-16, *A*) and assess urinary anatomy. Fluoroscopy captures are made of voiding as the Foley is removed (Fig. 24-16, *B*). VCUG teams often include an attending fellow or resident, a radiographer, and a child life specialist with access to a registered radiologist assistant (RRA) as required. The parents are encouraged to participate, as this can help soothe and calm the infant or child. Age-appropriate distraction devices are employed as required.

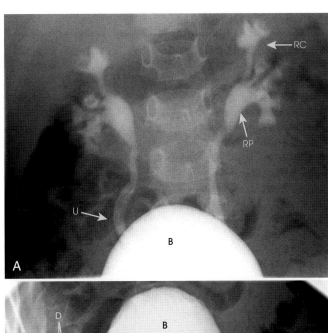

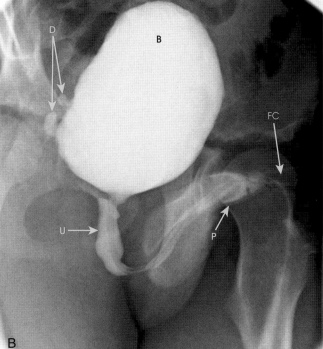

Fig. 24-16 A, VCUG, 33-month-old female with bilateral grade 3 reflux as seen in the AP projection under fluoroscopy. Bladder (B), ureter (U), renal pelvis (RP), and renal calyce (RC). **B,** VCUG, 8-year old male with bladder diverticula (D) as seen in the LPO projection. Voiding shows moderate dilatation of the posterior urethra (U). Foley catheter (FC), bladder (B), and uncircumcised penis (P).

Barium sulfate–based contrast agents are not water soluble and are for oral or rectal administration to rule out malrotation, investigate esophageal problems, perform swallow studies, or rule out Hirschsprung disease. The patient should be advised to drink plenty of liquids after the study, as the body does not break down barium. Barium is contraindicated for suspected perforations, instances of lower bowel obstructions, or attempted reduction of meconium ileus or meconium plug (Table 24-3).

CHEST

The most frequently ordered and one of the most challenging imaging exams in pediatric imaging is the chest x-ray. Patients between 1 and 4 years can be difficult to immobilize and position because they are strong and in an unfamiliar setting they are scared. The anxiety level created in this situation can be high for parents, students, and the experienced radiographer. Take the time to adequately explain to the parents the goals of the exam and how to correctly hold the child for the exam. Even though you are assured the parent can hold properly, it is essential that you remain vigilant in your transition from the patient to the exposure control station, ensuring that the parents continue to immobilize correctly and effectively. If the parent is struggling and frustrated, consider using the Pigg-O-Stat (Fig. 24-17) or, as a last resort, a radiographer may have to hold the child. Radiation delivered to the patient must always be as low as diagnostically achievable, and every attempt must be made to acquire the image on the first attempt. Quite simply, if you think the positioning is compromised or the immobilization ineffective, do not make the exposure.

TABLE 24-3

Gastrointestinal/Genitourinary Studies

Indications	Procedure	Contrast agent
Gastrointestinal studies		
R/O esophageal atresia	Swallow	LOMC
Dysphasia	Swallow	Barium
Stridor, R/O retropharyngeal abscess	Airway fluoroscopy	Air
R/O malrotation	UGI	Barium
R/O irritable bowel syndrome	UGISB	Barium
R/O Hirschsprung, low bowel obstruction	Contrast enema	Cysto Conray 17.2%
CF cleanout	Contrast enema	Cysto Conray 17.2% w/Gastrografin
Meconium ileus	Contrast enema	Gastrografin w/Water 1:1
Intussusception reduction	Air enema	Air
R/O swallowing dysfunction	MBSW	Barium
Genitourinary		
Febrile UTI, R/O reflux, hydronephrosis	VCUG	Cysto Conray 17.2%
Megaureter	VCUG, IVP	Cysto Conray 17.2%
Ectopic ureter	VCUG	Cysto Conray 17.2%
Ureterocele, ureteral duplication	IVP	LOMC, Optiray 320
Neurogenic bladder Bladder diverticula	VCUG	Cysto Conray 17.2%

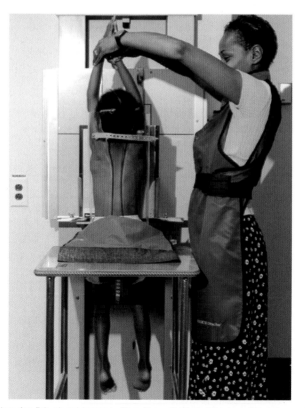

Fig. 24-17 Position for PA chest image. The Pigg-O-Stat (Modern Way Immobilizers, Clifton, TN) is a pediatric positioner and immobilization tool. The IR is held in the metal extension stand.

The central ray for PA and lateral projections is directed to the level of T6-7 (nipple line), but the collimated field should extend from and include the mastoid tips to 13 cm (2 inches) above the iliac crests. Inclusion of the mastoid tips shows the upper airway; narrowed or stenotic airways are a common source of respiratory problems in pediatric patients. By collimating just above the iliac crests, the radiographer will be sure to include the inferior costal margins. Numerous children arrive in the imaging department with long lung fields resulting from hyperinflation (e.g., patients with cardiac disorders and asthma).

Most radiologists will agree that upright chest images yield a great deal more diagnostic information than supine images. It is important, however, that you be able to achieve diagnostic quality in both positions. Infants needing supine and cross-table lateral images can be immobilized using Velcro straps around the knees and a Velcro band across the legs. The patient is supine on a radiolucent pad with the arms held above the head for both the AP and the cross-table lateral. This technique is particularly useful for patients with chest tubes, delicately positioned gastrostomy tubes, or soft tissue swellings or protrusions that may be compromised by the sleeves of the Pigg-O-Stat.

Chest (<1 Year)

At Boston Children's Hospital (BCH), all non-bedside, two-view chest x-rays and most decubitus views of infants, 0 to 365 days, are performed using a "baby box" invented by our technical director, Linda Poznauskis (Fig. 24-18). This device has proven invaluable for immobilizing and positioning the infant with minimal discomfort and helping to ensure a diagnostic and reproducible exam in a timely manner. The patient must be nude from the waist up with all heart monitor leads removed (when safe), and lines and tubes (especially nasogastric tubes) positioned away from the chest anatomy. The baby is placed supine on the box, shielded, and the lower

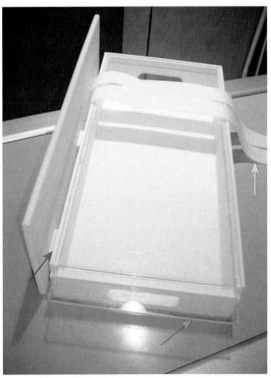

Fig. 24-18 The baby box aids in the immobilization of an infant (0 to 12 months) for AP and cross-table lateral chest x-rays, soft tissue neck and C-spine imaging. There is a sliding tray *(orange arrow)* that holds the CR IR for supine positions, a slot on the side *(blue arrow)* holds the IR for cross-table work, and Velcro straps *(yellow arrow)* are used to immobilize.

torso immobilized with the attached Velcro (Velcro USA, Inc., Manchester, NH) strap and sandbag as necessary. The parent is directed to slowly raise the baby's arms up and alongside its head. While holding the arms at the level of the elbows, the parent places his or her thumbs at the sides of the head or on the forehead to assure that the baby's head is in a true supine position with no rotation or obliquity (Fig. 24-19). A small rotation of the head will cause distortion of the infant's lung fields, and if the baby arches its back the image will be rendered lordotic. Special attention should be paid to the tendency of parents to pull

the arms and baby toward them rather than simply holding the arms and head together. This results in the patient being slowly pulled from under the Velcro and off the IR, causing the lung apices to be clipped. Collimate, ensure that the parent continues to immobilize effectively, and expose when the baby's belly is fully distended indicating a full inspiration. Do not be in a hurry here—activate the rotor, pick up the rhythm of the infants breathing, and time your exposure. If the infant is hyperventilating, an inspiratory image will be obtained, although it may not be at full inspiration.

The left, cross-table, lateral projection (Fig. 24-20) is obtained by placing the IR in the baby box's shallow groove on the left side of the baby box. Using the same holding technique, the Velcro is released and the patient is moved closer to the IR, thus minimizing OID (magnification); the Velcro is then refastened. Collimation should allow the x-ray beam to overlap onto the side of the box closest to the x-ray tube to prevent clipping the posterior lung fields. It is imperative, especially for medicolegal reasons, that all first-time AP images and all subsequent images contain the correct marker placement.

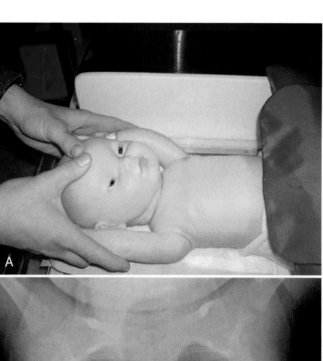

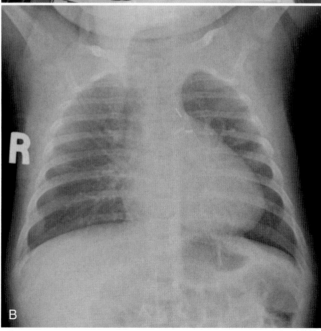

Fig. 24-19 A, Supine AP chest x-ray for an infant younger than 12 months. Parent immobilizes at the elbows with thumbs at or on sides of forehead. **B,** AP chest image of infant younger than 12 months.

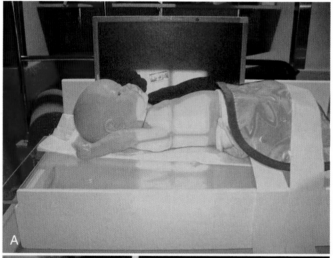

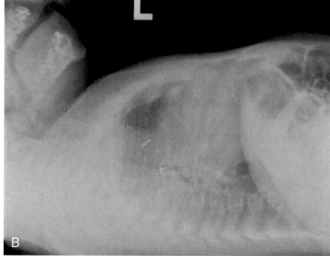

Fig. 24-20 A, Left, cross-table, lateral chest projection: same immobilization as for AP, but infant must be moved closer to the IR to reduce OID and avoid clipping the spine. **B,** Lateral projection chest image of an infant younger than 12 months.

Chest (>1 Year)

This population of little patients will resist any positioning the radiographer attempts by wiggling, twisting, crying, contorting, or all of the above in what appears to be an effort to force a repeat image. The biggest reason for repeats in this age group is that the patient pulls away from the image receptor, resulting in a lordotic image. Properly positioning this age group requires good communication between the radiographer and parents. Parents can be tentative about holding their child firmly. If the child is allowed to twist or lean away from the IR, the image will be non-diagnostic. If the parents are unsuccessful in immobilization, use the Pigg-O-Stat (if age appropriate) or use a radiographer as a last resort.

Chest x-rays (for children 1 to 6 years old) can be obtained by seating the child at the end of the exam table using a custom-made frame that supports the IR and aids in the positioning of the child. The PA chest x-ray is accomplished with the child's arms raised next to the head with instructions to the parent that the child's head and arms be held as a unit (Fig. 24-21). A slight upward pull on the child's body will keep a straight torso. Do not let the patient lean away from the IR, as this will produce a lordotic image; this can be prevented either by moving the patient's bottom away from the IR or by placing a 15-degree positioning sponge between the patient and the IR at the level of the patient's abdomen, with the thicker portion at the level of the pelvic ilia. Patients should be nude from the waist up in order to visualize and time the inspiration.

For the sitting left lateral, patients are held from behind or the front, with arms in the same position as used for the PA (Fig. 24-22). A large firm positioning sponge can be placed between the parent's chest and the patient's back, or the positioning can be done without the sponge on older children. While holding the child's head and arms as a unit, the parent is instructed to exert a slight upward pull while keeping the patient's back against the sponge and perpendicular to the IR. If the patient is unruly, a second person will be required to hold down on the child's knees. Make sure you have a clear view of the patient's belly to check for inspiration. Older patients are done standing using an upright bucky.

Image evaluation

The criteria used to evaluate the image are inclusion of the full lung fields, airway, visibility of peripheral lung markings, rotation, inspiration, cardiac silhouette, mediastinum, and bony structures. In the PA chest image, the ideal technical factor is a selection that permits visualization of the intervertebral disk spaces through the heart (the most dense area), while showing the peripheral lung markings (the least dense area). Rotation should be assessed by evaluating midline structures (sternum, trachea, spinous processes, etc.). These anterior and posterior midline structures should be superimposed. Similar to chest radiography in adults, the visualization of eight to nine posterior ribs is a reliable indicator of an image taken with good inspiration (Table 24-4).

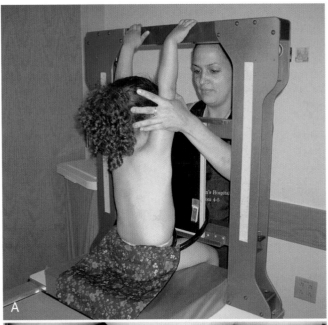

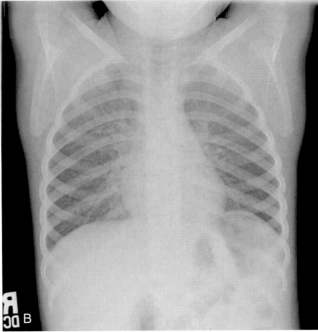

Fig. 24-21 A, Parent holding for a PA chest on a child older than 1 year. B, Resultant chest image. Care should be taken to tie up textured hair, as it can show as an artifact on digital images.

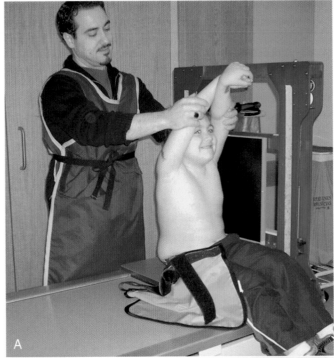

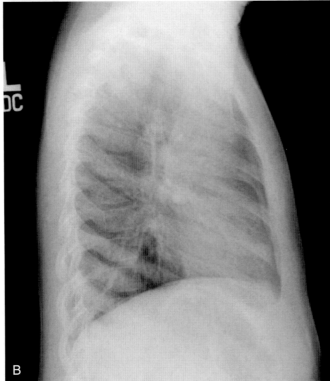

Fig. 24-22 A, Parent holding for a lateral chest on child older than 1 year. B, Resultant chest image.

TABLE 24-4

Quick reference guide for image assessment

	Density		Recorded detail	Contrast		Anatomy	Rotation check
	Most dense	Least dense		Long scale >3 shades	Short scale >3 shades		
PA chest	Midline; intervertebral disk spaces, heart	Peripheral lung markings	Peripheral lung markings	Airway, heart, apices, bases, mediastinum, lung markings behind diaphragm and heart		Airway to bases	Airway position, SC joints, lung field measurement, cardiac silhouette
PA chest	Heart	Retrocardiac space	Peripheral lung markings	Airway, heart, apices, bases		Airway to bases, spinous process to sternum	Superimposition of ribs, spinous processes on profile
Abdomen	Lumbar spine	Peripheral edges, soft tissue above the iliac crests	Organ silhouettes	Diaphragm, liver, kidney, spine, gas shadows		Right and left hemidiaphragm, pubic symphysis, right and left skin edges	
Limbs	Bone	Soft tissue	Bony trabecular patterns		Bone, muscle, soft tissue	Joints above and below injury, all soft tissue	AP and lateral images must not resemble obliques
Hips	Hip joints	Iliac crests	Bony trabecular patterns		Bone, soft tissue	Iliac crests, lesser trochanter	Symmetric iliac crests
Lateral lumbar spine	L5-S1	Spinous processes	Bony trabecular patterns		Bone	T12 to coccyx, spinous processes to vertebral bodies	Alignment of posterior surfaces of vertebral bodies

Evaluating the image to determine its diagnostic quality is a practiced skill. This chart, designed as a quick reference guide, outlines the five important technical criteria and the related anatomic indicators used in critiquing images.

AP, Anteroposterior; *posteroanterior* (PA); *SC,* sternoclavicular.

Chest (3 to 18 Years)

Upright

Upright images on children 3 to 18 years old are easily obtained by observing the following steps:

- Help the child sit on a large wooden box, a wide-based trolley with brakes, or a stool, with the IR supported using a metal extension stand. Young children are curious and have short attention spans. By having them sit, the radiographer can prevent them from wiggling from the waist down.
- For the PA position, have the child hold onto the side supports of the extension stand, with the chin on top of or next to the IR. This prevents upper body movement.
- When positioning for the lateral image, have the parent (if his or her presence is permitted) assist by raising the child's arms above the head and holding the head between the arms (Fig. 24-23).

Supine

Infants needing supine and cross-table lateral images can be immobilized using Velcro straps around the knees and a Velcro ban across the legs (Fig. 24-24). The patient is elevated on a sponge with the arms held up, and a cross-table lateral is performed. This technique is particularly useful for patients with chest tubes, delicately positioned gastrostomy tubes, or soft tissue swellings or protrusions that may be compromised by the sleeves of the Pigg-O-Stat.

Image evaluation

As in adult chest radiography, the use of kVp is desirable in pediatric chest imaging; however, this is relative. In adult imaging, high kVp generally ranges from 110 to 130, but for pediatric PA projections, kVp ranges from 80 to 90. The use of a higher kVp is not always possible because the corresponding mAs are too low to produce a diagnostic image.

The criteria used to evaluate recorded detail include the resolution of peripheral lung markings. Evaluating any image for adequate density involves assessing the most and least dense areas of the anatomy that is shown. In the PA chest image, the ideal technical factor is a selection that permits visualization of the intervertebral disk spaces through the heart (the most dense area) while showing the peripheral lung markings (the least dense area). Rotation should be assessed by evaluating the position of midline structures. Posterior and anterior midline structures (i.e., sternum, airway, and vertebral bodies) should be superimposed. The anatomic structures to be shown include the airway (trachea) to the costophrenic angles. Similar to chest radiography in adults, the visualization of 8 to 9 posterior ribs is a reliable indicator of an image taken with good inspiration (see Table 24-4).

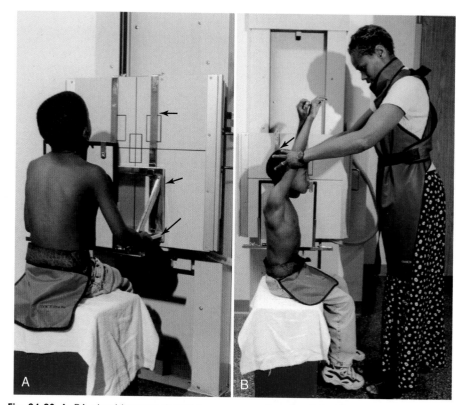

Fig. 24-23 A, PA chest images should be performed on the 3- to 18-year-old with the child sitting. **B,** The parent, if present, can assist with immobilization for the lateral image by holding the child's head between the child's arms. Metal extension stands (arrows on **A** and **B**) are commercially available from companies that market diagnostic imaging accessories.

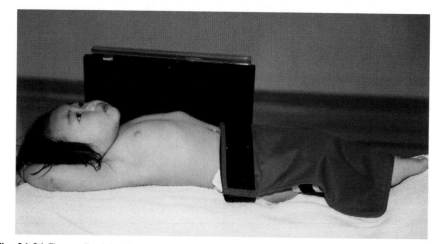

Fig. 24-24 The patient is raised on a sponge with arms held up by the head, and the legs are immobilized using Velcro straps. The IR is in place for the horizontal lateral beam (cross-table lateral).

PELVIS AND HIPS

General principles

The initial radiography examination of the pelvis and hips is routinely done for children older than 1 year. Ultrasonography is used for infants younger than 1 year. With a basic comprehension of the most common pediatric pelvic positions, pathologies, and disease processes, the radiographer can provide the radiologist with the superior diagnostic images required to make an accurate diagnosis.

Despite the importance of radiation protection, little written literature is available to guide radiographers on the placement of gonadal shields and when to use shielding. The radiographer should observe the following guidelines:

- *Always* use gonadal shielding on boys. Take care, however, to prevent potential lesions of the pubic symphysis from being obscured.
- In girls, use gonadal protection on all images *except* the first AP projection of the *initial* examination of the hips and pelvis.
- After sacral abnormality or sacral involvement has been ruled out, use shielding on subsequent images in girls.
- Before proceeding, check the girl's records or seek clarification from the parents regarding whether this is the child's first examination.
- Because the female reproductive organs are located in the mid-pelvis with their exact position varying, ensure that the shield covers the sacrum and part or all of the sacroiliac joints, making sure it does not cover the hip joints or pubic symphysis.

NOTE: Many children have been taught that no one should touch their "private parts." Radiographers need to be sensitive and use discretion when explaining and carrying out the procedure.

- *Never touch the pubic symphysis in a child,* regardless of whether you are positioning the patient or placing the gonadal shield.
- The superior border of the pubic symphysis is always at the level of the greater trochanters. Use the trochanters as a guide for positioning and shield placement. The CR should be located midline at a point midway between the anterior superior iliac spine (ASIS) and the symphysis.
- In boys, keep the gonadal shield from touching the scrotum by laying a 15-degree sponge or a cloth over the top of the femora. The top of the shield can be placed 3 cm below the level of the trochanters, and the bottom half of the shield can rest on top of the sponge or cloth (Fig. 24-25).
- In girls, place the top, widest part of the shield in the midline, level with the ASIS.

Initial images

Hip examinations on children are most often ordered to assess for Legg-Calvé-Perthes disease (aseptic avascular necrosis of the femoral head), developmental dysplasia of the hip (DDH), slipped capital femoral epiphyses (SCFE), and to diagnose nonspecific hip pain. These conditions require the evaluation of the symmetry of the acetabula, joint spaces, and soft tissue, therefore symmetric positioning is crucial. The initial examination of the hips and pelvis in children older than 1 year includes a well-collimated AP projection and a lateral projection commonly referred to as a frog lateral. This position is more correctly described as a coronal image of the pelvis with the thighs in abduction and external rotation, or the Lauenstein position (see Chapter 7). This bilateral imaging serves as a baseline for future imaging and allows comparison of right to left hips.

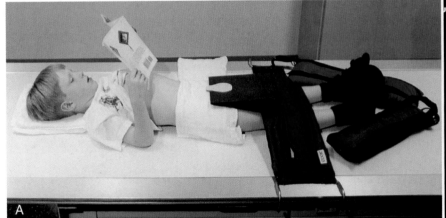
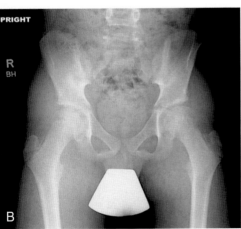

Fig. 24-25 A, The male gonadal shield should cover the scrotum without obscuring the pubic symphysis. The greater trochanters indicate the upper border of the pubic symphysis; the top of the shield should be placed approximately ½ inch below this level. The gonadal shield rests on a 15-degree sponge, which prevents the radiographer's hands from coming close to or touching the scrotal area.
B, A 3½-year-old normal pelvis; note the shielding.

Preparation and communication

All images of the abdomen and pelvic girdle should be performed with the child's underwear or diaper removed. Buttons, silk screening, and metal on underwear as well as wet diapers produce significant artifacts on images, often rendering them nondiagnostic. The radiographer should have all required positioning devices on the table prior to the patient's arrival.

Positioning and immobilization

As described previously, *symmetric positioning* is crucial. As in many examinations, the hip positions that are the most uncomfortable for the patient are often the most crucial. When a child has hip pain or dislocation, symmetric positioning is difficult to achieve because the patient often tries to compensate for the discomfort by rotating the pelvis. The radiographer should observe the following steps when positioning the patient:

- As with hip examinations in any patient, check that the ASISs are equidistant from the table.
- After carefully observing and communicating with the patient to discover the location of pain, use sponges to compensate for rotation. Sponges should routinely be used to support the thighs in the frog-leg position. This can help prevent motion artifacts.

- Do not accept poorly positioned images. Repeat instructions as necessary to achieve optimal positioning.

Because *immobilization techniques* should vary according to the aggressiveness of the patient, the radiographer can follow these additional guidelines:

- Make every effort to use explanation and reassurance as part of the immobilization method. A child may require only a Velcro band placed across the legs as a safety precaution.
- For an active child, wrap a Velcro strip around the knees and place large sandbags over the arms (see Fig. 24-12). The Velcro strip over the knees keeps the child from wiggling one leg or both legs out from under the Velcro band and possibly rolling off the table.
- If the child has enough strength to free his or her arms from the sandbags, ask a parent to stand on the opposite side of the table from the radiographer and hold the child's arms. The parent's thumbs should be placed directly over the child's shoulders (Fig. 24-26). This method of immobilization is used extensively. It also works well for supine abdominal images, intravenous urograms (IVUs), overhead GI procedures, and spinal radiography.

Leg-length-discrepancies, which can cause hip problems, are diagnosed using a *Scanogram,* a technique in which three exposures of the lower limbs (single exposures centered over the hips, knees, and ankles) are made on a single 35 × 43 cm IR (see Chapter 11). Two radiolucent rulers with radiopaque numbers are included bilaterally and within the collimated field, making it possible for the orthopedic surgeon to then calculate the difference in leg lengths.

Evaluating images

Rotation or symmetry can be evaluated by ensuring that midline structures are in the midline and that the ilia appear symmetric. Depending on the degree of skeletal maturation, visualization of the trochanters can indicate the position of the legs when the image was taken. Symmetry in the skin folds is also an important evaluation criterion for the diagnostician. The anatomy to be shown includes the crests of the ilia to the upper quarter of the femora. The image should demonstrate the bony trabecular pattern in the hip joints, which is the thickest and most dense area within the region. The visualization of the bony trabecular pattern is used as an indicator that sufficient recorded detail has been shown; this should not be at the expense of showing the soft tissues—the muscles and skin folds (see Table 24-4).

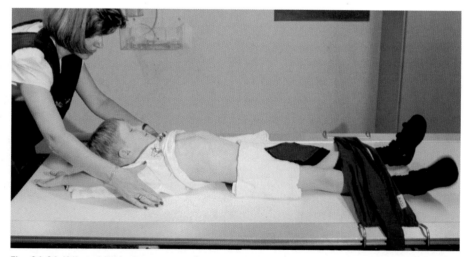

Fig. 24-26 If the child is strong enough or aggressive enough to remove the sandbags (see Fig. 24-12), the parent can hold the child's humeri by placing the thumbs directly over the child's shoulders.

LIMB RADIOGRAPHY

Limb radiography accounts for a high percentage of pediatric general radiographic procedures in most clinics and hospitals. Producing a series of diagnostic images will require you to assess the child's age-appropriate development, behavior, and age in order to determine which forms of immobilization you will employ. This is best accomplished in consultation with the parents; an active 3-year-old may require that you use immobilization techniques that are one or two age groups below the patient's chronologic age group.

Immobilization
Newborn to 2 years old
Depending on the exam, swaddling the child in a blanket, towel, or pillowcase will make the child manageable when performing upper limb radiography. This wrapping technique, a modification of the "bunny" method (Fig. 24-27), keeps the infant warm and allows one parent to concentrate on immobilizing the injured limb. When imaging small hands, a piece of Plexiglas can be used to firmly hold the hand while making the exposure. Lower extremities are best imaged with the help of swaddling, a Velcro band, or parent holding over the abdomen with a large sandbag placed over the unaffected leg (Fig. 24-28).

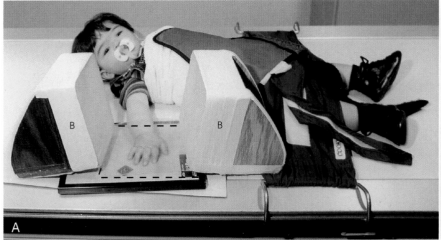
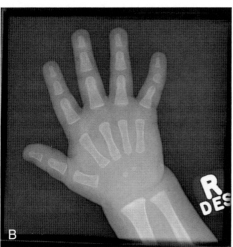

Fig. 24-27 A, With a simple modification of the "bunny" technique using a towel (or pillowcase), the child can be immobilized for upper limb radiography. Plexiglas *(dashed lines)* and "bookends" *(B)* can be used to immobilize the hands of children 2 years old and younger. Note that after the child is wrapped, a Velcro band is used for safety, and a small apron is placed diagonally over the body to protect the sternum and gonads. The IR is placed on a lead mat, which prevents the image receptor from sliding on the table. **B,** Nine-month-old normal right hand.

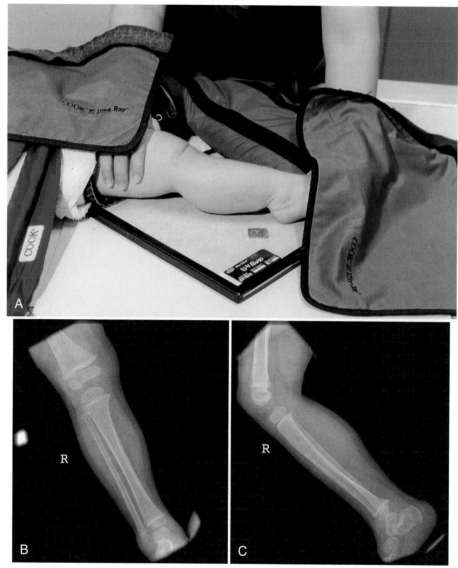

Fig. 24-28 A, The challenges of immobilizing lower limbs are greater than those of immobilizing upper limbs. After wrapping both of the patient's arms in a towel and placing a Velcro band over the abdomen, the radiographer can place a large sandbag over the unaffected leg. With careful collimation and proper instruction, the parent can hold the limb as demonstrated. Normal 21-month-old AP **(B)** and lateral **(C)** tibia and fibula.

Preschool age

The upper limbs of preschoolers are best imaged with the child sitting on the parent's lap as shown in Fig. 24-29. If the parent is unable to participate, these children can be immobilized as described previously.

With parental participation, radiography of the lower limbs can be accomplished with the child sitting or lying on the table. Preventing the patient from falling from the table is always a primary concern with preschoolers. Instruct the parent to remain by the child's side if the child is seated on the table or stool. If the examination is performed with the child lying on the table, a Velcro band over the abdomen or parent holding should be employed.

NOTE: The child's ankle should be in flexion, not extension.

School age

School-age children generally can be managed in the same way as adult patients for upper and lower limb examinations.

Radiation protection

The upper body should be protected from scatter radiation in all examinations of the upper limbs because of the close proximity of the thymus, sternum, and breast tissue. Child-sized lead aprons with cartoon characters are both popular and practical (Fig. 24-30).

Fractures

Fractures in children's bones occur under two circumstances: abnormal stresses in normal bone and normal stresses in abnormal bone. A fracture is defined as the breaking or rupture of a bone caused by mechanical forces either applied to the bone or transmitted directly along the line of the bone. Children's bone fractures differ from those of adults because growth is active and favors rapid repair and remodeling. In general, children's bones are less dense than those of adults, and the ability to visualize soft tissue and bony detail are of utmost importance, in particular small linear fractures are difficult to discern without good soft tissue detail. Fat pad displacement and tissue swelling may be the only radiographic signs of injury. Such subtle findings can disguise an epiphyseal growth plate fracture, which if left untreated could result in irregular or cessation of growth in the affected bone. Overriding and distraction deformities may correct without residual deformity, but rotational deformities will not. Consequently, images of the fractured bone showing the relative position of the two ends of the bone (AP, lateral, oblique) are necessary for evaluation of rotation; preliminary assessment may require the *contralateral* side to be examined for comparison.

The earlier in a child's life this epiphyseal fracture occurs, the better the chances of spontaneous correction of angulation fractures.

Here is an abbreviated list of some of the more common pediatric extremity fractures.

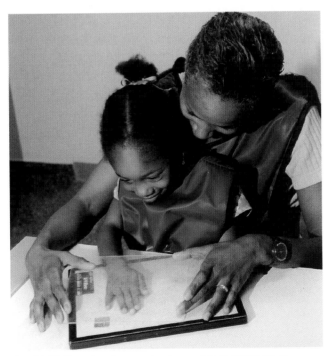

Fig. 24-29 Preschoolers are best managed sitting on a parent's lap. A lead mat is used to keep the IR from sliding. Note the use of Plexiglas to immobilize fingers. (The parent's hands are shown without lead gloves and not draped in lead for illustration purposes only.)

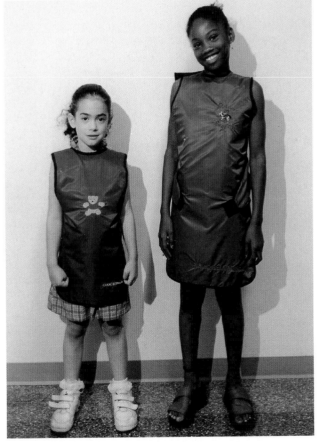

Fig. 24-30 The teddy bear on this full-length apron *(left)* makes it appropriate for young children.

Salter-Harris

About a third of all skeletal injuries to children are at the epiphyseal growth plates, especially in the ankle and wrist. Salter and Harris described these fractures in 1963 as Salter-Harris types I through V (Fig. 24-31).

Plastic or bow

The bones of children, as compared to those of adults, can absorb and deflect more energy without breaking due to a lower bending resistance. Plastic or bowing fractures occur in children when this bending resistance is exceeded and the bone or bones bow without breaking. The bowing fracture is a bending deformity, which usually occurs in the forearm. There is no grossly visible fracture in the tubular structure of the bone; however,

microfractures are visible using microscopy. The bowing is appreciable on plain images and often requires a comparison view to confirm the deformation. A bowing fracture is usually reduced under general anesthesia, as the force required to reduce the bowing is substantial.

Greenstick

A green stick fracture occurs when one cortex of the bone's diaphysis breaks and the side remains intact.

Torus

The torus fracture is a type of greenstick fracture in which the load on the bone is in the same direction as the diaphysis, causing the cortex to fold back on itself.

Toddler's fracture

A toddler's fracture is described as a subtle, nondisplaced, oblique fracture of the distal tibia in children 9 months to 3 years of age; the fracture may only be seen on one view of the lower shaft of the tibia. If AP, lateral, and oblique projections are radiographically negative, but there is strong suspicion of a toddler's fracture, a radionuclide scan may be indicated. The child's age and the presentation are significant to this diagnosis. It is important to realize that this is a common accidental injury, which the parents may not have witnessed. If the onset of symptoms (pain, non-weight-bearing) is rapid and the patient's age is within the noted range, a toddler's fracture has a high index of suspicion. Remember, however, that a similar fracture in a very young infant who is not yet a "toddler" cannot be ascribed to accidental falls and, therefore, would be suspicious of abuse.

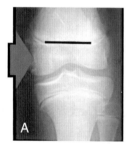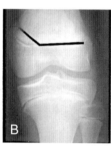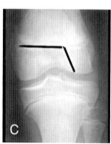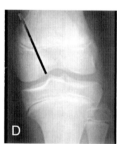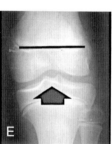

Fig. 24-31 Salter-Harris fractures. The black lines represent the fracture lines. **A,** A type I fracture occurs directly through the growth plate. **B,** A type II fracture extends through the growth plate and into the metaphyses. **C,** A type III fracture line extends through the growth plate and into the epiphyses. **D,** A type IV fracture line extends through the metaphyses, across or sometimes along the growth plate, and through the epiphyses. **E,** A type V fracture involves a crushing of all or part of the growth plate. Fractures that occur through the epiphyses are significant injuries because they can affect growth if not recognized and treated properly. Proper radiographic technique is required for the demonstration of both soft tissue and bone. This is especially important with type I fractures, in which the growth plate is separated as a result of a lateral blow, and type V fractures, in which the growth plate has sustained a compression injury. Types I and V fractures do not occur through the bone.

Supracondylar fracture

More severe than the toddler's fracture, the supracondylar fracture is the most common elbow fracture in children, accounting for 60% of all pediatric elbow fractures (Fig. 24-32). Occurring frequently in children between the ages of 3 and 10, it is caused by the child falling on an outstretched hand with hyperextension of the elbow. The most extensively displaced of these fractures can cause serious vascular and nerve damage. Great care should be taken when positioning for this fracture.

Image evaluation

Among the many striking differences in radiographic appearance between adult and pediatric patients are the bone trabeculae and the presence of epiphyseal lines or growth plates in pediatric patients. As they gain experience in evaluating pediatric images, radiographers develop a visual appreciation for these differences. To the uneducated eye, a normally developing epiphysis, for example, may mimic a fracture. For this reason, and because fractures can occur through the epiphyseal plate, physicians, and to a certain degree radiographers, must learn to recognize epiphyseal lines and their appearance at various stages of ossification. Fractures that occur through the epiphysis are called *growth plate fractures* (Salter-Harris). Because the growth plates are composed of cartilaginous tissue, the *density* of the image must be such that soft tissue is shown in addition to bone (see Table 24-4). Visualization of the bony trabecular pattern is used as an indicator that sufficient *recorded detail* has been achieved. Because of the small size of pediatric extremities, an imaging system with superior resolution is required. Generally, the speed of the imaging system should be half that used for spines and abdomens.

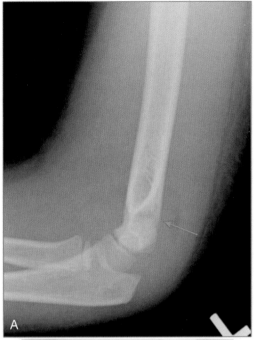

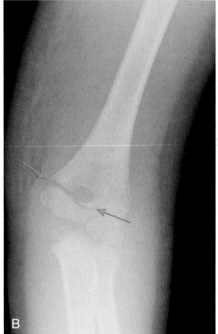

Fig. 24-32 A-B, AP and lateral projections of a supracondylar fracture.

SKULL AND PARANASAL SINUSES
Skull

The two most common indications for a pediatric, radiographic skull series are to rule out craniosynostosis and fracture. Synostosis is the fusion of two bones, and it can be normal or abnormal. The term *craniosynostosis,* or *premature cranial suture synostosis,* describes the premature closure of one or more of the cranial sutures and may be isolated or part of a craniofacial syndrome; both result in the deformity of the calvaria's shape. Etiologically, abnormal synostosis is described as either primary or secondary. Primary craniosynostosis is characterized by some type of defect in one or more of the cranial sutures and can be intrinsic or familial. The familial form manifests as a component of a craniofacial syndrome (Pfeiffer, Apert, Crouzon, Beare-Stevenson) and may be the result of one of several genetic mutations. Secondary craniosynostosis is the result of some underlying medical condition, which can be systemic or metabolic (hyperthyroidism, hypercalcemia, vitamin D deficiency, sickle cell, or thalassemia). Microcephaly, encephalocele, and shunted hydrocephalus can diminish the growth stretch at sutures, which can lead to craniosynostosis secondarily.

Calvarial growth takes place perpendicular to the suture lines. The suture lines involved, time of onset, and the sequence in which individual sutures fuse will determine the nature of the deformity. When sutures fuse prematurely, calvarial growth occurs along the axis of the fused suture. The altered skull shape is diagnostic. Restoring growth is dependent on the early release of all fused sutures.

The birth prevalence of craniosynostosis ranges from approximately 3 to 5 cases per 10,000 live births. The isolated variety (only one suture affected) constitutes 80% to 90% of cases, and the sutures most commonly involved, in descending order of frequency, are the sagittal, coronal, metopic, and lambdoid. The syndromic variety accounts for up to 10% to 20% of cases. Coronal synostosis is more frequently seen in females, whereas sagittal synostosis is more common in males. Most cases are diagnosed early in life. Skull images of infants are obtained in the supine position. Radiographic views include (1) a supine AP projection obtained to demonstrate the calvaria, (2) one or both lateral projections obtained to demonstrate the calvaria and skull base (both lateral projections are indicated in trauma and focal lesion evaluation), and (3) an AP axial Towne projection, but only with a 30-degree caudad angle (due to differing skull morphology in pediatric patients younger than age 10 years) is obtained to demonstrate the occipital bone and foramen magnum.

Skull fractures occurring in children are usually the result of blunt force trauma and include both accidental and nonaccidental trauma, as well as those sustained from forceps extraction at birth. Fractures can occur with minimal force in the abnormally fragile bone associated with osteogenesis imperfecta. Diastatic fracture lines (breaks along the sutures) present as more lucent, more linear, and exhibit no interdigitations, which distinguish them from sutures. Depressed skull fractures appear dense due to the overlapping bone fragments. Skull radiography will demonstrate horizontal linear fracture lines that may not be visible on computed tomography (CT) when the fracture is parallel to the CT axis. All skull imaging is done with a grid, large focal spot, using a set technique (can use AEC for AP), and with no clothing from the waist up. Immobilizing an infant for a skull series is accomplished most efficiently by using the "bunny immobilization" technique (Fig. 24-33), as all three projections can be accomplished with minimal help, or the parents can be drafted to immobilize the shoulders, torso, and legs (sand bags will work if the patient is younger than 2 years); this technique, however, requires a lot more instruction and is less reliable.

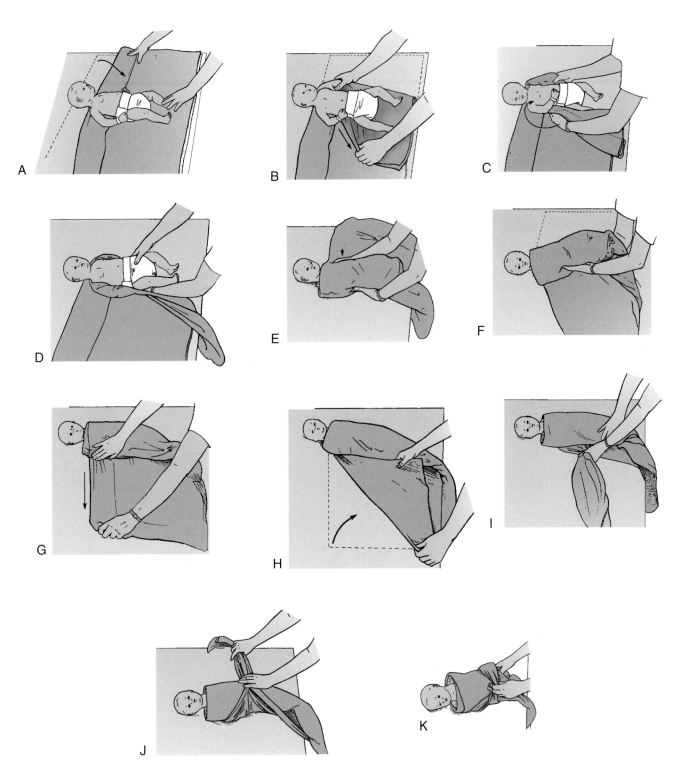

Fig. 24-33 The "bunny" method used to immobilize the patient for cranial radiography. **A** to **D** focus on immobilization of the shoulders, **E** to **G** concentrate on the humeri, and **H** to **K** illustrate the way the sheet is folded and wrapped to immobilize the legs. **A,** Begin with a standard hospital sheet folded in half lengthwise. Make a 6-inch fold at the top, and lay the child down about 2 feet from the end of the sheet. **B,** Wrap the end of the sheet over the left shoulder, and pass the sheet under the child. **C,** This step makes use of the 6-inch fold. Reach under, undo the fold, and wrap it over the right shoulder. (Steps **B** and **C** are crucial to the success of this immobilization technique because they prevent the child from wiggling the shoulders free.) **D,** After wrapping the right shoulder, pass the end of the sheet under the child. Pull it through to keep the right arm snug against the body. **E,** Begin wrapping, keeping the sheet snug over the upper body to immobilize the humeri. **F,** Lift the lower body and pass the sheet underneath, keeping the child's head on the table. Repeat steps **E** and **F** if material permits. **G,** Make sure the material is evenly wrapped around the upper body. (Extra rolls around the shoulder and neck area produce artifacts on 30-degree fronto-occipital and submentovertical images.) **H,** Make a diagonal fold with the remaining material (approximately 2 feet). **I,** Roll the material together. **J,** Snugly wrap this over the child's femora. (The tendency to misjudge the location of the femora and thus wrap too snugly around the lower legs should be avoided.) **K,** Tuck the end of the rolled material in front. (If not enough material remains to tuck in, use a Velcro strip or tape to secure it.)

(From the Michener Institute for Applied Health Sciences, Toronto.)

The AP skull (Fig. 24-34, *A*) is positioned with the orbitomeatal line (OML) perpendicular to the IR using two round, 10-cm, radiolucent sponges, one on either side of the head. It is important when using these sponges to use your palms rather than pressing your fingers into the sponge (which will appear on the image). The axial Townes method (Fig. 24-34, *B*) is also done supine using the "mouse ears" sponges to bring the chin toward the chest so that the OML is perpendicular to the exam table and IR. The central ray is directed 30 degrees caudad and enters 2.5 to 5 cm above the glabella. The lateral skull can be imaged using one of two methods. The first projection is a left, cross-table lateral (Fig. 24-34, *C*) with the infant supine and elevated on a radiolucent pad and positioned supine. The grid holder with IR is parallel to the skull and extends to the tabletop (below the pad) to avoid clipping of the posterior skull. The infant's shoulder is in contact with IR (Fig. 24-35). The central ray is perpendicular and enters 1 cm superior to the external auditory meatus (EAM). Use the flat surface of the hand to position one round "mouse ear" sponge just superior to the vertex of the skull and the other hand to hold the mental protuberance of the mandible. Leave the infant supine and rotate the skull to a lateral position with the side of interest down. The central ray enters 1 cm superior to EAM. Position one "mouse ear" sponge just posterior to

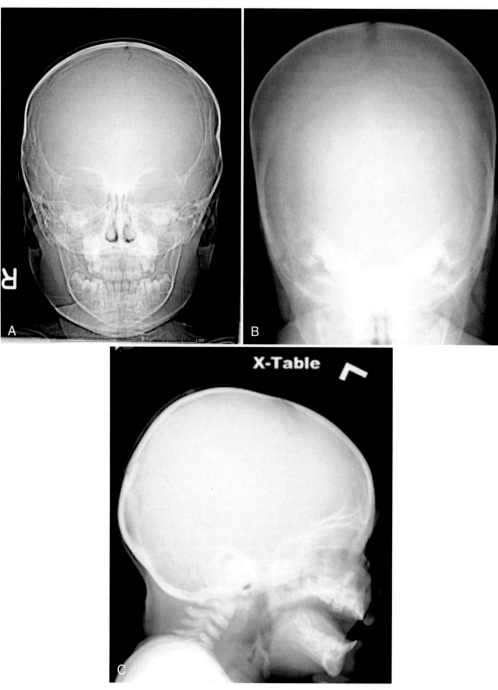

Fig. 24-34 A, AP skull. **B,** Townes 30 degrees. **C,** Lateral (method 1 as mentioned previously).

the vertex of the skull (use a flat hand) and the other hand will hold the mental protuberance of the mandible. This is an awkward position for infants so expect them to struggle (Table 24-5).

Paranasal sinuses

The main indication for performing a paranasal sinus series on the pediatric patient is to rule out sinusitis. However, radiographic opacification is not a clear indication of sinus disease; incidental findings of mucosal thickening with magnetic resonance imaging (MRI) are common in children younger than 5 years when examined for other indicated reasons according to Caffey. Because errors in positioning may simulate pathologic change in this age group, demonstrating air-fluid level in an upright exam with compelling clinical and laboratory support would probably warrant the diagnosis of sinusitis without resorting to CT. The maxillary, ethmoid, and sphenoid sinuses are present and aerated at birth, whereas the frontal sinuses do not usually appear until the second year.

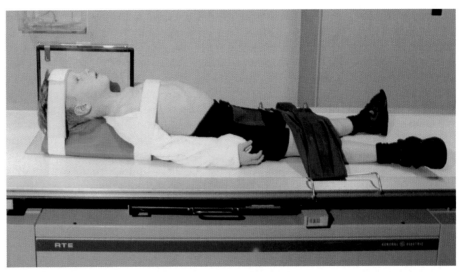

Fig. 24-35 Effective immobilization for lateral skull images with a horizontal beam can be achieved using the infant head and neck immobilizer.

TABLE 24-5
Summary of skull projections

AP skull	No angle on central ray, which enters at the nasion with the OML perpendicular to the imaging plate
AP axial Townes	Central ray 30-degree caudad, enters at the nasion.
Lateral 1	Dorsal decubitus projection (cross-table lateral); central ray enters superior to EAM
Lateral 2	Supine with side of interest down; central ray enters superior to EAM

The paranasal sinus protocol may include three views: Caldwell (Fig. 24-36), Waters (Fig. 24-37), and a left lateral projection (Fig. 24-38), which should include frontal sinus anatomy, C-spine, and airway to the thoracic inlet. Proper collimation to the area of interest is the single most common shortcoming. To preserve image quality, consider precollimating before moving the patient into position; collimate to the area of interest only. Adjusting your light field on the back of the head does not allow for divergence of the central ray, thus too much of the skull is included. Experience has shown that in children younger than 8 years, the Caldwell method requires no central ray angulation and can be positioned with forehead and nose against the bucky. This is possibly due to the immature and varying morphology of the pediatric skull (Fig. 24-39).

The central ray is horizontal and exits at the nasion for the Caldwell method. For the Waters method, the child's nose and chin touch the bucky and the central ray remains horizontal exiting at the acanthion, projecting the petrous ridges below the maxillary sinuses. The major pitfall is too much central ray angulation, which causes the sinuses to either not be visualized or falsely appear to be obliterated. The left lateral is really a soft tissue neck that includes the vertical plate of the frontal bone (where frontal sinuses will be seen, but not usually prior to 2 years), nasal shadow, the C-spine, and the thoracic inlet. With both the Waters and Caldwell methods, ask the patient to move away from the bucky or upright grid once you have determined the appropriate receptor height, precollimate to the area of interest, and then place the patient back in the light field. The image quality will be improved and radiation to the patient will be reduced. This technique takes some getting used to because the projected light field on the back of the head will appear too small; trust science, the beam will diverge. Place your marker so it will not appear over an area of interest.

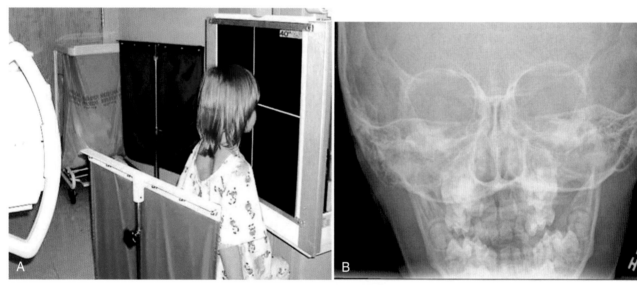

Fig. 24-36 A, Caldwell without 15-degree angle. Note that both nose and forehead touch the grid at this age. **B,** Caldwell image.

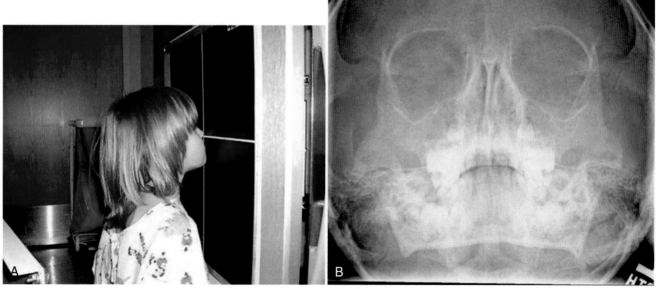

Fig. 24-37 A, Waters method with chin and nose touching grid. **B,** Waters image.

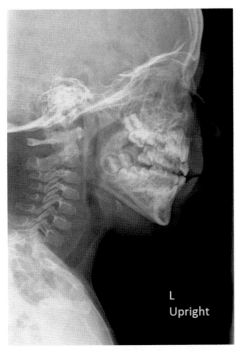

Fig. 24-38 Lateral projection for sinus series. The indication for the exam is normally noisy breathing with suspected adenoid hypertrophy. Often collimation includes from the frontal sinus to the thoracic inlet on inspiration through the nose in cases of other possible causes such as foreign bodies and retropharyngeal space anomalies (e.g., abscess). This collimation is also used for STN for similar reasons.

SOFT TISSUE NECK

Indications for the soft tissue neck (STN) include foreign bodies, stridor, laryngo- and tracheal malacia, laryngotracheal bronchitis, epiglottitis, and adenoid hypertrophy. The diagnostic quality of this exam requires careful instructions, neck extension, an inspiratory exposure, and complete immobilization. These requirements are more easily achieved with the infant or child in the supine position, although the exam can be done successfully with the patient in the upright position depending on how much the child will cooperate. The only contraindication to the supine position is the presence of epiglottitis (Fig. 24-40); these patients must always be imaged in the sitting or upright position. *Never place these patients in the supine position as a swollen epiglottis can block the airway.* A "baby box" can be used for soft tissue neck exams with infants and small children (6 months to 3 years). A 15-degree radiolucent sponge is placed under the infant/child's shoulders to achieve a slight extension of the neck and airway (shielding and immobilization are identical to the chest x-ray). A parent will hold the patient at the shoulders, pulling down slightly. The second holder, using two round, Mickey Mouse ear sponges (using flat hands), one on either side of the head and above the sella turcica, will hold the head in a true lateral position in extension and without rotation (Fig. 24-41). Collimation should be from the nasion (including complete nasal passage) to the thoracic inlet, including the entire C-spine. The head in flexion or an expiratory image may cause a false positive for enlargement of the retropharyngeal soft tissues. The lateral projection should be done with a set technique, no grid, at 182 cm SID.

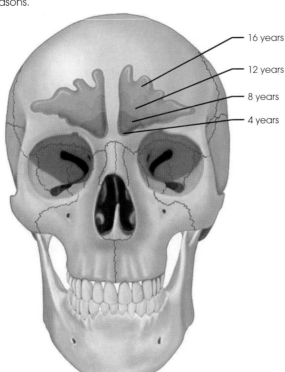

Fig. 24-39 Frontal sinus development correlated with age—green, 4 years; blue, 8 years; purple, 12 years; pink, 16 years.

(From Fonseca RJ et al: *Oral and maxillofacial trauma*, ed 4, St. Louis, 2013, Elsevier.)

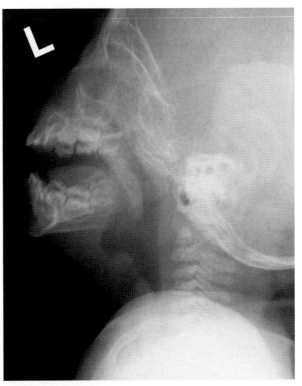

Fig. 24-40 There is diffuse swelling of the epiglottis, aryepiglottic folds, and the retropharyngeal soft tissues. These findings are consistent with epiglottitis.

The AP soft tissue neck projection must be performed with a 102-cm SID grid. Patients from infants to adolescents should be positioned with the patient's occlusal plane perpendicular to the image receptor (exact positioning will vary with age) to prevent the occipital bone from superimposing the airway (overextension). Flexion will also cause superimposition of the airway. The thick part of a 15-degree radiolucent sponge placed under the patient's shoulders will help position the skull for the AP supine extension (Fig. 24-42; using a 15-degree extension of the skull). A small cephalad angle can also be used with the AP projection to better visualize C-1 and C-2.

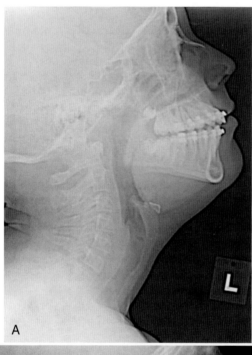

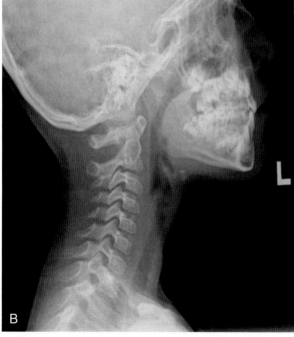

Fig. 24-41 A, Soft tissue neck (STN) with a Fuji Synapse soft tissue preset. **B,** STN without preset.

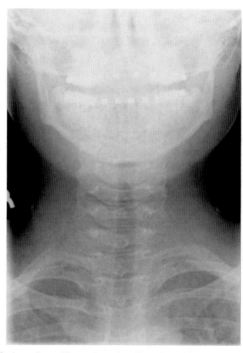

Fig. 24-42 A well positioned and collimated AP projection with a 15-degree wedge radiolucent sponge placed under the patient's shoulders and a small cephalad angle.

Foreign Bodies
AIRWAY FOREIGN BODY

Airway foreign bodies (FB) occur with frequency in children ages 6 months to 3 years, although it is not uncommon in teenagers. Radiolucent objects include firm vegetables, peanuts, hard candy, peas, carrots, and raisins. Round-shaped foods are the most frequently aspirated. Radiopaque FBs (Fig. 24-43) include coins (most common), hair clips, safety pins, and small toys. Splintered wood and glass have also been discovered, usually as the result of traumatic injury. Balloons are most likely to result in death. A young child with a persistent cough but without a fever carries a high index of suspicion for FB aspiration. Clinical presentations may also include stridor, a wheezing cough, recurrent pneumonia, or hemoptysis. If a radiolucent FB is in the trachea, the chest image may be normal, requiring a CT, or it may demonstrate bilateral over or under inflation (air trapping). More commonly, the FB is found in the bronchial tree, and most frequently the right main stem bronchus,

which is larger and more in line with the trachea. On images the FB presents most commonly as a unilateral hyperlucent lung (see Fig. 24-43, A).

The soft tissue neck is accomplished with the help of an infant head and neck immobilizer (see Fig. 24-43). If an FB is suspected clinically, inspiratory and expiratory images may be obtained to rule out air trapping, as younger children will be unable to cooperate with inhalation and expiration commands; right and left decubitus views would then be indicated. The hyperinflated lung will not deflate when the patient is lying on the affected side. A routine protocol for imaging FB includes an AP chest to include the full airway, an abdomen to include lung bases and pubic symphysis, and a lateral soft tissue neck (nasion to thoracic inlet including C-spine). All images must overlap. This survey ensures that multiple objects are not missed and provides a complete imaging of the airway and alimentary tract. If the FB is suspected of being in the airway, then bilateral decubitus views would be indicated.

INGESTED FOREIGN BODY

Whereas older children and parents might provide a history of FB ingestion, young children may simply present with unexplained drooling or inability to swallow solids. The image readily demonstrates a radiopaque object, of which coins are the most common. A coin in the esophagus will usually lie in the coronal plane (Fig. 24-44), whereas a coin in the trachea will be visualized in the sagittal plane; a nonradiopaque FB may require an esophagogram for visualization. If a contrast study is indicated, a small amount of low-osmolar, nonionic, water-soluble contrast should be used like Iohexol (Omnipaque 350). Pica, or the compulsive ingestion of nonfood articles, may be common in those with serious mental impairment or developmental delay (Fig. 24-45). Pica is the Medieval Latin name for the bird called the magpie that, it is claimed, has a penchant for eating almost anything.

Foreign Bodies

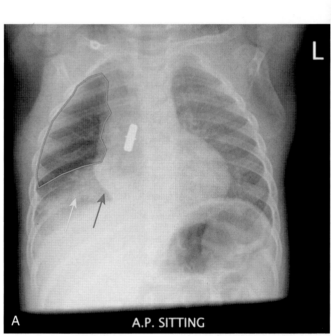
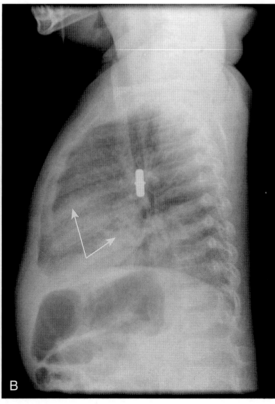

Fig. 24-43 A, A foreign body in the right main stem bronchus. There is atelectasis (collapse) predominantly affecting the right lower lobe *(yellow arrow)*. Note the distinct right heart border on the AP *(red arrow)* and unilateral hyperlucent lung *(green outline)*. **B,** Note the patchy opacities below the foreign body in the lateral view *(yellow arrows)*.

(Used with permission from Lifeinthefastlane.com at http://lifeinthefastlane.com/lower-airway-foreign-body/)

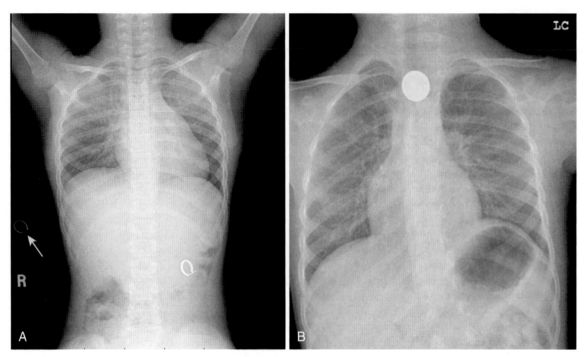

Fig. 24-44 A, Ingested earring. Reference earring placed lateral to the patient *(yellow arrow)* to assist in confirmation. **B,** Coin in the coronal plane.

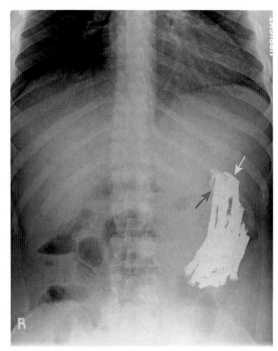

Fig. 24-45 Gastrointestinal pica with paper clip *(green arrow)* and coin *(yellow arrow).*

Selected Pediatric Conditions and Syndromes

CYSTIC FIBROSIS

Cystic fibrosis (CF) is an autosomal recessive disorder of the exocrine system caused by mutations located on chromosome 7. Generally speaking, these mutations affect the sodium and chloride ion transport system, which operates at the surface level of epithelial cells, resulting in thick mucus that cannot be cleared. These cells line the airways, sweat glands, gastrointestinal tract (GI), and the genitourinary system. The organ systems most impacted are the lungs, sinuses, pancreas, intestines, hepatobiliary tree, the spermatic ducts in the male (vas deferens), and reduced fertility rates in the female. There are approximately 30,000 CF patients in the United States and 70,000 worldwide. The median survival age as of 2010 was 37.4 years with 40% of patients older than 18. One of the earliest manifestations of CF is meconium ileus in the neonate. Most patients are diagnosed in the first year with 50% presenting with a chronic cough by 10 months.

Pulmonary complications are the leading cause of morbidity and mortality with CF. In a healthy person, the surfaces of the respiratory tract are bathed in a salty surfactant that traps and, with the help of cilia, removes pathogens and foreign substances from the lungs. This system is compromised in the CF patient, allowing microbes such as *Pseudomonas aeruginosa, Staphylococcus aureus,* and *Haemophilus influenza* to flourish in stagnant mucus leading to inflammation and bronchoconstriction, ultimately causing irreversible lung damage. Due to its low radiation dose, chest radiography is the modality of choice for evaluating respiratory complications resulting from CF. The earliest sign of irreversible lung disease in these patients is bronchiectasis. Radiographic findings include bronchial thickening and dilation, peribronchial cuffing, mucoid impaction, and cystic radiolucencies (Fig. 24-46).

Nonrespiratory manifestations include a whole range of GI complications from meconium ileus in neonates to adult gastroesophageal reflux and rectal mucosal prolapse. As the patient ages, GU complications include renal compromise, nephrolithiasis (3% to 6% of patients), and diabetic nephropathy. Musculoskeletal disorders include abnormal bone mineralization of unknown etiology and metabolic bone disease due to malnutrition and decreased lung function. Reproductive manifestations include late onset puberty (1 to 4 years), a 95% to 99% infertility rate in male patients due to blockage or absence of the spermatic ducts (vas deferens), and incomplete epididymides.

Depending on the course and severity of the disease, CF can develop into one of the most debilitating illnesses of adolescence. It is important that radiographers understand the challenges facing these teenagers.

Standard precautions for CF patients include the following:
1. Departments sending a CF for imaging must call ahead to place a room on hold.
2. Check-in sends the arriving patient immediately to the room on hold.
3. The patient is assigned a "fast pass," which pushes him or her to the front of the imaging cue.
4. The patient is changed appropriately (chest or KUB).
5. The radiographer is gowned and gloved and should attempt to maintain a 3-foot separation from the patient.
6. The radiographer, in the presence of the patient, should clean all surfaces that the patient will contact during the exam.
7. Gown and gloves must be replaced if the radiographer must leave the room.
8. Upon completion of the exam, the patient is sent back to the ordering department and all horizontal surfaces that were within 6 feet of the patient as well as surfaces the patient contacted must be disinfected.

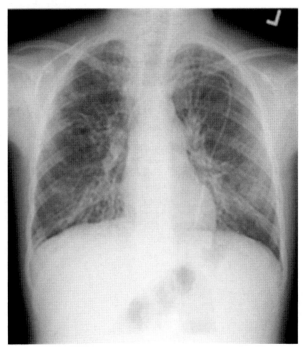

Fig. 24-46 AP chest of patient with CF.

DEVELOPMENTAL DYSPLASIA OF THE HIP

Developmental dysplasia of the hip (DDH) is the malformation of the acetabulum in utero and is usually the result of fetal positioning or a breech birth. The acetabulum fails to form completely and the femoral head(s) are displaced superiorly and anteriorly. The ligaments and tendons responsible for proper alignment are often affected. Females are affected at a rate five times more than males, the left hip is involved more than the right, and 5% to 20% of cases occur bilaterally. The clinical diagnosis is made when there is partial or complete displacement of femoral head from the acetabulum relative to the pelvis. With infants younger than 6 months of age, the modality of choice is ultrasound (US) due to its lack of radiation and because the cartilaginous nature of the hip is better visualized at this stage of development. US is used for infant follow-up until 6 months, at which time images can be used to confirm placement of the femoral head(s).

Radiographic exams used to diagnose DDH include the frog lateral and von Rosen method. There is some discussion among radiologists that because the frog lateral position is used to reduce the dysplasia, the von Rosen should be the preferred position. Treatment of DDH varies with the diagnosis. Subluxation of the hip in the neonate may be stabilized in weeks if the femora are abducted in flexion, aided by double and triple diapering. A dislocated or dislocatable hip may be reduced and immobilized by the use of a Pavlik harness worn for 1 to 2 months; more complex cases may require surgery and a spica cast. During follow-up imaging, care should be taken when the spica cast is removed to keep the legs abducted to ensure hip stability. Later interventions include periacetabular osteotomy (PAO) surgery to correct the developmental dysplasia (Fig. 24-47).

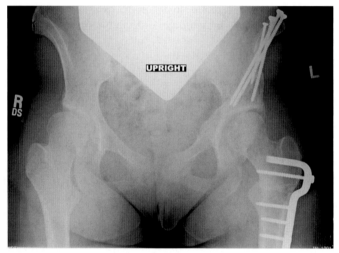

Fig. 24-47 Follow-up image post left periacetabular osteotomy (PAO) surgery to correct developmental dysplasia of the left hip (DDH). The right femur also suffers from a lack of acetabular coverage due to a malformed acetabulum.

Nonaccidental Trauma (Child Abuse)

Although no *universal* agreement exists on the definition of child abuse, the radiographer should have an appreciation of the all-encompassing nature of this problem. *Child abuse* has been described as "the involvement of physical injury, sexual abuse or deprivation of nutrition, care or affection in circumstances, which indicate that injury or deprivation may not be accidental or may have occurred through neglect."[1] Although diagnostic imaging staff members are usually involved only in cases in which physical abuse is a possibility, they should realize that sexual abuse and nutritional neglect are also prevalent.

It is mandatory in all states and provinces in North America for health care

[1]Robinson MJ: *Practical pediatrics,* ed 6, New York, 2007, Churchill Livingstone.

professionals to *report suspected cases of abuse or neglect.* The radiographer, while preparing or positioning the patient, may be the first person to suspect abuse or neglect (Fig. 24-48). The first course of action for the radiographer should be to consult a radiologist (when available) or the attending physician. After this consultation, the radiographer may no longer have cause for suspicion because some naturally occurring skin markings mimic bruising. *If the radiographer's doubts persist, the suspicions must be reported to the proper authority, regardless of the physician's opinion.* Recognizing the complexity of child abuse issues, many health care facilities have developed a multidisciplinary team of health care workers to respond to these issues. Radiographers working in hospitals have access to this team of physicians, social workers, and psychologists for the purposes of reporting their concerns.

The American College of Radiology (ACR) defines a skeletal survey as "a sys-

tematically performed series of radiographic images that encompasses the entire skeleton or those anatomic regions appropriate for the clinical indications." There are three indications for a skeletal survey according to the ACR: suspected nonaccidental trauma (abuse), skeletal dysplasias, syndromes and metabolic disorders, and neoplasms. Fractures in the first year of life are relatively rare, so their occurrence might warrant a skeletal survey to rule out child abuse. Although 64% of all reported cases of maltreatment with major physical injury occur in patients 0 to 5 years of age, those with radiologic evidence of abusive injury will be younger than 2 years of age. Pediatric imaging departments have specific protocols that protect the patient when there is a suspicion or evidence of child abuse. The diagnosis of abuse becomes more likely when there is a discrepant history of minor trauma in a child with complex, multiple fractures. Although policies vary from institution to institution, the goal is

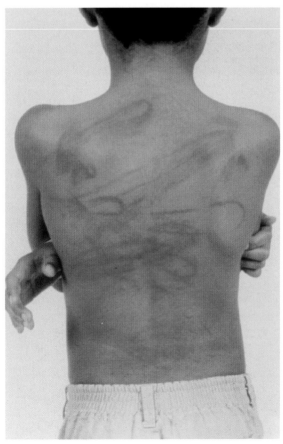

Fig. 24-48 Seven-year-old with loop marks representative of forceful blows by a looped belt.

always protection of the child. The nonaccidental traumas often present in the emergency room for other indications and when imaged are found to have fractures of a suspicious nature. A scenario may go something like this:

1. Parent and 9-month infant are seen in the emergency room (ER) where infant presents with shortness of breath, wheezing, and low-grade fever for 2 days.
2. Patient is assigned to an exam room for nurse/doctor interview, assessment, and physical examination.
3. Routine standard-of-care chest x-rays are ordered to rule out pneumonia.
4. Radiographer alerts radiologist to the presence of what appears to be two healing posterior rib fractures (Fig. 24-49) and corner fractures (Fig. 24-50).
5. Radiologist consults with a child protection team and ER attending.
6. Hospital social services are called to conduct an interview with the parent.
7. The hospital's child protection team, ER attending, and social worker explain the findings to the parent. The family is then escorted, by security, to radiology for an immediate skeletal survey.

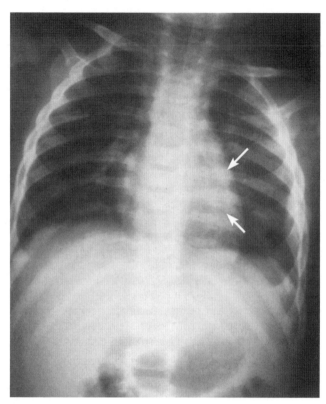

Fig. 24-49 Chest radiograph showing different stages of healing posterior rib fractures.

Depending on the findings, the infant may be admitted for care or removed from the home by Child Protective Services. Children presenting with emergent head trauma would be admitted and transferred to a surgical ICU. The abuse of a child is so repugnant that the urge to judge the parents will almost be reflexive; try to resist this temptation and stay focused on the very difficult and emotional task of providing medical care to the patient. Give a thorough explanation of what the skeletal survey entails: the time involved, the special accommodations that are provided for their infant, and inform them that the infant will cry. Allowing the parents to participate in the exam is a judgment call; overly emotional parents may be more of a hindrance, whereas calm parents may help to sooth their infant. The parents who will not be helping should be escorted to a nearby waiting room. The survey can be accomplished quickly and efficiently with experienced radiographers.

Due to the medicolegal sensitivity of the skeletal survey and to expedite the exam, it is always best to have three radiographers working the exam: one immobilizes and positions; the second sets technique, positions, shields, collimates, and makes the exposure; the third supplies the two-person team with image plates if CR, immobilization devices, processes, and assesses the quality of each image. A skeletal survey for nonaccidental trauma on infants younger than 1 year should be done on high-resolution mammography imaging plates using a dedicated processor. The table should have a pad with sheet, chucks, positioning sponges, pacifier, Sweeties (if not contraindicated), and gonadal shield. Have all supplies at the table or readily accessible within the room. The room should be warmed as appropriate and warming lights used as required. The radiology nurse should be aware that a survey is ongoing. All images are made with the infant lying on the IR (nothing is placed between the IR and patient). The patient can stay in a diaper, which will be removed when the abdomen/pelvis/femurs are imaged. Imaging should be timely, efficient, and repeats avoided. The radiologist accesses the images when the imaging is complete and will request additional images as needed.

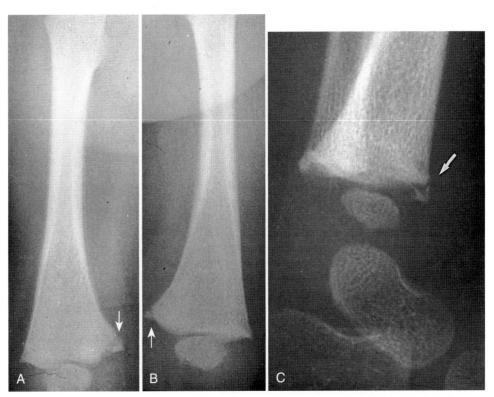

Fig. 24-50 Images demonstrating physical abuse. Left and right corner fractures (*arrows,* **A** and **B**) and bucket-handle fractures (*arrow,* **C**) are considered classic indicators of physical abuse in children. The bucket-handle appearance is subtle and demonstrated only if the "ring" is seen on profile (*arrow*).

Imaging Protocol at Boston Children's Hospital (BCH)

- For efficiency and for medicolegal reasons, two radiographers should be in the room when imaging.
- Only AP projections are required for long bones unless there is a positive finding (Tables 24-6 and 24-7)
- Equivocal findings in a long bone may necessitate a lateral projection.
- Hand images should be slightly obliqued rather than PA.
- Use mammography-imaging plates (increased resolution) and expose one body part per plate.
- Reduce motion by using the large focal spot, exposing only on expiration, with complete immobilization.
- All skeletal survey images should be done with 60 kVp (increased bony detail for CR-based systems).
- The 2-week follow-up exam does not require skull images.
- There should be nothing between the IR and the body part.
- Chest and abdominal images should overlap.

Table 24-6 is a skeletal survey protocol for nonincidental traumas of infants younger than 12 months is tabletop at 102 cm SID, using a large focal spot with bone technique and mammography imaging plates. Table 24-7 lists radiologic findings.

TABLE 24-6

Survey skeletal projections

AP and lateral skull (a positive finding may require right and left laterals and Townes)
AP and lateral chest
Bilateral shallow obliques of chest to show ribs
Abdomen (to overlap with chest)
AP bilateral femurs
AP bilateral tibias
AP bilateral feet
AP bilateral humeri
AP bilateral forearms
Bilateral hands, oblique 20 degrees
Lateral C spine
Lateral L spine

A positive finding may require laterals of extremities.

TABLE 24-7

Specificity of radiologic findings

High specificity
Metaphyseal lesions
Rib fractures, especially posterior
Scapular fractures
Spinous process fractures
Sternal fracture

Moderate specificity*
Multiple fractures, especially bilateral
Fractures of different ages
Epiphyseal separations
Vertebral body fractures and subluxations
Fractures of the digits
Complex skull fractures

Low specificity (but common)*
Clavicle fractures
Long bone shaft fractures
Linear skull fractures
Subperiostial new bone formation

*Moderate and low-specificity lesions become high when history of trauma is absent or inconsistent with injuries. Used with permission of Dr. Paul Kleinman, Boston Children's Hospital, Boston, MA.

Childhood Pathologies
OSTEOGENESIS IMPERFECTA

Osteogenesis imperfecta (OI) means "imperfectly formed bone." It is a serious but rare heritable or congenital disease of the skeletal system (20,000 to 50,000 cases in the United States). It results from a genetic defect on two genes that encode for type 1 collagen, the main collagen of osseous tissue, tendons, teeth, skin, inner ear, and sclera of the eyeballs. Although people with OI may have different combinations of symptoms, they all have weaker bones. Some common symptoms of OI include the following:

1. Short stature
2. Triangular-shaped face
3. Breathing problems
4. Hearing loss
5. Brittle teeth
6. Bone deformities, such as bowed legs or scoliosis

There are several types of OI, which vary in severity and symptoms and are classified as types I to IV.

Type I

Type I is the most common and mildest form. In this type the collagen is normal but is produced in reduced quantities. There is little or no bone deformity, although the bones remain fragile and easily broken. Teeth are prone to carries and are easily broken. The sclera of the eyes may have a purple, blue, or gray tint.

Type II

Type II is the most severe form of the disease, and many infants do not survive. The collagen suffers from the genetic defect, and bones may break in utero (Fig. 24-51).

Type III

Type III patients have improperly formed collagen, often with severe bone deformities, as well as other complications. The infant is often born with numerous fractures and tinting of the sclera. Children are generally shorter and have spinal deformities, respiratory complications, and brittle teeth.

Type IV

Type IV is moderately severe, and the collagen defect and bones, although easily fractured, are only mildly to moderately deformed. Some people may be shorter than average with brittle teeth.

Use verbal communication when imaging the patient with OI, being careful not to physically move or position the body. Let the patient position him- or herself or with the help of a parent to avoid causing new fractures. The caregiver or parent should do the transfer, changing, and aid in positioning. The exam table will require a radiolucent pad with sheet, a pillow, or towel under the patient's head, and radiolucent positioning devices to help support the patient. The radiographer should communicate the exact positioning required and then review the position before exposure. Positioning devices may be employed, but the family should place them. The radiographer will use his or her positional skills with the radiographic tube (move tube not patient) to obtain two projections differing by 90 degrees, thereby avoiding manipulating the part of interest. One of the reasons it is so important to ask the patient, "Is there anything I should know about your medical condition that would help me to help you?" is because the patient might have OI and it may not be indicated on the exam requisition. Although the omission of such critical information is hard to believe, it does happen; this is why we have "time-outs" before invasive procedures.

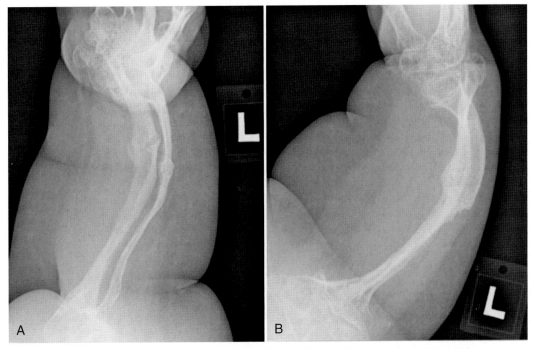

Fig. 24-51 Patients with OI are not only fragile, but their anatomy can be misshaped, making it difficult to determine what the correct position is for AP and lateral projections. AP and lateral projections of the left tibia and fibula.

PATHOLOGIC FRACTURES AND BENIGN AND MALIGNANT NEOPLASMS

Long bones, ribs, and facial bones are susceptible to fibrous displacement of their osseous tissue creating a benign condition called fibrous dysplasia. As these neoplasms grow, they erode the bone causing the cortices to thin and weaken, which may lead to pathologic fracture. These dysplasias can become filled with fluid and are then known as bone cysts, often occurring in the upper ends of the humeri, femurs, and tibias of children, which are usually located beneath the epiphysis traveling down the metaphysis as they grow. The cysts often appear as incidental findings from another exam or following a pathologic fracture. Radiographically they present as thin-walled lucencies with sharp boundaries.

Osteochondroma

One of three types of chondromas, also known as osteochondromas, does not appear in the fetal skeleton and is virtually nonexistent until the second year of life. Growing from the bone's shaft, the tumor widens the bone, weakening the cortex (Fig. 24-52). Covered in periosteum that is continuous with the bone shaft and with its tip covered by a proliferative cartilage cap, the exostosis usually grows away from the joint using a similar mechanism to that of the epiphysis; there is no involvement of the bone's epiphyseal ossification center. When the person reaches maturity, bone growth ceases as it does in the tumor. There can be secondary vascular and neural manifestations, the patient can present with pain and swelling, or, alternately, the patient may be asymptomatic.

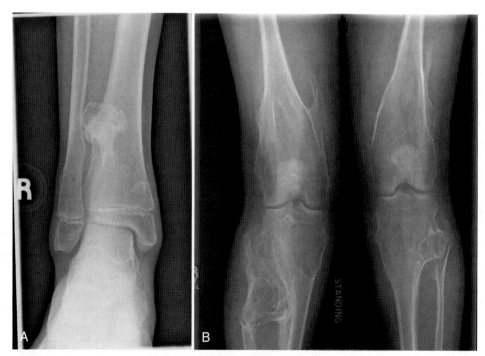

Fig. 24-52 A, A 14-year-old with a right, distal, tibial, pedunculated osteochondroma and deformation of distal fibula. **B,** Bilateral osteochondromas.

(Courtesy of Dr. George Taylor, Radiology, Boston Children's Hospital.)

Aneurysmal Bone Cyst (ABC)

Aneurysmal bone cyst (ABC) occurs in children and young adults and has an unknown etiology. Secondary ABCs make up about 50% of all cases, and there is preponderance in females. The most commonly affected sites are both long and short tubular bones (Fig. 24-53), neural arches of the vertebral bodies, pelvic, and facial bones. The cyst is composed of blood and connective tissue with connective tissue predominating as the ABC ages (see Fig. 26-34, B). The most characteristic radiologic finding is a thin shell of bone containing the dilated cyst. ABCs are classified into five types, I through V, and should be removed immediately due to their potential for rapid and extensive damage.

Osteoid Osteoma

A small, benign, ovoid tumor rarely exceeding 1 cm in diameter, osteoid osteomas occur most commonly in the tibia, femur, and the tubular bones of the hands (basal phalanges) and feet including their respective epiphyses (Fig. 24-54, A). About 90% of these lesions occur in the first 2 decades of life. Radiographically they appear as a well-circumscribed radiolucency with a density at the center (nidus) in the midst of extensive bony thickening and sclerosis. These tumors are hard to penetrate radiographically and may require an increased technique. Although the lesion rarely exceeds 1 cm in diameter, the sclerosis that accompanies it can reach to 2 cm. A lesion larger than 2 cm is most likely an osteoblastoma. Treatment of osteoid osteomas includes, but is not limited to, tetracycline localization in the nidus. Radio frequency ablation (RF) is another treatment option, in which an electrode tip at 90-degree centigrade is placed into the nidus for 6 minutes (Fig. 24-54, B).

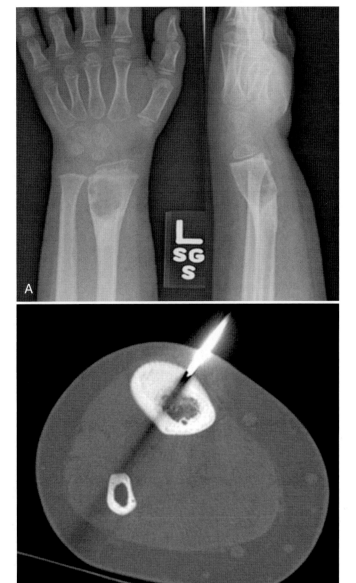

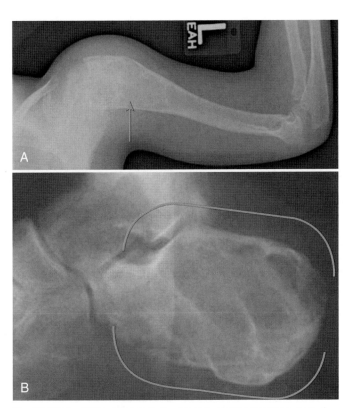

Fig. 24-53 A, ABC of the left proximal humerus *(orange arrow).* **B,** ABCs in the tarsus *(orange parentheses).*

Fig. 24-54 A, AP and lateral views of distal radial osteoid osteoma. **B,** Radio frequency ablation (RF) of an osteoid osteoma of the right tibia.

Malignant Neoplasms
Osteosarcoma

Alternatively known as osteogenic sarcoma, it is the most common of the primary malignant tumors. Usually appearing in the second decade of life, it usually begins in the center of the metaphysis, enlarges, and destroys the bone. Males seem to have a slight preponderance. The most common sites are the metaphysis of the proximal humeri and proximal tibias, and the femurs. The earliest presentations of this rapidly growing tumor are pain and swelling at the site. Pathologic fractures are not uncommon, and systemic signs attesting to its rapid growth are weight loss, anemia, and dilated surface veins at the site. The chief radiologic finding is an increase in ossification of the tumor tissue, which may present as an irregularly radiolucent, multiloculated mass. Metastases occur early, usually in the lungs, and chemotherapy increases the risk of secondary tumors, both sarcomas and osteosarcomas, after the treatment of the primary tumor. Bone sarcomas show a chromosome band that supports a recessively transmitted predisposition for this tumor and for retinoblastomas.

Ewing sarcoma

Occurring usually at the end of the first decade or beginning of the second, Ewing sarcoma is the second most common malignant tumor in children, and almost any bone in the body may be affected. These tumors grow most frequently in the ilium, femurs, humeri (Fig. 24-55), and tibias. Unlike most of the primary malignancies, Ewing sarcoma does present with fever, weakness, pallor, and lassitude in contrast to most of the primary malignancies. It is not an osteogenic tumor, and the distinctive radiographic findings are the normally opaque spongiosa and cortical bone replaced by more radiolucent tumor tissue with bone destruction, layered periosteal new bone (onion-skin), and overlying large and swollen soft-tissue mass.

PNEUMONIA

Pneumonia is the most frequent type of lung infection, resulting in inflammation with compromised pulmonary function. It ranks sixth among the leading causes of mortality in the United States and is the most lethal nosocomial infection. Viruses are the most common cause of both upper and lower respiratory tract infections, whereas bacteria account for about 5% of all childhood pneumonias. In children younger than 2 years old, 90% of cases are viral, with the respiratory syncytial virus (RSV) responsible for about a third of these cases. Viral or interstitial pneumonias are more common, usually less severe than bacterial pneumonia, and frequently caused by influenza. Radiographic findings are minimal, and the infection is usually confirmed clinically or through serologic tests.

Although chest images are important in determining the location of the inflammation, they are not definitive as to whether the causative agent is viral or bacterial; some knowledge of the suspected pathogens and their radiographic appearances can offer clues (Fig. 24-56). Pneumonias appear as soft, patchy, ill-defined alveolar infiltrates or pulmonary densities. The inflammation may affect the entire lobe of a lung (lobar pneumonia), a segment of a lung (segmental pneumonia), the bronchi and associated alveoli (bronchopneumonia), or the interstitial lung tissue (interstitial pneumonia).

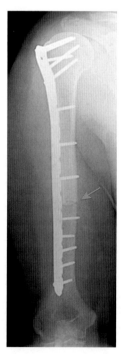

Fig. 24-55 Neutral view of right humerus postosteotomy and plating for Ewing osteosarcoma. (*Orange arrow* points to osteotomy site.)

The single most common pneumonia-producing bacterial agent in school-age children is *Mycoplasma pneumonia* (present in 40% to 60% of cases). Pneumococcal (lobar) pneumonia is the most common bacterial pneumonia, probably because the bacteria are present in our healthy throats. It presents on the image as a collection of fluid in one or more lobes; the degree of segmental involvement can usually be identified with a lateral view. Staphylococcal and streptococcal bacterial pneumonias are far less common. Staphy-

lococcal pneumonia occurs infrequently except during an epidemic of influenza, when it can be common and life threatening especially in infants. Streptococcal pneumonias are even more rare, accounting for less than 1% of all hospital admissions for acute bacterial pneumonia. Radiographic findings are localized around the bronchi, usually of the lower lobes.

Mycoplasma pneumonia is caused by mycoplasmas and is most common in older children and young adults. This disease appears as a fine reticular pattern

in a segmental distribution, followed by patchy areas of air space consolidation. In severe cases, the radiographic appearance may mimic tuberculosis. The morbidity rate associated with mycoplasma pneumonia is very low, even when the disease is not treated. Aspiration (chemical) pneumonia or chemical pneumonitis is caused by aspirated vomitus and appears on the image as densities radiating from either hila.

One of the most common challenges facing the radiologist is to rule out pneumonia. In most cases, the PA and lateral positions of the chest will suffice. In equivocal cases, the decubitus views are helpful in clarifying a suspected pulmonary abnormality. Images should be made with short exposure times (large focal spot) and must be inspiratory. Artifacts, possibly leading to a false positive, can be avoided with careful patient positioning, a peak inspiratory image, and ensuring the neonate's head is midline without any rotation. Pathologic conditions such as cystic fibrosis and asthma with atelectasis will distort the lung fields and could lead to an erroneous finding of pneumonia. Comparison to earlier images is essential to rule out residual or recurrent problems that might suggest an underlying abnormality. A pneumatocele (a thin-walled, radiolucent, air-containing cyst) is the characteristic radiographic lesion and is more typically seen in children. In later stages of the disease, these can enlarge, forming empyemas.

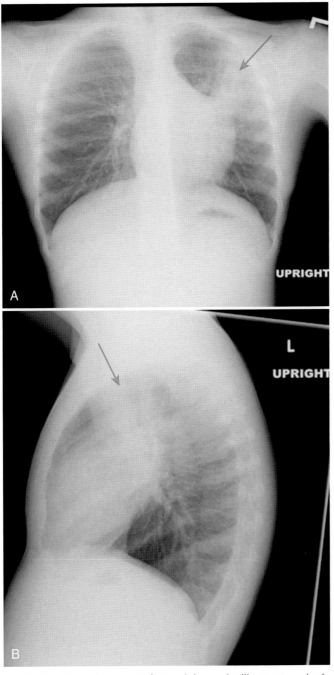

Fig. 24-56 PA and lateral chest images of an adolescent with pneumonia (*orange arrows*).

PROGERIA

Progeria is a rare combination of dwarfism and premature aging also known as Hutchison-Gilford syndrome. It is one of the many genetically based premature aging disorders that occur sporadically, with an incidence of 1 in 8 million births and a male-to-female ratio of 1.5:1. There is a strong racial susceptibility for Caucasians who represent 97% of patients. Derived from the Greek, meaning "prematurely old," the progeria patient ages up to 7 years for every year of life. These children fall within the expected growth percentile at birth, but after the first decade they have only achieved the stature of a 3 year old. The child's average life span is 13 years (range 7 to 27 years).

There is no cure for progeria, and death is mainly due to cardiovascular complications like myocardial infarction or congestive heart failure. Symptoms include scleroderma, loss of hair and subcutaneous fat, short stature (average 100 cm), low weight (12 to 15 kg), abnormal dentition, an increased prominence of scalp veins, coxa valga, and osteopenia (Fig. 24-57). Progeria is probably an autosomal recessive syndrome affecting the *LMNA* gene that produces a defective lamina A protein resulting in a weakened cell nucleus. This unstable nucleus apparently results in premature aging.

SCOLIOSIS

Scoliosis is an abnormal lateral curvature of the spine in excess of 10 degrees, which has a component of rotation, bringing the ribs anteriorly in the direction of the rotation, and affecting lung function in more serious cases (Fig. 24-59). The scoliotic curve may be simple or involve a compensating curve resulting in an "S" shape; the spinal curvature may occur on the right, the left, or both sides. In the greater population, between 3 and 5 children out of every 1000 develop a scoliosis that requires treatment. It affects girls about seven times more than boys, and idiopathic scoliosis tends to run in families, although no genetic link has been found. Scoliosis occurs, and is treated, as three main types.

Idiopathic

The most common type occurs mostly in preadolescent and adolescent girls; however, most cases either remain asymptomatic or the curves are too small to require treatment. Idiopathic scoliosis is comprised of three subtypes:

Adolescent. Represents the majority of cases, mostly in girls between 10 to 13 years old, and often requires no treatment.

Juvenile. Represents about 10% of cases in the age range of 3 to 9 years.

Infantile (early onset). Accounts for about 5% of cases, occurring in boys from birth to 3 years old and is mostly self-resolving.

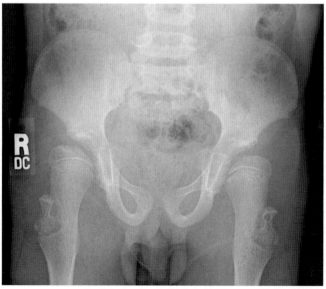

Fig. 24-57 A Progeria patient with osteopenia.

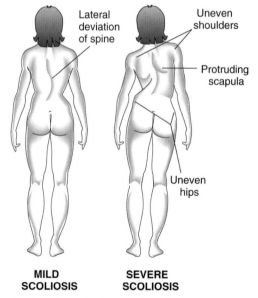

Fig. 24-58 Symptoms that suggest scoliosis.

(From VanMeter: *Gould's Pathophysiology for the Health Professions,* ed 5, St. Louis, 2014, Elsevier.)

Neuromuscular

This refers to scoliosis that is associated with disorders of the nerve or muscular systems (e.g., cerebral palsy, spina bifida, muscular dystrophy, or spinal cord injury).

Congenital

This is the least common form and occurs in utero between 3 and 6 weeks causing partial, missing, or fused vertebrae.

Scoliosis imaging

Usually indicated are standing *erect* AP and lateral images of the entire spine from the external auditory meatus (EAM) to the sacroiliac (SI) joints at 182 cm (see Volume I, Chapter 8, scoliosis projections, for references). The first PA image is without breast shields to allow for visualization of the ribs and spine in their entirety. The lateral view should always be protected, whether the patient is male or female, by the use of a shadow shield to cover the face and breast tissue, while being careful to avoid clipping the anterior C-spine and the anterior L-spine in lordotic patients, and must include the EAM. In subsequent PAs, breast tissue should be protected for both male and female patients by using a shadow shield; the inexperienced radiographer should consult the patient's previous PA images to determine the location and severity of the curve before shielding (Fig. 24-59).

Filtration should always be used to compensate for thickness and density differences of the C-spine and thoracic cavity, respectively. The C-spine filter is placed at the x-ray tube window, and its projection should begin at the top of the shoulders and extend superiorly. The thoracic filter, again mounted at the x-ray tube window, begins at the mid-horizontal line and extends superiorly. A hypersthenic patient will dictate the need for additional C-spine compensating filters. The patient should remove all piercings, be undressed, wearing only underwear or boxers (check to make sure females have removed their bras), a hospital gown, and socks. Posture should be as the patient normally carries himself or herself and erect. Sitting images are more involved and require care in patient transfer to the special scoliosis-imaging chair. Holding help will most likely be required, and the lateral position should have a positioning sponge between the patient's back and the holder for support. The patient's pelvis should be as close to the grid or sponge as possible. This can be difficult with cerebral palsy (CP) patients, as they tend to slide away from a support and may require that their knees be held so they cannot slide forward. If the patient's wheelchair has removable sides, some patients can be imaged in their chairs, but great care should be made to maintain *erect* posture. Make every attempt to shield these patients, although breast protection may not be possible due to the severity of the curve(s) and pelvic structure. A more advanced modality is the slot-scan EOS system (Biospace Med, Paris, France), which is covered later under "Advances in Technology."

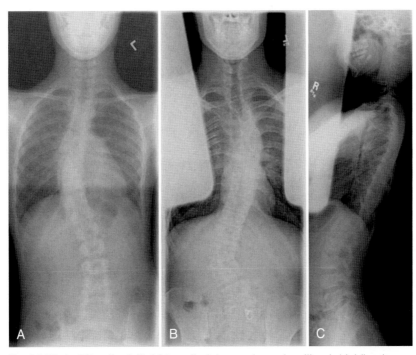

Fig. 24-59 A, Often the initial PA scoliosis image is made without shielding to reveal relationships of spine, ribs, and pelvis. **B,** Follow-ups (FU) require breast shields. **C,** Shadow shields for breast tissue and eyes and a secondary stand-shield are used with all lateral views unless ordered otherwise.

Cobb angle, patterns of scoliosis, and estimation of rotation

The degree of curvature is measured from the PA view using the Cobb method. The image is examined to see what type of curve is present—acute (fracture?), smooth and arcuate, lumbar or thoracic, single or double—and whether there are any rib or vertebral anomalies. To measure the Cobb angle, one identifies the curve's superior and inferior end vertebrae, which are the two vertebrae that tilt most severely toward the concavity of the curve. Straight lines are then drawn across the superior and inferior end plates of the curve's upper and lower end vertebrae; the lines extend toward the concavity. These lines will intersect off the image, making the Cobb angle impossible to measure, so to the right of the spine from each end plate line extend a perpendicular line until they both intersect. The angle superior to the intersection represents the Cobb angle. Once the Cobb angle is determined, an estimation of the degree of rotation can be determined with reference to the vertebrae at the apex of the curve.

Lateral bends

Pediatric patients scheduled for surgery will have bending images to assess the rigidity and flexibility of the curve(s). A left thoracolumbar curve would be considered the major curve (structural) if it failed to correct with either right or left bends. The lumbar curve on the same patient would be considered a compensatory curvature (nonstructural) if it corrects on the right bend. Once the patient has reached skeletal maturity, curves of less than 30 degrees will not progress.

Skeletal maturity

In pediatric radiology, evaluation of skeletal maturity is made on the basis of bone growth in an image of the left hand and wrist. In children with endocrine abnormalities and growth disorders, the determination of skeletal maturation (bone age) is important in their diagnosis and treatment. In clinical practice, bone age is most often obtained by comparing the image with a set of reference hand images from the atlas by Greulich and Pyle. This reference work is the result of a 1950s survey of a healthy, white, middle to upper class population. A study by Zhang[1] questioned the validity of using the Greulich and Pyle atlas for an ethnically diverse population and found that ethnic and racial differences in growth patterns exist at certain ages with both Asians and Hispanics; this was seen in both male and female subjects, especially in girls ages 10 to 13 years and boys ages 11 to 15 years.

Treatment options

Options for treatment of scoliosis range from observation and monitoring to physical therapy, bracing, casting, and surgery. Invasive treatments may include spinal fusion/instrumentation, dual posterior growing rods to control spinal deformity, rod lengthening for infantile scoliosis, thoracoscopic anterior spinal surgery and instrumentation, osteotomy, or a combination of surgical procedures.

---

[1]Zhang A: Racial differences in growth patterns of children assessed on the basis of bone age, *Radiology* 250:228, 2009.

Advances in Technology

RADIOGRAPHY

Although this technology has been available in Europe for some time, it has been approved in North America more recently. The EOS system (Biospace Med, Paris, France) (Figs. 24-60 and 24-61) for orthopedic imaging has three advantages over conventional x-ray–based systems according to the company:

1. Greatly reduced dose to patient
2. Allows three-dimensional modeling for evaluation of rotation, torsion, and orientation
3. Imaging is always on-axis and distortion free

EOS allows the slot-scan–based image to be made weight bearing, sitting (without assistance), and without the need for stitching. Various clinical parameters useful in evaluating and developing a patient's path to recovery are calculated automatically, including a patient report with images. Lower limb modeling is not adapted for patients younger than 15 years. Spine modeling is not adapted for patients 7 and younger or for the following pathologies: supernumerary vertebrae, congenital deformities, and spondylolisthesis.

MAGNETIC RESONANCE IMAGING

Many imaging centers routinely sedate young children before an MRI, incurring anesthesia costs, overnight admissions for infants, costs associated with sedation, anesthesia preparation, and recovery, and reduced patient and family satisfaction. To this end, BCH conducted two pilot studies during 2009 and 2010 to assess the feasibility of pediatric scans without sedation ("Try Without," unpublished); in the initial pilot, children between the ages of 5 and 7 were assessed, and in the second pilot children from 4 to 6 years and infants 0 to 6 months of age were assessed. With adequate preparation and age-appropriate distractions, some children under the age of 7 remained still without sedation for 20 to 60 minutes. Results showed that 88% of children between the ages of 5 and 7 and 82% of children 4 to 6 years old including infants 0 to 6 months completed their scans without sedation. Since 2010, 3300 children have completed their MRI scans without sedation. You will see more of this cost/benefit/patient satisfaction analysis in the future of health care.

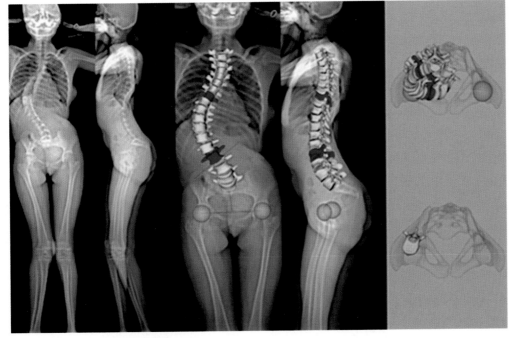

Fig. 24-60 EOS slot-scan standing scoliosis images of a 13-year-old female CP patient, with 3D remodeling showing axial rotation of individual vertebrae (e) and large lateral ejection of the apical vertebrae (f).

(Image courtesy of EOS Imaging, Cambridge, MA.)

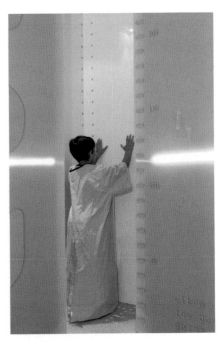

Fig. 24-61 Patient positioned for simultaneous acquisition of PA and lateral full spine views for scoliosis.

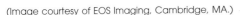

A "noiseless" MRI system (Silent Scan, GE Healthcare, Waukesha, WI) that scans at a noise level of about 4 dB, as compared to 86 to 110 dB with current technology, is available commercially; the reduced noise is the result of 3D MR acquisition, in combination with proprietary high-fidelity gradient and RF system electronics according to the company (Fig. 24-62). If this technology meets expectations, it could offer the potential for further reductions in sedation for younger patients.

ULTRASOUND

A wireless transducer (Siemens) is available that will transmit over a distance of 3 meters, which may assist with imaging infants and children. Called a point-of-care system, the transducer will expand the use of US in both interventional radiology and therapeutic applications. US has made huge advances through the years, but it is still largely constrained by bandwidth (0 to 50 MHz) and sensitivity. In a collaborative effort to overcome these limitations, Texas A&M University, King's College London, the Queen's University of Belfast, and the University of Massachusetts, Lowell, have developed a new meta-material that converts ultrasound waves into optical signals, making possible images with greater detail (0 to 150 MHz), maintaining sensitivity, and allowing one to see deeper into tissues.

COMPUTED TOMOGRAPHY

In pediatric patients, CT has been useful in diagnosing congenital anomalies, assessing metastases, and diagnosing bone sarcomas and sinus disease. Young children have difficulty following the instructions needed for a diagnostic scan. Suggestions regarding approach and atmosphere are presented at the beginning of this chapter. As in the care of any pediatric patient, the role of the CT radiographer is essential to the success of the examination; the radiographer must gain the respect and confidence of the young patient and the caregiver, if present. The CT scanner itself is an imposing piece of equipment that needs careful explanation to help allay the patient's fears. One of the most significant fears is claustrophobia, which can be reduced by the use of distraction devices like virtual goggles and music and creative room décor (Fig. 24-63).

Toshiba has unveiled its Aquilion One Vision 640-slice CT scanner. This new system is equipped with a gantry rotation of 0.275 seconds, a 100-kw generator, and 320 detector rows (640 unique slices) covering 16 cm in a single rotation, with the industry's thinnest slices at 500 microns (0.5 mm). The One Vision uses an alternating focal spot that allows 16-cm z-axis coverage to be sampled twice, generating 640 slices in one rotation. The system can accommodate larger patients with its 78-cm bore and fast rotation, including bariatric patients and patients with high heart rates. More slices and shorter scan times reduce the possibility of patient motion (cardiac CT) and allow for scanning bariatric patients or larger anatomy. The faster scan times should reduce the number of patients requiring sedation. The Image Gently campaign has suggested CT protocols for reducing CT dose to patients.

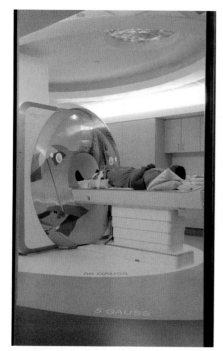

Fig. 24-62 MRI suite with Siemens Skyra scanner. This machine can be used for adults and children.

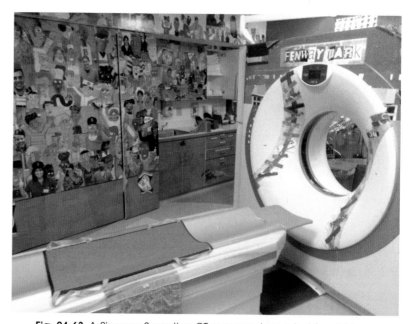

Fig. 24-63 A Siemens Sensation CT scanner decorated for children.

INTERVENTIONAL RADIOLOGY

Image-guided, minimally invasive interventional radiography (IR) has dramatically changed the role of the radiology department in teaching and nonteaching hospitals and clinics. In the past, the justifications and rationales for radiology departments were diagnostic ones. Radiology departments with interventional staff now offer hospitals therapeutic services in addition to diagnostic procedures. This heightened awareness has largely resulted from the nature and efficacy of interventional procedures. Therapeutic procedures performed in IR provide an attractive alternative to surgery for the patient, parent, hospital, and society. A procedure performed in IR is much less invasive and expensive than one performed in the operating room. Shortened inpatient stays for IR procedures translate into economic savings for the parents and hospital.

For simplicity, interventional radiology can be divided into vascular and nonvascular procedures. Vascular procedures are generally performed in angiographic suites. During these therapeutic interventions, angiography and ultrasonography are also performed for diagnostic and guidance purposes. Angiography can be arterial or venous; pediatric vasculature is well suited to both. IV injection of contrast media is favored in infants because their relatively small blood volume and rapid circulation allow for good vascular imaging. In infants, hand injections are often preferred over power injections to help avoid extravasation. Intraarterial digital subtraction angiography (DSA) (see Chapter 23) has become a valuable tool. DSA is performed using a diluted contrast medium, which can reduce pain. Road mapping is a software tool, available on newer angiographic equipment, that uses the intraarterial contrast injection and fluoroscopy to display arterial anatomy—a useful tool for imaging tortuous vessels.

Vascular procedures can be neurologic, cardiac, or systemic in nature. Nonvascular procedures often involve the digestive and urinary systems; examples include the insertion of gastrostomy tubes to supplement the nutrition of pediatric patients and insertion of cecostomy tubes in chronically constipated patients with spina bifida. Vascular access devices are of three types: nontunneled, tunneled, and implanted. The selection of device is often determined by a combination of factors, including the purpose of the access and estimated indwelling time. The physician or patient may choose a particular device after assessing issues of compliance or underlying clinical factors.

Nontunneled catheters are commonly referred to as *peripherally inserted central catheters (PICCs)*. They are available with single or multiple lumens. The insertion point is usually the basilic or cephalic vein, at or above the antecubital space of the nondominant arm. Multiple lumens are desirable when a variety of medications (including total parenteral nutrition) are to be administered (Fig. 24-64). These devices must be strongly anchored to the skin because children often pull on and displace the catheters, resulting in damage to the line and potential risk to themselves.

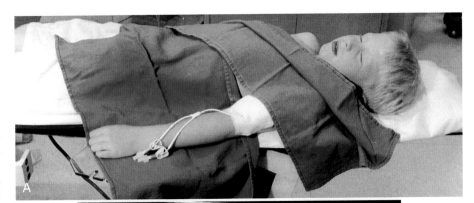

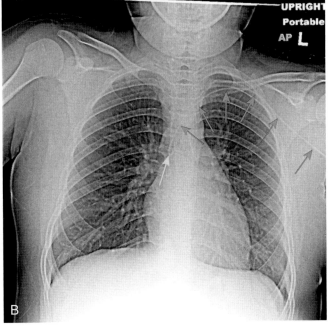

Fig. 24-64 A, Postinsertion image of a double-lumen PICC in a 7-year-old boy (shown in the interventional suite). Conscious sedation was used for this procedure. **B,** Left-sided PICC. Orange arrows track the double lumen PICC to its terminus (yellow arrow) in the superior vena cava (SVC).

Tunneled catheters, as with PICCs, can have multiple lumens. In contrast to PICCs they are not inserted into the peripheral circulation; rather, they are inserted via a subcutaneous tunnel into the subclavian or internal jugular veins. The tunneling acts as an anchoring mechanism for the catheter to facilitate long-term placement (Fig. 24-65). Tunneled catheters are used to administer chemotherapy, antibiotics, fluids, and hemodialysis and are referred to as Hickman lines when placed in subclavian or internal jugular veins.

Implanted devices are often referred to as ports. These are titanium or polysulfone devices with silicone centers attached to catheters. The whole device is implanted subcutaneously with the distal end of the catheter tip advanced to the superior vena cava or right atrium. A port is the device of choice for noncompliant patients, and children and adults who are undergoing chemotherapy and for aesthetic purposes or long-term use would rather not have the limb of a catheter protruding from their chest (Fig. 24-66).

Vascular access devices have dramatically changed the course of treatment for many patients in a positive way. Patients who would have previously been hospitalized for antibiotic therapy can now go home with the device in place and resume normal activity. The increased prevalence of these devices means that patients with vascular access devices are in the community and visiting radiology departments everywhere. PICCs have a smaller likelihood of introducing catheter-related infections; tunneled lines present a greater risk.

Radiographers must recognize vascular access devices and treat them with utmost care. They should report dislodged bandages and sites showing signs of infection (i.e., redness, exudate immediately). Catheter-related infections constitute the largest nosocomial source of infection; they can be life threatening and cost hospitals hundreds of thousands of dollars each year.

Postprocedural care vascular access devices currently represent a significant and ongoing challenge for all personnel who treat, manage, and come in contact with these patients.

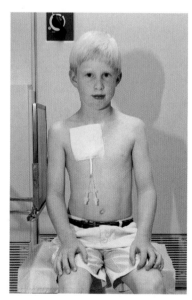

Fig. 24-65 External appearance of tunneled, double-lumen central venous access device. These catheters are used for long-term therapy. Their short track to the heart can increase the risk of infection, necessitating proper care for maintenance.

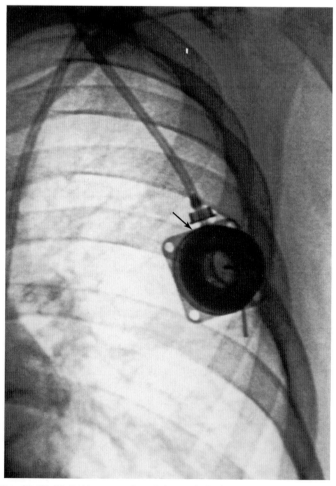

Fig. 24-66 Digital image of port (arrow). Ports are vascular devices that must be accessed subcutaneously. They are preferred for active children and for aesthetic reasons.

ACKNOWLEDGMENTS

To all who came before us and shared their knowledge and the many people who gave willingly of their time, experience, and expertise: George Taylor, MD, Department of Radiology, Boston Children's Hospital (BCH); Jeanne Chow, MD, Department of Radiology, BCH; Carol Barnewolt, MD, Department of Radiology, BCH; Alison Ames, RT(R), outpatient supervisor, Department of Radiology, BCH; Judith Santora, RT(R), inpatient supervisor, Department of Radiology, BCH; Richard Cappick, RT(R), CT, CT modality operations manager, Department of Radiology, BCH; Diane Biagiotti, BS, RT(R), MRI modality operations manager, Department of Radiology, BCH.

Selected bibliography

Coley BD: *Caffey's Pediatric Diagnostic Imaging,* ed 12, St. Louis, MO, 2013, Elsevier.

Centers for Disease Control, Autism Spectrum Disorders, Available at: http://www.cdc.gov/ncbddd/autism/facts.html. Accessed 2014.

Erikson EH: *Childhood and society,* New York, 1993, WW Norton & Company.

Godderidge C: *Pediatric imaging,* Philadelphia, 1985, WB Saunders.

Gray C, White AL: *My social stories book,* 2002, Jessica Kingsley.

Hudson J: *Prescription for success: supporting children with ASD in the medical environment,* 2006, Autism Asperger Publishing Company.

Kleinman PK: *Diagnostic imaging of child abuse,* Baltimore, 1987, Williams & Wilkins, p 2.

Kreiborg S: Postnatal growth and development of the craniofacial complex in premature craniosynostosis. In Cohen MM Jr, MacLean RE, editors: *Craniosynostosis: diagnosis, evaluation and management,* New York, 2000, Oxford University Press, pp 158-170.

Kwan-Hoong Ng, Cameron JR: *Using the BERT Concept top promote public understanding of radiation.* International conference on the radiological protection of patients. Organized by the International Atomic Energy Agency, Malaga, Spain, March 26-30, 2001, C&S Paper Series 7, pp 784-787.

Mace JD, Kowalczyk N: *Radiographic pathology for technologists,* ed. 4, St. Louis, MO, 2004, Mosby, pp 23-24.

Morton-Cooper A: *Health care and the autism spectrum: a guide for health professionals, parents and careers,* 2004, Jessica Kingsley. Available from the NAS Publications Department.

Silverman F et al: The limbs. In *Caffey's pediatric X-ray diagnosis: an integrated approach,* vol 2, ed 9, St. Louis, MO, 1993, Mosby, pp 1881-1884.

Volkmar FR, Wiesner LA: *Healthcare for children on the autism spectrum: a guide to medical, nutritional and behavioural issues,* Bethesda, MD, 2004, Woodbine House.

Advances in Technology

25

GERIATRIC RADIOGRAPHY

SANDRA J. SELLNER-WEE
CHERYL MORGAN-DUNCAN

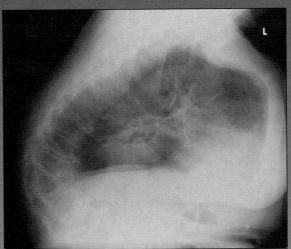

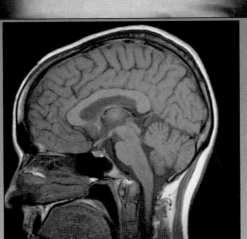

OUTLINE

Demographics and Social Effects of Aging, 162

Elder Abuse, 165

Attitudes toward the Older Adult, 165

Physical, Cognitive, and Psychosocial Effects of Aging, 166

Physiology of Aging, 168

Patient Care, 175

Performing the Radiograph Procedure, 176

Radiographic Positioning for Geriatric Patients, 177

Conclusion, 182

Geriatrics is the branch of medicine dealing with the aged and the problems of aging individuals. The field of *gerontology* includes illness prevention and management, health maintenance, and promotion of quality of life for aging individuals. The ongoing increase in the number of people older than age 65 in the U.S. population is well known. An even more dramatic aging trend exists among people older than 85 years. The number of people 100 years old is approximately 100,000 and increasing. Every aspect of the health care delivery system is affected by this shift in the general population. The 1993 Pew Health Commission Report noted that the "aging of the nation's society and the accompanying shift to chronic care that is occurring foretell major shifts in care needs in which allied health professionals are major providers of services." As members of the allied health professions, radiographers are an important component of the health care system. As the geriatric population increases, so does the number of medical imaging procedures performed on older adult patients. Students and practitioners must be prepared to meet the challenges that this dramatic shift in patient popula-tion represents. An understanding of geri-atrics can foster a positive interaction between the radiographer and the older adult patient.

Demographics and Social Effects of Aging

The acceleration of the "gray" American population began when individuals born from 1946 to1964 (known as the "baby boomers") began to turn age 50 in 1996. The number in the age 65 and older cohort is expected to reach 70.2 million by 2030 (Fig. 25-1). The U.S. experience regard-ing the increase in the older adult popula-tion is not unique; it is a global one. As of 1990, 28 countries had more than 2 million persons older than 65, and 12 additional countries had more than 5 million people older than 65. The entire older adult population of the world has begun a pre-dicted dramatic increase for the period 1995-2030.

Research on a wide variety of topics ranging from family aspects of aging, eco-nomic resources, and the delivery of long-term care states that gender, race, ethnicity, and social class have consistently influ-enced the quality of the experience of aging. The experience of aging results from the interaction of physical, mental, social, and cultural factors. Aging varies across cultures. Culturally, aging and the treatment of health problems in older adults are often determined by the values of an ethnic group. Culture also may determine the way the older person views the process of aging and the manner in which he or she adapts to growing older. A more heterogeneous older adult popula-tion than any generation that preceded it can be expected as a result of increasing immigration from nonwhite countries and a lower fertility and reproductive rate among the white population. This group will contain a mix of cultural and ethnic backgrounds. The United States is a mul-ticultural society in which a generalized view of aging would be difficult. *Health care professionals need to know not only diseases and disorders common to a spe-cific age group but also the disorders common to a particular ethnic group.* An appreciation of diverse backgrounds can help the health care professional provide a personal approach when dealing with and meeting the needs of older adult patients. Many universities are incorporat-ing cultural diversity into their curricula.

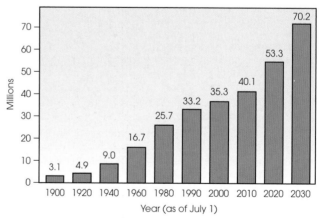

Fig. 25-1 Number of persons older than 65 years in millions, 1900-2030.

(Reprinted from U.S. Department of Commerce, Economics and Statistics Administration: *65+ in the United States,* Washington, DC, 1996, U.S. Bureau of the Census.)

The *economic status* of older adults varies and has an important influence on their health and well-being (Fig. 25-2). Most older adults have an adequate income, but many minority patients do not. Single older adults are more likely to be below the poverty line. Economic hardships increase for single older adults, especially women. Of the population older than age 85, 60% is composed of women, making women twice as likely as men to be poor. By age 75, nearly two thirds of women are widows. Financial security is extremely important to an older adult. Many older adults are reluctant to spend money on what others may consider necessary for their well-being. A problem facing aging Americans is health care finances. Older adults often base decisions regarding their health care not on their needs but exclusively on the cost of health care services.

An increase in health care and the aging population go hand in hand. Heart disease, cancer, and stroke account for 7 of every 10 deaths among people older than 65. By 2025, an estimated two thirds of the U.S. health care budget will be devoted to services for older adult patients.

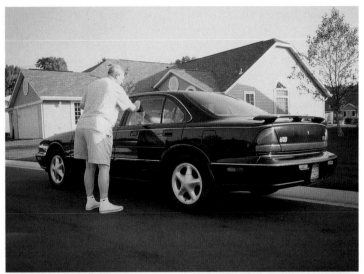

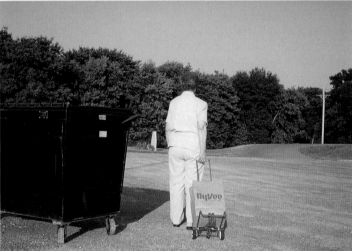

Fig. 25-2 The economic status of older adults varies and is an important influence on their health and well-being.

Aging is a broad concept that includes physical changes in people's bodies over adult life; psychological changes in their minds and mental capacities; social psychological changes in what they think and believe; and social changes in how they are viewed, what they expect, and what is expected of them. Aging is a constantly evolving concept. Notions that biologic age is more critical than chronologic age when determining health status of the older adult are valid. Aging is an individual and extremely variable process. The functional capacity of major body organs varies with advancing age. Environmental and lifestyle factors affect the age-related functional changes in the body organs. Advancements in medical technology have extended the average life expectancy in the United States by nearly 20 years since the 1960s, which has allowed senior citizens to be actively involved in every aspect of American society. People are healthier longer today because of advanced technology; the results of health promotion and secondary disease prevention; and lifestyle factors, such as diet, exercise, and smoking cessation, which have been effective in reducing the risk of disease (Fig. 25-3). Most older adult patients seen in the health care setting have been diagnosed with at least one chronic condition. Individuals who in the 1970s would not have survived a debilitating illness such as cancer or a catastrophic health event such as a heart attack can now live for more extended periods, sometimes with various concurrent debilitating conditions. Although age is the most consistent and strongest predictor of risk for cancer and for death from cancer, management of an older adult cancer patient becomes complex because other chronic conditions, such as osteoarthritis, diabetes, chronic obstructive pulmonary disease, and heart disease, must also be considered in their care. Box 25-1 lists the top 10 chronic conditions for people older than 65 years.

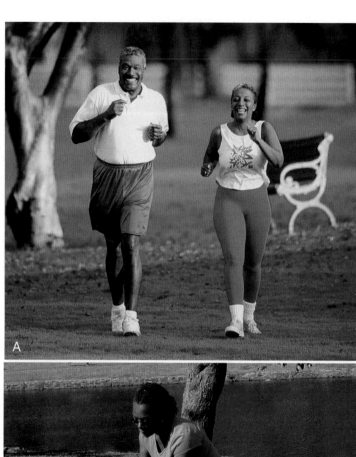

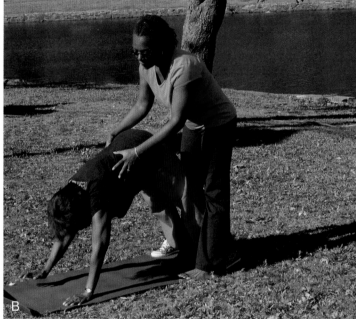

Fig. 25-3 A, Lifestyle factors—such as diet, exercise, and smoking cessation—reduce the risk of disease and increase life span. **B,** Yoga emphasizes breathing and slow, low-impact motion, which are good for those with arthritis.

BOX 25-1

Top 10 chronic conditions of people older than 65 years

Arthritis
Hypertension
Hearing impairment
Heart disease
Cataracts
Deformity or orthopedic impairment
Chronic sinusitis
Diabetes
Visual impairment
Varicose veins

Elder Abuse

Another emerging worldwide issue of older adults is elder abuse. It has been estimated that 2.1 million cases of elder abuse are reported each year. These numbers may be suspect, however, because studies estimate that only one in five cares is reported to the authorities. It is thought that elder abuse is approximately as common as child abuse. Elder abuse is defined as the knowing, intentional, or negligent act by a caregiver or any other person that causes harm or a serious risk of harm to a vulnerable adult. Box 25-2 lists the various types of abuse. The typical victim of abuse is older than 75 years. Most studies of elder abuse show the incidence to be gender neutral. Physical abuse is usually received from the victim's spouse (50%), less often from the victim's children (23%), and only in 17% of cases is the abuse from nonfamily caregivers.

The radiologic technologist should be aware that the presence of injury is not proof of abuse. It is important to be watchful for the warning signs of abuse or neglect listed in Box 25-3. The older adult is often embarrassed by the situation and may be hesitant to communicate his or her concerns for fear of retaliation. The technologist needs to employ excellent communication skills, accurate documentation, and quality radiographs, and the technologist should report any suspicions of neglect or abuse. Injuries sustained by older adult victims are typically to the head, face, and neck as well as defensive injuries.

Attitudes toward the Older Adult

The attitudes of health care providers toward older adults affect their health care. Research indicates that health care professionals have significantly more negative attitudes toward older patients than younger ones. This attitude must change if health care providers are to have positive interactions with older adult patients. These attitudes seem to be related to the pervasive stereotyping of the older adult, which serves to justify avoiding care and contact with them, as well as the older adults being reminders of one's own mortality. *Ageism* is a term used to describe the stereotyping of and discrimination against older adults and is considered to be similar to that of racism and sexism. Ageism emphasizes that frequently older adults are perceived to be repulsive and that distaste for the aging process itself exists. Ageism suggests that most older adults are senile, miserable most of the time, and dependent rather than independent individuals. The media have also influenced ongoing stereotypic notions about older adults. Commercials target older adults as consumers of laxatives and wrinkle creams and other products that promise to prolong their condition of being younger, more attractive, and desirable. Television sitcoms portray the older adult as stubborn and eccentric. Health care providers must learn to appreciate the positive aspects of aging so that they can assist older adult patients in having positive experiences with imaging procedures.

BOX 25-2

Forms of elder abuse

Physical: inflicting physical pain or injury
Sexual: nonconsensual sexual contact of any kind
Neglect: failure by those responsible to provide food, shelter, health care, or protection
Exploitation: illegal taking, misuse, or concealment of funds, property, or assets of a senior
Emotional: inflicting mental pain, anguish, or distress through verbal or nonverbal acts
Abandonment: desertion of a vulnerable older adult by anyone who has assumed the responsibility for care or custody of that person
Self-neglect: failure of a person to perform essential, self-care tasks, which threatens his or her own health or safety

---

BOX 25-3

Warning signs of elder abuse

- Bruises, pressure marks, broken bones, abrasions, and burns may be an indication of physical abuse, neglect, or mistreatment
- Unexplained withdrawal from normal activities, sudden change in alertness, and unusual depression may be indicators of emotional abuse
- Bruises around the breasts or genital area may occur from sexual abuse
- Sudden changes in financial situations may be the result of exploitation
- Bedsores, unattended medical needs, poor hygiene, and unusual weight loss may be indicators of possible neglect
- Behavior such as belittling, threats, and other uses of power and control by a caregiver may be an indicator of verbal or emotional abuse
- Strained or tense relationships, frequent arguments between caregiver and older adult

A 1995 study by Rarey concluded that most of 835 radiographers surveyed in California were not well informed about gerontologic issues and were not prepared to meet the needs of their patients older than age 65.[1] Reuters Health reported from a Johns Hopkins study that medical students generally have poor knowledge and understanding of older adults, and this translates to an inferior quality of care for older patients. More education in gerontology is necessary for radiographers and physicians. Education would enable health care providers to adapt imaging and therapeutic procedures to accommodate mental, emotional, and physiologic alterations associated with aging and to be sensitive to cultural, economic, and social influences in the provision of care for older adult patients.

Physical, Cognitive, and Psychosocial Effects of Aging

The human body undergoes a multiplicity of physiologic changes second by second. Little consideration is given regarding these changes unless they are brought on by sudden physical, psychological, or cognitive events. Each older adult is a unique individual with distinct characteristics. These individuals have experienced a life filled with memories and accomplishments.

Young or old, the definition of quality of life is an individual and personal one. Research has shown that health status is an excellent predictor of happiness. Greater social contact, health satisfaction, low vulnerable personality traits, and fewer stressful life events have been linked to successful aging. *Self-efficacy* can be defined as the level of control one has over one's future. Many older adults feel they have no control over medical emergencies and fixed incomes. Many have fewer choices about their personal living arrangements. These environmental factors can lead to depression and decreased self-efficacy. An increase in illness usually parallels a decrease in self-efficacy.

Older adults may experience changing roles from a life of independence to dependence. The family dynamic of a parent caring for children and grandchildren may evolve into the children caring for the aging parent. Older adulthood is also a time of loss. Losses may include the death of a spouse and friends and loss of income owing to retirement. Loss of health may be the reason for the health care visit. The overall loss of control may lead to isolation and depression in the older adult. Death and dying are also imminent facts of life.

A positive attitude is an important aspect of aging. Many older people have the same negative stereotypes about aging that young people do.[1] For them, feeling "down" and depressed becomes a common consequence of aging. One of five people older than age 65 in a community shows signs of clinical depression. Yet health care professionals know that depression can affect young and old. Research has shown most older adults rate their health status as good to excellent. How older adults perceive their health status depends largely on their successful adaptation to disabilities.

Radiographers need to be sensitive to the fact that an older adult may have had to deal with many social and physical losses in a short period. More important, they must recognize symptoms resulting from these losses to communicate and interact effectively with these patients.

Although as a health care provider the radiographer's contribution to a patient's quality of life may be minimal, it is not insignificant. The radiographer must remember that each older adult is unique and deserves respect for his or her own opinions.

---

[1]Rarey LK: Radiologic technologists' responses to elderly patients, *Radiol Tech* 69:566, 1996.

[1]Rowe JW, Kahn RL: *Successful aging*, New York, 1999, Dell.

The aging process alone does not likely alter the essential core of the human being. Physical illness is not aging, and age-related changes in the body are often modest in magnitude. As one ages, the tendencies to prefer slower-paced activities, take longer to learn new tasks, become more forgetful, and lose portions of sensory processing skills increase slowly but perceptibly. Health care professionals need to be reminded that *aging and disease are not synonymous.* The more closely a function is tied to physical capabilities, the more likely it is to decline with age, whereas the more a function depends on experience, the more likely it will increase with age. Box 25-4 lists the most common health complaints of older adults.

Joint stiffness, weight gain, fatigue, and loss of bone mass can be slowed through proper nutritional interventions and low-impact exercise. The importance of exercise cannot be overstated. Exercise has been shown to increase aerobic capacity and mental speed. Exercise programs designed for older adults should emphasize increased strength, flexibility, and endurance. One of the best predictors of good health in later years is the number and extent of healthy lifestyles that were established in earlier life.

An older adult may show decreases in attention skills during complex tasks. Balance, coordination, strength, and reaction time all decrease with age. Falls associated with balance problems are common in the older adult population, resulting in a need to concentrate on walking. *Not overwhelming older adults with instructions is helpful.* Their hesitation to follow instructions may be a fear instilled from a previous fall. Sight, hearing, taste, and smell all are sensory modalities that decline with age. Older people have more difficulty with bright lights and tuning out background noise. Many older adults become adept at lip reading to compensate for loss of hearing. For radiographers to assume that all older adult patients are hard of hearing is not unusual; they are not. Talking in a normal tone, while making volume adjustments only if necessary, is a good rule of thumb. Speaking slowly, directly, and distinctly when giving instructions allows older adults an opportunity to sort through directions and improves their ability to follow them with better accuracy (Fig. 25-4).

Cognitive impairment in older adults can be caused by disease, aging, and disuse. *Dementia* is defined as progressive cognitive impairment that eventually interferes with daily functioning. It includes cognitive, psychological, and functional deficits including memory impairment. With normal aging comes a slowing down and a gradual wearing out of bodily systems, but normal aging does not include dementia. Yet the prevalence of dementia increases with age. Persistent disturbances in cognitive functioning, including memory and intellectual ability, accompany dementia. *Fears of cognitive loss, especially Alzheimer's disease, are widespread among older people.*

Alzheimer's disease is the most common form of dementia. Health care professionals are more likely to encounter people with this type. Most older adults work at maintaining and keeping their mental functions by staying active through mental games and exercises and keeping engaged in regular conversation. When caring for patients with any degree of dementia, verbal conversation should be inclusive and respectful. One should never discuss these patients as though they are not in the room or are not active participants in the procedure.

BOX 25-4

Most common health complaints of older adults

Weight gain
Fatigue
Loss of bone mass
Joint stiffness
Loneliness

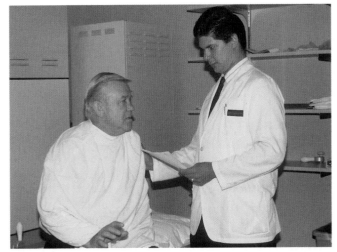

Fig. 25-4 Speaking slowly, directly, and distinctly when giving instructions allows older adults an opportunity to sort through directions and improves their ability to follow them with better accuracy.

One of the first questions asked of any patient entering a health care facility for emergency service is, "Do you know where you are and what day it is?" Health care providers need to know just how alert the patient is. Although memory does decline with age, this is experienced mostly with short-term memory tasks. Long-term memory or subconscious memory tasks show little change over time and with increasing age. There can be various reasons for confusion or disorientation. Medication, psychiatric disturbance, or retirement can confuse the individual. For some older people, retirement means creating a new set of routines and adjusting to them. Most older adults like structure in their lives and have familiar routines for approaching each day.

Physiology of Aging

Health and well-being depend largely on the degree to which organ systems can successfully work together to maintain internal stability. With age, there is apparently a gradual impairment of these homeostatic mechanisms. Older adults experience nonuniform, gradual, ongoing organ function failure in all systems. Many of the body organs gradually lose strength with advancing age. These changes place older adults at risk for disease or dysfunction, especially in the presence of stress. At some point, the likelihood of illness, disease, and death increases. Various physical diseases and disorders affect the mental and physical health of people of all ages. They are more profound among older adults because diseases and disorders among older people are more likely to be chronic in nature. *Although aging is inevitable, the aging experience is highly individual and is affected by heredity, lifestyle choices, physical health, and attitude.* A great portion of usual aging risks can be modified with positive shifts in lifestyle.

AGING OF THE ORGAN SYSTEMS
Integumentary system disorders
Disorders of the integumentary system are among the first apparent signs of aging.

The most common skin diseases among older adults are herpes zoster (shingles), malignant tumors, and decubitus ulcers. With age comes flattening of the skin membranes, making it vulnerable to abrasions and blisters. The number of melanocytes decreases, making ultraviolet light more dangerous, and the susceptibility to skin cancer increases. Wrinkling and thinning skin are noticeable among older adults; this is attributable to decreases in collagen and elastin in the dermis. A gradual loss of functioning sweat glands and skin receptors occurs, which increases the threshold for pain stimuli, making an older adult vulnerable to heat strokes. With age comes atrophy or thinning of the subcutaneous layer of skin in the face, back of the hands, and soles of the feet. Loss of this "fat pad" can cause many foot conditions in older adults.

The most striking age-related changes to the integumentary system are the graying, thinning, and loss of hair. With age, the number of hair follicles decreases, and the follicles that remain grow at a slower rate with less concentration of melanin, causing the hair to become thin and white. A major problem with aging skin is chronic exposure to sunlight. The benefits of protecting one's skin with sunscreen and protective clothing cannot be overemphasized and become more evident as one grows older. The three most common skin tumors in older adults are basal cell carcinoma, malignant melanoma, and squamous cell carcinoma.

Nervous system disorders
The nervous system is the principal regulatory system of all other systems in the body. It is probably the least understood of all body systems. Central nervous system disorders are among the most common causes of disability in older adults, accounting for almost 50% of disability in individuals older than age 65. Loss of myelin in axons the nervous system contributes to the decrease in nerve impulse velocity that is noted in aging. One such condition of the nervous system decline is Alzheimer's disease, which is known to be the most common form of dementia. More than 5 million Americans currently suffer from the disease, and it is estimated that this number will rise to about 13 million by 2050. Though there exist drug remedies and therapies, and lifestyle modification to stifle its progress, there is no cure for the disease.

In the healthy brain, an intricate network of billions of nerve cells communicate using electrical signals that regulate thoughts, memories, sensory perception, and movement. In Alzheimer's patients, brain cells die when genes and other factors cause the formation of an amyloid protein, which eventually breaks up and forms plaques—the hallmark of Alzheimer's disease. These plaques ultimately lead to the destruction of brain cells. Once the brain cells are destroyed, neural connections are shut down, causing decreased cognitive functions. Other known risk factors of this disease are, of course, age and family history. The greatest risk factor for this disease is increasing age. After age 65, the risk doubles every 5 years. After age 85, the risk is nearly 50%.

Although family history increases the risk for getting the disease, there are a large number of Alzheimer's patients with no family history, suggesting that there are other factors influencing the development of the disease. In addition to the Alzheimer's gene, there is some evidence that some forms of the disease may be due to a "slow virus"; it is also possible that the disorder is caused by an accumulation of toxic metals in the brain or by the absence of certain kinds of endogenous brain chemicals.

Health experts inarguably propose that as the baby boomers become closer to the age where they may contract the disease, Medicare will become burdened with an estimated $626 billion dollars more in Alzheimer's-related health care cost. There is also the considerable psychological burden that is attached to this debilitating disease: adults are becoming more concerned that the disease will affect them or someone they know.

Current attempts to detect Alzheimer's disease include imaging procedures such as structural imaging with magnetic resonance imaging (MRI) or computed tomography (CT). These tests are currently used to rule out other conditions that may cause symptoms similar to Alzheimer's but require different treatment options. As for functional imaging of Alzheimer's disease, position emission tomography (PET) scans show diminished brain cell activity in the regions affected. Molecular imaging research studies are aggressively being pursued, because they promise to detect biologic cues indicating early stage Alzheimer's before it alters the brain's structure or function and causes irreversible loss of memory or the ability to reason and think.

Similar to any other organ system, the nervous system is vulnerable to the effects of atherosclerosis with advancing age. When blood flow to the brain is blocked, brain tissue is damaged. Repeated episodes of cerebral infarction can eventually lead to multi-infarct dementia. The changes in the blood flow and oxygenation to the brain slow down the time to carry out motor and sensory tasks requiring speed, coordination, balance, and fine motor hand movements. This decrease in the function of motor control puts the older adult at a higher risk for falls. Healthy changes in lifestyle can reduce the risk of disease. High blood pressure is a noted risk and can be decreased with medication, weight loss, proper nutritional diet, and exercise.

Sensory system disorders

All of the sensory systems undergo changes with age. Beginning around age 40, the ability to focus on near objects becomes increasingly difficult. The lens of the eye becomes less pliable, starts to yellow, and becomes cloudy, resulting in farsightedness *(presbyopia)*. Distorted color perception and cataracts also occur. Changes in the retina affect the ability to adapt to changes in lighting, and the ability to tolerate glare decreases, making night vision more difficult for older adults.

Hearing impairment is common in older adults. The gradual progressive hearing loss of tone discrimination is called *presbycusis*. Men are affected more often than women, and the degree of loss is more severe for high-frequency sounds. Speech discrimination is problematic when in noisy surroundings, such as a room full of talking people.

There is a decline in sensitivity to taste and smell with age. The decline in taste is consistent with a decreased number of taste buds on the tongue, decreased saliva, and dry mouth that accompany the aging process.

Hyposmia is the impairment of the ability to smell. It accounts for much of the decreased appetite and irregular eating habits that are noted consistently in older adults. Similar to taste, the degree of impairment varies with a particular odor, and the ability to identify odors in a mixture is gradually lost with age.

Musculoskeletal system disorders

Musculoskeletal dysfunction is the major cause of disability in older adults. Osteoporosis, the reduction in bone mass and density, is one of the most significant age-related changes. Women are four times as likely as men to develop this disease. Risk factors for osteoporosis include estrogen depletion, calcium deficiency, physical inactivity, testosterone depletion, alcoholism, and cigarette smoking. The rate of new bone resorption surpasses the rate of new bone formation at approximately age 40. This accounts for a subsequent loss of 40% of bone mass in women and 30% of bone mass in men over the course of the life span. Osteoporosis is associated with an increased risk of fractures. Common fracture sites are the vertebral bodies, distal radius, femoral neck, ribs, and pubis. Changes in the shape of the vertebral bodies can indicate the degree and severity of osteoporosis. Advanced cases may show complete compression fractures of the vertebral bodies. Compression fractures can result in severe kyphosis of the thoracic spine (Fig. 25-5).

The incidence of degenerative joint disease, osteoarthritis, increases with age. Osteoarthritis is the chronic deterioration of the joint cartilage, and the weight-bearing joints are the most commonly affected. Obesity is probably the most important risk factor. Osteoarthritis of the joint cartilage causes pain, swelling, and a decrease in range of motion in the affected joint. Osteoarthritis is the second most common cause of disability in the United States, affecting more than 50 million Americans. At age 40, most adults have osteoarthritic changes visible on radiographic images of the cervical spine. The most progressive changes occur in weight-bearing joints and hands as age increases (Fig. 25-6).

Total joint replacement or arthroplasty procedures are common among older adult patients. Joint replacement may offer pain relief and improve joint mobility. Joint replacements can be performed on any joint including the hip, knee, ankle, foot, shoulder, elbow, wrist, and fingers. Hip and knee replacements are the most common and the most effective (Fig. 25-7).

With age, women are more likely to store fat in their hips and thighs, whereas men store fat in their abdominal area. Without exercise, muscle mass declines, resulting in decreased strength and endurance, prolonged reaction time, and disturbed coordination. It cannot be overemphasized that regular physical training can improve muscle strength and endurance, along with cardiovascular fitness, even in the oldest individuals.

Cardiovascular system disorders

The cardiovascular system circulates the blood, which delivers oxygen and nutrients to all parts of the body and removes waste products. Damage to this system can have negative implications for the entire body. Decreased blood flow to the digestive tract, liver, and kidneys affects the absorption, distribution, and elimination of substances, such as medications and alcohol.

Cardiovascular disease is the most common cause of death worldwide. The maximum heart rate during exercise decreases with age; older adults become

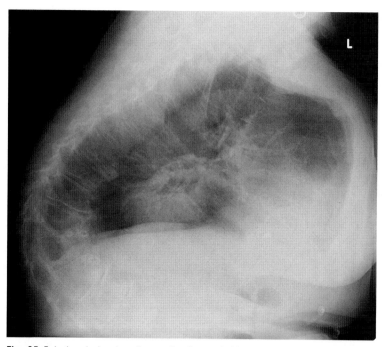

Fig. 25-5 Lateral chest radiograph of a geriatric patient with kyphosis and compression fractures.

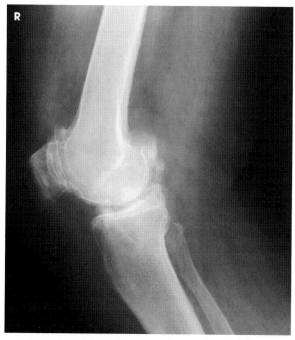

Fig. 25-6 Lateral knee radiograph showing severe arthritis.

short of breath and tire quickly. Loss of arterial elasticity results in elevated systolic blood pressure, increasing the risk for heart disease and stroke. Another prevalent problem is postural hypertension, in which there is a decrease in systemic blood pressure when rising from a supine to a standing position. The predominant change that occurs in the blood vessels with age is atherosclerosis, a development of fatty plaques in the walls of the arteries. These fatty plaques within the artery wall can lead to ulcerations of the artery wall, subsequently making the artery prone to the formation of blood clots. The plaques also cause destruction of the artery wall, causing it to balloon, increasing the risk of an aneurysm. Complications can lead to an embolism, heart attack, or stroke.

Congestive heart failure is due to an inability of the heart to propel blood at a sufficient rate and volume. This pathology is more common in older adults, particularly individuals 75 to 85 years old. People who are most at risk for developing congestive heart failure include individuals who have been diagnosed with coronary artery disease, heart attack, cardiomyopathy, untreated hypertension, and chronic kidney disease. Radiographically, the heart is enlarged, and the hilar region of the lungs is congested with increased vascular markings. Exposure factors must be adjusted to visualize the heart borders despite the pulmonary edema.

Preventive health measures, such as control of high blood pressure, diet, exercise, and smoking cessation, decrease the risk of cardiovascular disease. These interventions are more effective if initiated earlier in life.

Gastrointestinal system disorders

Gastrointestinal disorders in older adults include malignancies, peptic ulcer disease, gastrointestinal bleeding, pancreatitis, difficulty swallowing, diverticulitis, gastric outlet obstruction, esophageal foreign bodies, constipation, and fecal incontinence. Mouth and teeth pain, side effects of medication, decreased saliva, and dry mouth can lead to nutritional deficiencies, malnutrition, and dehydration problems. Most gastrointestinal disorders are related to an age-related decrease in the rate of gastric acid production and secretions and decreased motility of the smooth muscle in the large intestine. A decrease in acid production and secretion can lead to iron-deficiency anemia, peptic ulcers, and gastritis. Diverticulosis, a common problem in older adults, develops when the large intestine herniates through the muscle wall. Gallstone disease, hepatitis, and dehydration tend to be more common in older adults. Healthy lifestyle habits, such as smoking cessation, low alcohol intake, a high fiber–low sugar diet, and regular exercise, can decrease the risk of gastrointestinal problems. Gastrointestinal malignancies are second only to lung cancer as a cause of cancer mortality. Survival after colon and rectal cancer is increased with inexpensive early detection. Stool samples and rectal examinations are effective in detecting early cancer (Fig. 25-8).

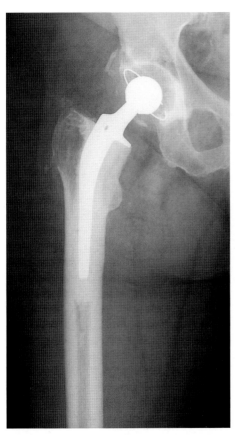

Fig. 25-7 AP proximal femur radiograph showing a total hip arthroplasty procedure.

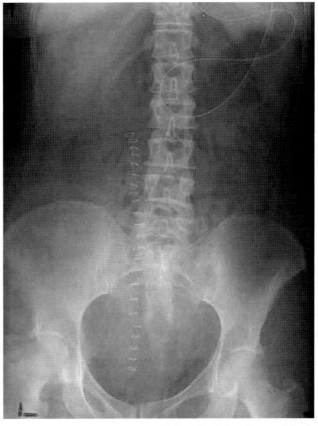

Fig. 25-8 Postoperative image of an older adult patient showing an AP abdomen with surgical staples and nasogastric tube.

Immune system decline

Age takes its toll on the immune system. To be immune to an infection implies protection from that infection. The ability of one's body to remain free of infections requires the immune system to distinguish healthy cells from invading microorganisms or altered cancer cells. The age-related decline of immune system function makes older adults more vulnerable to diabetes mellitus, pneumonia, and nosocomial infections. The incidence of infectious disease increases. Influenza, pneumonia, tuberculosis, meningitis, and urinary tract infections are prevalent among older adults. The three general categories of illness that preferentially affect older adults are infections, cancer, and autoimmune disease.[1]

---

[1]Chop WC, Robnett RH: *Gerontology for the health care professional,* ed 2, Philadelphia, 2009, Davis.

Respiratory system disorders

Throughout the aging process, the lungs lose some of their elastic recoil, trapping air in the alveoli. This reduced elasticity decreases the rate of oxygen entering the bloodstream and the elimination of carbon dioxide. The muscles involved in breathing become a little more rigid, which can account for shortness of breath with physical stress. In the wall of the thorax, the rib cage stiffens, causing kyphotic curvature of the thoracic spine. Respiratory diseases that increase in frequency with aging include emphysema, chronic bronchitis, pneumonia, and lung cancer.

Chronic obstructive pulmonary disease refers to a variety of breathing disorders that cause a decreased ability of the lungs to perform ventilation. Emphysema is the permanent destruction and distention of the alveoli. Cigarette smoking is the most significant risk factor in the development of emphysema and is the leading cause of chronic bronchitis. Chronic bronchitis is an inflammation of the mucous membrane of the bronchial tubes. These two conditions are considered irreversible. Chest radiographs may show hyperinflation of the lungs (Fig. 25-9).

Pneumonia is the most frequent type of lung infection and among the leading causes of death in older adults. This population is also at an increased risk for aspiration pneumonia secondary to slower swallowing reflexes and other health conditions. Radiographically, pneumonia may appear as soft, patchy alveolar infiltrates or pulmonary densities (Fig. 25-10).

Lung cancer is the second most common cancer and the most common cause of cancer-related death in men and women. More Americans die each year from lung cancer than from breast, prostate, and colorectal cancers combined.

There is a strong association between low lung function and the future development of coronary heart disease. Research has shown that the total amount of air inhaled in one's deepest breath and the fastest rate at which one can exhale are powerful predictors of how many more years one will live. Sedentary lifestyle is the greatest risk factor in lung function, and lifestyle habits are the crucial factors over which one has control.

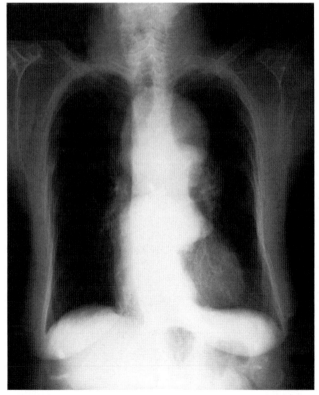

Fig. 25-9 PA chest radiograph showing emphysema.

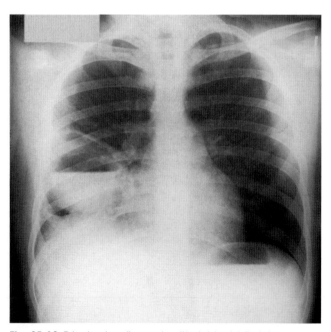

Fig. 25-10 PA chest radiograph with right middle lobe pneumonia and accompanying abscess.

Hematologic system disorders

A major hematologic concern in older adults is the high prevalence of anemia. Individuals with anemia often have pale skin and shortness of breath, and they fatigue easily. As bone ages, the marrow of the bone has a harder time maintaining blood cell production than young bone marrow when the body is stressed. The high incidence of anemia in older adults is believed to be a result not of aging per se, but rather of the high frequency of other age-related illnesses that can cause anemia. Anemia is not a single disease but a syndrome that has several causes. Insufficient dietary intake and inflammation or destruction of the gastrointestinal lining leading to inability to absorb vitamin B_{12} causes a type of anemia that affects older adults. Because of other physiologic stresses affecting marrow production, older adults have an increased incidence of various blood disorders.

Genitourinary system disorders

Familiar age-related genitourinary changes are those associated with incontinence. Changes in bladder capacity and muscle structure predispose older adults to this problem. Urinary and bowel incontinence can also lead to social and hygiene concerns. Along with structural changes in the genitourinary system, the number of nephrons in the kidneys decreases dramatically after the onset of adulthood. This decreased reserve capacity of the kidneys could cause what would otherwise be a regularly prescribed dose of medication to be an overdose in an older adult. The role of the kidneys to maintain the body's water balance and regulate the concentration according to the body's need diminishes with age. Acute and chronic renal failure affects many older adults.

Benign prostatic hyperplasia can affects 70% of men older than age 70. Benign prostatic hyperplasia is enlargement of the prostate gland, which can cause obstruction of the flow of urine. Surgical resection of the prostate may be necessary. Prostate cancer is primarily a disease of later life, and more than 80% of tumors are found in men older than 65 years. Prostate cancer is the most common cancer in men and the third most common cause of cancer deaths in men. Radiographic imaging of the male reproductive system comprises ureterograms, intravenous urography, and computed tomography. Ultrasound is commonly used to evaluate testicular masses and prostate nodules.

Endocrine system disorders

The endocrine system is another principal regulatory system of the body. Age-related changes in thyroid function result from inadequate responses of target cells to thyroid hormone. The most common age-related disease associated with the endocrine system is diabetes mellitus. Non–insulin-dependent diabetes mellitus increases in frequency with age and accounts for about 90% of all cases. Regular exercise and weight loss can significantly reduce the risk and delay the onset of non–insulin-dependent diabetes.

SUMMARY

Aging is the one certainty in life. It starts at conception and continues throughout the life cycle. No two people age in the same way. As stated earlier, aging is individualized and is affected by heredity, lifestyle choices, physical health, and attitude. Despite the changes that occur in the body systems observed with aging, most older adults view themselves as healthy. They learn to adapt, adjust, and compensate for the disabilities secondary to aging. *Older people are stereotyped into two groups: diseased and normal.* The normal group is at high risk of disease but is just not there yet. By categorizing these older adults as normal, health professionals tend to underestimate their vulnerability. Modest increases in blood pressure, blood sugar, body weight, and low bone density are common among normal older adults. These risk factors promote disease, and yet they can be modified. They may be age related in industrial societies, but they are not age determined or harmless. Positive lifestyle changes, such as diet, exercise, and smoking cessation, reduce the risk of disease and improve the quality of life. Good health cannot be left to chance, and staying healthy depends to a large degree on lifestyle choices and attitude.

SUMMARY OF PATHOLOGY: GERIATRIC RADIOGRAPHY

Condition	Definition
Alzheimer's disease	Progressive, irreversible mental disorder with loss of memory, deterioration of intellectual functions, speech and gait disturbances, and disorientation
Atherosclerosis	Condition in which fibrous and fatty deposits on the luminal wall of an artery may cause obstruction of the vessel
Benign prostatic hyperplasia	Enlargement of prostate gland
Chronic obstructive	Chronic condition of persistent obstruction of bronchial airflow pulmonary disease
Compression fracture	Fracture that causes compaction of bone and decrease in length or width
Congestive heart failure	Heart is unable to propel blood at sufficient rate and volume
Contractures	Permanent contraction of a muscle because of spasm or paralysis
Dementia	Broad impairment of intellectual function that usually is progressive and interferes with normal social and occupational activities
Emphysema	Destructive and obstructive airway changes leading to increased volume of air in the lungs
Geriatrics	Branch of medicine dealing with the aged and the problems of aging individuals
Gerontology	Branch of medicine dealing with illness prevention and management, health maintenance, and promotion of quality of life for older adults
Kyphosis	Abnormally increased convexity in the thoracic curvature
Osteoarthritis	Form of arthritis marked by progressive cartilage deterioration in synovial joints and vertebrae
Osteoporosis	Loss of bone density
Renal failure	Failure of the kidney to perform essential functions
Urinary incontinence	Absence of voluntary control of urination

Patient Care

Box 25-5 lists quick tips for working with older adult patients. These tips are discussed in the following pages.

PATIENT AND FAMILY EDUCATION

Educating all patients, especially older adult patients, about imaging procedures is crucial to obtain their confidence and compliance. More time with older adult patients may be necessary to accommodate their decreased ability to process information rapidly. Most older adults have been diagnosed with at least one chronic illness. They typically arrive at the clinical imaging environment with a natural anxiety because they are likely to have little knowledge of the procedure or the highly technical modalities employed for their procedures. A fear concerning consequences resulting from the examination exacerbates their increased levels of anxiety. Taking time to educate patients and their families or significant caregivers in their support system about the procedures makes for a less stressful experience and improved patient compliance and satisfaction.

BOX 25-5

Tips for working with older adult patients

Take time to educate the patient and the family

Speak lower and closer

Treat the patient with dignity and respect

Give the patient time to rest between projections and procedures

Avoid adhesive tape: older adult skin is thin and fragile

Provide warm blankets in cold examination rooms

Use table pads and handrails

Always access the patient's medical history before contrast medium is administered

---

COMMUNICATION

Good communication and listening skills create a connection between the radiographer and the patient. Older people are unique and should be treated with dignity and respect. Examples of appropriate communication may include addressing the patient by his or her title and last name. It is inappropriate to call someone "honey" or "dear." Each older adult is a wealth of cultural and historical knowledge that becomes a learning experience for the radiographer. If it is evident that the patient cannot hear or understand verbal directions, it is appropriate to speak lower and closer. Background noise can be disrupting to an older person and should be eliminated if possible when giving precise instructions. Giving instruction individually provides the older adult time to process a request. An empathetic, warm attitude and approach to a geriatric patient result in a trusting and compliant patient.

TRANSPORTATION AND LIFTING

Balance and coordination of an older adult patient can be affected by normal aging changes. The patient's anxiety about falling can be diminished by assistance in and out of a wheelchair and to and from the examination table. Many older adult patients have decreased height perception resulting from some degree of vision impairment. Hesitation of the older adult patient may be due to previous falls. Assisting an older patient when there is a need to step up or down throughout the procedure is more than a reassuring gesture. Preventing opportunities for falls is a responsibility of the radiographer. The older adult patient often experiences vertigo and dizziness when moving from a recumbent position to a sitting position. Giving the patient time to rest between positions mitigates these disturbing, frightening, and uncomfortable sensations. The use of table handgrips and

proper assistance from the radiographer create a sense of security for an older adult patient. A sense of security results in a compliant and trusting patient throughout the imaging procedure.

SKIN CARE

Acute age-related changes in the skin cause it to become thin and fragile. The skin becomes more susceptible to bruising, tears, abrasions, and blisters. All health care professionals should use caution in turning and holding an older adult patient. Excessive pressure on the skin causes it to break and tear. *Adhesive tape should be avoided because it can be irritating and can easily tear the skin of an older person.* The loss of fat pads makes it painful for an older adult patient to lie on a hard surface and can increase the possibility of developing ulcerations. Decubitus ulcers, or pressure sores, are commonly seen in bedridden people and people with decreased mobility. Bony areas such as the heels, ankles, elbow, and lateral hips are frequent sites for pressure sores. A decubitus ulcer can develop in 1 to 2 hours. Almost without exception, tables used for imaging procedures are hard surfaced and cannot be avoided. The use of a table pad can reduce the friction between the hard surface of the table and the patient's fragile skin. Sponges, blankets, and positioning aids make the procedure much more bearable and comfortable for the older adult patient.

Because skin plays a crucial role in maintaining body temperature, the increasing thinning process associated with aging skin renders the patient less able to retain normal body heat. The regulation of body temperature of an older adult varies from that of a younger person. To prevent hypothermia in rooms where the ambient air temperature is comfortable for the radiographer, it may be essential to provide blankets for the older adult patient.

CONTRAST AGENT ADMINISTRATION

Because of age-related changes in kidney and liver functions, the amount, but not the type, of contrast media is varied when performing radiographic procedures on an older adult patient. The number of functioning nephrons in the kidneys steadily decreases from middle age throughout the life span. Compromised kidney function contributes to the older adult patient being more prone to electrolyte and fluid imbalance, which can create life-threatening consequences. They are also more susceptible to the effects of dehydration because of diabetes and decreased renal or adrenal function. The decision of type and amount of contrast media used for the geriatric patient usually follows some sort of routine protocol. Assessment for contrast agent administration accomplished by the imaging technologist must include age; history of liver, kidney, or thyroid disease; history of hypersensitivity reactions and previous reactions to medications or contrast agents; sensitivity to aspirin; over-the-counter and prescription drug history including the use of acetaminophen (Tylenol); and history of diabetes and hypertension.[1]

The imaging technologist must be selective in locating an appropriate vein for contrast agent administration on the older adult patient. The technologist should consider the location and condition of the vein, decreased integrity of the skin, and duration of the therapy. Thin superficial veins, repeatedly used veins, and veins located in areas where the skin is bruised or scarred should be avoided. The patient should be assessed for any swallowing impairments, which could lead to difficulties with drinking liquid contrast agents. The patient should be instructed to drink slowly to avoid choking, and an upright position helps prevent aspiration.

[1]Norris T: Special needs of geriatric patients, *American Society of Radiologic Technologists Homestudy Series,* vol 4, no 5, 1999.

JOINT COMMISSION CRITERIA

The Joint Commission is the accrediting and standards-setting body for hospitals, clinics, and other health care organizations in the United States. Employees in institutions accredited by the Joint Commission must demonstrate age-based communication competencies, which include the older adult. The standards were adopted as a means of demonstrating competence in meeting the physiologic and psychological needs of patients in special populations. These populations include infants, children, adolescents, and older adults.

Age-related competencies

Standard HR 01.05.03 of the Human Resources section of the Joint Commission manual states: "When appropriate, the hospital considers special needs and behaviors of specific age groups in defining qualifications, duties, and responsibilities of staff members who do not have clinical privileges but who have regular clinical contact with patients (e.g., radiologic technologists and mental health technicians)." The intent of the standard is to ensure age-specific competency in technical and clinical matters but is not limited to equipment and technical performance. Age-specific competencies address the different needs people have at different ages. Examples of age-specific care for older adults may include the following: assessing visual or hearing impairments; assessing digestive and esophageal problems, such as reflux, bladder, and bowel problems; addressing grief concerns; providing warmth; and providing safety aids. Being able to apply age-specific care also includes the use of age-appropriate communication skills. Clear communication with the patient can be the key to providing age-specific care. Knowledge of age-related changes and disease processes assists all health care professionals, including those in the radiation sciences, in providing care that meets the needs of the older adult patient.

Performing the Radiographic Procedure
RADIOGRAPHER'S ROLE

The role of the radiographer is no different than that of all other health professionals. The whole person must be treated, not just the manifested symptoms of an illness or injury. Medical imaging and therapeutic procedures reflect the impact of ongoing systemic aging in documentable and visual forms. Adapting procedures to accommodate disabilities and diseases of geriatric patients is a crucial responsibility and a challenge based almost exclusively on the radiographer's knowledge, abilities, and skills. An understanding of the physiology and pathology of aging and an awareness of the social, psychological, cognitive, and economic aspects of aging are required to meet the needs of older adult patients. Conditions typically associated with older adult patients invariably require adaptations or modifications of routine imaging procedures. The radiographer must be able to differentiate between age-related changes and disease processes. Production of diagnostic images requiring professional decision making to compensate for physiologic changes, while maintaining the compliance, safety, and comfort of the patient, is the foundation of the contract between the older adult patient and the radiographer.

To know how to care for individuals with Alzheimer's disease, it is important to become familiar with some simple facts about the disease and behaviors that are associated with it. Alzheimer's disease is a progressive disease with no known cure. There are five stages: preclinical stage, mild cognitive impairment, mild dementia, moderate dementia, and severe dementia. The disease is often diagnosed in the mild stage of dementia. Box 25-6 lists these stages and a brief description of each.

The rate of progression of Alzheimer's disease varies widely. On average people with this disease live 8 to 10 years after diagnosis; however, some will live as long as 25 years after diagnosis. Pneumonia is a common cause of death because impaired swallowing allows food or beverages to enter the lungs, where an infection can begin. Other common causes of death include complications from urinary tract infections and falls.

It is important that the radiologic technologist becomes aware of and understands the various types of physical and cognitive impairments associated with Alzheimer's disease. It requires patience and compassion and attentiveness when dealing with this patient group. Patients who are at risk of falling must never be left alone whether in the radiology waiting room or in the examination room.

Caregivers should be encouraged to accompany the patient to appointments whenever possible. It is sometimes more comforting to the patient to have a familiar person with him or her in an unfamiliar setting. In addition, depending on the stage of the disease, some patients may tend to wander, often wanting to "go home." Home sometimes is their native town, state, or even country. So they can travel considerable distances before they are found. There have been cases where patients have wandered off, never to be found, or never to be found alive. For that reason the patient should never be left alone. Whenever possible, and whenever a caregiver has not accompanied the patient, a two-technologist team should be available to care for the patient while in the diagnostic radiology suite—one acquiring the images and one in the role of companion to the patient while the images are being processed and reviewed. The patient should be then handed off to the unit or responsible party upon completion of the exam.

It is not uncommon for Alzheimer's patients to ask repetitive questions or to become accusatory. The technologist should exercise a great deal of patience and use distraction techniques to eliminate the frustration this may cause. Simply changing the subject or asking an unrelated question may reduce the repetitive questioning or conversation. There may be occasions when the patient will require restraints to complete the exam. Note, however, that restraints should only be applied in cases where the patient can potentially cause harm to himself or to others.

Working quietly and smoothly around the patient and maintaining calm, relaxing, and noise-free surroundings is the preferred situation for Alzheimer's patients in the radiology department. The music, if any, should be soothing and relaxing. This will potentially benefit all types of patients.

Radiographic Positioning for Geriatric Patients

The preceding discussions and understanding of the physical, cognitive, and psychosocial effects of aging can help radiographers adapt to the positioning challenges of the geriatric patient. In some cases, routine examinations need to be modified to accommodate the limitations, safety, and comfort of the patient. Communicating clear instructions with the patient is important. The following discussion addresses positioning suggestions for various structures.

CHEST

The position of choice for the chest radiograph is the upright position; however, an older adult patient may be unable to stand without assistance for this examination. The traditional posteroanterior (PA) position is to have the "backs of hands on hips." This may be difficult for someone with impaired balance and flexibility. The radiographer can allow the patient to wrap his or her arms around the chest stand as a means of support and security. The patient may not be able to maintain his or her arms over the head for the lateral projection of the chest. The radiographer should provide extra security and stability while the patient is moving the arms up and forward (Fig. 25-11).

BOX 25-6

Stages and symptoms of Alzheimer's disease

Stages of Alzheimer's disease	Description of behaviors/symptoms
Preclinical stage	Symptoms usually go unnoticed during this stage. This stage of Alzheimer's disease can last for years, possibly even decades. Diagnostic imaging technologies can now identify deposits of the amyloidal beta substance that have been associated with Alzheimer's disease.
Mild cognitive impairment	Memory lapses, interrupted thought processes. Trouble with time management. Trouble making sound decisions.
Mild dementia	Memory loss of recent events. Difficulty with problem solving. Difficulty completing complex tasks and making sound judgments. Changes in personality—may become subdued, or withdraw from certain social situations. Difficulty organizing or expressing thoughts. Gets lost or wanders away from home. Misplaces belongings.
Moderate dementia	Displays increasingly poor judgment. Confusion deepens. Memory loss increases. Needs assistance with daily routine activities. Becomes suspicious or paranoid and accusatory to caregivers or family members. Rummaging, tapping feet, rubbing hands, banging. Outbursts of physical aggression.
Severe dementia (late stage)	Inability to hold coherent conversations. Inability to recognize some or all family members. Requires assistance with personal care. Decline in physical abilities—needs assistance walking or may experience uncontrollable bladder and bowel functions. Inability to swallow; rigid muscles; abnormal reflexes.

When the patient cannot stand, the examination may be done seated in a wheelchair, but some issues affect the radiographic quality. First, the radiologist needs to be aware that the radiograph is an anteroposterior (AP) instead of a PA projection, which may make comparison difficult. Hyperkyphosis can result in the lung apices being obscured, and the abdomen may obscure the lung bases. In a sitting position, respiration may be compromised, and the patient should be instructed on the importance of a deep inspiration.

Positioning of the image receptor (IR) for a kyphotic patient should be higher than normal because the shoulders and apices are in a higher position. Radiographic landmarks may change with age, and the centering may need to be lower if the patient is extremely kyphotic. When positioning the patient for the sitting lateral chest projection, the radiographer should place a large sponge behind the patient to lean him or her forward (Fig. 25-12).

SPINE

Radiographic spine examinations may be painful for a patient with osteoporosis who is lying on the x-ray table. Positioning aids such as radiolucent sponges, sandbags, and a mattress may be used as long as the quality of the image is not compromised (Fig. 25-13). Performing upright radiographic examinations may also be appropriate if a patient can safely tolerate this position. The combination of cervical lordosis and thoracic kyphosis can make positioning and visualization of the cervical and thoracic spine difficult. Lateral cervical projections can be done with the patient standing, sitting, or lying supine. The AP projection in the sitting position may not visualize the upper cervical vertebrae because the chin may obscure this anatomy. In the supine position, the head may not reach the table and result in magnification. The AP and open-mouth projections are difficult to do in a wheelchair.

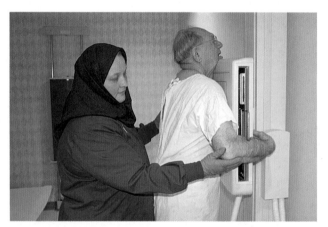

Fig. 25-11 Radiographer positioning patient's arms around the chest stand for a PA chest radiograph. Having the patient hold on in this way provides stability.

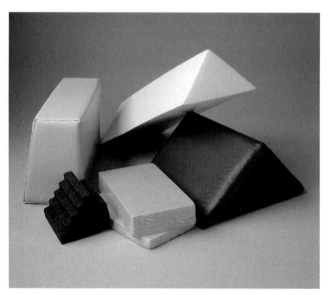

Fig. 25-13 Positioning sponges and sandbags are commonly used as immobilization devices.

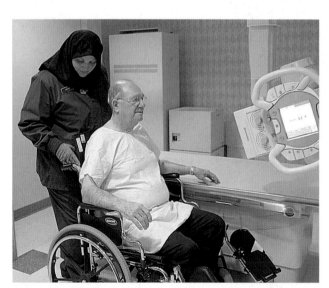

Fig. 25-12 Radiographer placing the IR behind a patient who is unable to stand. With careful positioning of the IR and x-ray tube, a quality image of the chest can be obtained.

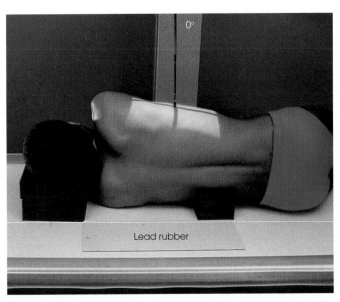

Fig. 25-14 Recumbent lateral thoracic spine. Support placed under lower thoracic region; perpendicular central ray.

The thoracic and lumbar spines are sites for compression fractures. The use of positioning blocks may be necessary to help the patient remain in position. For the lateral projection, a lead blocker or shield behind the spine should be used to absorb as much scatter radiation as possible (Fig. 25-14).

PELVIS AND HIP

Osteoarthritis, osteoporosis, and injuries as the result of falls contribute to hip pathologies. A common fracture in older adults is to the femoral neck. An AP projection of the pelvis should be done to examine the hip. If the indication is trauma, the radiographer should *not attempt to rotate the limbs.* The second view taken should be a cross-table lateral of the affected hip. If hip pain is the indication, assist the patient to internal rotation of the legs with the use of sandbags if necessary (Figs. 25-15 and 25-16).

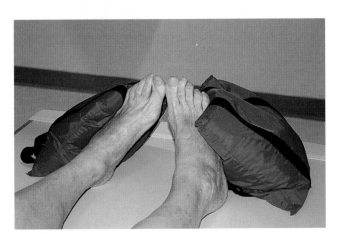

Fig. 25-15 Legs inverted for AP projection of the pelvis. Wrapping flexible sandbags around the feet can help the geriatric patient hold his or her legs in this position.

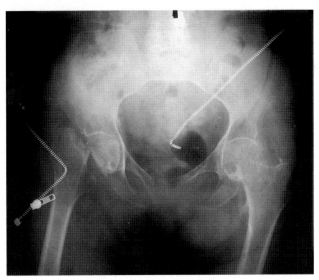

Fig. 25-16 An older adult patient with Alzheimer's disease was brought to the emergency department because he could not walk. The patient did not complain of pain. Note fracture of the right hip. Trauma radiograph was made with patient's pants on and the zipper is shown.

UPPER EXTREMITY

Positioning the geriatric patient for projections of the upper extremities can present its own challenges. Often the upper extremities have limited flexibility and mobility. A cerebrovascular accident or stroke may cause contractures of the affected limb. Contracted limbs cannot be forced into position, and cross-table views may need to be done. The inability of the patient to move his or her limb should not be interpreted as a lack of cooperation. Supination is often a problem in patients with contractures, fractures, and paralysis. The routine AP and lateral projections can be supported with the use of sponges, sandbags, and blocks to raise and support the extremity being imaged. The shoulder is also a site of decreased mobility, dislocation, and fractures. The therapist should assess how much movement the patient can do before attempting to move the arm. The use of finger sponges may also help with the contractures of the fingers (Fig. 25-17).

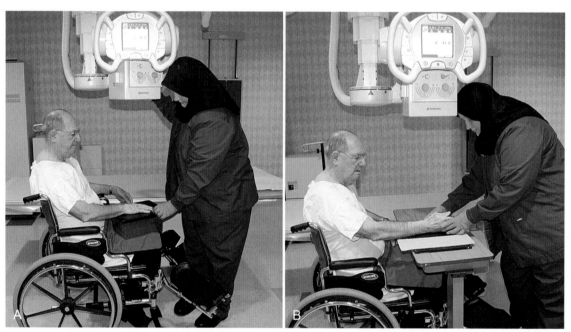

Fig. 25-17 Most projections of the upper limb can be obtained with the patient in a wheelchair and with some creativity. **A,** Patient being positioned for an AP hand radiograph. Note use of a 4-inch sponge to raise IR. **B,** Patient being positioned for a lateral wrist radiograph. A hospital food tray table provides a base for IR and for ease of positioning.

LOWER EXTREMITY

The lower extremities may have limited flexibility and mobility. The ability to dorsiflex the ankle may be reduced as a result of neurologic disorders. Imaging on the x-ray table may need to be modified when a patient cannot turn on his or her side. Flexion of the knee may be impaired and require a cross-table lateral projection. If a tangential projection of the patella, such as the Settegast method, is necessary, and the patient can turn on his or her side, the radiographer can place the IR superior to the knee and direct the central ray perpendicular through the patellofemoral joint.

Projections of the feet and ankles may be obtained with the patient sitting in the wheelchair. Positioning sponges and sandbags support and maintain the position of the body part being imaged (Fig. 25-18).

TECHNICAL FACTORS

Exposure factors also need to be taken into consideration when imaging the geriatric patient. The loss of bone mass and atrophy of tissues often require a lower kilovoltage (kVp) to maintain sufficient contrast. kVp is also a factor in chest radiographs when there may be a large heart and pleural fluid to penetrate.

Patients with emphysema require a reduction in technical factors to prevent overexposure of the lung field. Patient assessment can help with the appropriate exposure adjustments.

Time may also be a major factor. Geriatric patients may have problems maintaining the positions necessary for the examinations. A short exposure time helps reduce voluntary and involuntary motion and breathing. The radiographer needs to ensure that the geriatric patient clearly hears and understands the breathing instructions.

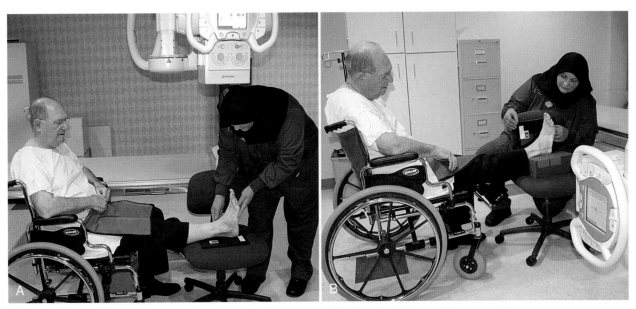

Fig. 25-18 Projections of the lower limb, especially from the knee and lower, can be obtained with the patient in a wheelchair. **A,** AP projection of the ankle with the patient's leg and foot resting on a chair. **B,** Lateral projection of the ankle performed by using a chair as a rest and a sponge to raise the IR.

Conclusion

Imaging professionals will continue to see a change in the health care delivery system with the dramatic shift in the population of people older than age 65. This shift in the general population is resulting in an ongoing increase in the number of medical imaging procedures performed on older adult patients. Demographic and social effects of aging determine the way in which older adults adapt to and view the process of aging. An individual's family size and perceptions of aging, economic resources, gender, race, ethnicity, social class, and availability and delivery of health care affect the quality of the aging experience. Biologic age is much more critical than chronologic age when determining the health status of the older adult.

Healthier lifestyles and advancements in medical treatment are creating a generation of successfully aging adults, which should decrease the negative stereotyping of older adults. Attitudes of all health care professionals, whether positive or negative, affect the care provided to the growing older adult population. Education about the mental and physiologic alterations associated with aging, along with the cultural, economic, and social influences accompanying aging, enables the radiographer to adapt imaging and therapeutic procedures to the older adult patient's disabilities resulting from age-related changes.

The human body undergoes a multiplicity of physiologic changes and failure in all organ systems. The aging experience is affected by heredity, lifestyle choices, physical health, and attitude, making it highly individualized. No individual's aging process is predictable and is never exactly the same as that of any other individual. Radiologic technologists must use their knowledge, abilities, and skills to adjust imaging procedures to accommodate for disabilities and diseases encountered with geriatric patients. Safety and comfort of the patient are essential in maintaining compliance throughout imaging procedures. Communication, listening, sensitivity, and empathy lead to patient compliance. The Joint Commission, recognizing the importance of age-based communication competencies for older adults, requires the employees of accredited health care organizations to document their achievement of these skills. Knowledge of age-related changes and disease processes enhances the radiographer's ability to provide care that meets the needs of the increasing older adult patient population.

Selected bibliography

Campbell PR: *U.S. population projections by age, sex, race and Hispanic origin: 1995 to 2025*, Washington, DC, 1996, U.S. Bureau of the Census, Population Division, PPL-47.

Chop WC, Robnett RH: *Gerontology for the health care professional,* ed 2, Philadelphia, 2009, Davis.

Ferrara MH: *Alzheimer's Disease: Human Diseases and Conditions,* ed 2, vol 1, Detroit, 2010, Charles Scribner's Sons, pp 70-76. Copyright 2010 Charles Scribner's Sons, a part of Gale, Engage Learning.

Garfein AJ, Herzog AR: Robust aging among the young-old, old-old, and oldest-old, *J Gerontol Soc Sci* 50B(Suppl):S77, 1995.

Health professions in service to the nation, San Francisco, 1993, Pew Health Professions Commission.

Hobbs FB, Danion BL: *65+ in the United States,* 1996, Washington, DC, U.S. Department of Commerce and U.S. Department of Health and Human Service, pp 23-190.

Mazess RB: On aging bone loss, *Clin Orthop* 165:239, 1982.

Norris T: Special needs of geriatric patients, *American Society of Radiologic Technologists Homestudy Series,* vol 4, no 5, 1999.

Park A: Alzheimer's unlocked. *Time [serial online],* October 25:176:53, 2010. Available from: Academic Search Premier, Ipswich, MA. Accessed November 4, 2012.

Rarey LK: Radiologic technologists' responses to elderly patients, *Radiol Technol* 69:566, 1996.

Rimer BK et al: Multistrategy health education program to increase mammography use among women ages 65 and older, *Public Health Rep* 107:369, 1992.

Spencer G: *What are the demographic implications of an aging U.S. population from 1990 to 2030?* Washington, DC, 1993, American Association of Retired Persons and Resources for the Future.

Thali M et al: *Brogdon's forensic radiology,* ed 2, Boca Raton, FL, 2011, CRC Press, pp 287-288.

Thibodeau GA, Patton KT: *Anatomy & Physiology,* ed 8, VitalSource Bookshelf, Mosby, 032012, November 04, 2012. http:// pageburstls.elsevier.com/books/978-0-323-08357-7/id/B9780323083577500128_f21.

University of Pittsburgh Schools of the Health Sciences: New compound identifies Alzheimer's disease brain toxins, study shows, *Science Daily,* March 28, http://www.sciencedaily.com, 2008. Retrieved November 7, 2012, from

U.S. Department of Commerce, Economics and Statistics Administration: *65+ in the United States,* Washington, DC, 2000, U.S. Bureau of the Census.

http://www.alz.org/research/science/alzheimers_disease_causes.asp#age. Accessed November 4, 2012.

http://www.alz.org/research/science/earlier_alzheimers_diagnosis.asp#Brain. Accessed November 4, 2012.

http://www.sciencedaily.com/releases/2008/03/080326114855.htm. Accessed November 7, 2012.

http://go.galegroup.com/ps/retrieve.do?sgHitCountType=None&sort=RELEVANCE&inPS=true&prodId=GVRL&userGroupName=passaicc&tabID=T003&searchId=R1&resultListType=RESULT_LIST&contentSegment=&searchType=AdvancedSearchForm&currentPosition=11&contentSet=GALE%7CCX2830200023&&docId=GALE|CX2830200023&docType=GALE. Accessed July 13, 2013.

Alzheimer's disease: *The Encyclopedia of the Brain and Brain Disorders,* Available at: http://go.galegroup.com/ps/retrieve.do?sgHitCountType=None&sort=RELEVANCE&inPS=true&prodId=GVRL&userGroupName=passaicc&tabID=T003&searchId=R1&resultListType=RESULT_LIST&contentSegment=&searchType=AdvancedSearchForm&currentPosition=15&contentSet=GALE%7CCX1692600038&&docId=GALE|CX1692600038&docType=GALE *Turkington, Carol, and Harris, Joseph R.* 3rd ed. *Facts on File Library of Health and Living* New York: Facts on File, 2009. p16-22. COPYRIGHT 2009 Carol Turkington.

http://www.mayoclinic.com/health/alzheimers-stages/AZ00041. Accessed December 11, 2012.

http://www.alz.org/care/alzheimers-early-mild-stage-caregiving.asp. Accessed November 4, 2012.

http://www.aoa.gov/AoA_programs/Elder_Rights/EA_Prevention/whatIsEA.aspx. Accessed July 10, 2013.

http://wwwpreventelderabuse.org/elderabuse/professionals/medical.html. Accessed July 10, 2013.

http://www.asrt.org/docs/educators/forensic_radiography_white_paperfin.pdf. Accessed July 10, 2013.

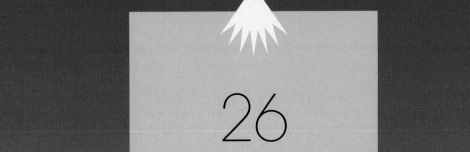

26

MOBILE RADIOGRAPHY

KARI J. WETTERLIN

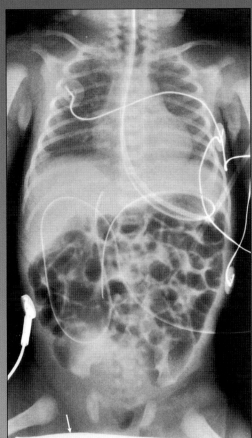

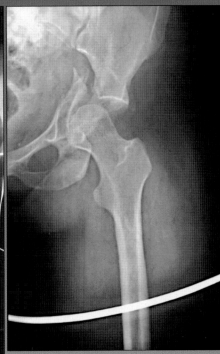

OUTLINE

Principles of Mobile
  Radiography, 184
Mobile X-Ray Machines, 184
Technical Considerations, 184
Radiation Safety, 188
Isolation Considerations, 189
Performing Mobile
  Examinations, 190
RADIOGRAPHY, 192
Chest, 192
Abdomen, 196
Pelvis, 200
Femur, 202
Cervical Spine, 206
Chest and Abdomen: Neonate, 208

Principles of Mobile Radiography

Mobile radiography using transportable radiographic equipment allows imaging services to be brought to the patient. In contrast to the large stationary machines found in radiographic rooms, compact mobile radiography units can produce diagnostic images in virtually any location (Fig. 26-1). Mobile radiography is commonly performed in patient rooms, emergency departments, intensive care units, surgery, recovery rooms, and nursery and neonatal units. Some machines are designed for transport by automobile or van to extended care facilities or other off-site locations requiring radiographic imaging services.

Mobile radiography was first used by the military for treating battlefield injuries during World War I. Small portable units were designed to be carried by soldiers and set up in field locations. Although mobile equipment is no longer "carried" to the patient, the term *portable* has persisted and is often used in reference to mobile procedures.

This chapter focuses on the most common projections performed with mobile radiography machines. The basic principles of mobile radiography are described and helpful hints are provided for successful completion of the examina-tions. An understanding of common projections enables the radiographer to perform most mobile examinations ordered by the physician.

Mobile X-Ray Machines

Mobile x-ray machines are not as sophisticated as the larger stationary machines in the radiology department. Although mobile units are capable of producing images of most body parts, they vary in their exposure controls and power sources (or generators).

A typical mobile x-ray machine has controls for setting kilovolt (peak) (kVp) and milliampere-seconds (mAs). The mAs control automatically adjusts milli-amperage (mA) and time to preset values. Maximum settings differ among manufacturers, but mAs typically range from 0.04 to 320 and kVp from 40 to 130. The total power of the unit ranges from 15 to 25 kilowatts (kW), which is adequate for most mobile projections. By comparison, the power of a stationary radiography unit can reach 150 kW (150 kVp, 1000 mA) or more.

Some mobile x-ray machines have preset anatomic programs (APRs) similar to stationary units. The anatomic programs use exposure techniques with predetermined values based on the selected examination. The radiographer can adjust these settings as needed to compensate for differences in the size or condition of a patient. The much wider dynamic range available with CR or DR and the ability to manipulate the final image with computer software results in images of proper density.

Some mobile units have direct digital capability, where the image is acquired immediately on the unit. These machines have a flat panel detector, similar to those found in a DR table Bucky. The detector either is connected to the portable unit by a tethered cord or communicates through wireless technology (Fig. 26-2).

Technical Considerations

Mobile radiography presents the radiographer with challenges different from those associated with performing examinations with stationary equipment in the radiology department. Although the positioning of the patient and placement of the central ray are essentially the same, three important technical matters must be clearly understood to perform optimal mobile examinations: the *grid,* the *anode heel effect,* and the *source–to–image receptor distance (SID).* In addition, exposure technique charts must be available (see Fig. 26-5).

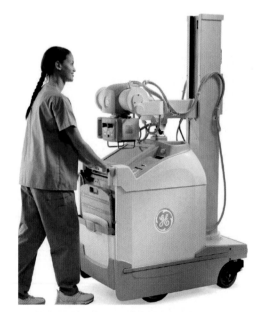

Fig. 26-1 Radiographer driving a battery-operated mobile radiography machine to a patient's room.

GRID

Because the phosphor material used in CR imaging plates has higher absorption in the scattered x-ray energy range compared with screen-film, image quality degradation from scatter is more pronounced when using CR. Grid use is crucial in portable CR imaging.

For optimal imaging, a *grid* must be level, centered to the central ray, and correctly used at the recommended focal distance, or radius. When a grid is placed on an unstable surface such as the mattress of a bed, the weight of the patient can cause the grid to tilt "off level." If the grid tilts transversely while using a longitudinal grid, the central ray forms an angle across the long axis. Image density is lost as a result of grid "cutoff" (Fig. 26-3). If the grid tilts longitudinally, the central ray angles through the long axis. In this case, grid cutoff is avoided, but the image may be distorted or elongated.

A grid positioned under a patient can be difficult to center. If the central ray is directed to a point transversely off the midline of a grid more than 1 to 1½ inches (2.5 to 3.8 cm), a cutoff effect similar to that produced by an off-level grid results. The central ray can be centered longitudinally to any point along the midline of a grid without cutoff. Depending on the procedure, beam-restriction problems may occur. If this happens, a portion of the image is "collimated off," or patient exposure is excessive because of an oversized exposure field.

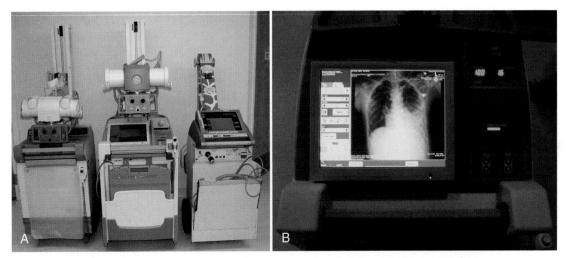

Fig. 26-2 A, The machine on the left is an analog mobile unit, and the other two are digital units. Notice the two digital mobile units have a computer screen. **B,** Mobile digital screen with a chest image.

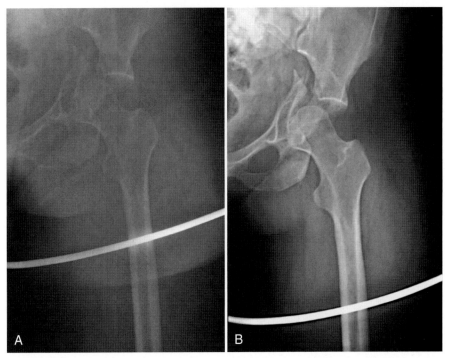

Fig. 26-3 Mobile radiograph of proximal femur and hip, showing comminuted fracture of left acetabulum. **A,** Poor-quality radiograph resulted when grid was transversely tilted far enough to produce significant grid cutoff. **B,** Excellent-quality repeat radiograph on the same patient, performed with grid accurately positioned perpendicular to central ray.

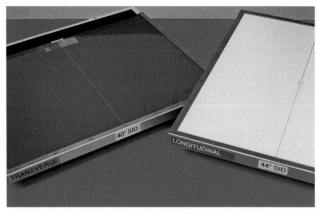

Fig. 26-4 Transverse and longitudinal grids mounted on rigid holder, many times referred to as "slip-on." Focal ranges are clearly identified for proper use.

Table 26-1

Cathode placement for mobile projections

Part	Projection	Cathode placement
Chest	AP	Diaphragm
	AP—decubitus	Down side of chest
Abdomen	AP	Diaphragm
	AP—decubitus	Down side of abdomen
Pelvis	AP	Upper pelvis
Femur	AP	Proximal femur
	Lateral	Proximal femur
Cervical spine	Lateral	Over lower vertebrae (40-inch [102-cm] SID only)
Chest and abdomen in neonate	All	No designation*

Note: The cathode side of the beam has the greatest intensity.
*Not necessary because of small field size of the collimator.

Grids used for mobile radiography are often of the focused type. Some radiology departments continue to use the older, parallel-type grids, however. All focused grids have a recommended focal range, or radius, that varies with the grid ratio. Projections taken at distances greater or less than the recommended focal range can produce cutoff in which image density is reduced on lateral margins. Grids with a lower ratio have a greater focal range, but they are less efficient for cleaning up scatter radiation. The radiographer must be aware of the *exact* focal range for the grid used. Most focused grids used for mobile radiography have a ratio of 6:1 or 8:1 and a focal range of about 36 to 44 inches (91 to 112 cm). This focal range allows mobile examinations to be performed efficiently. Inverting a focused grid causes a pronounced cutoff effect similar to that produced by improper distance.

Today most grids are mounted on a protective frame, and the image receptor (IR) is easily inserted behind the grid (Fig. 26-4). A final concern regarding grids relates to the use of "tape-on" grids. If a grid is not mounted on an IR holder frame but instead is manually fastened to the surface of the IR with tape, care must be taken to ensure that the tube side of the grid faces the x-ray tube. The examinations described in this chapter present methods of ensuring proper grid and IR placement for projections that require a grid.

ANODE HEEL EFFECT

Another consideration in mobile radiography is the *anode heel effect*. The heel effect causes a decrease of image density under the anode side of the x-ray tube. The heel effect is more pronounced with the following:
- Short SID
- Larger field sizes
- Small anode angles

Short SIDs and large field sizes are common in mobile radiography. In mobile radiography, the radiographer has control of the anode-cathode axis of the x-ray tube relative to the body part. Correct placement of the anode-cathode axis with regard to the anatomy is essential. When performing a mobile examination, the radiographer may not always be able to orient the anode-cathode axis of the tube to the desired position because of limited space and maneuverability in the room. For optimal mobile radiography, the anode and cathode sides of the x-ray tube should be clearly marked to indicate where the high-tension cables enter the x-ray tube, and the radiographer should use the heel effect maximally (Table 26-1).

SOURCE–TO–IMAGE RECEPTOR DISTANCE

The SID should be maintained at 40 inches (102 cm) for most mobile examinations. A standardized distance for all patients and projections helps to ensure consistency in imaging. Longer SIDs—40 to 48 inches (102 to 122 cm)—require increased mAs to compensate for the additional distance. The mA limitations of a mobile unit necessitate longer exposure times when the SID exceeds 40 inches (102 cm). Despite the longer exposure time, a radiograph with motion artifacts may result if the SID is greater than 40 inches (102 cm). In addition, motion artifacts may occur in the radiographs of critically ill adult patients and infants or small children who require chest and abdominal examinations but may be unable to hold their breath.

RADIOGRAPHIC TECHNIQUE CHARTS

A radiographic technique chart should be available for use with every mobile machine. The chart should display, in an organized manner, the standardized technical factors for all the radiographic projections done with the machine (Fig. 26-5). A caliper should also be available; this device is used to measure the thickness of body parts to ensure that accurate and consistent exposure factors are used. Measuring the patient also allows the radiographer to determine the optimal kVp level for all exposures (Fig. 26-6).

MOBILE RADIOGRAPHIC TECHNIQUE CHART

AMX—4   40-inch SID   CR IP   8:1 grid

Part	Projection	Position	cm—kVp	mAs	Grid
Chest	AP	Supine/upright	21—120	3.2	Yes
	AP	Lateral decubitus	21—85	6.25	Yes
Abdomen	AP	Supine	23—74	25	Yes
	AP	Lateral decubitus	23—74	32	Yes
Pelvis	AP	Supine	23—74	32	Yes
Femur (distal)	AP	Supine	15—70	10	Yes
	Lateral	Dorsal decubitus	15—70	10	Yes
C-spine	Lateral	Dorsal decubitus	10—62	20	Yes
NEONATAL					
Chest/abdomen	AP	Supine	7—64	0.8	No
	Lateral	Dorsal decubitus	10—72	1	No

Fig. 26-5 Sample radiographic technique chart showing manual technical factors used for the 10 common mobile projections described in this chapter. The kVp and mAs factors are for the specific centimeter measurements indicated. Factors vary depending on the actual centimeter measurement.

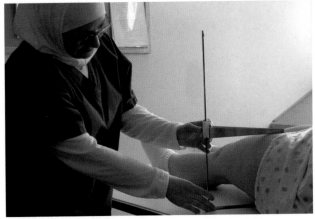

Fig. 26-6 Radiographer measuring the thickest portion of the femur to determine the exact technical factors needed for the examination.

Radiation Safety

Radiation protection for the radiographer, others in the immediate area, and the patient is of paramount importance when mobile examinations are performed. *Mobile radiography produces some of the highest occupational radiation exposures for radiographers.* The radiographer should wear a lead apron and stand as far away from the patient, x-ray tube, and useful beam as the room and the exposure cable allow. The recommended *minimal* distance is 6 ft (2 m). For a horizontal (cross-table) x-ray beam or for an upright anteroposterior (AP) chest projection, the radiographer should stand at a right angle (90 degrees) to the primary beam and the object being radiographed. The least

amount of scatter radiation occurs at this position (Fig. 26-7). Shielding and distance have a greater effect on exposure reduction, however, and should always be considered first.

The most effective means of radiation protection is *distance.* The radiographer should inform all persons in the immediate area that an x-ray exposure is about to occur so that they may leave to avoid exposure. Lead protection should be provided for any individuals who are unable to leave the room and for individuals who may have to hold a patient or IR.

The patient's gonads should be shielded with appropriate radiation protection devices for any of the following situations:

- X-ray examinations performed on children
- X-ray examinations performed on patients of reproductive age
- Any examination for which the patient requests protection
- Examinations in which the gonads lie in or near the useful beam
- Examinations in which shielding would not interfere with imaging of the anatomy that must be shown (Fig. 26-8)

In addition, the source-to-skin distance (SSD) cannot be less than 12 inches (30 cm), in accordance with federal safety regulations.[1]

---

[1]National Council on Radiation Protection: Report 102: medical x-ray, electron beam and gamma ray protection for energies up to 50 MeV, Bethesda, MD, 1989.

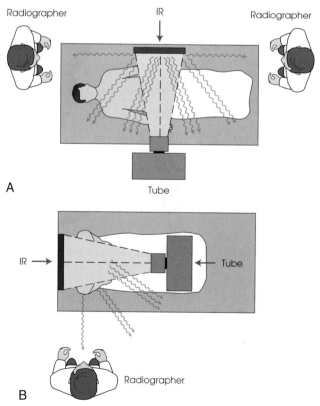

Fig. 26-7 Whenever possible, the radiographer should stand at least 6 feet (2 m) from the patient and useful beam. The lowest amount of scatter radiation occurs at a right angle (90 degrees) from the primary x-ray beam. **A,** Note radiographer standing at either the head or the foot of the patient at a right angle to the x-ray beam for dorsal decubitus position lateral projection of the abdomen. **B,** Radiographer standing at right angle to the x-ray beam for AP projection of the chest. *IR,* Image receptor.

Isolation Considerations

Two types of patients are often cared for in isolation units: (1) patients who have infectious microorganisms that could be spread to health care workers and visitors and (2) patients who need protection from potentially lethal microorganisms that may be carried by health care workers and visitors. Optimally, a radiographer entering an isolation room should have full knowledge of the patient's disease, the way it is transmitted, and the proper way to clean and disinfect equipment before and after use in the isolation unit. Because of the confidentiality of patient records, the radiographer may be unable to obtain information about a patient's specific disease, however. All patients must be treated with universal precautions. If isolation is used to protect the patient from receiving microorganisms (reverse isolation), a different protocol may be required. Institutional policy regarding isolation procedures should be available and strictly followed.

When performing mobile procedures in an isolation unit, the radiographer should wear the required protective apparel for the specific situation: gown, cap, mask, shoe covers, and gloves. All of this apparel is not needed for every isolation patient. All persons entering a strict isolation unit wear a mask, a gown, and gloves, but only gloves are worn for drainage secretion precautions. Radiographers should always wash their hands with warm, soapy water before putting on gloves. The x-ray machine is taken into the room and moved into position. The IR is placed into a clean, protective cover. Pillowcases would not protect the IR or the patient if body fluids soak through them. A clean, impermeable cover should be used in situations in which body fluids may come into contact with the IR. For examinations of patients in strict isolation, two radiographers may be required to maintain a safe barrier (see Chapter 1).

After finishing the examination, the radiographer should remove and dispose of the mask, cap, gown, shoe covers, and gloves according to institutional policies. All equipment that touched the patient or the patient's bed must be wiped with a disinfectant according to appropriate aseptic technique. The radiographer should wear new gloves, if necessary, while cleaning equipment. Handwashing is repeated before the radiographer leaves the room.

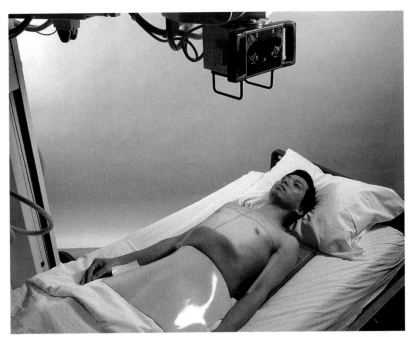

Fig. 26-8 Patient ready for mobile chest examination. Note lead shield placed over the patient's pelvis. This shield does not interfere with the examination.

Performing Mobile Examinations

INITIAL PROCEDURES

The radiographer should plan for the trip out of the radiology department. Ensuring that all of the necessary devices (e.g., IR, grid, tape, caliper, markers, blocks) are transported with the mobile x-ray machine provides greater efficiency in performing examinations. Many mobile x-ray machines are equipped with a storage area for transporting IRs and supplies. If a battery-operated machine is used, the radiographer should check the machine to ensure that it is acceptably charged. An inadequately charged machine can interfere with performance and affect the quality of the radiograph.

Before entering the patient's room with the machine, the radiographer should follow several important steps (Box 26-1). The radiographer begins by checking that the correct patient is going to be examined. After confirming the identity of the patient, the radiographer enters, makes an introduction as a radiographer, and informs the patient about the x-ray examinations to be performed. While in the room, the radiographer observes any medical appliances, such as chest tube boxes, catheter bags, and intravenous (IV) poles, that may be positioned next to or hanging on the sides of the patient's bed. The radiographer should ask family members or visitors to step out of the room until the examination is finished. If necessary, the nursing staff should be alerted that assistance is required.

Communication and cooperation between the radiographer and nursing staff members are essential for proper patient care during mobile radiography. In addition, communication with the patient is *imperative,* even if the patient is or appears to be unconscious or unresponsive.

EXAMINATION

Chairs, stands, IV poles, wastebaskets, and other obstacles should be moved from the path of the mobile machine. Lighting should be adjusted if necessary. If the patient is to be examined in the supine position, the base of the mobile machine should be positioned toward the middle of the bed. If a seated patient position is used, the base of the machine should be toward the foot of the bed.

For lateral and decubitus radiographs, positioning the base of the mobile machine parallel to or directly perpendicular to the bed allows the greatest ease in positioning the x-ray tube. Room size can also influence the base position used.

The radiographer sometimes may have difficulty accurately aligning the x-ray tube parallel to the IR while standing at the side of the bed. When positioning the tube above the patient, the radiographer may need to check the x-ray tube and IR alignment from the foot of the bed to ensure that the tube is not tilted.

For all projections, the primary x-ray beam must be collimated no larger than the size of the IR. When the central ray is correctly centered to the IR, the light field coincides with or fits within the borders of the IR.

A routine and consistent system for labeling and separating exposed and unexposed IRs should be developed and maintained. It is easy to "double expose" IRs during mobile radiography, particularly if many examinations are performed at one time. DR radiography in which one detector is used for every exposure helps eliminate the chance of double exposure. Most institutions require additional identification markers for mobile examinations. Typically the time of examination (especially for chest radiographs) and technical notes such as the position of the patient are indicated. A log may be maintained for each patient and kept in the patient's room. The log should contain the exposure factors used for the projections and other notes regarding the performance of the examination.

PATIENT CONSIDERATIONS

A brief but total assessment of the patient must be conducted before and during the examination. Some specific considerations to keep in mind are described in the following sections.

Assessment of the patient's condition

A thorough assessment of the patient's condition and room allows the radiographer to make necessary adaptations to ensure the best possible patient care and imaging outcome. The radiographer assesses the patient's level of alertness and respiration and determines the extent to which the patient is able to cooperate and the limitations that may affect the procedure. Some patients may have varying degrees of drowsiness because of their medications or medical condition. Many mobile examinations are performed in patients' rooms immediately after surgery; these patients may be under the influence of various anesthetics. It is always important to communicate with the patient even if he or she is not alert.

BOX 26-1

Preliminary steps for the radiographer before mobile radiography is performed

- Announce your presence to the nursing staff, and ask for assistance if needed.
- Determine that the correct patient is in the room.
- Introduce yourself to the patient and family as a radiographer and explain the examination.
- Observe the medical equipment in the room and other apparatus and IV poles with fluids. Move the equipment if necessary.
- Ask family members and visitors to leave.*

*A family member may need to be present for the examination of a small child.

Patient mobility

The radiographer must never move a patient or part of the patient's body without assessing the patient's ability to move or tolerate movement. *Gentleness* and *caution* must prevail at all times. If unsure, the radiographer should always check with the nursing staff or physician. Many patients who undergo total joint replacement may be unable to move the affected joint for many days without assistance, but this may not be evident to the radiographer. Some patients may be able to indicate verbally their ability to move or their tolerance for movement. *The radiographer should never move a limb that has been operated on or is broken, unless the nurse, the physician, or sometimes the patient grants permission.* Inappropriate movement of the patient by the radiographer during the examination may harm the patient.

Fractures

Patients can have various fractures and fracture types, ranging from one simple fracture to multiple fractures of many bones. A patient lying awake in a traction bed with a simple femur fracture may be able to assist with a radiographic examination. Another patient may be unconscious and have multiple broken ribs, spinal fractures, or a severe closed head injury.

Few patients with multiple fractures are able to move or tolerate movement. The radiographer must be cautious, resourceful, and work in accordance with the patient's condition and pain tolerance. If a patient's trunk or limb must be raised into position for a projection, the radiographer should have ample assistance so that the part can be raised safely without causing harm or intense pain.

Interfering devices

Patients who are in intensive care units or orthopedic beds because of fractures may be attached to various devices, wires, and tubing. These objects may be in the direct path of the x-ray beam and consequently produce artifacts on the image. Experienced radiographers know which of these objects can be moved out of the x-ray beam. When devices such as fracture frames cannot be moved, it may be necessary to angle the central ray or adjust the IR to obtain the best radiograph possible. In many instances, the objects have to be radiographed along with the body part (Fig. 26-9). The radiographer must exercise caution when handling any of these devices and should never remove traction devices without the assistance of a physician.

Positioning and asepsis

During positioning, the patient often perceives the IR (with or without a grid) as cold, hard, and uncomfortable. Before the IR is put in place, the patient should be warned of possible discomfort and assured that the examination will be for as short a time as possible. The patient appreciates the radiographer's concern and efficiency in completing the examination as quickly as possible.

If the surface of the IR inadvertently touches bare skin, it can stick, making positioning adjustments difficult. *The skin of older patients may be thin and dry and can be torn by manipulation of the IR if care is not taken.* A cloth or paper cover over the IR can protect the patient's skin and alleviate some of the discomfort by making it feel less cold. The cover also helps to keep the IR clean. IRs should be wiped off with a disinfectant for asepsis and infection control after each patient.

The IR must be enclosed in an appropriate, impermeable barrier in any situation in which it may come in contact with blood, body fluids, and other potentially infectious material. A contaminated IR can be difficult and sometimes impossible to clean. Approved procedures for disposing of used barriers must be followed.

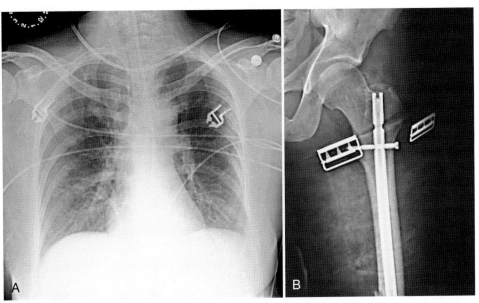

Fig. 26-9 A, Mobile radiograph of chest. Note various objects in the image that could not be removed for the exposure. **B,** Mobile radiograph of proximal femur and hip. Metal buckles could not be removed for the exposure.

ANTEROPOSTERIOR PROJECTION*
Upright or supine

Image receptor: The image receptor should be 14 × 17 inches (35 × 43 cm) lengthwise or crosswise, depending on body habitus.

Position of patient
Depending on the condition of the patient, the projection should be performed with the patient in the upright position or to the greatest angle the patient can tolerate, whenever possible. Use the supine position for critically ill or injured patients.

---

*The nonmobile projection is described in Chapter 10.

Position of part
- Center the midsagittal plane to the IR.
- To include the entire chest, position the IR under the patient with the top about 2 inches (5 cm) above the *relaxed* shoulders. The exact distance depends on the size of the patient. When the patient is supine, the shoulders may move to a higher position relative to the lungs. Adjust accordingly.
- Ensure that the patient's shoulders are relaxed; then internally rotate the patient's arms to prevent scapular superimposition of the lung field, if not contraindicated.
- Ensure that the patient's upper torso is not rotated or leaning toward one side (Fig. 26-10).
- *Shield gonads.*
- *Respiration:* Inspiration, unless otherwise requested. If the patient is receiving respiratory assistance, carefully watch the patient's chest to determine the inspiratory phase for the exposure.

Central ray
- Perpendicular to the long axis of the sternum and the center of the IR. The central ray should enter about 3 inches (7.6 cm) below the jugular notch at the level of T7.

Collimation
- Adjust to at least 14 × 17 inches (35 × 43 cm) on the collimator, less for smaller patients.

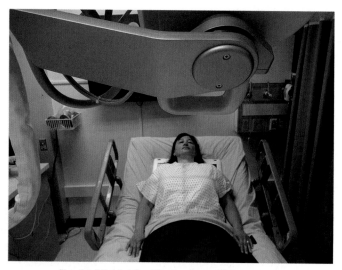

Fig. 26-10 Mobile AP chest: partially upright.

DIGITAL RADIOGRAPHY

A grid must be used for all mobile computed radiography chest examinations if the exposure technique is more than 90 kVp. (Review the manufacturer's protocol for the exact kVp levels for the unit being used.) When a crosswise-positioned longitudinal grid is used, the central ray must be perpendicular to the grid to prevent grid cutoff.

Structures shown

This projection shows the anatomy of the thorax, including the heart, trachea, diaphragmatic domes, and, most importantly, the entire lung fields, including vascular markings (Fig. 26-11).

EVALUATION CRITERIA

The following should be clearly shown:
- Evidence of proper collimation
- No motion; well-defined (not blurred) diaphragmatic domes and lung fields
- Lung fields in their entirety, including costophrenic angles
- Pleural markings
- Ribs and thoracic intervertebral disk spaces faintly visible through heart shadow
- No rotation, with medial portion of clavicles and lateral border of ribs equidistant from vertebral column

NOTE: To ensure the proper angle from the x-ray tube to the IR, the radiographer can double-check the shadow of the shoulders from the field light projected onto the IR. If the shadow of the shoulders is thrown far above the upper edge of the IR, the angle of the tube must be corrected.

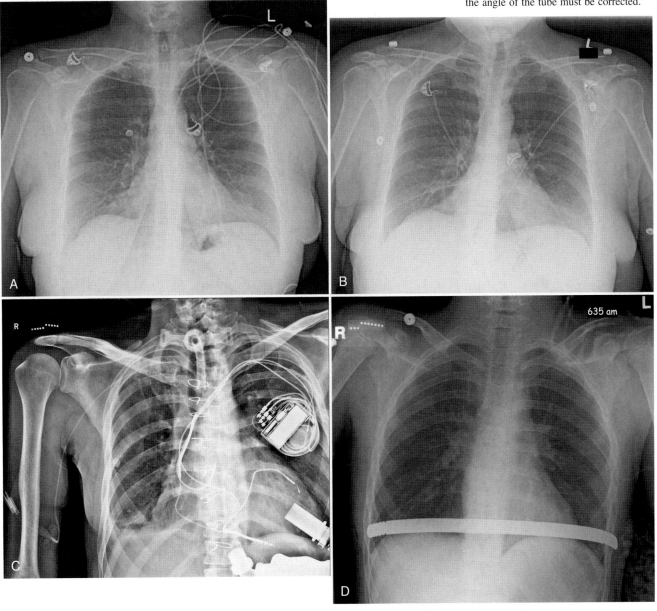

Fig. 26-11 Mobile AP chest radiographs. **A,** AP chest image with incorrect cephalic tube angle resulting in an apical lordotic image in which the ribs appear boxy, the clavicles are projected too high, and the heart has a distorted silhouette. A tangle of lead wire is seen over the upper left chest. **B,** Repeat image with the correct angle central ray perpendicular to the long axis of the sternum. The radiographer has also positioned the lead wires appropriately. **C,** Mobile PICC placement image to visualize the PICC line from entrance to tip. Also seen are the tracheostomy, pacemaker, sternal wires, and ventricular assist device. **D,** Adolescent postoperative patient with strut placed for pectus excavatum repair. Ice pack is seen in the lower right corner of the image.

AP OR PA PROJECTION*
Right or left lateral decubitus position

> **Image receptor:** The image receptor should be a 14- × 17-inch (35- × 43-cm) lengthwise grid IR.

Position of patient
- Place the patient in the lateral recumbent position.
- Flex the patient's knees to provide stabilization, if possible.
- Place a firm support under the patient to elevate the body 2 to 3 inches (5 to 8 cm) and prevent the patient from sinking into the mattress.
- Raise both of the patient's arms up and away from the chest region, preferably above the head. An arm lying on the patient's side can imitate a region of free air.
- Ensure that the patient cannot roll off the bed.

*The nonmobile projection is described in Chapter 10.

Position of part
- Position the patient for the AP projection whenever possible. It is much easier to position an ill patient (particularly the arms) for an AP.
- Adjust the patient to ensure a lateral position. The coronal plane passing through the shoulders and hips should be vertical.
- Place the IR behind the patient and below the support so that the lower margin of the chest is visible.
- Adjust the grid so that it extends approximately 2 inches (5 cm) above the shoulders. The IR should be supported in position and not leaning against the patient to avoid distortion (Fig. 26-12).
- *Shield gonads.*
- *Respiration:* Inspiration unless otherwise requested.

Central ray
- Horizontal and perpendicular to the center of the IR, entering the patient at a level of 3 inches (7.6 cm) below the jugular notch

Collimation
- Adjust to 14 × 17 inches (35 × 43 cm) on the collimator.

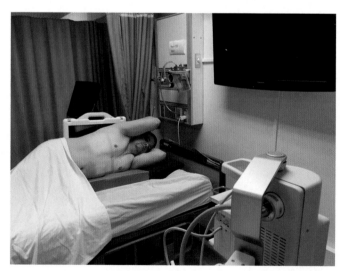

Fig. 26-12 Mobile AP chest: left lateral decubitus position. Note gray pad placed under the chest to elevate it. The block is necessary to ensure that the left side of chest is included on image.

Structures shown

This projection shows the anatomy of the thorax, including the entire lung fields and any air or fluid levels that may be present (Fig. 26-13).

EVALUATION CRITERIA

The following should be clearly shown:
- Evidence of proper collimation
- No motion
- No rotation
- Affected side in its entirety (upper lung for free air and lower lung for fluid)
- Patient's arms out of region of interest
- Proper identification to indicate that decubitus position was used

NOTE: Fluid levels in the pleural cavity are best visualized with the affected side down, which also prevents mediastinal overlapping. Air levels are best visualized with the unaffected side down. The patient should be in position for at least 5 minutes before the exposure is made to allow air to rise and fluid levels to settle.

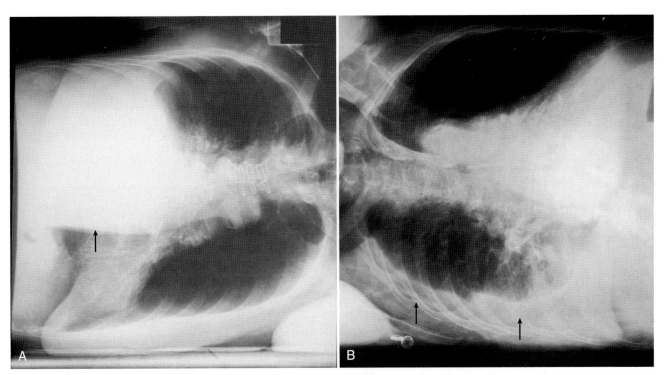

Fig. 26-13 Mobile AP chest radiographs performed in lateral decubitus positions in critically ill patients. **A,** Left lateral decubitus position. The patient has a large right pleural effusion (*arrow*) and no left effusion. Complete left side of thorax is visualized because of elevation on a block. **B,** Right lateral decubitus position. The patient has right pleural effusion (*arrows*), cardiomegaly, and mild pulmonary vascular congestion. Complete right side of thorax is visualized because of elevation on a block.

AP PROJECTION*

Image receptor: The image receptor should be a 14- × 17-inch (35- × 43-cm) lengthwise grid.

Position of patient
- If necessary, adjust the patient's bed to achieve a horizontal bed position.
- Place the patient in a supine position.

Position of part
- Position the grid under the patient to show the abdominal anatomy from the pubic symphysis to the upper abdominal region.
- Keep the grid from tipping side to side by placing it in the center of the bed and stabilizing it with blankets or towels if necessary.
- Use the patient's draw sheet to roll the patient; this makes it easier to shift the patient from side to side during positioning of the IR, and it provides a barrier between the patient's skin and the grid.

---

*The nonmobile projection is described in Chapter 16.

- Center the midsagittal plane of the patient to the midline of the grid.
- Center the grid to the level of the iliac crests. If the emphasis is on the upper abdomen, center the grid 2 inches (5 cm) above the iliac crests or high enough to include the diaphragm.
- Adjust the patient's shoulders and pelvis to lie in the same plane (Fig. 26-14).
- Move the patient's arms out of the region of the abdomen.
- *Shield gonads.* This may not be possible in a female patient.
- *Respiration:* Expiration.

Central ray
- Perpendicular to the center of the grid along the midsagittal plane and at the level of the iliac crests or the 10th rib laterally

Collimation
- Adjust to 14 × 17 inches (35 × 43 cm) on the collimator.

Structures shown

This projection shows the following: the inferior margin of the liver; the spleen, kidneys, and psoas muscles; calcifications; and evidence of tumor masses. If the image includes the upper abdomen and diaphragm, the size and shape of the liver may be seen (Fig. 26-15).

EVALUATION CRITERIA

The following should be clearly shown:
- Evidence of proper collimation
- No motion
- Outlines of the abdominal viscera
- Abdominal region, including pubic symphysis or diaphragm (both may be seen on some patients)
- Vertebral column in center of image
- Psoas muscles, lower margin of liver, and kidney margins
- No rotation
- Symmetric appearance of vertebral column and iliac wings

NOTE: Hypersthenic patients may require two separate projections using a crosswise grid. One grid is positioned for the upper abdomen, and the other is positioned for the lower abdomen.

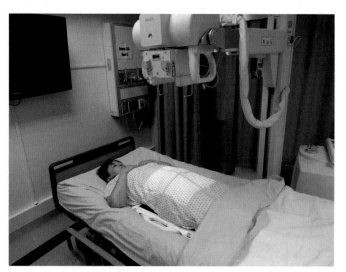

Fig. 26-14 Mobile AP abdomen.

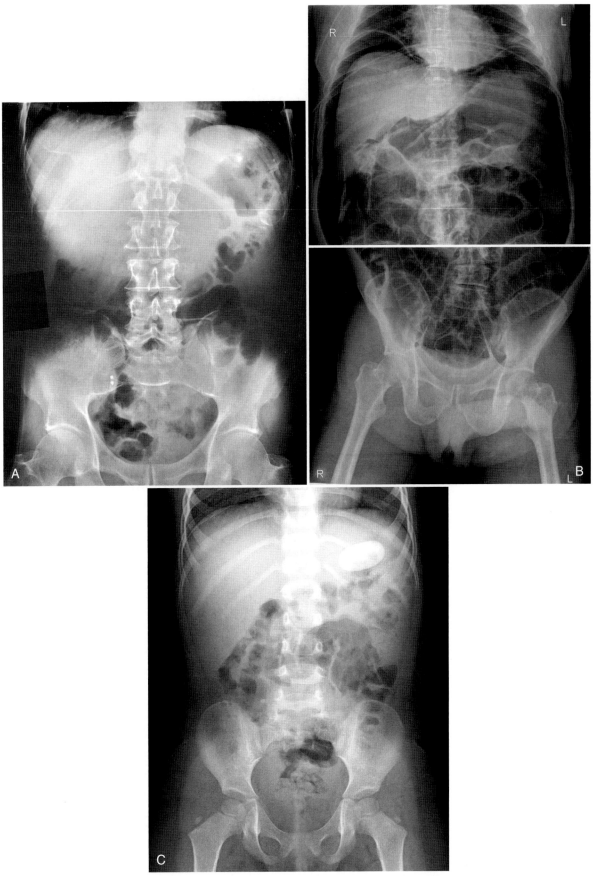

Fig. 26-15 Mobile AP abdomen radiographs. **A,** Abdomen without pathology. The entire abdomen is seen in this patient. **B,** Because of this patient's increased body habitus, two crosswise (landscape) images of the abdomen were necessary to include all abdominal structures. Counting vertebral bodies ensures adequate overlap. Note the large amount of free air indicative of a perforated bowel. **C,** Mobile AP abdomen image of a pediatric patient. Ingested jewelry bead is seen in the fundus of the stomach.

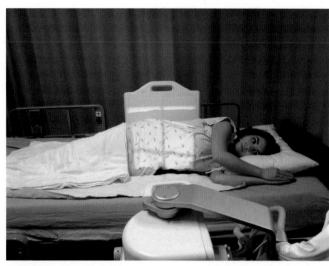

Fig. 26-16 Mobile AP abdomen: left lateral decubitus position. Note black blocks placed under the abdomen to level the abdomen and keep the patient from sinking into the mattress.

ANTEROPOSTERIOR OR POSTEROANTERIOR PROJECTION*
Left lateral decubitus position

> **Image receptor:** The image receptor should be a 14- × 17-inch (35- × 43-cm) lengthwise grid.

Position of patient
- Place the patient in the left lateral recumbent position unless requested otherwise.
- Flex the patient's knees slightly to provide stabilization.
- If necessary, place a firm support under the patient to elevate the body and keep the patient from sinking into the mattress.
- Raise both of the patient's arms away from the abdominal region, if possible. The right arm lying on the side of the abdomen may imitate a region of free air.
- Ensure that the patient cannot fall out of bed.

Position of part
- Use the posteroanterior (PA) or AP projection, depending on the room layout.
- Adjust the patient to ensure a true lateral position. The coronal plane passing through the shoulders and hips should be vertical.
- Place the grid vertically in front of the patient for a PA projection and behind the patient for an AP projection. The grid should be supported in position and not leaned against the patient; this position prevents grid cutoff.
- Position the grid so that its center is 2 inches (5 cm) above the iliac crests to ensure that the diaphragm is included. The pubic symphysis and lower abdomen do not have to be visualized (Fig. 26-16).
- Before making the exposure, ensure that the patient has been in the lateral recumbent position for at least 5 minutes to allow air to rise and fluid levels to settle.
- *Shield gonads.*
- *Respiration:* Expiration.

---

*The nonmobile projection is described in Chapter 16.

Central ray

- Horizontal and perpendicular to the center of the grid, entering the patient along the midsagittal plane

Collimation

- Adjust to 14 × 17 inches (35 × 43 cm) on the collimator.

Structures shown

Air or fluid levels within the abdominal cavity are shown. These projections are especially helpful in assessing free air in the abdomen. The right border of the abdominal region must be visualized (Fig. 26-17).

EVALUATION CRITERIA

The following should be clearly shown:
- Evidence of proper collimation
- No motion
- Well-defined diaphragm and abdominal viscera
- Air or fluid levels, if present
- Right and left abdominal wall and flank structures
- No rotation
- Symmetric appearance of vertebral column and iliac wings

NOTE: Hypersthenic patients may require two projections with the 14- × 17-inch (35- × 43-cm) grid positioned crosswise to visualize the entire abdominal area. A patient with a long torso may require two projections with the grid lengthwise to visualize the entire abdominal region.

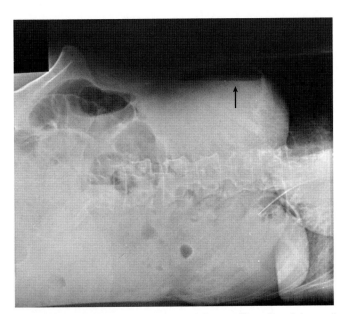

Fig. 26-17 Mobile AP abdomen: left lateral decubitus position. Free intraperitoneal air is seen on the upper or right side of the abdomen (*arrow*). The radiograph is slightly underexposed to show free air more easily.

AP PROJECTION*

Image receptor: The image receptor should be a 14- × 17-inch (35- × 43-cm) grid crosswise.

Position of patient
- Adjust the patient's bed horizontally so that the patient is in a supine position.
- Move the patient's arms out of the region of the pelvis.

*The nonmobile projection is described in Chapter 7.

Position of part
- Position the grid under the pelvis so that the center is midway between the anterior superior iliac spine (ASIS) and the pubic symphysis. This is about 2 inches (5 cm) inferior to the ASIS and 2 inches (5 cm) superior to the pubic symphysis.
- Center the midsagittal plane of the patient to the midline of the grid. The pelvis should not be rotated.
- Rotate the patient's legs medially approximately 15 degrees when not contraindicated (Fig. 26-18).
- *Shield gonads:* This may not be possible in female patients.
- *Respiration:* Suspend.

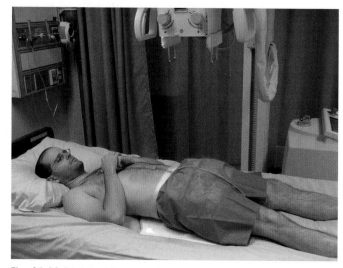

Fig. 26-18 Mobile AP pelvis. Grid is placed horizontal and perpendicular to central ray.

Central ray

- Perpendicular to the midpoint of the grid, entering the midsagittal plane. The central ray should enter the patient 2 inches (5 cm) above the pubic symphysis and 2 inches (5 cm) below the ASIS.

Collimation

- Adjust to 14 × 17 inches (35 × 43 cm) on the collimator.

Structures shown

This projection shows the pelvis, including the following: both hip bones; the sacrum and coccyx; and the head, neck, trochanters, and proximal portion of the femora (Fig. 26-19).

EVALUATION CRITERIA

The following should be clearly shown:

- Evidence of proper collimation
- Entire pelvis, including proximal femora and both hip bones
- No rotation
- Symmetric appearance of iliac wings and obturator foramina
- Both greater trochanters and ilia equidistant from edge of radiograph
- Femoral necks not foreshortened and greater trochanters in profile

NOTE: It is common for the patient's weight to cause the bottom edge of the grid to tilt upward. The x-ray tube may need to be angled caudally to compensate and maintain proper grid alignment, preventing grid cutoff. The exact angle needed is not always known, however, or easy to determine. The radiographer may want to lower the foot of the bed slightly (Fowler position), shifting the patient's weight more evenly on the grid and allowing it to be flat. A rolled-up towel or blanket placed under the grid also may be useful to prevent lateral tilting. If the bed is equipped with an inflatable air mattress, the maximum inflate mode is recommended. Tilting the bottom edge of the grid downward is another possibility. Check the level of the grid carefully and compensate accordingly.

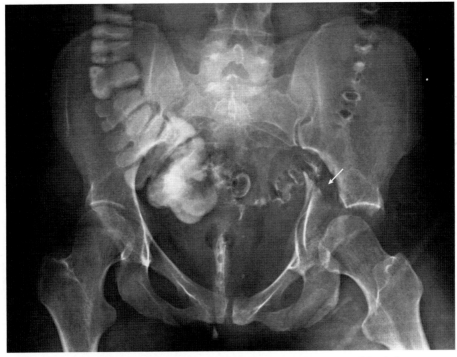

Fig. 26-19 Mobile AP pelvis. This patient has a comminuted fracture of the left acetabulum with medial displacement of medial acetabular wall (*arrow*). Residual barium is seen in the colon, sigmoid, and rectum.

AP PROJECTION*

Most mobile AP and lateral projections of the femur may be radiographs of the middle and distal femur taken while the patient is in traction. The femur cannot be moved, which presents a challenge to the radiographer.

Image receptor: The image receptor should be a 14- × 17-inch (35- × 43-cm) grid lengthwise.

Position of patient

- The patient is in the supine position.

*The nonmobile projection is described in Chapter 6.

Position of part

- *Cautiously* place the grid lengthwise under the patient's femur, with the distal edge of the grid low enough to include the fracture site, pathologic region, and knee joint.
- Elevate the grid with towels, blankets, or blocks under each side, if necessary, to ensure proper grid alignment with the x-ray tube.
- Center the grid to the midline of the affected femur.
- Ensure that the grid is placed parallel to the plane of the femoral condyles (Fig. 26-20).
- *Shield gonads.*
- *Respiration:* Suspend.

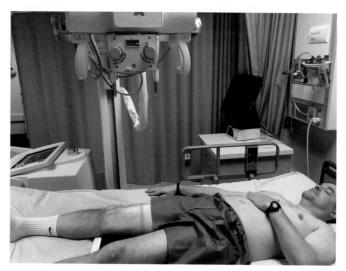

Fig. 26-20 Mobile AP femur.

Central ray

- Perpendicular to the long axis of the femur and centered to the grid
- Ensure that the central ray and grid are aligned to prevent grid cutoff.

Collimation

- Adjust to top at ASIS for hip, bottom at tibial tuberosity for knee, 1 inch (2.5 cm) on side of the shadow of the femur, and 17 inches (43 cm) in length.

DIGITAL RADIOGRAPHY

The thickest portion of the femur (proximal area) must be carefully measured, and an appropriate kVp must be selected to penetrate this area. The computer cannot form an image of the anatomy in this area if penetration does not occur. A light area of the entire proximal femur would result. Positioning the cathode over the proximal femur would improve CR image quality.

Structures shown

The distal two thirds of the femur, including the knee joint, are shown (Fig. 26-21).

EVALUATION CRITERIA

The following should be clearly shown:
- Evidence of proper collimation
- Most of femur, including knee joint
- No knee rotation
- Adequate penetration of proximal portion of femur
- Any orthopedic appliance, such as plate and screw fixation

NOTE: If the entire length of the femur needs to be visualized, an AP projection of the proximal femur can be performed by placing a 14- × 17-inch (35- × 43-cm) grid lengthwise under the proximal femur and hip. The top of the grid is placed at the level of the ASIS to ensure that the hip joint is included. The central ray is directed to the center of the grid and long axis of the femur (see Fig. 26-3).

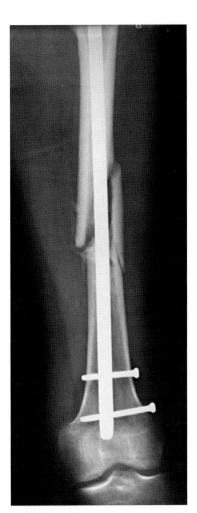

Fig. 26-21 Mobile AP femur radiograph showing a fracture of the midshaft with femoral rod placement. The knee joint is included on the image.

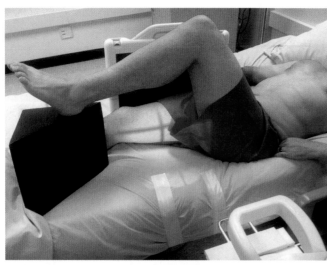

Fig. 26-22 Mobile mediolateral left femur. An assistant wearing a lead apron holds and positions the right leg and femur and steadies the grid.

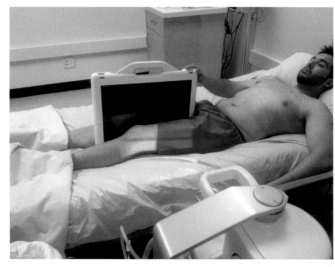

Fig. 26-23 Mobile lateromedial left femur. Grid is placed between the legs and steadied by the patient.

LATERAL PROJECTION*
Mediolateral or lateromedial projection
Dorsal decubitus position

The femur may not be able to be moved, which presents a challenge to the radiographer. The *mediolateral* projection is generally preferred because more of the proximal femur is demonstrated.

> **Image receptor:** The image receptor should be a 14- × 17-inch (35- × 43-cm) grid lengthwise.

Position of patient
- The patient is in the supine position.

Position of part
- Determine whether a mediolateral or lateromedial projection is to be performed.

Mediolateral projection
- Visualize the optimal length of the patient's femur by placing the grid in a vertical position next to the lateral aspect of the femur.
- Place the distal edge of the grid low enough to include the patient's knee joint.
- Have the patient, if able, hold the upper corner of the grid for stabilization; otherwise, support the grid firmly in position.
- Support the unaffected leg by using the patient's support (a trapeze bar if present) or a support block.
- Elevate the unaffected leg until the femur is nearly vertical. An assistant may need to elevate and hold the leg of a critically ill patient. The assistant may also steady the grid and must wear a lead apron for protection (Fig. 26-22).

Lateromedial projection
- Place the grid next to the medial aspect of the affected femur (between the patient's legs), and ensure that the knee joint is included (Fig. 26-23).
- Ensure that the grid is placed *perpendicular* to the epicondylar plane.
- *Shield gonads.*
- *Respiration:* Suspend.

---

*The nonmobile projection is described in Chapter 6.

Central ray

- Perpendicular to the long axis of the femur, entering at its midpoint.
- Ensure that the central ray and grid are aligned to prevent grid cutoff; the central ray is centered to the femur and not to the center of the grid.

Collimation

- Adjust to top at ASIS for hip, bottom at tibial tuberosity for knee, 1 inch (2.5 cm) on side of the shadow of the femur, and 17 inches (43 cm) in length.

The thickest portion of the femur (proximal area) must be measured carefully, and an appropriate kVp must be selected to penetrate this area. The computer cannot form an image of any anatomy in this area if penetration does not occur. A light area of the entire proximal femur would result. Positioning the cathode over the proximal femur would improve CR image quality.

Structures shown

This projection shows the distal two thirds of the femur, including the knee joint, without superimposition of the opposite thigh (Fig. 26-24).

EVALUATION CRITERIA

The following should be clearly shown:
- Evidence of proper collimation
- Most of femur, including knee joint
- Patella in profile
- Superimposition of femoral condyles
- Opposite femur and soft tissue out of area of interest
- Adequate penetration of proximal portion of femur
- Orthopedic appliance, if present

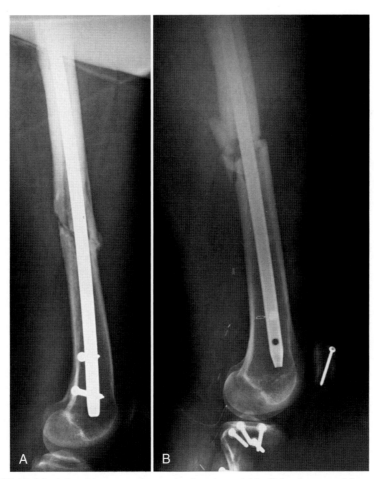

Fig. 26-24 Mobile lateral femur radiographs showing midshaft fractures and femoral rod placement. The knee joints are included on the image. **A,** Mediolateral. **B,** Lateromedial.

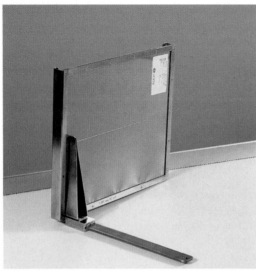

Fig. 26-25 Measuring caliper used to hold a 10- × 12-inch (24- × 30-cm) grid in place for mobile lateral cervical spine radiography.

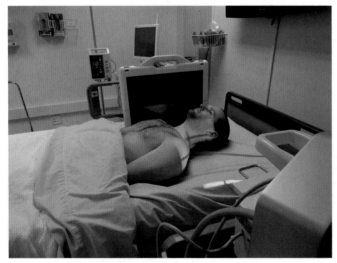

Fig. 26-26 Mobile lateral cervical spine.

LATERAL PROJECTION*
Right or left dorsal decubitus position

> **Image receptor:** The image receptor should be a 10- × 12-inch (24- × 30-cm) grid lengthwise; may be performed with a nongrid IR on smaller patients.

Position of patient
- Position the patient in the supine position with arms extended down along the sides of the body.
- Observe whether a cervical collar or another immobilization device is being used. *Do not remove the device without the consent of the nurse or physician.*

Position of part
- Ensure that the upper torso, cervical spine, and head are not rotated.
- Place the grid lengthwise on the right or left side, parallel to the neck.
- Place the top of the grid approximately 1 inch (2.43 cm) above the external acoustic meatus (EAM) so that the grid is centered to C4 (upper thyroid cartilage).
- Raise the chin slightly. *If the patient has a new trauma, suspected fracture, or known fracture of the cervical region, check with the physician before elevating the chin. Improper movement of a patient's head can disrupt a fractured cervical spine.*
- Immobilize the grid in a vertical position. The grid can be immobilized in multiple ways if a holding device is unavailable. The best method is to use the measuring caliper. Slide the long portion of the caliper under the shoulders of the patient, with the short end of the caliper pointing toward the ceiling and the grid held between the ends of the caliper (Fig. 26-25). Another method is to place pillows or a cushion between the side rail of the bed and the IR, holding the IR next to the patient. Tape also works well in many instances (Fig. 26-26).
- Have the patient relax the shoulders and reach for the feet, if possible.
- *Shield gonads.*
- *Respiration:* Full expiration to obtain maximum depression of the shoulders.

---

*The nonmobile projection is described in Chapter 8.

Central ray
- Horizontal and perpendicular to the center of the grid. This should place the central ray at the level of C4 (upper thyroid cartilage).
- Ensure that proper alignment of the central ray and grid is maintained to prevent grid cutoff.
- Because of the great object-to-image receptor distance (OID), SID of 60 to 72 inches (158 to 183 cm) is recommended. This also helps show C7.

Collimation
- Adjust top at top of ear attachment (TEA), bottom to jugular notch, and 1 inch (2.5 cm) on sides of neck.

DIGITAL RADIOGRAPHY

To ensure that the lower cervical vertebrae are fully penetrated, the kVp must be set to penetrate the C7 area.

Structures shown
This projection shows the seven cervical vertebrae, including the base of the skull and the soft tissues surrounding the neck (Fig. 26-27).

EVALUATION CRITERIA

The following should be clearly shown:
- Evidence of proper collimation
- All seven cervical vertebrae, including interspaces and spinous processes
- Neck extended when possible so that rami of mandible are not overlapping C1 or C2
- C4 in center of grid
- Superimposed posterior margins of each vertebral body

NOTE: It is essential that C6 and C7 be included on the image. To accomplish this, the radiographer should instruct the patient to relax the shoulders toward the feet as much as possible. If the examination involves pulling down on the patient's arms, the radiographer should exercise extreme caution and evaluate the patient's condition carefully to determine whether pulling of the arms can be tolerated. Fractures or injuries of the upper limbs, including the clavicles, must be considered. Applying a strong pull to the arms of a patient in a hurried or jerking manner can disrupt a fractured cervical spine. If the lateral projection does not adequately visualize the lower cervical region, the Twining method, sometimes referred to as the "swimmer's" position, which eliminates pulling of the arms, may be recommended for patients who have experienced trauma or have a known cervical fracture. One arm must be placed above the patient's head (the Twining method is described in Chapter 8).

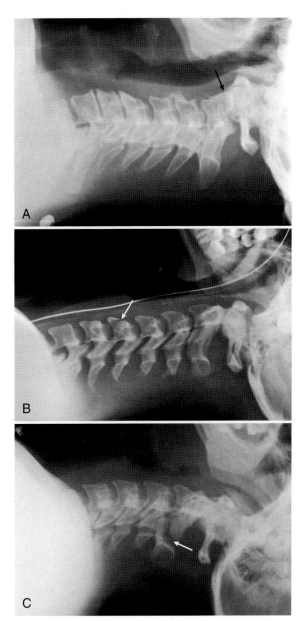

Fig. 26-27 Mobile lateral cervical spine radiographs performed at the patient's bedside several weeks after trauma. **A,** Entire cervical spine shows slight anterior subluxation of the dens on the body of C2 (*arrow*). **B,** Entire cervical spine shows nearly vertical fracture through the body of C5 with slight displacement (*arrow*). **C,** First five cervical vertebrae show vertical fractures through posterior aspects of C2 laminae (*arrow*) with 4-mm displacement of the fragments. Earlier radiographs showed that C6 and C7 were unaffected and did not need to be included in this follow-up radiograph.

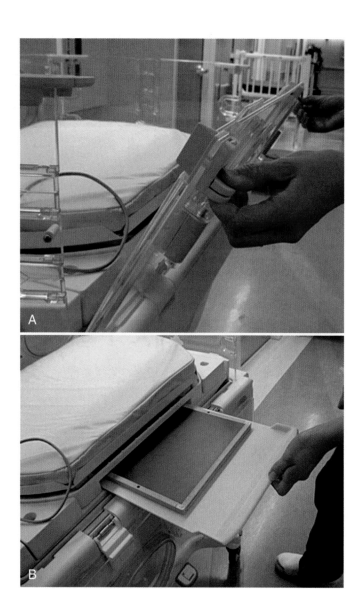

Fig. 26-28 A, Side panel of the isolette being lowered to gain access to the IR tray. **B,** IR being placed on a special tray for placement below the infant.

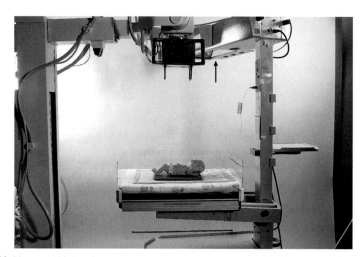

Fig. 26-29 Neonatal intensive care unit bassinet with a premature infant. Overhead heating unit (*arrow*) is moved out of the way to accommodate mobile x-ray machine tube head.

AP PROJECTION

The chest and abdomen combination described here is typically ordered for premature newborns who are in the neonatal intensive care unit. If a chest or abdomen projection is ordered separately, the radiographer should adjust the central ray and collimator accordingly.

> **Image receptor:** The image receptor should be an 8- × 10-inch (20- × 24-cm) or 10- × 12-inch (24- × 30-cm) grid lengthwise.

Position of patient

Position the infant supine in the center of the IR. Some bassinets have a special tray to hold the IR. Positioning numbers along the tray permits accurate placement of the IR (Fig. 26-28). If the IR is directly under the infant, cover the IR with a soft, warm blanket.

Position of part

- *Carefully* position the x-ray tube over the infant (Fig. 26-29).
- Ensure that the chest and abdomen are not rotated.
- Move the infant's arms away from the body or over the head and bring the legs down and away from the abdomen. The arms and legs may have to be held by a nurse, who should wear a lead apron.
- Leave the head of the infant rotated. (See note at end of this section.)
- Adjust the collimators closely to the chest and abdomen (Fig. 26-30).
- *Shield gonads.*
- *Respiration:* Inspiration. Neonates have an extremely fast respiratory rate and cannot hold their breath. Make the best attempt possible to perform the exposure on full inspiration (Fig. 26-31).

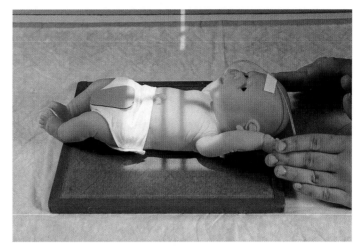

Fig. 26-30 Mobile chest and abdomen radiograph of a neonate. Note the male gonadal shield. (In actual practice, the IR is covered with a soft, warm blanket.)

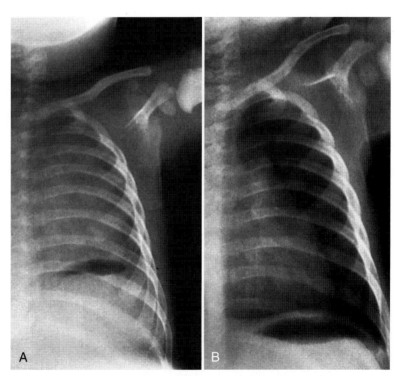

Fig. 26-31 Radiographs on inspiration and expiration in a neonate. **A,** Left side of chest is shown at full expiration. Note the lack of normal lung markings and the illusion of massive pulmonary disease. Diaphragm is not seen, and heart appears enlarged. **B,** Repeat radiograph of the same patient performed correctly at full inspiration. Diaphragm may be seen correctly at the level of the 10th posterior rib. The same technical factors were used for both exposures.

(Courtesy Department of Radiology, Rochester General Hospital, Rochester, NY. From Cullinan AM, Cullinan JE: *Producing quality radiographs,* ed 2, Philadelphia, 1994, Lippincott.)

Central ray

- Perpendicular to the midpoint of the chest and abdomen along the midsagittal plane

Collimation

- Adjust top to 1 inch (2.5 cm) above shoulders, bottom at lower rib margins for chest or to pubic symphysis if chest and abdomen requested, and 1 inch (2.5 cm) on sides.

Structures shown

The anatomy of the entire chest and abdomen is shown (Fig. 26-32).

EVALUATION CRITERIA

The following should be clearly shown:

- Evidence of proper collimation
- Anatomy from apices to pubic symphysis in the thoracic and abdominal regions
- No motion
- No blurring of lungs, diaphragm, and abdominal structures
- No rotation of patient

NOTE: When performing an AP or lateral projection of the chest, the radiographer should keep the head and neck of the infant straight so that the anatomy in the upper chest and airway is accurately visualized. Straightening the head of a neonate in the supine position can inadvertently advance an endotracheal tube too far into the trachea, however. It is sometimes more important to leave the head of an intubated neonatal patient rotated in the position in which the infant routinely lies to obtain accurate representation of the position of the endotracheal tube on the radiograph.

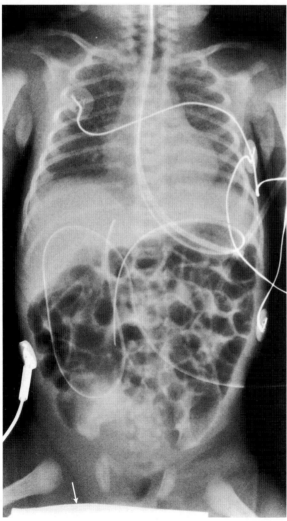

Fig. 26-32 Mobile AP chest and abdomen radiograph of a neonate. Exposure technique shows the anatomy of entire chest and abdomen. Note gonadal shield accurately positioned on this male infant (*arrow*).

LATERAL PROJECTION
Dorsal decubitus position

Image receptor: The image receptor should be an 8- × 10-inch (20- × 24-cm) or 10- × 12-inch (24- × 30-cm) grid lengthwise. Most premature neonates cannot be turned on their sides or placed upright for a lateral projection.

Position of patient
- *Carefully* place the x-ray tube on the side of the bassinet.
- Position the infant supine on a radiolucent block covered with a soft, warm blanket. If a radiolucent block is not readily available, an inverted box of tissues works well.

Position of part
- Ensure that the infant's chest and abdomen are centered to the IR and not rotated.
- Move the infant's arms above the head. The infant's arms have to be held up by a nurse, who should wear a lead apron.
- Place the IR lengthwise and vertical beside the patient and immobilize it.
- Leave the head of the infant rotated. (See note on p. 210.)
- Adjust the collimators closely to the chest and abdomen (Fig. 26-33).
- *Shield gonads.*
- *Respiration:* Inspiration. Neonates have an extremely fast respiratory rate and cannot hold their breath. Make the best attempt possible to perform the exposure on full inspiration.

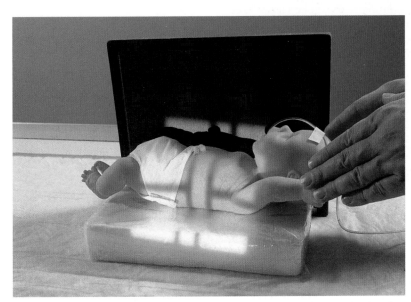

Fig. 26-33 Mobile lateral chest and abdomen radiograph of a neonate in dorsal decubitus position. The infant is positioned on a raised block with the IR below the block.

Central ray

- Horizontal and perpendicular to the midpoint of the chest and abdomen along the midcoronal plane

Collimation

- Adjust top to 1 inch (2.5 cm) above shoulders, bottom at lower rib margins for chest or to pubic symphysis if chest and abdomen requested, and 1 inch (2.5 cm) on sides.

Structures shown

This projection shows the anatomy of the entire chest and abdomen, with special attention to the costophrenic angles in the posterior chest. If present, air and fluid levels are visualized (Fig. 26-34).

EVALUATION CRITERIA

The following should be clearly shown:
- Evidence of proper collimation
- Anatomy of chest and abdomen from apices to pubic bone
- No motion
- No blurring of lungs, diaphragm, and abdominal structures
- No rotation of patient
- Air and fluid levels, if present

Selected bibliography

Adler AM, Carlton RR: *Introduction to radiography and patient care*, ed 4, Philadelphia, 2007, Saunders.

Bontrager KL: *Textbook of radiographic positioning*, ed 7, St Louis, 2010, Mosby.

Bushong SC: *Radiologic science for technologists*, ed 9, St Louis, 2008, Mosby.

Ehrlich RA, McClosky ED: *Patient care in radiography*, ed 7, St Louis, 2009, Mosby.

Hall-Rollins J, Winters R: Mobile chest radiography: improving image quality, *Radiol Technol* 71:5, 2000.

Statkiewicz-Sherer MA et al: *Radiation protection in medical radiography*, ed 6, St Louis, 2011, Mosby.

Tucker DM, et al: Scatter in computed radiography, *Radiology* 188:271, 1993.

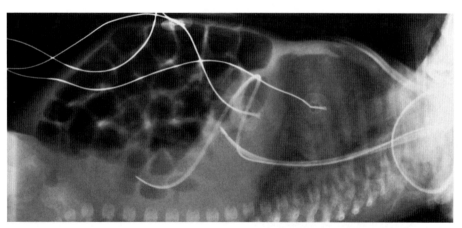

Fig. 26-34 Mobile lateral chest and abdomen radiograph of a neonate in dorsal decubitus position. Exposure technique shows the anatomy of the entire chest and abdomen.

27

SURGICAL RADIOGRAPHY

KARI J. WETTERLIN

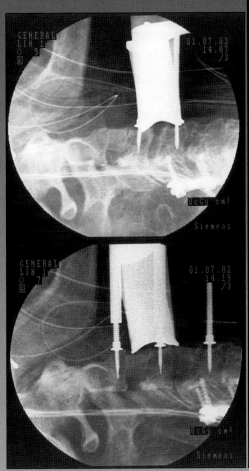

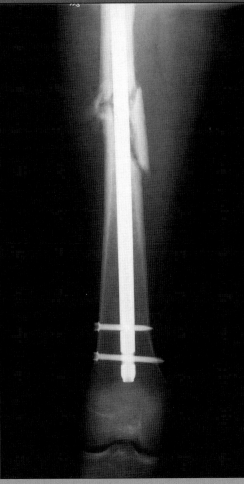

OUTLINE

Surgical Team, 214
Proper Surgical Attire, 216
Operating Room Attire, 217
Personal Hygiene, 217
Dance of the Operating
Room, 218
Equipment, 221
Cleaning of Equipment, 222
Radiation Exposure
Considerations, 223
Fluoroscopic Procedures for
the Operating Room, 223
Mobile Radiography
Procedures for the
Operating Room, 242

Surgical radiology is a dynamic experience. The challenges a radiographer encounters in the surgical suite are unique. Knowing the machinery and its capabilities and limitations is most important; in that regard, the radiographer can enter any operating room (OR) case, whether routine or extraordinary, and, with good communication, be able to perform all tasks well. An understanding of common procedures and familiarity with equipment enables the radiographer to perform most mobile examinations ordered by the physician. Surgical radiography can be a challenging and exciting environment for the radiographer but can also be intimidating and stressful. Surgical radiology requires educated personnel familiar with specific equipment routinely used during common surgical procedures. It requires expertise in teamwork. Preparedness and familiarity with equipment are key. Standard health and safety protocols must be followed to avoid contamination and to ensure patient safety. These are the basics, and the pieces come together in surgical radiology in distinctive ways.

This chapter focuses on the most common procedures performed in the surgical area. The basic principles of mobile imaging are detailed, and helpful suggestions are provided for successful completion of the examinations. This chapter is not intended to cover every possible combination of examinations or situations that a radiographer may encounter; rather it provides an overview of the surgical setting and a summary of common examinations. The scope of radiologic examinations in a surgical setting is vast and may differ greatly among health care facilities (Box 27-1). The goals of this chapter are to (1) provide an overview of the surgical setting and explain the role of the radiographer as a vital member of the surgical team, (2) assist the radiographer in developing an understanding of the imaging equipment used in surgical situations, and (3) present common radiographic procedures performed in the OR. The radiographer should review the surgery department protocols because they vary from institution to institution.

Surgical Team

At no other time is a patient so well attended as during a surgical procedure. A surgeon, one or two assistants, a surgical technologist, an anesthesia provider, a circulating nurse, and various support staff surround the patient. These individuals, each with specific functions to perform, form the OR team. This team literally has the patient's life in its hands. The OR team has been described as a symphony orchestra, with each person an integral entity in unison and harmony with his or her colleagues for the successful accomplishment of the expected outcomes. The OR team is subdivided, according to the functions of its members, into sterile and nonsterile teams.

BOX 27-1

Scope of surgical radiography

Surgical fluoroscopic procedures
- Abdomen: cholangiogram
- Chest-line placement: bronchoscopy
- Cervical spine: anterior cervical discectomy and fusion
- Lumbar spine
- Hip: cannulated hip screws or hip pinning, decompression hip screw
- Femoral and tibial nailing
- Extremity fluoroscopy
- Humerus: shoulder in beach chair position
- Femoral/tibial arteriogram

Mobile surgical radiography procedures
- Localization examinations of cervical, thoracic, and lumbar spine
- Mobile extremity examinations in OR

STERILE TEAM MEMBERS

Sterile team members scrub their hands and arms, don a sterile gown and gloves over proper surgical attire, and enter the sterile field. The sterile field is the area of the OR that immediately surrounds and is specially prepared for the patient. To establish a sterile field, all items necessary for the surgical procedure are sterilized. After this process, the scrubbed and sterile team members function within this limited area and handle only sterile items (Fig. 27-1). The sterile team consists of the following members:

- *Surgeon:* The surgeon is a licensed physician who is specially trained and qualified by knowledge and experience to perform surgical procedures. The surgeon's responsibilities include preoperative diagnosis and care, selection and performance of the surgical procedure, and postoperative management of care. The surgeon assumes full responsibility for all medical acts of judgment and for the management of the surgical patient.

- *Surgical assistant:* The first assistant is a qualified surgeon or resident in an accredited surgical educational program. The assistant should be capable of assuming responsibility for performing the procedure for the primary surgeon. Assistants help to maintain visibility of the surgical site, control bleeding, close wounds, and apply dressings. The assistant's role varies depending on the institution and with the type of procedure or surgical specialty.

- *Physician assistant:* The physician assistant is a nonphysician allied health practitioner who is qualified by academic and clinical training to perform designated procedures in the OR and in other areas of surgical patient care.

- *Scrub nurse:* The scrub nurse is a registered nurse (RN) who is specially trained to work with surgeons and the medical team in the OR.

- *Certified surgical technologist (CST):* The CST is responsible for maintaining the integrity, safety, and efficiency of the sterile field throughout the surgical procedure. The CST prepares and arranges instruments and supplies and assists the surgical procedure by providing the required sterile instruments and supplies. In some institutions, a licensed practical nurse (LPN) or RN may assume this role.

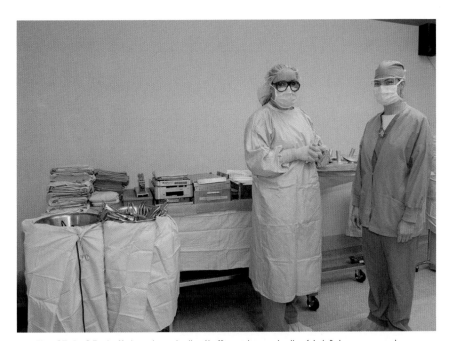

Fig. 27-1 OR staff showing sterile (*left*) and nonsterile (*right*) team members.

NONSTERILE TEAM MEMBERS

Nonsterile team members do not enter the sterile field; they function outside and around it. They assume responsibility for maintaining sterile techniques during the surgical procedure, but they handle supplies and equipment that are not considered sterile. Following the principles of aseptic technique, they keep the sterile team supplied, provide direct patient care, and respond to any requests that may arise during the surgical procedure.

- *Anesthesia provider:* The anesthesia provider is a physician (anesthesiologist) or certified RN anesthetist who specializes in administering anesthetics. Choosing and applying appropriate agents and suitable techniques of administration, monitoring physiologic functions, maintaining fluid and electrolyte balance, and performing blood replacements are essential responsibilities of the anesthesia provider during the surgical procedure.

- *Circulator:* The circulator is preferably an RN. The circulator monitors and coordinates all activities within the OR, provides supplies to the CST during the surgical procedure, and manages the care of the patient.
- *Radiographers:* The radiographer's role in the OR is to provide intraoperative imaging in a variety of examinations and with various types of equipment.
- *Others:* The OR team may also include biomedical technicians, monitoring technologists, and individuals who specialize in the equipment or monitoring devices necessary during the surgical procedure.

Proper Surgical Attire

Surgical attire protocols may change from institution to institution but should be available for review, understood, and followed by all staff members. Although small variances in protocol exist among institutions, there are common standards.

Large amounts of bacteria are present in the nose and mouth, on the skin, and on the attire of personnel who enter the restricted areas of the surgical setting. Proper facility design and surgical attire regulations are important ways of preventing transportation of microorganisms into surgical settings, where they may infect patients' open wounds. Infection control practices also involve personal measures, including personal fitness for work, skin disinfection (patient and personnel), preparation of personnel hands, surgical attire, and personal technique (surgical conscience).

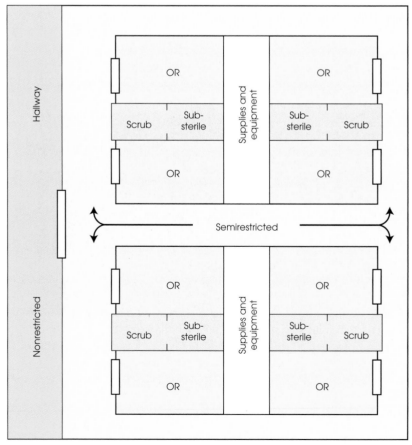

Fig. 27-2 OR suite layout showing restricted, nonrestricted, and semirestricted areas. ORs are "restricted."

Operating Room Attire

The OR should have specific written policies and procedures for proper attire to be worn within the semirestricted and restricted areas of the OR suite. The dress code should include aspects of personal hygiene important to environmental control. Protocol is strictly monitored so that everyone conforms to established policy.

Street clothes should never be worn within semirestricted or restricted areas of the surgical suite (Fig. 27-2). Clean, fresh attire should be donned at the beginning of each shift in the OR suite and as needed if the attire becomes wet or soiled. Blood-stained or soiled attire, including shoe covers, is unattractive and can also be a source of cross-infection or contamination. Soiled attire is not worn outside of the OR suite, and steps should be taken to remove soiled clothing immediately on exiting. OR attire should not be hung in a locker for wearing a second time. Under-clothing should be clean and totally covered by the scrub suit (Fig. 27-3). Other aspects of proper attire include the following:

- *Protective eyewear:* Occupational Safety and Health Administration (OSHA) regulations require eyewear to be worn when contamination from blood or body fluids is possible.
- *Masks:* Masks should be worn at all times in the OR but are not necessary in all semirestricted areas.
- *Shoe covers:* Shoe covers should be worn when contamination from blood or body fluids can be reasonably anticipated. Shoe covers should be changed whenever they become torn, soiled, or wet and should be removed before leaving the surgical area.
- *Caps:* Caps should be worn to cover and contain hair at all times in the restricted and semirestricted areas of the OR suite. Hoods are also available to cover hair, such as facial hair, that cannot be contained by a cap and mask.
- *Gloves:* Gloves should be worn when contact with blood or body substances is anticipated.
- *Radiation badge and identification:* A radiation badge and proper identification should be worn at all times.

PERSONAL HYGIENE

A person with an acute infection, such as a cold, open cold sore, or sore throat, is known to be a carrier of transmittable conditions and should not be permitted within the OR suite. Daily body cleanliness and clean hair are also important because good personal hygiene helps to prevent transportation of microbial fallout that can cause open wound infections. Daily body cleanliness and clean, dandruff-free hair help prevent superficial wound infections.

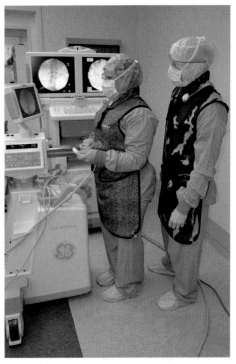

Fig. 27-3 Properly attired radiographers with protective eyewear and additional headwear to cover facial hair or long hair.

Dance of the Operating Room

The concepts of sterile and aseptic technique date back to Hippocrates, who boiled wine and water to pour into open wounds in an attempt to prevent infection. Galen changed the technique a bit and began boiling the instruments instead, and shortly thereafter Semmelweis noted a dramatic decline in postoperative infection by having the staff wash their hands and change gowns between surgical procedures.

Maintaining the sterile field in an OR suite can be like a well-choreographed dance when the team works well together. Certain moves and rules must be followed. Proper adherence to aseptic technique eliminates or minimizes modes and sources of contamination. Basic principles must be observed during the surgical procedure to provide the patient with a well-defined margin of safety. Everyone who cares for patients must carry out effective hospital and OR infection control programs. Infection control involves a wide variety of concepts including methods of environmental sanitation and maintenance of facilities; cleanliness of the air and equipment in the OR suite; cleanliness of the skin and apparel of patients, surgeons, and personnel; sterility of surgical equipment; strict aseptic technique; and careful observance of procedural rules and regulations.

Up to 10,000 microbial particles can be shed from the skin per minute. Nonsterile team members should not reach over a sterile field. When working over the sterile field (e.g., performing a posteroanterior [PA] lumbar spine), the sterile field should be covered with a sterile drape to protect the field (Fig. 27-4). The technologist cannot move the radiographic equipment into position over the sterile field until after the sterile cover is in place. A sterile team member should fold over the sterile drape on itself, and then a nonsterile team member should carefully remove the covering drape, being careful not to compromise the sterile field. If a sterile field is compromised, the OR staff should be notified immediately.

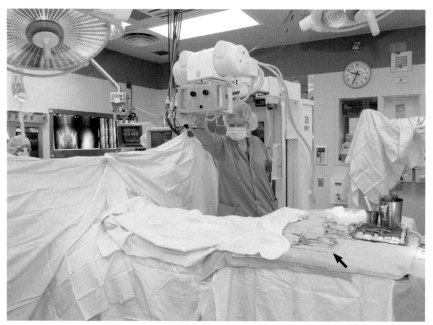

Fig. 27-4 Radiographer leaning over the sterile field while positioning the x-ray tube. The sterile incision site over which the radiographer works is properly covered to maintain a sterile field. Note the sterile instruments in the foreground (*arrow*). The radiographer should never move radiographic equipment over uncovered sterile instruments or an uncovered surgical site.

Communication is of utmost importance. As a result of the surgical sterile field, the radiographer is unable to help position the image receptor (IR) or the patient. Good, professional communication is essential while using sound, basic knowledge of anatomy and positioning. The radiographer may have to instruct the surgeon or resident on the proper position to visualize the desired portion of the anatomy best.

PROPER IMAGE RECEPTOR HANDLING IN THE STERILE FIELD

To maintain proper universal precautions, the radiographer must follow specific steps when handling an IR in the OR.

- *Surgical technologist (CST) taking the IR:* The CST holds a sterile IR cover open toward the radiographer. The radiographer should hold one end of the IR while placing the other end of the IR into the sterile IR cover. The CST grasps the IR and wraps the protective cover securely (Fig. 27-5).

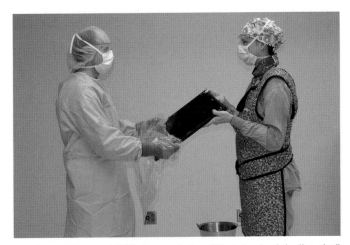

Fig. 27-5 Radiographer and CST place wireless DR detector into the sterile drape.

• *Radiographer accepting the IR after exposure:* After the exposure has been made, the radiographer needs to retrieve the IR. The CST should carefully open the sterile drape, exposing the detector for the technologist to grasp (Fig. 27-6). The CST would then dispose of the drape. In the event of an urgent situation in which the CST needs to hand the detector over, the radiographer must be wearing gloves to accept a covered IR that has been in the sterile field or under an open incision. The protective cover is possibly contaminated with blood or body fluids and should be treated accordingly. The radiographer should grasp the IR, open the protective cover carefully away from himself or herself or others so as not to spread blood or body fluids, and then ask another nonsterile person to remove the detector from the cover. The radiographer should dispose of the sterile cover in a proper receptacle and remember to remove gloves before handling the IR or any other equipment because the gloves are now considered contaminated. If contamination of the IR occurs, the radiographer should use hospital-approved disinfectant for cleaning before leaving the OR (Box 27-2).

ENEMIES OF THE STERILE FIELD

Lengthy or complex procedures increase the chance of sterile field contamination. Physical limitations, such as crowding, poor lighting, and staffing levels, are also a consideration. The floor is always considered contaminated. The radiographer should not place IRs, lead aprons, and shields on the floor.

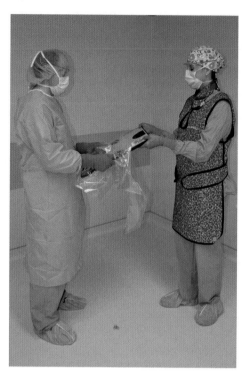

Fig. 27-6 CST correctly opens the sterile drape for the radiographer to remove the IR from the now-contaminated bag, being careful not to brush contaminants from bag onto self or others.

BOX 27-2

Principles of aseptic techniques

- Only sterile items are used within the sterile field.
- Only sterile persons handle sterile items or touch sterile areas.
- Nonsterile persons touch only nonsterile items or areas.
- Movement within or around a sterile field must not contaminate the sterile field.
- Items of doubtful sterility must be considered nonsterile.
- When a sterile barrier is permeated, it must be considered contaminated.
- Sterile gowns are considered sterile in front from the shoulder to the level of the sterile field and at the sleeves from the elbow to the cuff.
- Tables are sterile only at table level.
- Radiographers should not walk between two sterile fields if possible.
- Radiographers should avoid turning their backs toward the sterile field in compromised spaces.
- The radiographer should watch the front of clothing when it is necessary to be next to the patient.
- The radiographer must be aware of machinery close to the sterile field, including lead aprons hanging from the portable machine that may swing toward the sterile field.
- The lead apron needs to be secured if it is being worn next to the sterile field. The apron can easily slip forward when raising one's arms up to position the tube. A properly worn apron does not compromise the sterile field or jeopardize proper body mechanics.
- When positioning an IR under the OR table, the radiographer should not lift the sterile drapes above table level because this would compromise the sterile field.

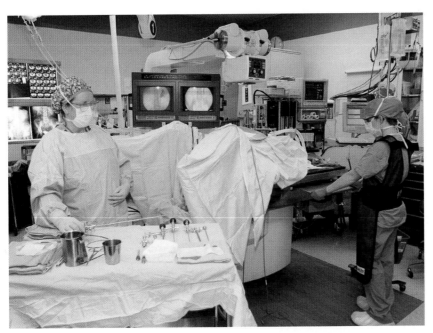

Fig. 27-7 In-room urologic radiographic equipment used for retrograde ureterograms.

Equipment

The radiographer must be well acquainted with the radiologic equipment. Some procedures may seldom occur. The radiographer should not fear a rare procedure if good communication and equipment knowledge are in place. IR holders enable the radiographer to perform cross-table projections on numerous cases and eliminate the unnecessary exposure of personnel who may volunteer to hold the IR. In mobile radiography, exposure times may increase for larger patients, and a holder eliminates the chance of motion from handheld situations.

Some OR suites, such as those used for stereotactic or urologic cases, have dedicated radiologic equipment (Fig. 27-7). Most radiographic examinations in the OR are performed with mobile equipment, however.

Mobile image machines are not as sophisticated as larger stationary machines in the radiology department. Mobile fluoroscopic units, often referred to as *C-arms* because of their shape (Fig. 27-8), are commonplace in the surgical suite. Mobile radiography is also widely used in the OR.

Good communication is imperative when providing safe and efficient imaging during a surgical case. It is important to establish a common language of terms between the surgeon and the technologist for C-arm operation (Fig. 27-9).

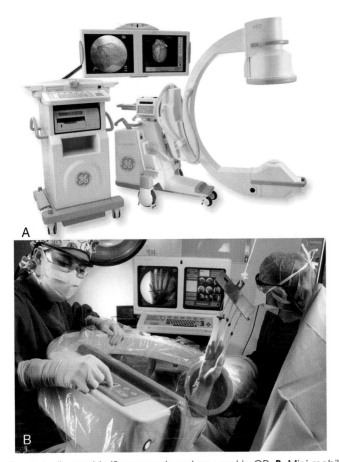

Fig. 27-8 **A,** C-arm radiographic/fluoroscopic system used in OR. **B,** Mini-mobile C-arm used for extremity examinations in OR.

Cleaning of Equipment

The x-ray equipment should be cleaned after each surgical case. If possible, the radiographer should clean the mobile image machine, including the base, in the OR suite, especially when the equipment is obviously contaminated with blood or surgical scrub solution. Cleaning within the OR helps reduce the possibility of cross-contamination. The x-ray equipment must be cleaned with a hospital-approved cleaning solution. Cleaning solutions should not be sprayed in the OR suite during the surgical procedure. If cleaning is necessary during the surgical procedure, opening the cleaning container and pouring the solution on a rag for use prevents possible contamination from scattered spray. Gloves should always be worn during cleaning. The underside of the image machine should be checked to ensure contaminants that might have splashed up from the floor are removed. Cleaning the equipment after an isolation case is necessary to prevent the spread of contaminants. All equipment that is used less frequently should undergo a thorough cleaning at least once a week and just before being taken into the OR.

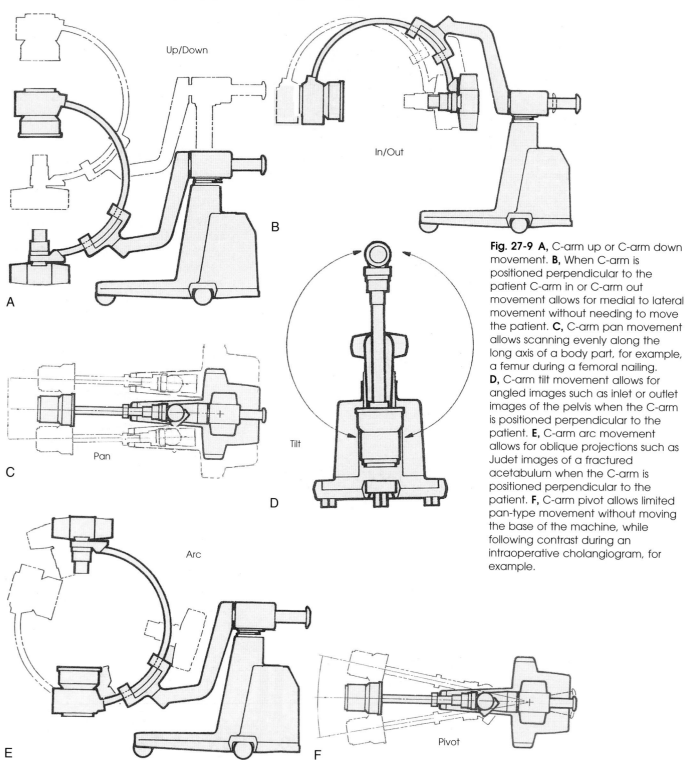

Fig. 27-9 A, C-arm up or C-arm down movement. **B,** When C-arm is positioned perpendicular to the patient C-arm in or C-arm out movement allows for medial to lateral movement without needing to move the patient. **C,** C-arm pan movement allows scanning evenly along the long axis of a body part, for example, a femur during a femoral nailing. **D,** C-arm tilt movement allows for angled images such as inlet or outlet images of the pelvis when the C-arm is positioned perpendicular to the patient. **E,** C-arm arc movement allows for oblique projections such as Judet images of a fractured acetabulum when the C-arm is positioned perpendicular to the patient. **F,** C-arm pivot allows limited pan-type movement without moving the base of the machine, while following contrast during an intraoperative cholangiogram, for example.

Radiation Exposure Considerations

Radiation protection for the radiographer, others in the immediate area, and the patient is of paramount importance when mobile fluoroscopic examinations are performed. The radiographer should wear a lead, or lead equivalent, apron and stand as far away from the patient, x-ray tube, and useful beam as the procedure, OR, and exposure cable allow. The most effective means of radiation protection is *distance*. The recommended *minimal* distance is 6 ft (2 m). When possible, the radiographer should stand at a right angle (90 degrees) to the primary beam and the object being radiographed. The least amount of scatter radiation occurs at this position. The greatest amount of scatter radiation occurs on the tube side of the fluoroscopic machine. It is recommended that the x-ray tube always be placed *under*

the patient (Fig. 27-10). Because of the significant amount of exposure to the facial and neck region, the x-ray tube should never be placed above the patient unless absolutely necessary.

The OR may have signs posted outside the room warning of radiation in use, or "lead aprons required when entering this room." Lead or lead equivalent protection should be provided for individuals who are unable to leave the room.

The patient's gonads should be shielded with appropriate radiation protection devices during examinations in which shielding would not interfere with imaging of the anatomy that must be shown. When fluoroscopic equipment with the tube *under* the table is to be used, shielding should be placed under the patient. In addition, the source-to-skin distance (SSD) should not be less than 12 inches (29 cm).

Fluoroscopic Procedures for the Operating Room
OPERATIVE (IMMEDIATE) CHOLANGIOGRAPHY

Operative cholangiography, introduced by Mirizzi in 1932, is performed during biliary tract surgery. After the bile has been drained from the ducts, and in the absence of obstruction, this technique permits the major intrahepatic ducts and the extrahepatic ducts to be filled with contrast medium.

The value of operative cholangiography is such that it has become an integral part of biliary tract surgery. It is used to investigate the patency of the bile ducts and the functional status of the sphincter of the hepatopancreatic ampulla to reveal the presence of calculi that cannot be detected by palpation. Intraoperative cholangiography can also show such conditions as small intraluminal neoplasms and stricture or dilation of the ducts. When the pancreatic duct shares a common channel with the distal common bile duct before emptying into the duodenum, it is sometimes seen on operative cholangiograms because it has been partially filled by reflux.

After exposing, draining, and exploring the biliary tract, and frequently after excising the gallbladder, the surgeon injects the contrast medium. This solution is usually introduced into the common bile duct through a needle, small catheter, or (after cholecystectomy) an inlaying T tube. When the latter route is used, the procedure is referred to as *delayed operative* or *operative T-tube cholangiography.*

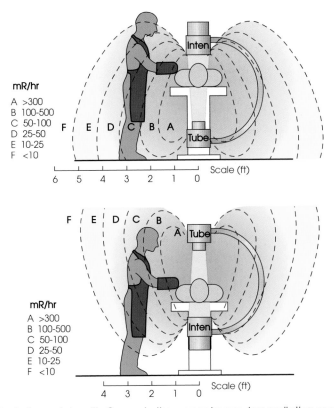

Fig. 27-10 Radiation safety with C-arm. In the *upper image,* less radiation reaches the facial and neck region when the x-ray tube is under the patient. This is the recommended position of the C-arm. In the *lower image,* there is a greater amount of radiation reaching the facial and neck regions.

(From Giese RA, Hunter DW: Personnel exposure during fluoroscopy, *Postgrad Radiol* 8:162, 1988.)

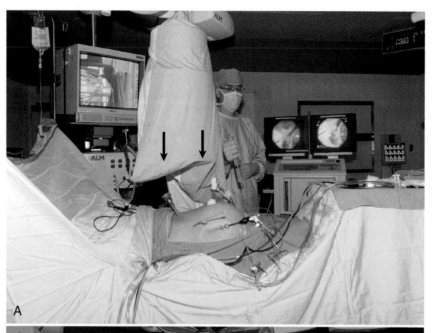

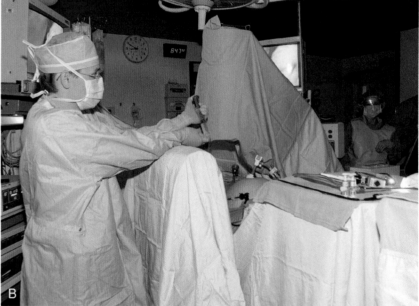

Fig. 27-11 A, C-arm in correct position for an abdominal cholangiogram. The assistant surgeon checks syringe for air bubbles before handing it to the surgeon for injection. The radiographer positioned fluoroscopic image intensifier (*arrows*) carefully to avoid hitting laparoscopic instruments protruding from the patient's abdomen. **B,** Surgeon, standing behind a sterile draped lead shield, injecting contrast media for an operative cholangiogram.

Position of patient

The patient is supine with the abdomen exposed. In laparoscopic cases, such as cholecystectomy, the abdomen is distended because air is injected into the abdominal cavity to allow adequate room for maneuvering of the camera and instruments. The radiographer should ensure no obstacles would impede the movement of the C-arm (Fig. 27-11).

NOTE: The radiographer should shield pregnant patients. The central ray comes from under the table, so appropriate shielding should be placed under the patient and placed so as not to obscure any pertinent anatomy.

Position of C-arm

Center the C-arm in the PA projection over the right side of the abdomen below the rib line. The patient may be tilted to the left or in the Trendelenburg position to aid in the flow of contrast medium to the complete biliary system. The C-arm should be tilted or canted until the PA projection is achieved. The C-arm may also have to be rotated to ensure that the spine does not obscure the biliary system. When the position is obtained, the surgeon injects contrast medium into the duct system under fluoroscopy. The radiographer should do the following:
- Provide radiation protection for all persons in the room.
- Remember that examination is optimal with suspended respiration.

Because of the length of time it may take for contrast medium to fill all ducts, respiration may be suspended at intervals throughout the examination.

Structures shown

This examination shows the biliary system full of contrast medium, including a portion of the cystic duct, the branches of the hepatic duct, the common bile duct, and often the pancreatic duct.

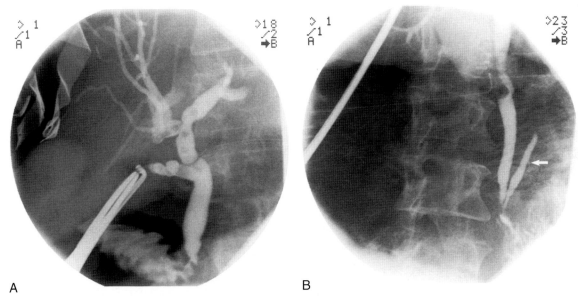

A   B

Fig. 27-12 Images of anatomy visualized during a cholangiogram using fluoroscopy. **A,** Intraoperative cholangiogram. **B,** Intraoperative cholangiogram showing pancreatic duct (*arrow*).

CHEST (LINE PLACEMENT, BRONCHOSCOPY)

Position of patient

The patient is supine with the arms secured at his or her sides. The radiographer should ensure there are no bars or supports in the table that would obscure the view of the chest. Allow room under the table for the C-arm to maneuver.

Position of C-arm

The C-arm should be covered with a sterile drape before entering the field. The C-arm enters the sterile field perpendicular to the patient and in position for a PA projection. If the surgeon prefers, the radiographer can reverse or invert the image to obtain anatomic position. Radiation protection should be provided for all persons in the room.

- *Line placement:* Find the point of insertion and follow the catheter to its end. This examination is done to ensure there are no kinks in the catheter and to show it is in proper position. Numerous catheters may be used in the OR. They are usually inserted to deliver medicines to chronically ill patients.
- *Rigid and flexible bronchoscopy:* Bronchoscopy may be done to perform biopsies, place stents, or dilate the bronchi.

Structures shown

Structures shown include all anatomy of the chest cavity, including the heart, lung fields, and ribs, and any instrumentation that may be introduced during the procedure. These instruments may include catheters, guidewires, bronchoscopes, stent devices, dilation balloons, or biopsy instruments.

EVALUATION CRITERIA

- Pertinent parts of the chest are distinguished easily (Fig. 27-13).
- Proper radiographic technique and contrast are maintained on the monitor.
- Image on the monitor is in true anatomic position or per the physician's preference.
- Sterile technique is maintained.

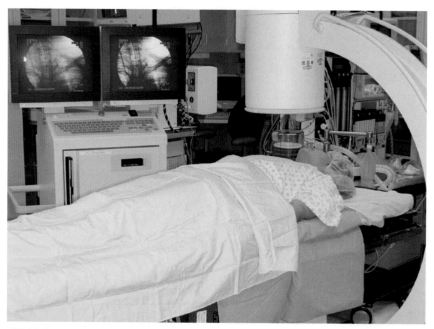

Fig. 27-13 Patient and C-arm in position for Hickman catheter placement. Introduction of catheter begins in the upper thorax and is completed with the catheter in the heart.

CERVICAL SPINE (ANTERIOR CERVICAL DISKECTOMY AND FUSION)

Position of patient

The patient is supine with the chin elevated and the neck in flexion. The patient's arms are at his or her sides.

Position of C-arm

PA projection

Cover the C-arm with sterile drape. Enter the sterile field perpendicular to the patient. Tilt the C-arm 15 degrees cephalad and center the beam over the cervical spine. Raise the C-arm to allow the surgeon to work if necessary. Ensure the spine is in the center of the monitor, and the top of spine and skull are at the top of the screen with no rotation.

Lateral projection

Rotate the C-arm under the table into lateral position with the beam parallel to the floor. Angle the C-arm either cephalad or caudal to obtain a true lateral view. Raise or lower the C-arm to bring the spine into the center of the field of view. Rotate the image on the monitor to the same plane as the patient with the spine parallel with the floor. Cases in which a PA projection is unnecessary may opt to have the C-arm positioned in "rainbow" fashion or arched over the patient (Fig. 27-14).

• Ensure there are no obstacles under the table that impede movement of the C-arm.
• The C-arm is often positioned before the patient is draped. In this case, the surgical team drapes the C-arm into the sterile field. Ensure that the C-arm can be moved out of the way without disturbing any instrumentation.

Structures shown

These positions show the affected area of the cervical spine and any hardware that may be introduced (Fig. 27-15). Because this surgery is most often performed to repair physiologic defects, abnormalities (e.g., osteophytes, degenerated disk spaces, subluxation) may be visible, especially in the lateral view.

EVALUATION CRITERIA

■ Cervical spine and its affected part are in the center of the monitor to maintain proper radiographic technique.
■ Image is rotated in the same plane as the patient.
■ PA projection should show spinous processes in the center of spinous bodies.
■ Lateral projection should show the bodies in profile and the interarticular facets aligned.
■ Sterile field is maintained.

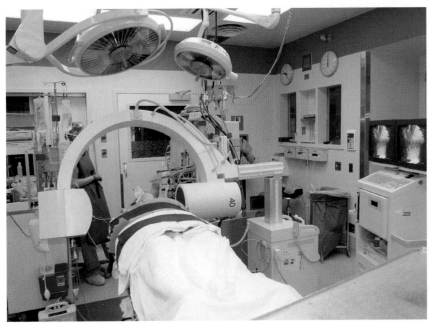

Fig. 27-14 C-arm placed in rainbow position for cervical procedures.

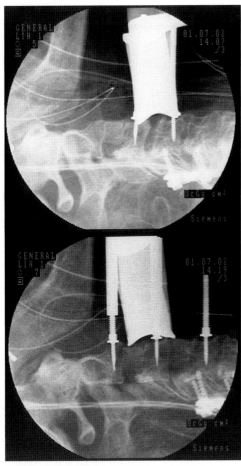

Fig. 27-15 Fluoroscopic image of cervical spine in lateral projection showing plate and screws used to fuse vertebrae.

LUMBAR SPINE
Position of patient

The patient is prone and positioned on chest rolls or a frame to flex the spine. His or her arms are placed on arm boards and located by the head of the table to bring them out of the field of view.

Position of C-arm
AP projection

Cover the C-arm with a sterile drape. The C-arm enters the field perpendicular to the patient. Center the beam in the anteroposterior (AP) projection over the affected area of the spine. Raise the C-arm to leave enough room between the IR and the patient so that the surgeon can work without being obstructed (Fig. 27-16). Ensure there is nothing in or under the table to impair the view of the spine.

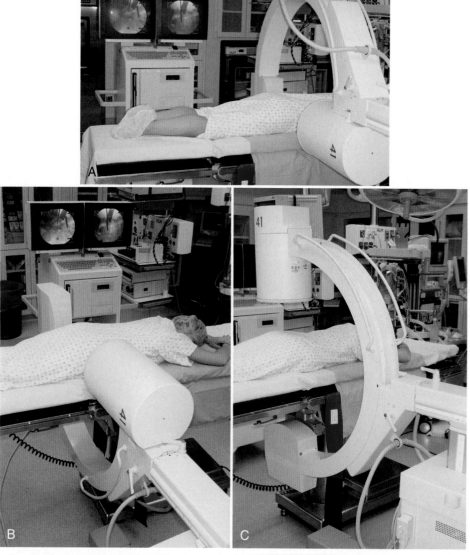

Fig. 27-16 A, C-arm correctly placed in rainbow position for lateral lumbar procedures. The rainbow position is used especially for larger patients in which the table size or size of the patient would not allow enough elevation of the C-arm to include the lumbar spine. **B,** C-arm positioned under the table. **C,** C-arm positioned for AP projection of lumbar spine.

Lateral projection

- Rotate the C-arm under the table into lateral position. Raise or lower the C-arm to bring the spine into the center of the monitor. The C-arm may need to be angled cephalad or caudal to obtain true lateral projection. Rotate the image on the monitor until the image is in same plane as the patient. The C-arm may be arched over the patient for the lateral projection, especially on hypersthenic patients because rotating the C-arm under the table would not allow a great enough height to visualize the lumbar region.
- The surgical team members place sterile drapes over both ends of the C-arm when they drape the patient.

Structures shown

These projections show the affected area of the spine, which includes the bodies, disk spaces, spinous processes, lamina, pedicles, and facets. When the case is completed, there is hardware in the spine, such as rods, plates, and screws, to hold the spine in alignment. A bone graft or interbody fusion device may also exist in the disk space to fuse the bones together (Fig. 27-17).

EVALUATION CRITERIA

- Affected area of the spine is viewed in its entirety (Fig. 27-18).
- Spine image is not rotated or angled on the monitor, showing true AP and lateral projections.
- Radiographic technique is maintained by properly centering the beam over the affected area.
- Image of the spine, whether AP or lateral, is rotated into the same plane as the patient. AP projection of the spine is in vertical axis, and the lateral view of the spine is in horizontal axis.
- Sterile field is maintained.
- Radiation protection is provided for the surgical team.

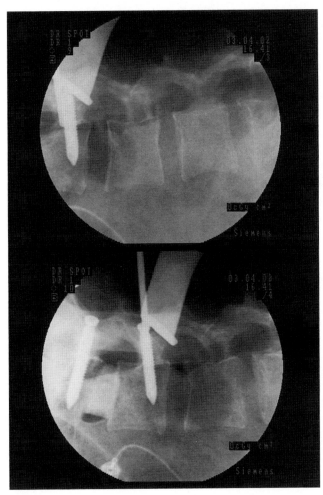

Fig. 27-17 Fluoroscopic lateral projection image of lumbar spine with instrumentation.

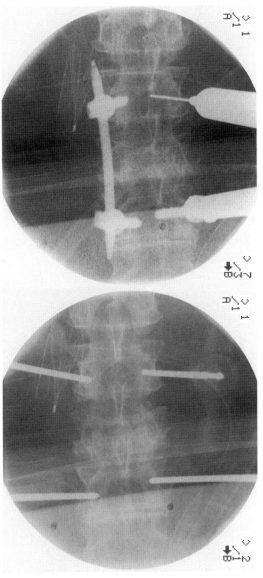

Fig. 27-18 AP projection fluoroscopic images during laparoscopic lumbar fusion.

HIP (CANNULATED HIP SCREWS OR HIP PINNING)

Position of patient

The patient is supine with the legs abducted and the affected leg held in traction. The patient's arm on the affected side is crossed over the body to be kept out of the field of view.

- These procedures are often done using an isolation drape or "shower curtain." In these cases, it is not necessary to cover the C-arm with a sterile drape; however, a nonsterile bag over the tube is recommended to prevent povidone-iodine (Betadine) staining of the C-arm.
- The radiographer is positioned between the patient's legs to ensure the patient is covered completely for privacy.

Position of C-arm

Position the C-arm between the patient's legs, and center the beam over the affected hip (Fig. 27-19). To obtain the lateral projection, rotate the C-arm under the leg and table to a lateral position (Fig. 27-20). Do not dislodge any instrumentation when rotating the C-arm.

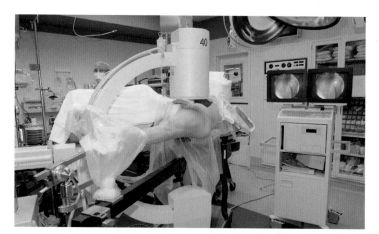

Fig. 27-19 C-arm positioned for PA projection of the hip.

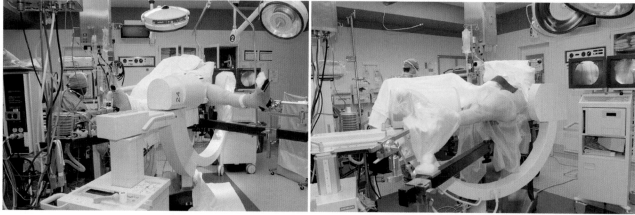

Fig. 27-20 C-arm properly positioned for lateral projection of the hip. After preliminary images are obtained, the hip is prepared for incision, and the C-arm is sterile draped.

- Before the procedure, the surgeon manipulates the leg under fluoroscopy to reduce the fracture (Fig. 27-21).
- The C-arm may have to be manipulated to achieve projections and may not be in true PA or lateral projection. Note the position of the C-arm on PA and lateral projections to return to this angle when necessary.
- When hardware is in the hip, rotate the C-arm under fluoroscopy to ensure that no hardware is in the hip joint space.

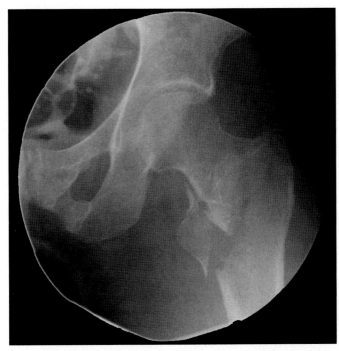

Fig. 27-21 PA projection of the hip with fracture of femoral neck.

Structures shown

This examination shows all parts of the proximal femur and hip joint, including the acetabular rim, femoral head and neck, and greater and lesser trochanters. Hardware may include cannulated screws or pins running parallel with the femoral neck used to reduce the fracture (Fig. 27-22).

- Hip is centered on monitor and in correct plane.
- Lateral side of femur and acetabular rim must be visualized to determine a starting point and to ensure no hardware enters the joint.
- Lesser trochanter is visible in profile on PA projection. Greater trochanter lies behind the femoral neck and shaft in lateral view.
- Proper radiographic technique is maintained.
- Sterile field is maintained.
- Radiation protection is provided.

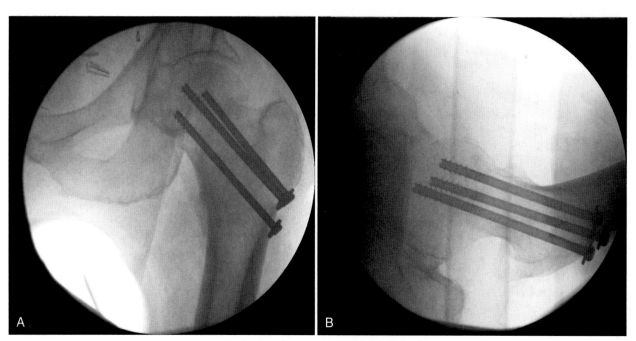

Fig. 27-22 A and **B,** PA projection (**A**) and lateral projection (**B**) fluoroscopic images of hip fracture reduction.

FEMUR NAIL

Position of patient and C-arm

During this procedure, a rod is inserted into the intramedullary (IM) canal to reduce a fracture of the shaft of the femur (Fig. 27-23). This rod or nail can be introduced either antegrade through the greater trochanter or retrograde through the popliteal notch.

Antegrade femoral nailing

During antegrade nailing, the patient is either supine or in the lateral position. In the supine position, the affected leg would most likely be in traction to help reduce the fracture. The legs would be abducted, and the unaffected leg would be flexed at the knee and hip and raised to allow the C-arm enough room to enter the sterile field. The patient's arm on the injured side is draped across the chest to keep it from obstructing the surgeon. With the patient in lateral position, the affected leg is extended forward to clear the opposite leg. If the patient is supine, the C-arm is posi-

tioned between the patient's legs, parallel to the unaffected leg, and centered over the hip. The C-arm may have to be rotated forward or backward to obtain a true PA projection. Rotate the C-arm under the table for a lateral projection.

Antegrade with the patient in the lateral position requires the radiographer to enter the sterile field and rotate the C-arm under the table to find a PA projection of the femur. Lateral projection is achieved with the tube starting in a true PA projection, rotating the C-arm forward 10 to 15 degrees, and tilting it 5 to 10 degrees cephalad.

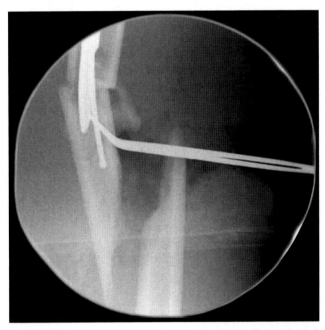

Fig. 27-23 Image of midshaft femoral fracture with guide rod being inserted to align fracture.

Retrograde femoral nailing

During the retrograde femoral nailing, the patient is supine with the injured leg exposed and the knee flexed and supported with a bump. This position allows the surgeon access to the popliteal notch without injuring the patella.

The sterile field is entered with the C-arm perpendicular to the patient. The C-arm is tilted cephalad to account for the flexed knee and to find the PA projection. The C-arm is rotated under the table for lateral position (Fig. 27-24).

Method

- Instruments or hardware may protrude from the operative site. Be sure to avoid disturbing these instruments or hardware or allowing them to puncture a sterile drape.
- Center the C-arm over the fracture site during canal reaming to ensure that the fracture remains reduced (Fig. 27-25).
- The table must allow for movement of the C-arm from the knee to the hip.
- Allow enough room between the patient and C-arm for the surgeon to work.

Screws are inserted into the femur and through the nail to fix the nail in place. When lining up the screw holes in the nail, the hole should be perfectly round and not oblong. Center the screw hole on the monitor. The magnification feature may be used to give the surgeon a better view. The C-arm may need to be tilted or rotated to obtain perfect circles. The surgeon also manipulates the leg to help align the screw holes. After the screws are inserted, check the length of the screws by placing the C-arm in PA projection. Screws should not protrude excessively from the cortical bone (Fig. 27-26).

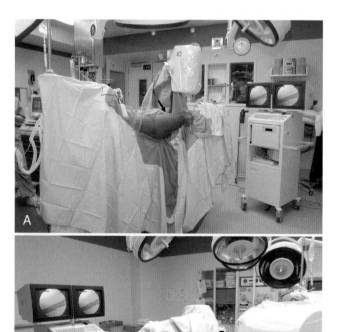

Fig. 27-24 A, C-arm positioned between patient's legs for PA projection during femoral nailing. *Arrow* is pointing to femur. **B,** C-arm rotated under femur (*arrow*) for lateral projection.

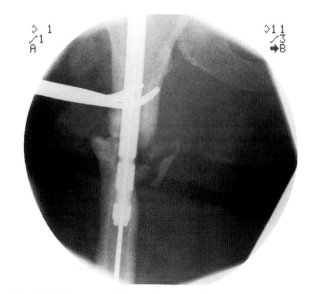

Fig. 27-25 Image of femur fracture during canal reaming.

Structures shown

All parts of the femur, including the greater and lesser trochanters, femoral neck, shaft, and condyles, are seen in the PA and lateral positions. Different instrumentation is in the IM canal beginning with a guide rod that is used to help reduce the fracture and provide a means for the canal reamers to pass through the fracture site (Fig. 27-27). After reduction, the nail and screws are seen.

EVALUATION CRITERIA

- Appropriate projections are seen unobstructed and in correct plane on the monitor.
- Screw holes are perfectly round and in the center of the monitor.
- Sterile field is maintained.
- Proper radiographic technique is maintained.
- Radiation protection is provided for the surgical team.

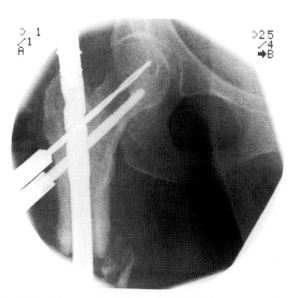

Fig. 27-26 PA projection of proximal screw in a femoral nail.

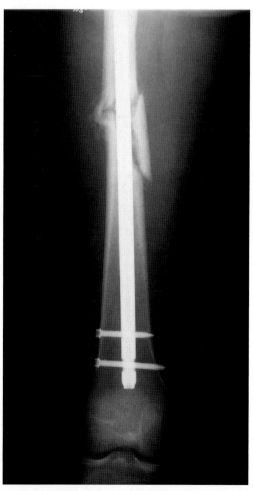

Fig. 27-27 PA projection of femur fracture reduced with guide rod and distal interlocking screws inserted.

Fluoroscopic Procedures for the Operating Room

TIBIA (NAIL)

Position of patient

The patient is supine with the affected leg exposed. The knee is flexed to allow access to the tibial tuberosity without injuring the patella. The injured leg is on the opposite side of the table so that the C-arm does not interfere with the surgical team.

Position of C-arm

Cover the C-arm with a sterile drape. Move the C-arm into the field perpendicular to the patient. Center the beam over the leg and tilt the tube to match the angle of the leg (Fig. 27-28). No obstructions should be under the table to avoid interfering with the C-arm movement. Rotate the C-arm under the table and into the lateral position, taking care not to disturb any instrumentation protruding from the operative site. Center the leg on the monitor by raising or lowering the C-arm. The surgeon manipulates the leg, and the radiographer tilts or rotates the C-arm to obtain round holes (Figs. 27-29 and 27-30). The magni-

fication feature can be used to enlarge the image if necessary. Advance the C-arm until its tube side is far enough from the injured leg to allow the surgeon to fit the drill and drill bit into the area.

- Along its shaft the tibia is triangular, so when checking the length of the screws the C-arm may have to be rotated forward or back to get a true length.
- Center the beam on the fracture site during canal reaming. When the leg is in the center of the monitor, turn the wheels of the C-arm horizontally to allow the machine to move longitudinally down the shaft of the leg without moving out of the field of view.

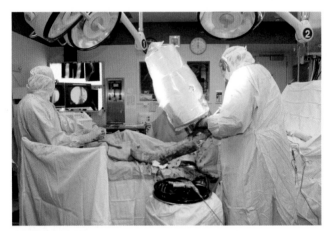

Fig. 27-28 C-arm positioned for tibial nailing. The radiographer tilted the fluoroscopic image intensifier to be parallel with the long axis of the leg.

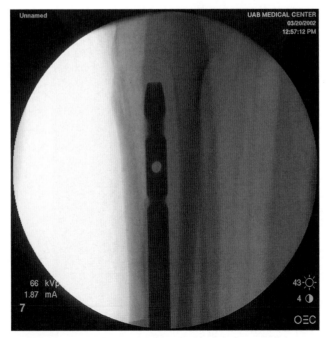

Fig. 27-29 Image of tibial nail screw holes in incorrect alignment and oblong in shape.

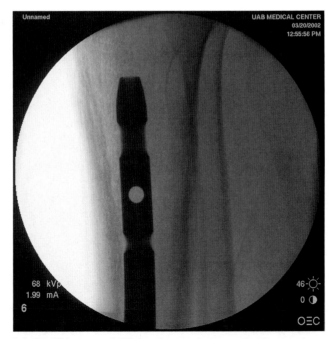

Fig. 27-30 Image of tibial nail screw holes perfectly round and magnified to assist proper alignment.

Structures shown

Structures shown include the tibia and fibula, the tibial shaft along with any fracture, the tibial plateau, tibial tuberosity, distal tibia, and ankle joint (Fig. 27-31). After hardware is inserted, the tibial nail fills the IM canal, with proximal and distal screws prominent.

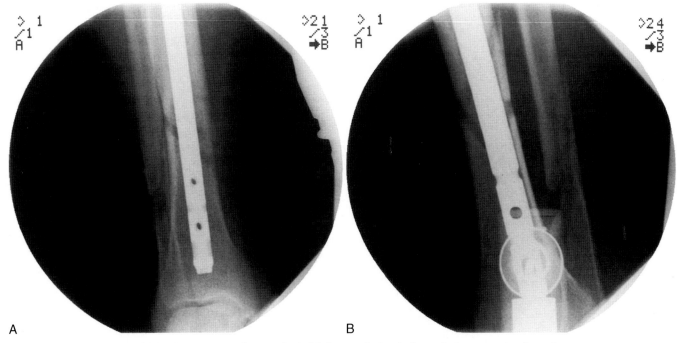

A

B

Fig. 27-31 A, Improper alignment of distal screw holes. **B,** Screw holes properly aligned with screwdriver over distal screw hole.

Fluoroscopic Procedures for the Operating Room

237

HUMERUS
Position of patient

The patient is supine or in a reclining or beach chair position (Fig. 27-32). The injured arm may be resting on a Mayo stand with the surgeon's assistant holding the arm to stabilize and align the humerus. The patient should be positioned with the shoulder off the side of the table. This position allows the humerus to be seen in its entirety without being obscured by the table.

Position of C-arm

Cover the C-arm with a sterile drape. Enter the field parallel to, or at a 45-degree angle to, the patient. The assistant rotates the arm medially with the elbow bent 90 degrees. The C-arm is tilted and rotated to obtain a true lateral projection, depending on the angle of patient position. The arm is held at the elbow to provide support, and the arm is rotated until the hand is pointing upward. The C-arm is tilted to obtain PA projection according to the patient's angle. Center the beam on the humerus.

- When installing a nail or rod into the humerus and trying to locate and center the distal screws, place a sterile drape over the tube or pull the sheets draping the patient over the tube. Touch only the underside of the sheets when placing them over the tube. Raise the tube to magnify the screw holes and to allow the surgeon to work.

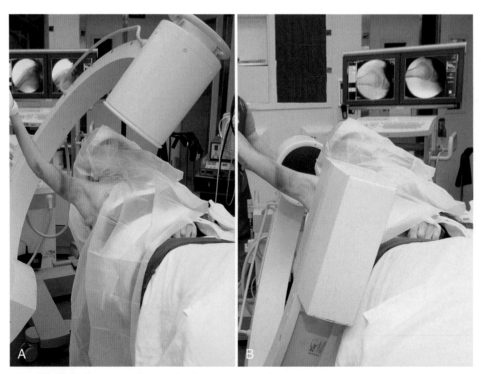

Fig. 27-32 A, C-arm positioned for PA projection of the shoulder with patient in beach chair position for preliminary imaging. **B,** C-arm positioned for axillary projection.

NOTE: Do not leave any drape over the tube for a long time to prevent unnecessary heat buildup in the tube.

• Be careful not to strike the patient's head with the image intensifier.

Structures shown

This procedure should show all parts of the humerus, including the head, neck, greater and lesser tubercles, shaft, and distal portion of the humerus. Any fractures and the hardware used for repair (Fig. 27-33) are also seen.

EVALUATION CRITERIA

■ Angle of humerus and C-arm coincide to obtain true PA and lateral projections.
■ When nailing the distal screws, holes should be perfectly round to allow screws to pass through the nail.
■ Humerus is in the center of the monitor to maintain radiographic technique.
■ Image is rotated in the same plane as the humerus.
■ Sterile field is maintained, especially with the proximity of possibly nonsterile portions of the tube to the sterile field.
■ Radiation protection is provided for surgical team.

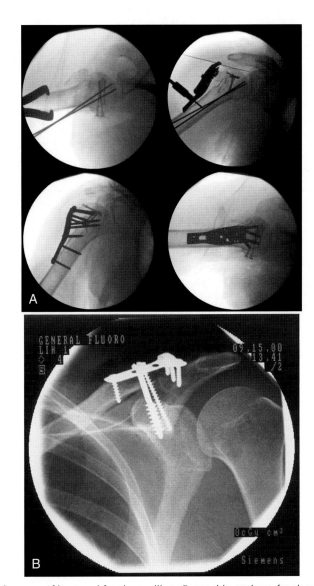

Fig. 27-33 A, Images of humeral fracture with nails used to reduce fracture of the humeral head. **B,** Image of clavicle fracture with plate and screw fixation.

FEMORAL/TIBIAL ARTERIOGRAM
Position of Patient

The patient is supine with the affected leg exposed from the groin area to the foot. There should be enough room under the table to allow the C-arm to move from the hip to the foot. The leg may be rotated medially or laterally to keep the femur or tibia from obscuring any vasculature (Fig. 27-34).

Position of C-arm

Cover the C-arm with a sterile drape and enter the field perpendicular to the patient. When the leg is in the center of the monitor, turn the wheels of the C-arm horizontally to allow the machine to move to the left or right without taking the leg out of the field of view. Use the subtraction or road-mapping feature to remove all structures except the contrast medium that is injected into the artery (Fig. 27-35). This feature shows any stenoses or injuries to the artery.

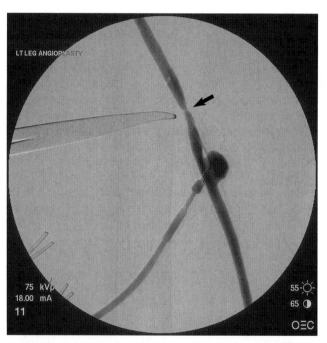

Fig. 27-34 Subtraction image of surgical femoral artery angiogram with stenosis (*arrow*).

Structures shown

The bones of the leg are seen before subtraction. After contrast medium is introduced, the femoral artery and its branches are seen, and, following the contrast medium down the leg, the popliteal and tibial arteries are seen. The contrast images show any pathologic defects in the arterial structures.

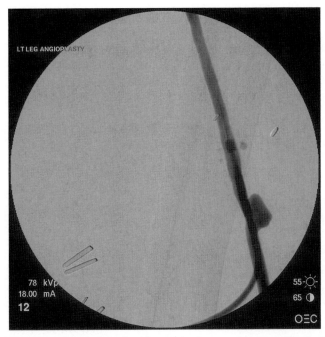

Fig. 27-35 Subtraction image of surgical femoral artery angiogram after balloon angioplasty.

Fluoroscopic Procedures for the Operating Room

Mobile Radiography Procedures for the Operating Room
CERVICAL SPINE

Image receptor: The image receptor should be a 10- × 12-inch (24- × 29-cm) grid IR crosswise.

Position of patient

The patient is upright, prone, or supine. In the upright and prone positions, the patient's head is held in a traction device to align the spine. In the supine position, the chin is elevated and held with a strap or tape.

Position of image receptor and portable machine

- Place the grid IR in the IR holder and cover with a sterile drape (Fig. 27-36).
- Position the IR holder on the opposite side of the patient. The surgical technician moves the sterile back table so that the radiographer does not compromise the sterile field.
- Direct the beam perpendicular to the IR and parallel to the floor.
- The beam enters perpendicular to the IR to eliminate grid cutoff.
- Raise or lower the tube and IR to center on the cervical spine.

Structures shown

- Cervical spine in lateral projection (Fig. 27-37).
- Degenerative or pathologic defects, such as osteophytes, fractures, or subluxation.
- Radiograph may be taken at the beginning of the case to verify the correct portion of the spine to be repaired. Instruments are placed to designate the level of the spine (Fig. 27-38).

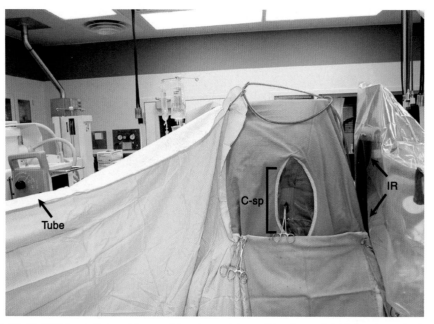

Fig. 27-36 Mobile radiographic machine (*arrow*) in position for upright lateral cervical spine. A surgical clamp, which is attached to the spinous process of interest, extends from the incision site. IR draped and in holder (*double arrow*) is centered to the patient.

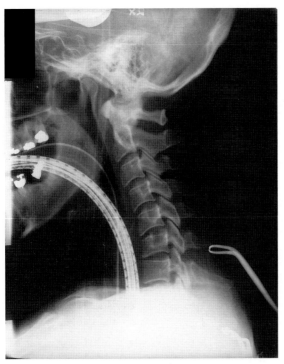

Fig. 27-37 Lateral cervical spine radiograph (patient in sitting position for surgery) showing localization marker in place on the spinous process of C6.

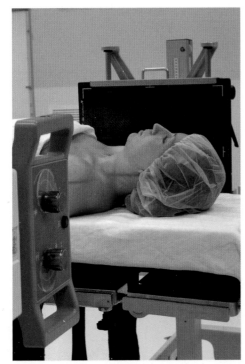

Fig. 27-38 Lateral projection of the cervical spine with patient supine. This was done to verify the correct position of instruments before continuing surgery. Often a spinal needle is placed in the disk space to show position. Note that even though a 14 × 17 wireless DR detector is used, the radiographer has properly coned to pertinent anatomy.

THORACIC OR LUMBAR SPINE

Image receptor: The image receptor should be a 14- × 17-inch (35- × 43-cm) grid IR crosswise.

Position of patient

The patient is prone or supine with the arms placed up by the head. The chest and abdomen are supported by a frame or chest roll to flex the spine into anatomic position. A radiograph may be done to verify that the surgeon is working on the correct vertebra or to show the position of hardware (Fig. 27-39).

Lateral projection

Place grid IR in IR holder and cover with a sterile drape. Position the holder next to the patient and move the IR up or down to center on the lumbar spine. Direct the beam perpendicular to the IR and parallel to the floor (Fig. 27-40). Respiration should be suspended during exposure.

PA projection

For the PA radiograph, slide IR in the slot under the table and center on the spine. Cover field with sterile drape. Center the beam to the IR and perpendicular to the long axis of the spine.

Structures shown

- The lumbar spine in PA and lateral projections.
- Vertebral bodies, spinous processes, facets, and lamina.

- Hardware to repair any defects. Bone grafts or interbody fusion devices may be used.
- Instrumentation is often seen on radiograph.
- PA projection may be obscured by the patient support.

EVALUATION CRITERIA

- Spine is in the center of the radiograph and in true PA or lateral projection.
- Spine bodies are seen without any rotation.
- All hardware used must be seen on radiograph.
- All unnecessary instrumentation is removed to avoid obscuring spine.
- Proper radiographic technique is used.
- Radiation protection is provided for the surgical team.

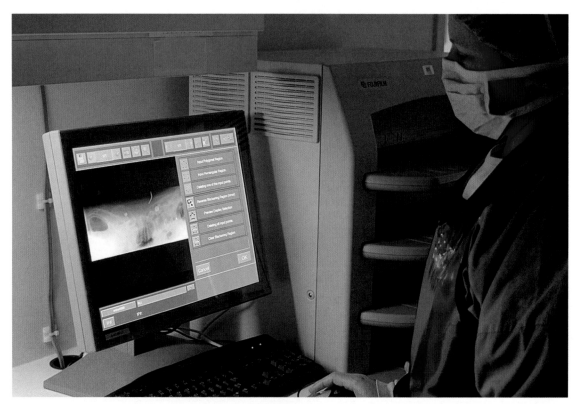

Fig. 27-39 Lateral lumbar spine with intraoperative marker to verify correct level of interest. CR and DR allows postprocessing adjustments.

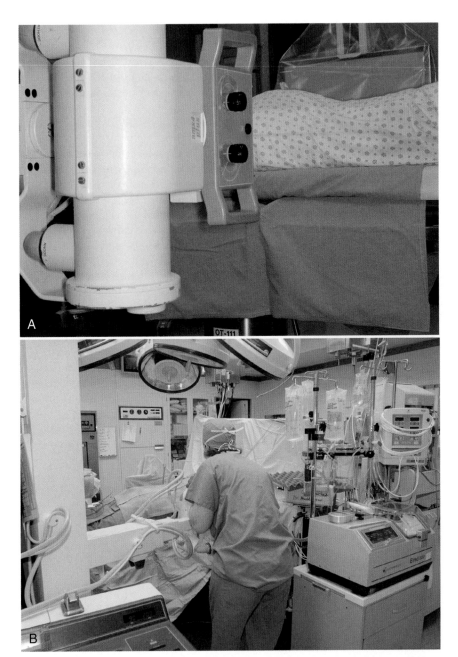

Fig. 27-40 A, Mobile x-ray machine correctly positioned for cross-table lateral lumbar spine. **B,** Radiographer positioning mobile unit intraoperatively for lateral lumbar spine procedure.

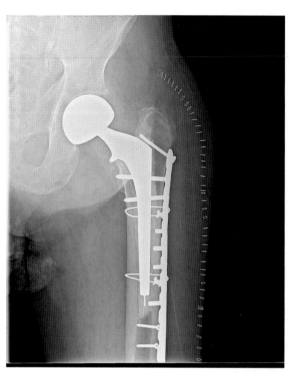

Fig. 27-41 PA projection of a hip joint replacement with plate and screw fixation following a periprosthetic femur fracture.

EXTREMITY EXAMINATIONS

Image receptor: Choose the appropriate-size IR to include all appropriate anatomy and hardware.

Position of patient

The patient is supine, prone, reclining, or in the beach chair position. Portable machines approach perpendicular to the patient. Institutions may cover the tube or sterile field, or both, with a sterile drape. Angle the tube to match the IR or desired projection. The surgeon may choose to hold the patient's limb in position during the exposure. To reduce exposure to the surgeon, positioning aids, such as sterile towels, sponges, or mallets, may be used.

The surgeon may also cover the field with a cloth sterile drape rather than a plastic sterile drape. If so, the surgeon marks the location of the part to ensure proper centering. Lighting may also need to be adjusted for better visualization of the field. For cross-table examinations, the beam is directed perpendicular to the IR and parallel to the floor. Center the beam to the IR and raise or lower the tube to the center of the part.

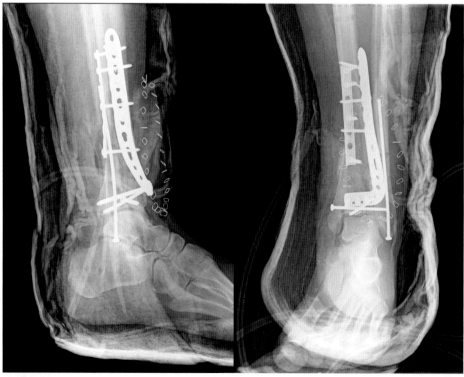

Fig. 27-42 AP and lateral postreduction images of a comminuted ankle fracture. Some casting materials require an increase in technical factors for correct penetration and image quality.

Structures shown

- All pertinent anatomy in correct alignment.
- Hardware including plates, wires, pins, screws, external fixation, and joint replacement components used to repair fractures or degenerative problems (Figs. 27-41 through 27-47).

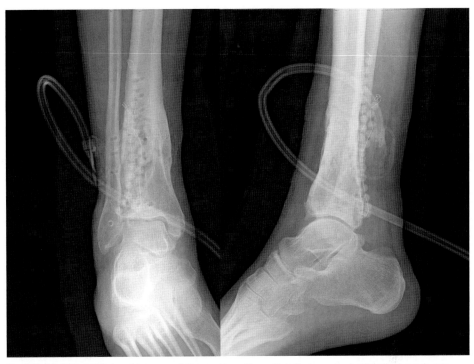

Fig. 27-43 AP and lateral image of the ankle with antibiotic beads. Antibiotic beads are placed at the site of infection to promote healing.

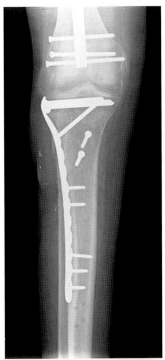

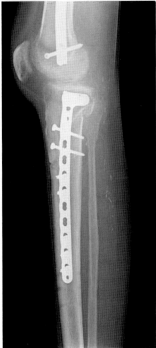

Fig. 27-44 AP projection of proximal tibia with plate and screw fixation used to repair tibial plateau fracture.

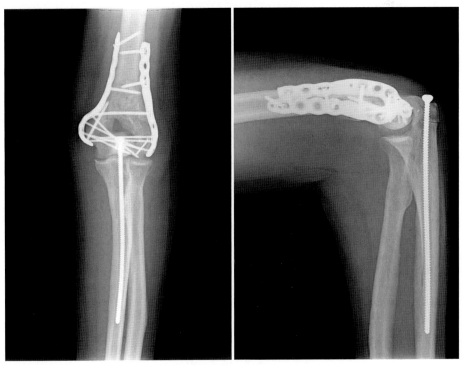

Fig. 27-45 Lateral projection of elbow with plate and screws used to reduce forearm fracture.

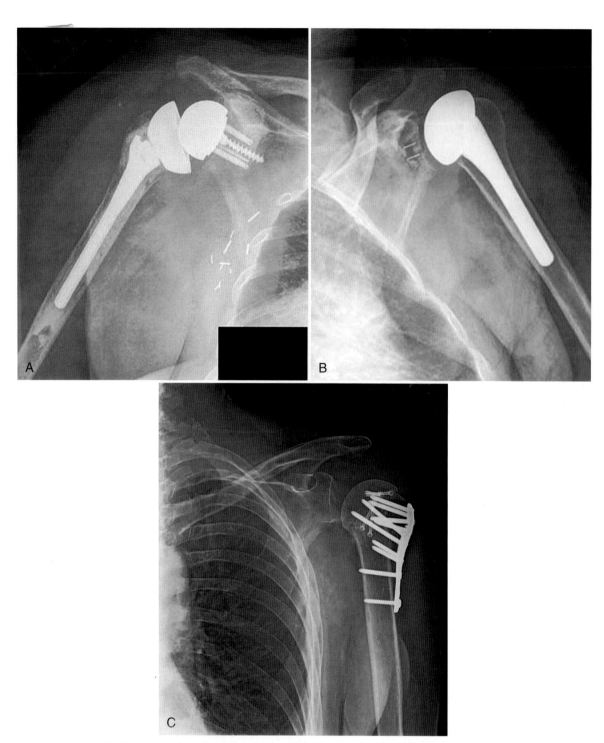

Fig. 27-46 A, Total shoulder arthroplasty with polyethelene glenoid component.
B, Reverse total shoulder arthroplasty. **C,** Shoulder with plate and screws fixation.
Creative patient positioning or tube angulation may be necessary to achieve optimal
images on complex comminuted fractures.

EVALUATION CRITERIA

- Complete joint including all hardware is seen on the image.
- Proper radiographic technique is used.
- Sterile field is maintained.
- Radiation protection is provided for surgical team.
- Collimation to include all hardware used.
- No unnecessary instruments are in field.

NOTE: Often to save time or cost, multiple projections are done on one imaging plate. Be careful not to superimpose any of the projections. Many surgeons request different projections depending on the individual case. When performing a wrist examination, the arm is positioned on one side of the imaging plate with the wrist in the AP or PA projection. Center the beam and collimate to the wrist to include all hardware. When the exposure is complete, the surgeon moves the arm to the other side of the imaging plate in the lateral position. Center the beam on the wrist and collimate (Fig. 27-48 and Fig. 27-49).

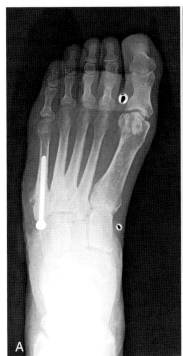
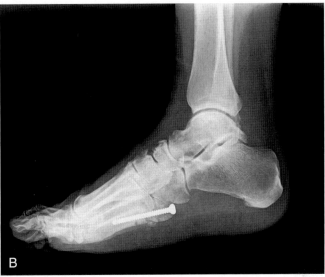

Fig. 27-47 AP (**A**) and lateral (**B**) postreduction images of a fifth metatarsal nonhealing fracture.

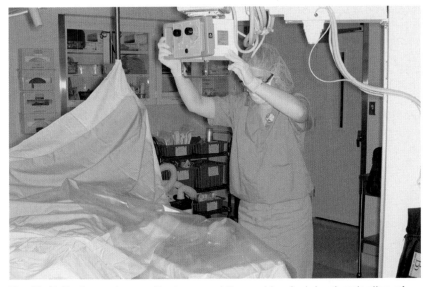

Fig. 27-48 Radiographer positioning a mobile machine for lateral projection of wrist.

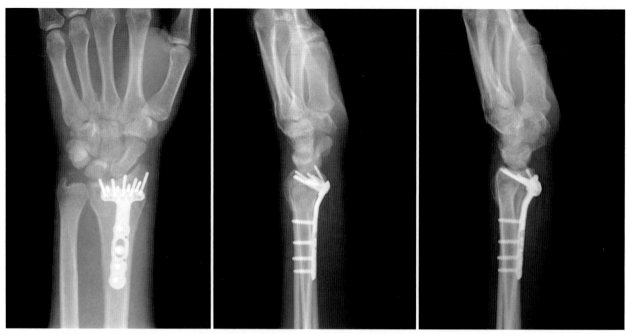

Fig. 27-49 PA, lateral, and tilt lateral projections of wrist. Note proper radial tilt of 22 degrees shows joint space clear of reduction screws.

Definition of Terms

antisepsis Chemical disinfection of the skin.

asepsis Absence of infection or germs or elimination of infectious agents.

aseptic technique Principles involved with manipulation of sterile and nonsterile items to prevent or minimize microbiologic contamination.

contamination Presence of pathogenic microorganisms.

microbial fallout Microorganisms normally shed from skin that can contaminate sterile surfaces or areas.

restricted area Operating rooms, clean core or sterile storage areas.

semirestricted area Area of peripheral support, such as hallways or corridors leading to restricted areas.

sterile Substance or object that is completely free of living microorganisms and is incapable of producing any form of organism.

strike-through Soaking through of moisture from nonsterile surfaces to sterile surfaces, or vice versa, allowing transportation of bacteria to sterile areas.

teamwork The Association of Surgical Technologists (AST) Standards of Practice Standard I states: "Teamwork is essential for perioperative patient care and is contingent on interpersonal skills. Communication is critical to the positive attainment of expected outcomes of care. All team members should work together for the common good of the patient, for the benefit of the patient and the delivery of actions with the health care team, the patient and family, superiors, and peers. Personal integrity and surgical conscience are integrated into every aspect of professional behavior."

unrestricted area Areas in which street clothes are permitted, such as outer hallways, family waiting areas, locker rooms, and employee lounges.

Selected bibliography

Anderson AC: *The radiologic technologist's handbook of surgical procedures*, Philadelphia, 2000, CRC Press.

Fortunato N: *Berry & Kohn's operating room technique*, ed 9, St Louis, 2000, Mosby.

Huth-Meeker M, Rothrock JC: *Alexander's care of the patient in surgery*, ed 10, St Louis, 1995, Mosby.

Huth-Meeker M, Rothrock JC: *Alexander's care of the patient in surgery*, ed 11, St Louis, 1999, Mosby.

Permar JA, Wetterlin KJ: Surgical radiography. In Frank ED et al, editors: *Merrill's atlas of radiographic positions and radiologic procedures*, ed 11, vol 3, St Louis, 2007, Mosby.

Wetterlin KJ: Mobile radiography. In Frank ED et al, editors: *Merrill's atlas of radiographic positions and radiologic procedures*, ed 9, vol 3, St Louis, 2007, Mosby.

28

SECTIONAL ANATOMY FOR RADIOGRAPHERS

TERRI BRUCKNER

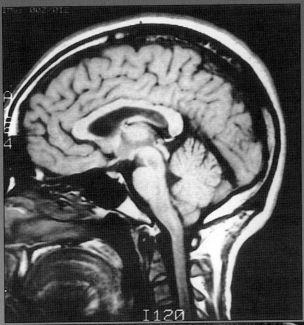

OUTLINE

Overview, 252
Cranial Region, 253
Thoracic Region, 269
Abdominopelvic Region, 282

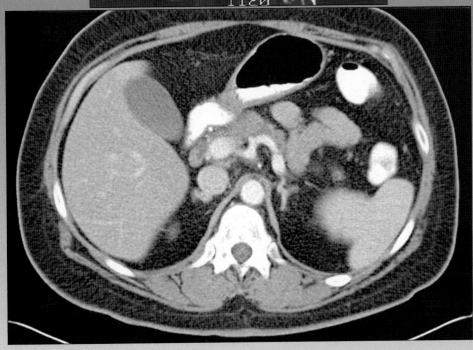

Overview

Imaging modalities, such as computed tomography (CT), magnetic resonance imaging (MRI), and diagnostic medical sonography, require the technologist to look at anatomy in the resultant images in a totally different way than they are used to with general radiographs. These technologies create cross-sectional imaging planes, in effect visualizing a slice through the body. Cross-sectional images have the advantage of visualizing anatomic structures without the sometimes confusing superimposition of other anatomic parts. Images are generated in various planes, which makes it crucial for the technologists working with these modalities to have a clear and complete understanding of general anatomic principles. Without a clear understanding of general anatomy, it is difficult to feel confident identifying normal and abnormal structures in cross section. This chapter provides the radiographer who possesses a background in general anatomy with an orientation to sectional anatomy and correlates that anatomy with structures shown on images from the various computer-generated imaging modalities.

Generally, three major imaging planes exist: axial, coronal, and sagittal. Axial planes (sometimes referred to as *transverse planes*) transect the body from anterior to posterior and from side to side. In effect, this type of horizontal plane divides the body into superior and inferior portions. Most images generated by CT are examples of axial or transverse planes. When looking at an axial image, it is helpful to imagine standing at the patient's feet and looking up toward the head. With this orientation, the patient's right side is to the viewer's left and vice versa. The anterior aspect of the patient is usually at the top of the image. Coronal planes divide the body into anterior and posterior portions. Coronal planes pass from superior to inferior and from side to side. Images viewed in the coronal plane are similar to radiographs in that the patient's

right side is on the technologist's left (one can imagine facing the patient while viewing this type of image). Sagittal planes divide the body into right and left portions. These planes pass from superior to inferior and from anterior to posterior. MR images frequently use the coronal and sagittal planes to present the desired anatomy. CT images may be obtained in the coronal or sagittal planes, or the computer may reformat information from axial images to obtain images in these planes. Any plane that does not fit the previous descriptions is referred to as an *oblique plane*. Ultrasonography and MRI of some structures, such as the heart, are generated using oblique planes.

CT uses x-rays to generate images, so the various shades on the images correspond to the gray scale that radiographers are accustomed to seeing. Bones and other dense materials are white, whereas air and lower density materials are closer to black. Fat, muscle, and organs are represented with various shades of gray. Hounsfield units or CT numbers represent the scale of white to black that is used in CT imaging. Lower numbers represent anatomic structures that are more easily penetrated by the x-ray and appear closer to black on the image. Higher numbers are related to more radiopaque structures and are lighter gray or white on the image. Similar to routine radiographs, blood vessels and organs of the digestive system are not easily distinguishable from other structures. To be able to identify these structures more accurately, patients are frequently given a radiopaque contrast medium. Intravascular contrast medium highlights vessels, making them appear radiopaque and whiter on the image. To visualize the gastrointestinal system, patients may be given a contrast agent by mouth or via the rectum. A full description of CT fundamentals is presented in Chapter 31.

MRI uses magnetic fields and radiofrequencies to generate images. Anatomic structures are represented on the image with regard to the signal generated from

their protons. Structures that produce a strong signal are generally lighter gray or white on the image, and structures that do not generate a strong signal tend to be darker on the image. The signal generated by these structures depends on many things, including the strength of the magnetic fields and the characteristics of the radiofrequencies used. Contrast medium may also be used when performing MRI to change the signal intensity of particular anatomic structures. Gadolinium, air, and fluid may be used as contrast agents depending on the organ of interest and the imaging sequences employed. MRI is discussed in depth in Chapter 30.

The cadaveric sections depicted in this chapter are representative of major organ structures for each of the body regions, and they *are depicted from the inferior surface to correspond to the images.* All relational terms are used in relation to the body in anatomic position (when a structure is described as being to the right of something, this refers to the *patient's* right, not the *viewer's* right). The major anatomic structures normally seen when using current imaging modalities are labeled. For each region of the body, a cadaveric section is presented, and representative images are included to provide an orientation to anatomic structures normally seen using the available imaging modalities. The cadaveric sections and diagnostic images do not match exactly; some structures are seen on only one of the illustrations for each body region. Major anatomic structures in each region of the body are reviewed in the following sections to make it easier to identify the images provided. Systematic review of the bones, vessels, major organs, and muscles begin each section. Selected images are presented in axial, sagittal, and coronal planes to show these structures. In practice, images should be examined collectively because the size, shape, and placement of these structures vary from slice to slice. "Following" a structure is frequently the ideal way to identify it.

Cranial Region

Fig. 28-1 is a cadaveric image that can be used to distinguish bone, muscle, and other soft tissue structures. Referring to this image should be helpful in identifying the sometimes confusing shadows on the images. The head can be thought of systematically as being composed of the skull, central nervous system structures, various sensory organs, cranial blood supply, and associated cranial and facial muscles. The bones of the skull are categorized as the 8 cranial bones and the 14 facial bones. The cranial bones include the frontal, occipital, and two parietal bones that surround and protect the external surface of the brain. The other four cranial bones include the ethmoid, sphenoid, and two temporal bones. The frontal bone forms the anterior surface of the skull, with a vertical portion that corresponds to the forehead and a horizontal portion that forms the roof of the orbits. Between the inner and outer layers of the vertical portion of the frontal bone, just superior to the level of the eyes, are the paired frontal paranasal sinuses. The vertex

(superiormost portion) of the skull is formed by the paired parietal bones. These roughly square-shaped bones articulate with the frontal bone at the coronal suture, with the temporal bones at the squamosal sutures, with the occipital bone at the lambdoidal suture, and with each other at the sagittal suture.

The posterior aspect of the skull is formed by the occipital bone, which is composed of a squamous (vertical) portion and a basilar portion. The foramen magnum is a large opening within the squamous portion that allows passage of the spinal cord into the brain. The external occipital protuberance is a large prominence on the posterior surface of this bone. Roughly corresponding in position to this landmark is the internal occipital protuberance. The ethmoid bone is found within the cranium and forms the medial walls of the orbits and part of the lateral walls of the nasal cavity. The ethmoid bone is divided into a horizontal portion called the *cribriform plate* and vertical portions called the *perpendicular plate* and *two labyrinths* or *lateral masses.*

The cribriform plate lies between the orbital plates of the frontal bone and supports the olfactory bulbs (cranial nerve I). The cribriform plate is perforated by many small foramina, which transmit nerves from the nose to this cranial nerve. Projecting superiorly from the cribriform plate is a small ridge of bone called the *crista galli,* which serves as the anterior attachment for the falx cerebri. Projecting inferiorly from the center of the cribriform plate is the perpendicular plate. This thin strip of bone forms the superior part of the bony nasal septum. Extending inferiorly from the lateral edges of the cribriform plate are the labyrinths or lateral masses. These are perforated by multiple air spaces, which are collectively called the *ethmoidal paranasal sinuses.* From the medial surface of each labyrinth, two scroll-shaped ridges of bone project into the nasal cavity. These are the superior and middle nasal conchae.

In the center of the base of the skull is the sphenoid bone. This bone is sometimes referred to as the *anchor bone of the cranium* because it articulates with all of

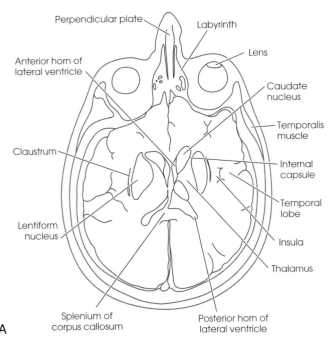
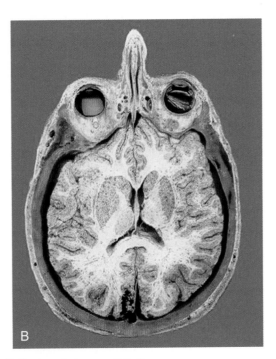

Fig. 28-1 A, Line drawing of gross anatomic section. **B,** Cadaveric image of skull.

Labels (A): Perpendicular plate, Labyrinth, Anterior horn of lateral ventricle, Lens, Caudate nucleus, Temporalis muscle, Claustrum, Internal capsule, Temporal lobe, Lentiform nucleus, Insula, Thalamus, Splenium of corpus callosum, Posterior horn of lateral ventricle

the cranial bones. Thinking of this bone as being composed of a body, two sets of wings, and a pterygoid portion is helpful. The body is the central portion of the bone and contains the easily identifiable landmark known as the *sella turcica.* The sella turcica forms a cup-shaped depression that surrounds and protects the pituitary gland. The anterior surface of the sella is called the *tuberculum sellae,* and the posterior portion is called the *dorsum sellae.* Two posterior clinoid processes project from the superior edge of the dorsum sellae and are attachments for dura mater partitions. Within the body of the sphenoid and inferior to the sella turcica are the paired sphenoidal paranasal sinuses. The lesser wings of the sphenoid are triangular ridges of bone found posterior to the orbital plates of the frontal bone. Directly inferior to the medial edge of each lesser wing is the optic canal, which transmits the optic nerve (cranial nerve II). The larger, greater wings support the temporal lobes of the cerebrum and extend from the body to the external surface of the skull. The pterygoid processes project inferiorly from the body of the sphenoid and form the posterior walls of the nasal cavity.

The temporal bones form part of the lateral walls of the cranium and extend internally to meet the sphenoid and the basilar portion of the occipital bone. Parts of the temporal bone include the squamous, tympanic, mastoid, and petrous portions. The squamous portion is the thin, fan-shaped external part of the bone superior to the external ear. It articulates with the parietal and several other cranial bones. Its articulation with the parietal bone is called the *squamous suture.* The tympanic portion is the area of the bone surrounding the external ear canal. The zygomatic process arches anteriorly from just superior to the external ear canal. Just inferior to the origin of the zygomatic process is the mandibular fossa, in which the condyle of the mandible is found. On the inferior surface of the tympanic portion of the bone is the styloid process, which serves as an attachment for muscles. Posterior to the ear is the mastoid portion, which is perforated by many small, air-filled cavities. The mastoid portion extends inferiorly to form the cone-shaped mastoid process. The petrous portion of the bone lies within the cranium, normally forming an angle of approximately 45 degrees to the median sagittal plane. This dense ridge of bone surrounds and protects the organs

of hearing and balance, the facial and vestibulocochlear nerves, and the internal carotid artery.

The organs associated with the face are surrounded and protected by 14 bones. Each of these bones is paired with the exception of the vomer and the mandible. The lacrimal bones are about the size of a fingernail and are found in the medial wall of the orbit between the maxilla and the labyrinth of the ethmoid bones. The nasal bones form the bridge of the nose and articulate superiorly with the frontal bone, laterally with the maxilla, and with each other in the midline. The zygomatic bones form the inferolateral walls of the orbits. Each of these bones articulates superiorly with the frontal bone, medially with the maxilla, and laterally with the zygomatic process of the temporal bone. The maxilla originates as two separate bones, which ultimately fuse along the midsagittal plane. This large bone forms the inferior surface of each orbit, the lateral walls of the nasal cavity, and the anterior portion of the roof of the mouth. On either side of the nasal cavity, large air-filled maxillary paranasal sinuses are embedded within the bone. The upper teeth are rooted within the alveolar process at the anteroinferior surface of the bone. The maxilla articulates with the nasal bones, the lacrimal bones, the frontal bone, the zygomatic bones, and the palatine bones. The inferior nasal conchae are scroll-shaped facial bones found in the nasal cavity, just inferior to the middle nasal conchae of the ethmoid bone. The L-shaped palatine bones form the posterior portion of the hard palate. The vertical portions of the palatines extend superiorly along the posterior nasal cavity to form a small part of the posterior orbit.

The vomer is an unpaired facial bone that rests on the hard palate and articulates with the inferior surface of the perpendicular plate of the ethmoid. It forms the inferior portion of the bony nasal septum. The mandible, which is also an unpaired facial bone, is formed by a body and two rami. The body comprises the anterior portion of the bone and presents an alveolar ridge in which the lower teeth are embedded. The rami extend superiorly from the body and end in anterior and posterior bony processes. The anterior process at the superior end of the ramus is the coronoid process, where muscles of mastication attach. The posterior process is the condyloid process, which rests in

the mandibular fossa of the temporal bone. This articulation, the temporomandibular joint, is the only movable articulation associated with the skull. (Refer to Chapter 20 for review of skull anatomy.)

The brain is surrounded by three layers of protective membranes called the *meninges.* From internal to external, they are the pia mater, arachnoid, and dura mater. The pia mater adheres directly to the brain and is composed of a fine network of capillaries and supporting tissue. The arachnoid is a delicate membrane that resembles a cobweb. The subarachnoid space lies between the arachnoid and pia mater. Cerebrospinal fluid (CSF) circulates in this space. The arachnoid does not closely adhere to cerebral structures. As it bridges the gap between various parts of the brain, enlarged regions or cisterns are formed in the subarachnoid space. Some of the more crucial cisterns include the cisterna magna, pontine, interpeduncular, and superior or *quadrigeminal cistern.* The cisterna magna is the largest of these and is found just inside the foramen magnum, between the cerebellum and the medulla oblongata. This cistern receives CSF from the fourth ventricle. The pontine cistern lies anterior to the pons and contains the basilar artery. The interpeduncular cistern is anterior to the midbrain. The infundibulum (stalk) of the pituitary and the vessels of the circle of Willis are seen here. The cistern found posterior to the midbrain is the superior cistern. It surrounds the pineal gland and the great cerebral vein. Ambient cisterns communicate with the superior cistern and extend laterally around the midbrain. The most external of the meninges is the double-layered dura mater. The outer layer of dura is attached to the inner surface of the cranial bones. The inner layer can be seen between cerebral structures and in large fissures. Dural sinuses are venous drainage channels formed where the inner dural layers separate from the outer layer. One of the largest dural flaps, the falx cerebri, is found in the longitudinal fissure between the cerebral hemispheres. It extends from the crista galli of the ethmoid to the occipital bone. The tentorium cerebelli extends between the cerebrum and the cerebellum. It attaches to the sella turcica and the internal surface of the occipital bones.

The structures of the central nervous system within the skull include the cerebrum, brain stem, and cerebellum. The cerebrum is the largest of these structures and is divided by the longitudinal fissure into two hemispheres. The hemispheres are connected to each other via a white matter tract called the *corpus callosum*. This arch-shaped structure is divided into the anterior genu, central body, and posterior splenium. Each cerebral hemisphere is divided into lobes that are named for the most adjacent cranial bone: frontal, parietal, temporal, and occipital. An additional lobe called the insula is buried deep to the temporal lobe. The cerebrum is thrown into numerous folds called *gyri,* which are separated by small fissures called *sulci.* The outer surface of the cerebrum consists of a thin layer of gray matter. The central portion of this part of the brain is mainly white matter (formed by myelinated nerve fibers). These fibers, referred to as the *corona radiata,* connect the gray matter of the cortex to deeper gray matter nuclei deep within each hemisphere. The buried gray matter centers are called *basal nuclei* or *basal ganglia* and include the claustrum, putamen, globus pallidus, and caudate nucleus. White matter tracts, or capsules, are found between these gray matter structures. Other gray matter structures found within the central cerebrum include the thalamus and hypothalamus. These form the walls of the third ventricle. Many of these gray and white matter structures are seen on the cadaveric section in Fig. 28-1.

The brain stem is formed by the midbrain, pons, and medulla oblongata. It lies between the cerebrum and cerebellum and serves as a relay for nerve impulses between the spinal cord and these two structures. The midbrain is the most superior of the three. White matter tracts called the cerebral peduncles extend from the anterior midbrain to the cerebrum. Toward the posterior aspect of the midbrain are the corpora quadrigemina, which are formed by two superior and two inferior colliculi that lie just inferior to the splenium of the corpus callosum. The cerebral aqueduct drains CSF from the third ventricle to the fourth ventricle and passes through the posterior portion of the midbrain. The central portion of the brain stem is formed by the pons. It communicates with the medulla, with the midbrain, and via white matter cerebellar peduncles to the cerebellum. The most inferior of the brain stem structures is the medulla oblongata, which is continuous with the spinal cord as it passes through the foramen magnum.

The cerebellum lies in the posteroinferior region of the cranium. Although smaller in size, it is similar in composition to the cerebrum. A midline fissure divides the cerebellum into hemispheres that are connected by a midline vermis. It is also thrown into numerous small folds, here called folia, which are separated by numerous small fissures. The outer surface of the cerebellum is composed of gray matter, with white matter constituting most of the central portion of this part of the brain. Gray matter nuclei can be found here also, although they are difficult to distinguish on images and are not discussed in this chapter.

Four large cavities called *ventricles* are found in the brain. The ventricles' major function is to produce CSF; this is accomplished as blood is filtered through capillary networks called *choroid plexuses* in each of the ventricles. The largest of these chambers are the lateral ventricles, one of which is found in each cerebral hemisphere. The lateral ventricles are divided into a body and anterior, posterior, and inferior horns. CSF from these chambers passes into the midline third ventricle through the interventricular foramina. The third ventricle is found between the cerebral hemispheres inferior to the lateral ventricles. The cerebral aqueduct drains CSF from here to the fourth ventricle. This ventricle is found between the cerebellum and the brain stem. Its walls are formed by white matter tracts called *cerebellar peduncles,* which connect the brain stem and cerebellum. A central aperture and two lateral apertures allow CSF to pass from the fourth ventricle into the subarachnoid space.

The brain is a highly metabolic organ, and to function well it needs a rich blood supply. Four major arteries supply the brain and its related structures: the two internal carotid arteries and the two vertebral arteries. The internal carotid arteries supply the anterior structures of the brain. After passing superiorly through the neck, these arteries enter the skull via the carotid canals in the petrous portion of the temporal bones. After exiting the petrous portion, the internal carotid arteries pass along the lateral aspect of the sella turcica, ultimately dividing into the anterior and middle cerebral arteries. The posterior communicating artery arises from the internal carotid just before this bifurcation. The anterior cerebral arteries pass anteriorly and superiorly to the longitudinal fissure, where they curl around the external aspect of the corpus callosum and supply the anterior portion of the brain. The middle cerebral arteries pass laterally to the lateral fissures, where their branches supply the middle portion of the brain. The posterior communicating arteries pass posteriorly to join with the branches from the vertebrobasilar arterial system. The vertebral arteries traverse the neck in the transverse foramina of the cervical spine and enter the posterior skull via the foramen magnum. These arteries pass superiorly along the anterior aspect of the medulla and at the base of the pons join to form the basilar artery. At the superior aspect of the pons, the basilar artery splits to form the posterior cerebral arteries. A unique arterial anastomosis exists in the brain to protect it from sudden loss of blood supply. This vascular connection is called the *circle of Willis.* The blood supply to the anterior brain is connected to the blood supply for the posterior brain as the posterior communicating arteries extend from the internal carotid arteries to the posterior cerebral arteries. This communication lies in the interpeduncular cistern, just anterior to the midbrain.

Venous drainage in the cranium is accomplished by two systems: cerebral veins and dural venous sinuses. The dural sinuses are created by gaps formed between the inner and outer layers of the dura mater. These gaps are found in the areas where the dura invaginates between the various structures of the brain. The superior sagittal sinus is found in the superior border of the falx cerebri, and the inferior sagittal sinus is found in its inferior margin. The channel formed where the falx cerebri meets the tentorium cerebelli is the straight sinus. This sinus is a continuation of the inferior sagittal sinus as it joins with the great cerebral vein. The transverse or lateral sinuses are found along the lateral aspect of the tentorium cerebelli as it meets the occipital bone. At the level of the petrous portions of the temporal bones, the transverse sinuses curl medially and inferiorly and become known as the *sigmoid sinuses.* As the sigmoid sinuses pass out of the cranium via the jugular foramina, these vessels change names again and become the internal jugular veins. One of the major veins within the skull is the great cerebral vein. This large venous structure is found in the superior cistern, and there it joins the inferior sagittal sinus to form the straight sinus.

Many muscles are associated with the face, only a few of which are referred to in the following sections. The temporalis muscle is found on the external surface of the squamous portion of the temporal bone. Its inferior attachment is to the coronoid process of the mandible. On the external surface of the mandibular rami are the masseter muscles, and on the internal surface of the rami are the pterygoid muscles. These muscles all are associated with moving the mandible and with swallowing.

A lateral skull radiograph is used here for localization of the imaging plane in this section (Fig. 28-2, *A*), and a sagittal MR image (Fig. 28-2, *B*) is used for localization of MRI cross sections of the brain. CT imaging for the cranium may be performed with the gantry parallel to or angled 15 to 20 degrees to the orbitomeatal line. Angling the gantry of the CT scanner allows for imaging of the brain without excess radiation to the eyes. MRI of the cranium generally results in images that are parallel to the orbitomeatal or infraorbitomeatal plane. More details on patient positioning for CT are provided in Chapter 29, and information on patient positioning for MRI is provided in Chapter 30. Because the imaging planes may be different for CT and MRI, some variation exists in the anatomic structures visualized on corresponding illustrations in this section. Seven identifying lines represent the approximate levels for each of the labeled images for this region.

The cranial CT image seen in Fig. 28-3 represents a CT slice obtained through the frontal and parietal bones, and Fig. 28-4 is a corresponding MR image. The *cortex,* or outer layer of gray matter, can be differentiated from the deeper *white matter.* The numerous *gyri,* or *convolutions,* and *sulci* are shown and are surrounded by the darker appearing CSF in the subarachnoid space. The *cerebral hemispheres* are separated by the *longitudinal cerebral fissure.* Invaginated in this fissure is a fold of *dura mater* called the *falx cerebri.* The *superior sagittal sinus,* which passes through the superior margin of the falx cerebri, follows the contour of the superior skull margin. In cross section, the anterior and posterior aspects of this sinus can normally be seen in the midline deep to the bony plates when the patient has been given an intravenous contrast agent and appear as triangular expansions near the bones easily seen on both the CT and MR images. Two of the five *cerebral lobes* are seen (frontal and parietal). The *corona radiata* is the central tract of white matter in the cerebrum and is darker than the cortex on the CT image; the white matter is lighter than

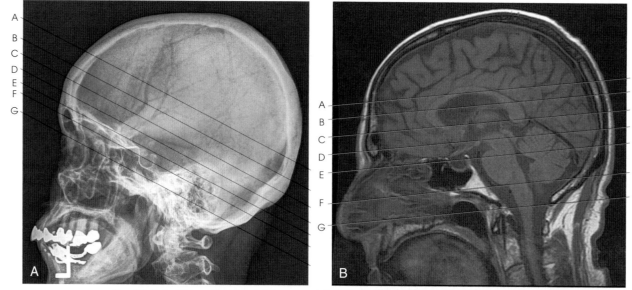

Fig. 28-2 A, CT localizer (scout) image of skull. **B,** Sagittal localizer for MRI of brain.

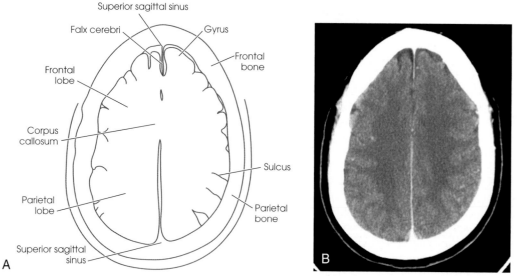

Fig. 28-3 A, Line drawing of CT section. **B,** CT image representing anatomic structures located at level *A* in Fig. 28-2, *A.*

the gray matter on the MR image. These sections were obtained at a level that passes through the superiormost portion of the *corpus callosum,* which separates the anterior and posterior portions of the falx cerebri.

Fig. 28-5 is an axial CT slice through the superior portions of the lateral ventricles; Fig. 28-6 is the corresponding MR image. Visualized bony structures on the CT scan include the *frontal bone* and the two *parietal bones.* The falx cerebri is seen within the *longitudinal fissure.* The *frontal lobes* and *parietal lobes* of the cerebrum are shown. In the center of each image, the *lateral ventricles* are easily seen because of the dark appearance of the CSF circulating within each. In the posterior portions of the ventricles, the contrast-filled capillary network of the *choroid plexuses* also is visualized. A thin membrane called the *septum pellucidum* can be seen separating the ventricles. The corpus callosum is an arch-shaped structure; in cross section at this level, only the anterior *genu* and the posterior *splenium* can be seen. The *caudate nuclei* lie along the lateral surfaces of the ventricles and tend to follow their curves. Because these nuclei are composed of gray matter, they are the same shade of gray as the cortex on MR images (see Fig. 28-6). Several contrast-filled vascular structures are visible. The *anterior cerebral arteries* lie within the longitudinal fissure just anterior to the genu of the corpus callosum. A few branches of the *middle cerebral arteries* are seen near the lateral aspect of the skull

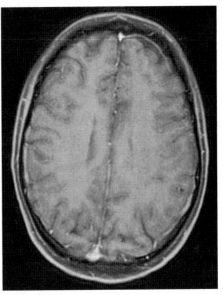

Fig. 28-4 MRI corresponding to level *A* in Fig. 28-2, *B.*

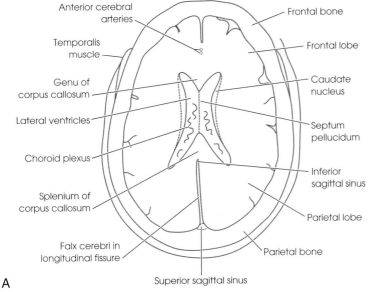

A

Fig. 28-5 A, Line drawing of CT section. **B,** CT image representing structures located at level *B* in Fig. 28-2, *A.*

Labels in drawing:
- Anterior cerebral arteries
- Temporalis muscle
- Genu of corpus callosum
- Lateral ventricles
- Choroid plexus
- Splenium of corpus callosum
- Falx cerebri in longitudinal fissure
- Superior sagittal sinus
- Frontal bone
- Frontal lobe
- Caudate nucleus
- Septum pellucidum
- Inferior sagittal sinus
- Parietal lobe
- Parietal bone

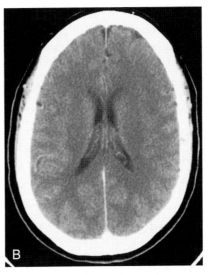

B

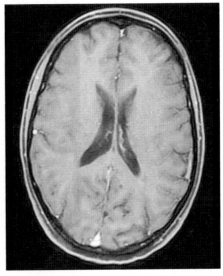

Fig. 28-6 MRI corresponding to level *B* in Fig. 28-2, *B.*

on the CT scan. The anterior and posterior portions of the superior sagittal sinus are seen in the periphery of the falx cerebri. The *inferior sagittal sinus* lies in the internal edges of the falx. The thin strips of muscle seen on the external surface of the frontal bone correspond to the superior edges of the *temporalis muscles*.

The axial sections through the midportion of the cerebrum show many of the central structures of the cerebral hemispheres (Fig. 28-7 is a CT image, and Fig. 28-8 is an MR image). Images at this level pass through the frontal bone, greater wing of the *sphenoid*, and squamous portion of the *temporal bones*. The poste-

rior portion of the skull comprises the top portion (squamous portion) of the *occipital bone* at this level. The falx cerebri is shown within the longitudinal fissure, with the superior sagittal sinus best shown in the midline of the anterior and posterior margins of this membrane. In the CT image, the genu of the corpus callosum is found between the anterior horns of the lateral ventricles; however, the posterior portion of this slice is inferior to the level of the splenium. The MR image shows the genu and the splenium. At this level, the MR image shows the *frontal, temporal, and occipital lobes* along with the *insula* (fifth lobe or island of Reil), which is deep

to the temporal lobe at the lateral fissure. Because of its orientation, the CT image shows the insula, frontal, and temporal lobes; the cerebellum occupies the posterior aspect of the skull in this image.

The anterior and temporal horns of the lateral ventricles are seen on the CT scan, whereas the anterior and posterior horns are visible on the MR image. Within each posterior horn is a portion of the choroid plexus, which appears bright owing to the presence of contrast medium in the capillaries. The heads of the caudate nuclei lie along the external surfaces of the anterior horns of each lateral ventricle. Several areas of gray matter can be seen faintly on

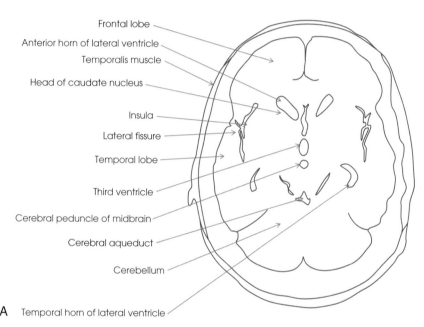

Frontal lobe
Anterior horn of lateral ventricle
Temporalis muscle
Head of caudate nucleus
Insula
Lateral fissure
Temporal lobe
Third ventricle
Cerebral peduncle of midbrain
Cerebral aqueduct
Cerebellum
A Temporal horn of lateral ventricle

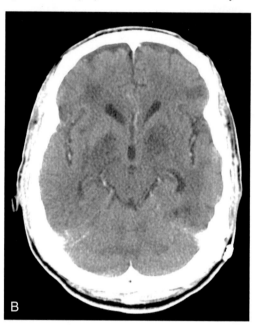
B

Fig. 28-7 A, Line drawing of CT section. **B,** CT image representing anatomic structures located at level *C* in Fig. 28-2, *A*.

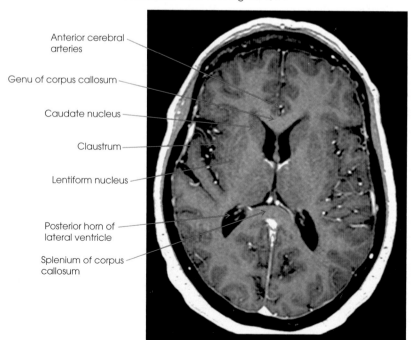

Anterior cerebral arteries
Genu of corpus callosum
Caudate nucleus
Claustrum
Lentiform nucleus
Posterior horn of lateral ventricle
Splenium of corpus callosum

Fig. 28-8 MRI representing anatomic structures located at level *C* in Fig. 28-2, *B*.

the CT image deep within the white matter of the cerebrum and constitute the basal nuclei. The MR image contrast has been enhanced so that the deep gray matter structures can be seen. The major components of the basal nuclei seen at this level are (from lateral to medial) the *claustrum, lentiform nucleus* (composed of the putamen and globus pallidus), and *caudate nucleus*. The lentiform nucleus is separated from the caudate nucleus and thalamus by a tract of white matter known as the *internal capsule*. These sections pass through the superior portion of the midline *third ventricle*. The *thalamus,* which serves as a central relay station for sensory impulses to the cerebral cortex, forms its lateral walls. The plane of the CT image passes through the structures of the midbrain. The anterior portions of the midbrain include the cerebral peduncles (white matter tracts that connect the cerebrum and the midbrain). The dark circular area at the posterior edge of the midbrain is the CSF-filled cerebral aqueduct. This passage connects the third and fourth ventricles and allows the circulation of CSF. A contrast-enhanced vessel, the great cerebral vein, is found just posterior to the third ventricle and the splenium of the corpus callosum on the MR image. It passes through the upper portion of the *superior cistern*. The pineal gland is also found in this cistern but is not clearly visualized in either image. This is an important radiographic landmark because of its tendency to calcify in adults. Branches of the middle cerebral artery are visible within the lateral fissures, and the anterior cerebral arteries can be seen in the anterior portion of the longitudinal fissure on the MR image.

Fig. 28-9 is a CT image that passes through the frontal lobe, pons, and cerebellum; Fig. 28-10 is the MR image, which

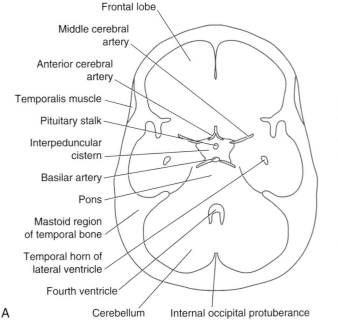
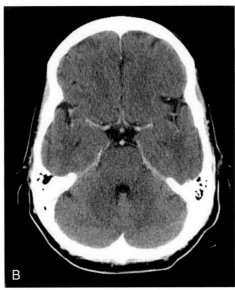

Frontal lobe
Middle cerebral artery
Anterior cerebral artery
Temporalis muscle
Pituitary stalk
Interpeduncular cistern
Basilar artery
Pons
Mastoid region of temporal bone
Temporal horn of lateral ventricle
Fourth ventricle

A   Cerebellum   Internal occipital protuberance

B

Fig. 28-9 A, Line drawing of CT section. **B,** CT image representing anatomic structures located at level *D* in Fig. 28-2, *A.*

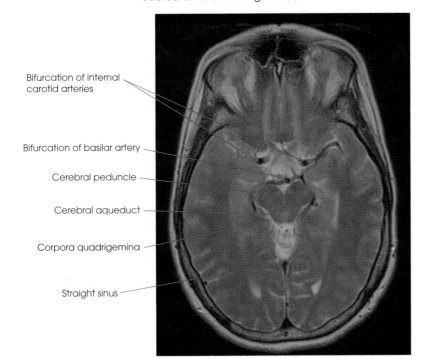

Bifurcation of internal carotid arteries
Bifurcation of basilar artery
Cerebral peduncle
Cerebral aqueduct
Corpora quadrigemina
Straight sinus

Fig. 28-10 MRI through circle of Willis corresponding to level *D* in Fig. 28-2, *B.*

259

passes through the superior portions of the orbits, the midbrain, and the occipital lobes. Bony structures visible in the CT image include the frontal bone, the temporal bones, and the occipital bone. Within the temporal bones, the black air-filled structures represent the mastoid air cells. The internal protrusion of bone in the center of the occipital bone is the internal occipital protuberance. The area of signal void between the eyes on the MR image corresponds to the frontal sinuses. Frontal and temporal lobes of the cerebrum are shown on the CT image, whereas the frontal, temporal, and occipital lobes of the cerebrum are shown on the MR image. The CT scan passes just inferior to the midbrain, and the MR image passes through the level of the midbrain. The large dark area in the center of the CT image is the interpeduncular cistern. This is an enlarged area in the subarachnoid space containing CSF. The optic chiasm and the circle of Willis normally lie within the interpeduncular cistern. The pituitary stalk and some of the vessels that contribute to the circle of Willis are visible on

this image. The pons lies posterior to the cistern. The cerebellum lies within the posterior fossa of the skull between the pons and the occipital bone. The large dark region between the pons and cerebellum is the CSF-filled fourth ventricle. The temporalis muscles are seen on the external surfaces on either side of the cranium. On the MR image, the *cerebral peduncles* form the anterior portions of the midbrain, and the *corpora quadrigemina* forms the posterior portion. The small light gray circle anterior to the colliculi is the CSF-filled *cerebral aqueduct.* Posterior to the midbrain is the *cerebellum,* which is surrounded by the *tentorium cerebelli.* The dark region anterior to the midbrain is the *interpeduncular cistern,* and the region posterior to the midbrain is the superior cistern. On the MR image, within and around the interpeduncular cistern are the *optic tracts, hypothalamus,* inferior portion of the third ventricle, and *mammillary bodies.*

The CT image is just superior to the internal carotid arteries and shows the origins of the left anterior and middle cerebral arter-

ies, at the anterior edge of the interpeduncular cistern. The anterior cerebral arteries pass from their origin toward the longitudinal fissure in the midline of the brain; the middle cerebral arteries course from their origins toward the lateral fissures. The CT image also shows the bifurcation of the basilar artery into the two posterior cerebral arteries. These vessels can be seen just anterior to the pons. The circle of Willis is an important vascular structure found in this region of the brain. Although it does not lie in the same plane as the imaging plane, much of the circle can be seen on the MR image. The bright anterior vascular structures represent the bifurcation of the internal carotid arteries into the anterior and middle cerebral arteries. The posterior cerebral arteries are seen here originating between the cerebral peduncles. The posterior and anterior communicating arteries are not seen in this image because they are not at the same level as the other vessels. The posterior portion of the superior sagittal sinus is located near the internal occipital protuberance; the *straight sinus* can be seen

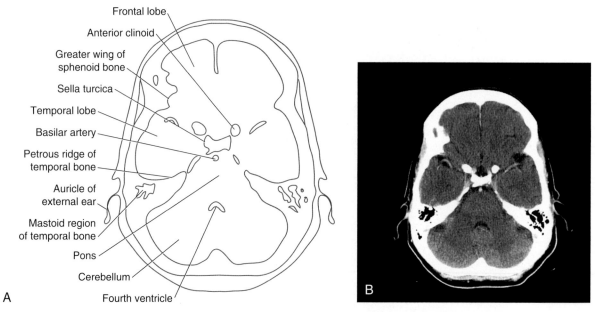

Frontal lobe
Anterior clinoid
Greater wing of sphenoid bone
Sella turcica
Temporal lobe
Basilar artery
Petrous ridge of temporal bone
Auricle of external ear
Mastoid region of temporal bone
Pons
Cerebellum
A   Fourth ventricle
B

Fig. 28-11 A, Line drawing of CT section. **B,** CT image representing anatomic structures located at level *E* in Fig. 28-2, *A.*

in the edge of the tentorium cerebelli, just posterior to the cerebellum on the MR image.

Fig. 28-11 is a CT image through the sella turcica and the posterior fossa. The MR image (Fig. 28-12) passes through the center of the orbits, the tops of the ears, the pituitary and center of the sella turcica, and the cerebellum. The MR image shows the *nasal bones,* visible in the anterior skull. Between the eyes the *ethmoidal sinuses* and the *cribriform plate* of the ethmoid bone is seen. The *sphenoidal sinuses* lie posterior to the ethmoidal sinuses. The *sella turcica* and *dorsum sellae* are seen surrounding the *pituitary gland.* Several cranial bones are visible on the CT scan. The anterior clinoids of the sella turcica and the greater wings of the sphenoid are seen. The roof of the sella is formed by the lesser wings, anterior clinoids, and posterior clinoids. The temporal bone constitutes most of the lateral portions

of the skull, and the *petrous ridges* can be seen on the CT image extending toward the median sagittal plane. The black air spaces near the lateral aspect of the petrous portions of these bones correspond to *mastoid air cells,* and the air spaces farther medial are associated with the internal structures of the ear. On the CT image, the frontal and temporal lobes of the cerebrum are visible, along with the pons and cerebellum. The dark region between the sella turcica and the pons is the pontine cistern, filled with CSF. The lower region of the fourth ventricle is seen between the pons and the cerebellum. On the MR image, both *globes* are visible within the orbits. Rectus muscles lie along the medial and lateral walls of each. The *optic nerves* are seen in the centers of the posterior orbits passing from the eyes toward the brain via the optic canal. The temporal lobes are found lateral to the sella turcica, resting in the middle cranial fossa. The *pons* lies posterior to the sella, and the

cerebellum is seen filling the posterior cranial fossa. The edges of the tentorium cerebelli can be seen faintly between the temporal lobes and the cerebellum. The dark region anterior to the pons corresponds to the CSF-filled *pontine cistern* in which the contrast-filled *basilar artery* is easily visualized on both the CT and MR images. The dark region between the pons and the cerebellum is the superior region of the *fourth ventricle.* On the CT image, the contrast-filled basilar artery lies between the sella and the pons. At this level in the MR image, the *internal carotid arteries* lie lateral to the body of the sphenoid bone in an almost horizontal orientation. The *confluence of sinuses* can be seen just anterior to the internal occipital protuberance on the MR image. The confluence is the region where the superior sagittal sinus and the straight sinus meet the transverse sinuses. The *transverse sinuses* are seen on the MR image at this level lying just internal to the

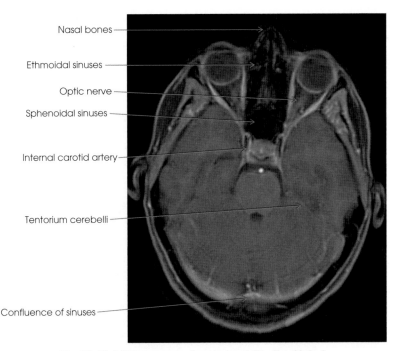

Nasal bones

Ethmoidal sinuses

Optic nerve

Sphenoidal sinuses

Internal carotid artery

Tentorium cerebelli

Confluence of sinuses

Fig. 28-12 MRI corresponding to level *E* in Fig. 28-2, *B.*

occipital bone. On the external surface of the skull in both images, the temporalis muscles lie along the temporal bones. The *auricle,* or cartilaginous portion of each ear, lies external to the temporal bone.

The sectional images through the lower cranium show the inferior portions of the cerebrum, brain stem, cerebellum, and associated major skeletal structures (Fig. 28-13 is a CT image, and Fig. 28-14 is an MR image). The CT image shows the frontal sinuses and the roofs of the orbits. The greater and lesser wings of the sphenoid bone are shown. The optic foramina (canals) can be seen between the greater and lesser wings. The optic chiasm and cavernous sinus can be seen posterior to the

optic foramen. The petrous and mastoid portions of the temporal bones are shown dividing the middle and posterior cranial fossae. The maxilla, *maxillary sinuses,* and nasal bones are seen in the anterior skull on the MR image (note the mass within the right maxillary sinus). The *zygomatic bones* form the lateral walls of the orbits, and the *maxillae* form the medial walls. The *perpendicular plate* and *vomer* form the bony nasal septum seen in the center of the nasal cavity. Posterior to the nasal cavity, the sphenoidal sinuses are seen between the lower aspects of the greater wings. Both petrous ridges extend toward the midline; these are seen as dark areas on the MR image because of the lack of signal

from this dense region of bone. Extending into the right petrous ridge is the *external auditory canal.* Just anterior to the canal is the *condyle of the mandible* resting in the mandibular fossa. Mastoid air cells lie posterior to the external acoustic meatus.

In the center of the skull, the greater wings of the sphenoid, petrous ridges, and basilar portion of the occipital bone meet. The CT image shows the lower portions of the frontal lobes and temporal lobes, along with the lower margin of the pons and the cerebellum. On the MR image, the most inferior folds of the temporal lobes are found in the middle cranial fossae resting on the greater wings of the sphenoid. The *medulla oblongata* lies posterior to the

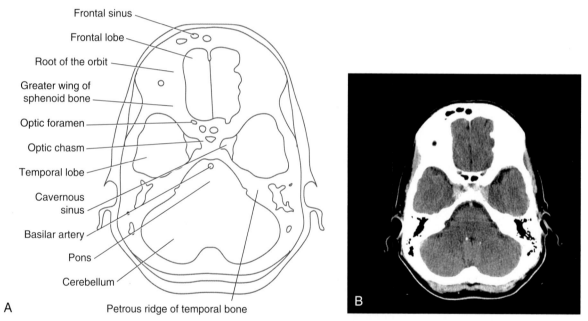

Fig. 28-13 A, Line drawing of CT section. **B,** CT image representing anatomic structures located at level *F* in Fig. 28-2, *A.*

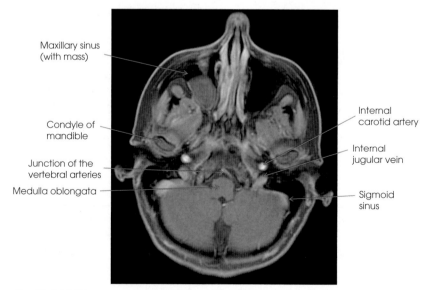

Fig. 28-14 MRI representing anatomic structures located at level *F* in Fig. 28-2, *B.*

basilar portion of the occipital bone. The cerebellum is seen within the posterior fossa. The small, dark space between the medulla and the cerebellum is the lower extent of the fourth ventricle. CSF in the *cisterna magna* circulates around the anterior and lateral reaches of the medulla. At the level of this image, the internal carotid arteries are found just posterior to the optic foramina, within the cavernous sinuses, on the CT scan; both are clearly visible as bright circles on the MR image. The *internal jugular veins* can also be seen on the MR image just posterior to the internal carotid arteries. The two *vertebral arteries* join, and lie anterior to the medulla on the

MR image. The CT image is just superior to the junction of the vertebral arteries and shows the lower part of the basilar artery. The transverse venous sinuses have passed anteriorly to the level of the petrous ridges and are seen on the MR image. At this point, they change position and change names to become the *sigmoid sinuses*.

Fig. 28-15 is a CT image and Fig. 28-16 is an MR image through the lower part of the skull. The plane of the CT image passes through the upper orbit, the sphenoidal sinuses, and the lower portion of the occipital bone. The frontal sinuses lie along the anterior skull. The crista galli is just posterior to these sinuses. This structure is a

superior projection of bone from the cribriform plate of the ethmoid bone; it functions as an attachment for the falx cerebri. On either side of the crista galli, the lowermost portions of the frontal lobes can be seen resting on the cribriform plate. The sphenoidal sinuses lie posterior to the crista galli, and the greater wings of the sphenoid extend laterally from the region of the sinuses. The external auditory canals extend into the petrous portions of the temporal bones, and mastoid air cells are visible posterior to the canals. The lower portion of the occipital bone forms the posteriormost region of the skull on this image.

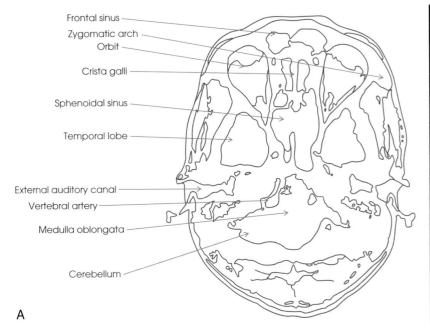

Frontal sinus
Zygomatic arch
Orbit
Crista galli
Sphenoidal sinus
Temporal lobe
External auditory canal
Vertebral artery
Medulla oblongata
Cerebellum

A

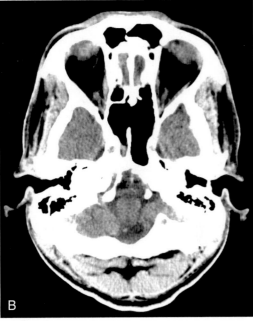

B

Fig. 28-15 A, Line drawing of CT section. **B,** CT image representing anatomic structures located at level *G* in Fig. 28-2, *A.*

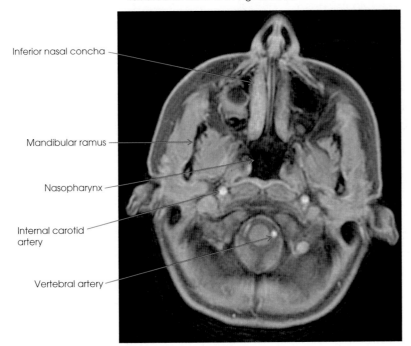

Inferior nasal concha
Mandibular ramus
Nasopharynx
Internal carotid artery
Vertebral artery

Fig. 28-16 MRI corresponding to level *G* in Fig. 28-2, *B.*

The MR image plane passes through the nose and the base of the skull. On the MR image, the large, air-filled maxillary sinuses lie on either side of the nose. The *inferior nasal conchae* and the vomer are seen within the nasal cavity. Posterior to the nasal cavity, the nasopharynx is seen on the MR image. Portions of the zygomatic arches are seen extending posteriorly from the sides of the sinuses on CT. The MR image is slightly inferior to the mandibular condyles and shows the rami of the mandible. The MR image passes through the mastoid processes and the top of the vertebral column. The CT shows the lower temporal lobes of the cerebrum, the *cerebellar tonsils,* and the medulla oblongata. The MR image shows the spinal cord because the structures in this image lie inferior to the foramen magnum. The contrast-filled internal carotid arteries lie anterior and lateral to the foramen magnum and spinal cord on the MR image but are not visible on the CT image. As the sigmoid venous sinuses pass through the jugular foramina, they become the internal jugular veins. These veins are visible on the MR image posterior and lateral to the internal carotid arteries. The contrast-filled vertebral arteries are seen along the anterolateral aspects of the medulla and spinal cord. Muscular structures on the external surface of the mandible are the *masseters,* and the structures on the internal surface are the *pterygoids.*

Finding images in sagittal, coronal, and oblique planes is increasingly common. CT scanners have the capability to generate images in the axial and coronal planes and to reconstruct the information in alternate planes. Magnetic resonance is capable of direct axial, sagittal, oblique, and coronal imaging. Representative images have been selected in the sagittal and coronal planes to help interpret the anatomy shown.

Fig. 28-17 is a posteroanterior (PA) skull (Caldwell method) image used to represent the locations of the following sagittal images of the brain. Fig. 28-18 is a midsagittal MR image of the cranium. The relationship between the cerebral hemisphere, cerebellum, and brain stem is shown. In this image, the frontal, parietal, and occipital lobes of the cerebrum are seen and correspond to the cranial bones. The corpus callosum is a white matter tract that connects the hemispheres and is found at the inferior aspect of the frontal and parietal lobes. CSF appears dark on this T1-weighted image, making it easy to trace the ventricular system. The anterior horn of the lateral ventricle is inferior to the genu of the corpus callosum. The third ventricle lies in the midline, between the two lateral ventricles. The lateral ventricles produce a great deal of CSF, which is transported to the third ventricle by way of the *intraventricular foramina (of Monro).* The third ventricle is not optimally visualized in this image. What is seen is the thalamus, which forms the lateral wall of the third ventricle. CSF drains from the third ventricle via the *cerebral aqueduct (of Sylvius),* which can be found within the midbrain (between the *corpora quadrigemina* and the *cerebral peduncles*). The *fourth ventricle* is also a midline structure and is situated between the pons and cerebellum. The large air-filled sphenoidal sinus is located anterior to the pons. Superior to this sinus, the pituitary gland rests within hypophyseal fossa formed by the sella turcica. Directly superior to the pituitary gland is the optic chiasm.

Several vascular structures are well shown in Fig. 28-18. The basilar artery appears between the clivus and pons.

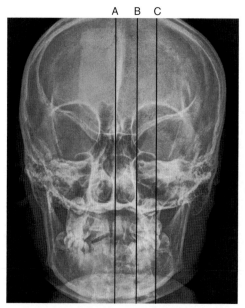

Fig. 28-17 PA projection of skull for localization of sagittal images.

Portions of the superior sagittal sinus can be seen between the cerebrum and the cranial bones. Between the cerebrum and cerebellum, the *straight sinus* (one of the dural venous sinuses) is noted within the tentorium cerebelli. This vessel is formed by the junction of the inferior sagittal sinus and the great cerebral vein (of Galen).

Fig. 28-19 is a sagittal MR image through the medial wall of the orbit. The dark, fluid-filled lateral ventricle is seen in the center of the cerebral hemisphere. Just inferior to it are the caudate nucleus and the thalamus. Because this image was obtained in a plane lateral to the midline, one of the cerebral peduncles is seen at the inferior border of the thalamus, and one of the cerebellar peduncles can be seen connecting the pons to the cerebel-

lum. At the floor of the cranium, a dark circle is seen that represents the internal carotid artery. Cerebral vertebral bodies and arches can be seen in the neck on either side of the vertebral canal. CSF is represented here by the dark shade of gray (this image is lateral to the cord). In the face, the nasal concha and tongue can be easily identified.

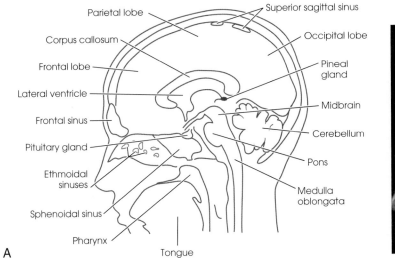

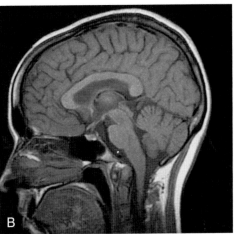

Fig. 28-18 A, Line drawing of MRI section. **B,** MRI through midsagittal plane, corresponding to level *A* in Fig. 28-17.

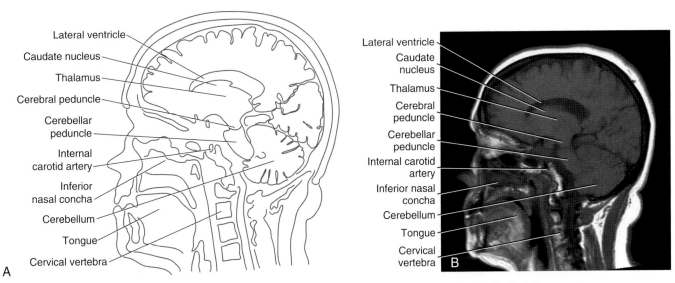

Fig. 28-19 A, Line drawing of MRI section. **B,** Sagittal MRI through medial wall of orbit corresponding to level *B* in Fig. 28-17.

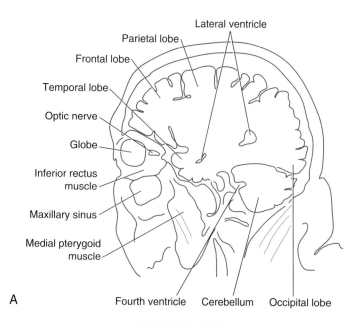

Lateral ventricle
Parietal lobe
Frontal lobe
Temporal lobe
Optic nerve
Globe
Inferior rectus muscle
Maxillary sinus
Medial pterygoid muscle

A

Fourth ventricle   Cerebellum   Occipital lobe

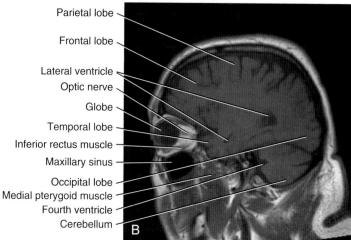

Parietal lobe
Frontal lobe
Lateral ventricle
Optic nerve
Globe
Temporal lobe
Inferior rectus muscle
Maxillary sinus
Occipital lobe
Medial pterygoid muscle
Fourth ventricle
Cerebellum

B

Fig. 28-20 A, Line drawing of MRI section. **B,** Sagittal MRI through midorbit corresponding to level *C* in Fig. 28-17.

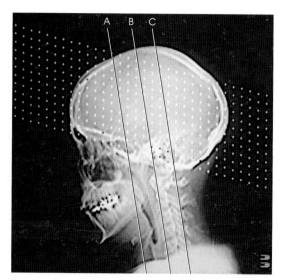

A B C

Fig. 28-21 CT localizer (scout) image of skull.

The sagittal MR image in Fig. 28-20 is sectioned through the center of the orbit. The frontal, parietal, occipital, and temporal lobes of the cerebrum all are visible. Within the cerebrum, CSF is seen within the temporal and posterior horns of the lateral ventricle (the fluid appears dark on this T1-weighted image). The cerebellum lies within the posterior fossa and is separated from the cerebrum by the tentorium cerebelli. Anterior to the cerebellum, the lateral aspect of the fourth ventricle can be seen. Within the orbit, several structures associated with the eye can be seen: the globe, a portion of the optic nerve, and the inferior rectus muscle. The dark area inferior to the orbit is the air-filled maxillary sinus. The medial pterygoid muscle, which lies on the internal aspect of the mandibular ramus, is visible inferior and posterior to the maxillary sinus.

A CT localizer, or scout, image (Fig. 28-21) is included as a reference for the next three coronal images. Fig. 28-22 is a coronal MR image through the anterior horns of the lateral ventricles and the pharyngeal structures. The anterior portions of the cerebral hemispheres are joined by the corpus callosum, which is immediately superior to the lateral ventricles. The membrane between the anterior horns of the lateral ventricles is the *septum pellucidum.* On the lateral aspect of each cerebral hemisphere is the *lateral fissure,* which divides the frontal lobe from the temporal lobe. The insula lies deep to this fissure.

Structures of the basal nuclei can be faintly identified. The caudate nucleus is lateral to the anterior horns. Inferolateral to the caudate nuclei are the internal capsules, white matter tracts that connect the cortex to deeper gray matter structures. The anterior portion of the third ventricle is found in the midline inferior to the lateral ventricles. Inferior to the third ventricle are the optic chiasm and pituitary gland (hypophysis cerebri). The *superior* and *inferior sagittal sinuses* occupy the margins of the falx cerebri in the longitudinal fissure between the hemispheres of the cerebrum. The internal carotid arteries occupy the *cavernous sinuses* along with several cranial nerves and are found lateral to the pituitary gland and sella turcica. Branches of the middle cerebral arteries occupy the lateral fissures of the cerebrum. Several air-filled structures are seen on this image; they are (from superior to inferior) the sphenoidal sinus and the *nasopharynx.* This image also shows the external carotid arteries within the parotid salivary glands.

Fig. 28-23 is a coronal MR image through the bodies of the lateral ventricles, the brain stem, and the bodies of the cervical vertebrae. The third ventricle is well shown and bordered laterally by the thalamus. The cartilaginous structures of the *external ear* surround the *external*

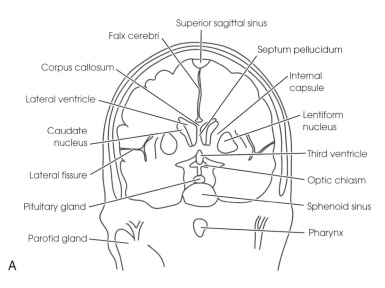

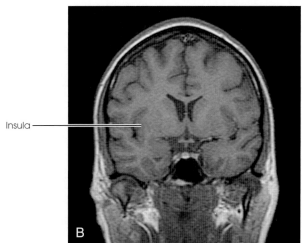

Fig. 28-22 A, Line drawing of MRI section. **B,** Coronal MRI corresponding to level *A* in Fig. 28-21.

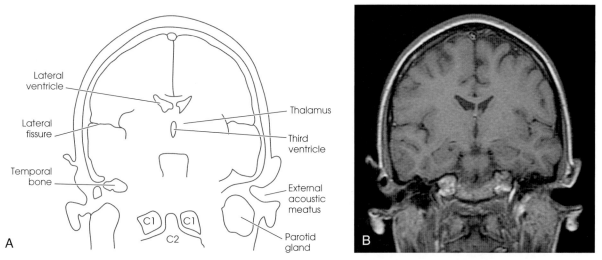

Fig. 28-23 A, Line drawing of MRI section. **B,** Coronal MRI corresponding to level *B* in Fig. 28-21.

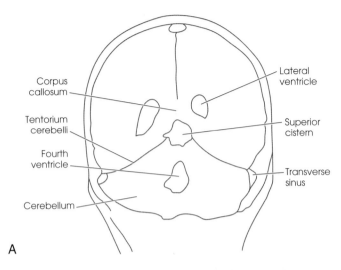

Corpus
callosum

Tentorium
cerebelli

Fourth
ventricle

Cerebellum

Lateral
ventricle

Superior
cistern

Transverse
sinus

A

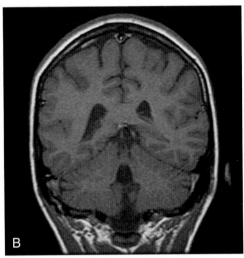

B

Fig. 28-24 A, Line drawing of MRI section. **B,** Coronal MRI corresponding to level *C* in Fig. 28-21.

acoustic meatus and *canal.* The dark region (low signal return) medial to the external acoustic canal corresponds to the *petrous portion of the temporal bone.* The first two cervical vertebrae are detailed in this section with the *dens* of the *axis* (C2) seen between the lateral masses of the *atlas* (C1). The large, whitish masses inferior to the external acoustic canals are the *parotid glands.*

Fig. 28-24 shows a coronal MR image through the lateral ventricles and cerebellum. The splenium of the corpus callosum is found between the lateral ventricles. Inferior to the splenium is the superior cistern. Portions of the cerebellum are visualized superior and inferior to the middle cerebellar peduncles. The large, dark area near the center of the cerebellum is the fourth ventricle. The dark line between the cerebellum and cerebrum represents the tentorium cerebelli. The transverse venous sinuses are visible in the lateral edges of the tentorium cerebella where it meets the occipital bone on each side. The large, dark areas (signal void) lateral to the cerebellum correspond to the bony mastoid portions of the temporal bone.

Thoracic Region

The thorax extends from the thoracic inlet to the diaphragm. The inlet is an imaginary plane through the first thoracic vertebra and the top of the manubrium. Sectional images of the thorax are obtained to include all structures between these boundaries. Two cadaveric images are included to assist in identifying some of the structures of the thorax. Fig. 28-25 is a cadaveric image that corresponds to a level just superior to the sternoclavicular joints. Fig. 28-30 (presented later) lies near the level of the sixth thoracic vertebra and shows the chambers of the heart and other surrounding structures.

The bones of the thorax include the thoracic vertebrae, ribs, sternum, clavicles, and scapulae. Each of the 12 thoracic vertebrae is subdivided into a body and a vertebral arch. The opening formed between these divisions is the vertebral foramen, through which the spinal cord travels. Two pedicles, two laminae, two transverse processes, and one spinous process constitute the arch. The pedicles are more anterior and unite with the body of the vertebra; the laminae form the posterior part of the arch and unite to give rise to the spinous process. Transverse processes arise from the lateral arch where pedicles and laminae meet. Two superior articular processes arise from the superior arch, and two inferior articular processes arise from the inferior arch. Superior and inferior articular processes from adjacent vertebrae articulate to form zygapophyseal joints. Notches between succeeding arches form the intervertebral foramina. These foramina transmit spinal nerves. Articular disks are found between the vertebral bodies. These disks are composed of a dense cartilaginous outer rim called the *annulus fibrosus* and a gelatinous central core called the *nucleus pulposus.* Twelve pairs of ribs curl around the lateral thorax to protect the lungs and heart. The head of each rib is posterior and articulates with the body of a thoracic vertebra. These joints are called *costovertebral joints.* Tubercles of the ribs are lateral to the heads and articulate with transverse processes of the vertebrae, forming costotransverse joints. Anteriorly, the first 10 pairs of ribs articulate with the sternum either directly or indirectly via costal cartilage. The sternum lies in the midline of the anterior chest wall. From superior to inferior, the parts are the manubrium, body, and xiphoid process. An indentation

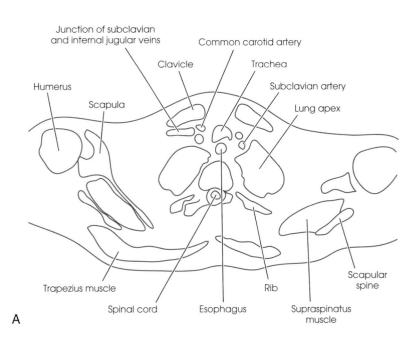

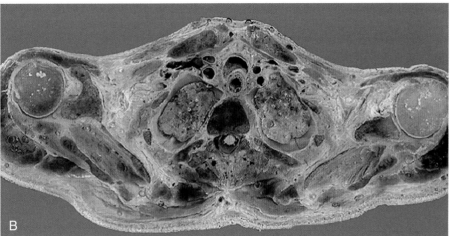

Fig. 28-25 A, Line drawing of gross anatomic section. **B,** Cadaveric image of superior thorax.

at the superior edge of the sternum, the jugular or sternal notch, lies at the level of the interspace between the second and third thoracic vertebrae. The manubrium joins the body of the sternum at the sternal angle, which corresponds to the interspace between the fourth and fifth thoracic vertebrae. The xiphoid process lies at approximately the level of the tenth thoracic vertebra. Familiarity with these vertebral levels can be helpful in orienting oneself when looking at thoracic sectional images.

The clavicles are slender, S-shaped bones that extend across the upper anterior thorax. The medial end of each clavicle articulates with the superolateral edge of the manubrium to form sternoclavicular joints. Acromioclavicular joints are formed where the lateral extremity of the clavicle articulates with the acromion process of the scapula. The scapulae are triangular bones in the superior posterior thorax. Thinking of the scapula as having two surfaces (anterior and posterior), three borders (superior, medial, and lateral), and three angles (superior, lateral, and inferior) is helpful. The posterior surface is divided into a superior fossa and an inferior fossa by the scapular spine. This bony ridge extends laterally and superiorly to end as the acromion process. The coracoid process projects from the superoanterior surface near the glenoid. The lateral angle is formed by the glenoid cavity, which articulates with the humeral head. Many of these bony structures are identifiable on Fig. 28-25.

Major components of the respiratory system are seen in the thorax. The trachea originates at the level of the sixth cervical vertebra (near the bottom of the thyroid cartilage). The trachea is formed by incomplete cartilage rings, which are open along its posterior surface. The trachea passes into the thorax and bifurcates into the right and left main bronchi near the level of the sternal angle (T4-5). The carina is the last cartilage ring of the trachea. The main bronchi pass through the hila of the lungs and branch to secondary bronchi, one for each lobe. The lungs are triangular organs enclosed in the thoracic cavity by the double-walled pleural membrane. The portion of the lung that lies superior to the clavicle is the apex; the part that rests on the diaphragm is the base. The most inferior and posterior reaches of the base constitute a region called the *costophrenic angle*. The bronchi and vascular structures enter and exit the center of the medial aspect of the lung at the hilum. Each lung is divided into superior and inferior lobes by an oblique fissure. The upper lobe of the right lung is divided further by a horizontal fissure to form a middle lobe that lies lateral to the heart. The portion of the left lung that corresponds in position to the right middle lobe is called the *lingula*.

The area between the lungs is the mediastinum. Within this cavity are the heart, trachea and bronchi, esophagus, major blood vessels, nerves, and lymphatic structures. The heart lies obliquely oriented in the lower mediastinum, surrounded by a double-walled fibrous sac called the *pericardium*. It rests on the diaphragm between the sternum and the thoracic spine. The superior surface is the base, and the inferior portion is the apex. The heart is divided into four chambers: two atria and two ventricles. The atria receive blood, and the ventricles pump blood away from the heart. The right atrium forms the right border of the heart and receives blood from the superior vena cava, inferior vena cava, and coronary sinus (the venous drainage channel for the heart muscle). Blood passes from here through the tricuspid (right atrioventricular) valve into the right ventricle. This chamber forms most of the anterior surface of the heart. As this ventricle contracts, blood passes through the infundibulum (pulmonary outflow tract), through the pulmonary semilunar valve, and into the main pulmonary artery toward the lungs. The left atrium forms the posterior border of the heart and receives blood from four pulmonary veins. Blood passes through the mitral (bicuspid or left atrioventricular) valve into the left ventricle. The most muscular of the chambers, the left ventricle forms the left side and inferiormost portion of the heart. Blood is pumped out through the aortic semilunar valve and into the aorta as this ventricle contracts. A muscular wall, the interventricular septum, can be seen between the ventricles. Chambers of the heart are seen in Fig. 28-26.

One portion of the digestive system is typically found in the thorax. The esophagus originates at the level of the sixth cervical vertebra as the posterior continuation of the pharynx. It continues into the thorax, at first posterior to the trachea, then posterior to the left atrium and ventricle of the heart. At the lower thorax, the esophagus pierces the diaphragm to continue into the abdomen.

The vascular system in the upper thorax can be confusing. To identify these structures, one must clearly understand the vascular anatomy. Tracing the paths of vessels through the scan can help alleviate some of the confusion. This discussion follows the path of circulation through the vessels. The discussion of arterial structures starts at the heart and follows the vessels toward the periphery. Veins are discussed from their peripheral origins and followed as they travel toward the heart.

The aorta originates from the left ventricle of the heart. Just distal to the aortic semilunar valve are the origins of the right and left coronary arteries, which supply the heart muscle. The aorta ascends along the posterior sternum, arches posterior and toward the left behind the sternal angle, and turns inferiorly to become the descending aorta. The descending aorta passes down the posterior thorax, resting against the left anterolateral surfaces of the vertebral bodies. The major vessels that supply the head and upper limbs arise from the aortic arch. From anterior to posterior, these are the brachiocephalic, left common carotid, and left subclavian arteries. The brachiocephalic artery passes superiorly and bifurcates into the right subclavian and right common carotid arteries posterior to the sternoclavicular joint. The right and left common carotid arteries ascend the neck along the lateral surface of the trachea. At approximately the level of the third cervical vertebra, each common carotid artery exhibits a dilation called the *carotid sinus* just proximal to bifurcating into internal and external carotid arteries. The subclavian arteries pass laterally across the upper thorax, just deep to the clavicles. At the outer edges of the first ribs, the subclavian arteries become the axillary arteries.

Venous drainage from the head is mainly through the jugular veins. The internal jugular veins accompany the carotid arteries down through the neck, lateral to the trachea. The subclavian veins are continuations of the axillary veins draining the upper limbs. These veins pass toward the midline deep to the clavicles. At the sternoclavicular joints, the internal jugular veins and the subclavian veins unite to form the brachiocephalic veins. The right brachiocephalic vein passes vertically downward; the left passes obliquely down, posterior to the manubrium. These two vessels unite to form the superior vena cava. The superior vena cava lies posterior to the right border of the sternum and enters the right atrium just below the level of the sternal angle. Venous drainage from the lower body is via the inferior vena cava. This vessel is found along the right anterior surface of the vertebral bodies and empties into the inferior aspect of the right atrium. The azygos vein is a small vessel that passes up the posterior thorax along the right anterior aspect of the vertebral bodies. It arches anteriorly (near the level of the aortic arch) to drain into the superior vena cava.

The pulmonary vascular system transports blood between the lungs and heart. The main pulmonary artery receives deoxygenated blood from the right ventricle. At the level of the sternal angle, this vessel gives rise to the right and left pulmonary arteries, which pass laterally toward the hila of the lungs. The bifurcation of the main pulmonary artery is just inferior to the aortic arch. Four pulmonary veins exit the hila, two from each lung, and pass medially to enter the superolateral aspect of the left atrium.

Many muscles can be seen in the thorax, especially in the shoulder region. The pectoralis major is a large, fan-shaped muscle superficially located along the anterior chest wall. The pectoralis minor lies just deep to the pectoralis major. The trapezius is the most superficial of the posterior thoracic muscles. The rhomboid major and minor muscles are deep to the trapezius and lie between the medial scapular borders and the spinous processes of the upper thoracic spine. The serratus anterior muscles attach to the medial side of the anterior scapula and blanket the external surface of the rib cage. Several muscles are associated with the scapula; many of these also attach to the humerus. The subscapularis muscle lines the anterior surface. Supraspinatus and infraspinatus muscles lie in the supraspinous and infraspinous fossae. The teres major and teres minor also lie along the infraspinous fossa. Four of these muscles are collectively known as the rotator cuff: subscapularis, supraspinatus, infraspinatus, and teres minor.

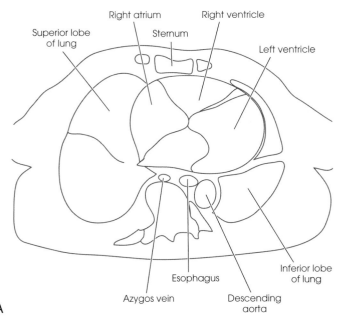

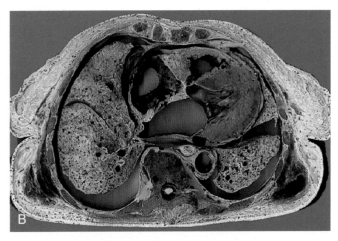

Fig. 28-26 A, Line drawing of gross anatomic section. **B,** Cadaveric image of central thorax.

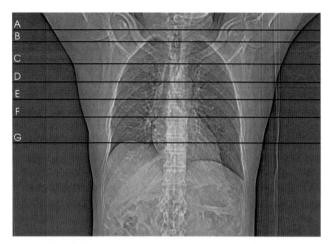

Fig. 28-27 CT localizer (scout) image of thorax.

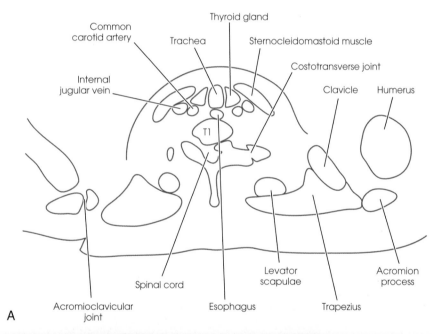

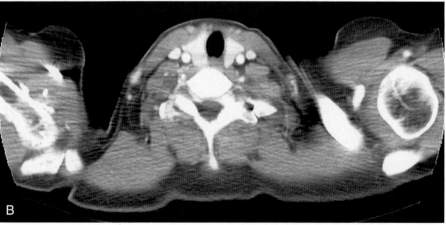

Fig. 28-28 A, Line drawing of CT section. **B,** CT image corresponding to level *A* in Fig. 28-27 through first thoracic vertebra.

The CT localizer, or scout, image represents an anteroposterior (AP) projection of the thoracic region with identifying lines (Fig. 28-27). These lines show the approximate levels for each of the labeled images for this region. Most of the images for this region are CT scans. When performing scans of the thorax, the patient's arms are extended above the head. This fact must be kept in mind when looking at upper thoracic scans because some anatomic structures do not correspond to the normal anatomic position. MR images are frequently degraded by motion artifact in the thorax, so only a few representative images are included.

Fig. 28-28 is a CT image at the level of T1 and show the relationship between the vertebral column, esophagus, and trachea. The body and *vertebral arch* of the first thoracic vertebra can be identified, and the spinal cord is seen in the vertebral foramen. The *costotransverse joint* between the first rib and the transverse process of the first thoracic vertebra is seen on the patient's left. The acromial extremity of the *clavicle* lies near the *acromion* on the left side, and the acromioclavicular joint is seen on the right. Because the patient's arms are raised, this scan passes through the surgical neck of the humerus. The inferior portion of the *thyroid gland,* which extends from C6 to T1, is positioned lateral to the *trachea.* The soft tissue shadow immediately posterior to the trachea is the *esophagus.* The *vertebral arteries* are positioned lateral to the vertebral column, and the *common carotid arteries* are found lateral to the trachea. At this level, the *internal jugular veins* are positioned to the lateral aspect of the carotid arteries. The contrast-filled axillary arteries can be seen in the medial aspect of the arms. The *sternocleidomastoid muscles* are found lateral to the thyroid gland. The *trapezius* is the most superficial muscle of the posterior thorax, with the levator scapulae muscles lying just anterior.

Fig. 28-29 is a CT image through the lower edge of T2. This scan passes through the *jugular notch* of the sternum and is just superior to the sternoclavicular joints. The costovertebral and costotransverse joints are seen between the ribs and the spine. On the right, the glenoid portion and the acromion process of the scapula are seen. The humerus is visible where it articulates with the glenoid cavity. On the left, the spine and the body of the scapula are seen. The *trachea* and esophagus are located anterior to the vertebral body. The major vessels of the superior thorax are visualized posterior to the clavicles. The right and left *brachiocephalic veins* are formed by the junction of the *subclavian veins* and the internal jugular veins. Because contrast medium was injected for this scan, the axillary and most of the right subclavian vein are filled with contrast medium. Posterior to the right clavicle, the right subclavian vein and internal jugular vein have joined. Because the image is slightly more inferior on the left, the image plane passes through the left brachiocephalic vein (below the junction of these two vessels). The brachiocephalic veins unite and form the *superior vena cava* at a more inferior level. The arterial branches to the head and upper limb are also visualized on this image. From the patient's right to left, they are the *right subclavian artery, right common carotid artery, left common carotid artery,* and *left subclavian artery.* The brachiocephalic artery gives rise to the right subclavian and right common carotid arteries and is inferior to this level. The *pectoralis major* and *pectoralis minor* lie along the anterior thoracic wall. The trapezius is the most superficial of the posterior muscles and is seen between the scapula and the spine on each side. The *subscapularis muscle* lines the left anterior scapula, the *infraspinatus* and *teres minor* line the posterior portion of this bone, and the *supraspinatus* is seen between the body and the scapular spine.

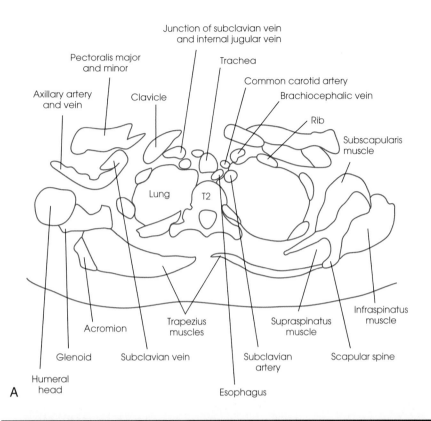

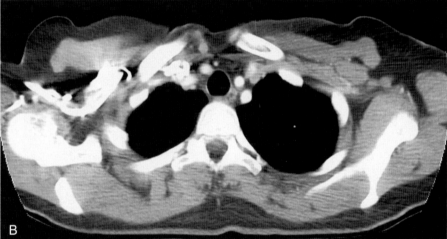

Fig. 28-29 A, Line drawing of CT section. **B,** CT image corresponding to level *B* in Fig. 28-27 through jugular notch.

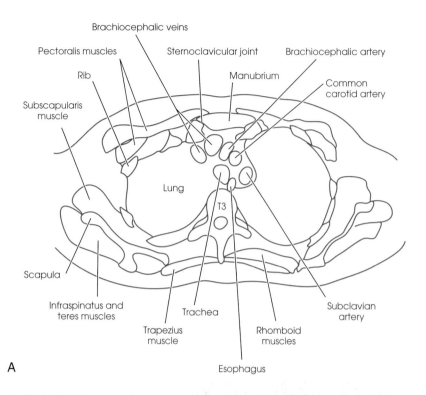

Brachiocephalic veins

Pectoralis muscles

Rib

Subscapularis muscle

Sternoclavicular joint

Manubrium

Brachiocephalic artery

Common carotid artery

Lung

T3

Scapula

Infraspinatus and teres muscles

Trapezius muscle

Trachea

Rhomboid muscles

Subclavian artery

Esophagus

A

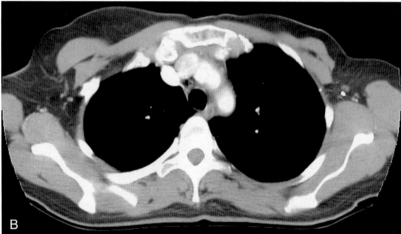

B

Fig. 28-30 A, Line drawing of CT section. B, CT image corresponding to level *C* in Fig. 28-27 just superior to aortic arch.

Fig. 28-30 is a CT image through the level of T3. Bony structures depicted in this image include the *manubrium* and sternoclavicular joints anteriorly, the ribs laterally, and the scapulae and vertebra posteriorly. The spine and the body of the right scapula are visible at this level. Costovertebral and costotransverse joints are noted along the right side of the vertebra. Several vascular structures, highlighted with contrast medium, are visible posterior to the manubrium. The right and left brachiocephalic veins are seen just posterior to the right sternoclavicular joint. This level is just superior to where the vessels join to form the superior vena cava. The brachiocephalic artery, left common carotid artery, and left subclavian artery curl around the left side of the trachea. This scan is just superior to the arch of the aorta and visualizes the origins of these three vessels. Posterior to the vessels are the trachea and esophagus. The upper lobes of each lung lie lateral to the mediastinal structures. The pectoralis major and pectoralis minor lie external to the anterior ribs. Rotator cuff muscles (subscapularis, infraspinatus, and teres minor) are shown anterior and posterior to the scapulae. The trapezius and *rhomboid muscles* lie between the scapulae and the spinous process of the vertebra in this image.

Fig. 28-31 is a CT scan obtained through the lower edge of T4. At this level, the brachiocephalic veins have joined to form the *superior vena cava*. The large contrast-filled structure in the left anterolateral mediastinum is the *aortic arch*.

Fig. 28-32 is a CT image at the level of T5 and shows the great vessels superior to the heart. (The heart is normally positioned between T7 and T11, with most of the organ lying left of the midline.) The *ascending aorta* is found anteriorly in the midline; the *descending aorta* is related to the left anterolateral surface of the vertebral bodies. (This relationship between the descending aorta and vertebral column is continuous through the thorax and

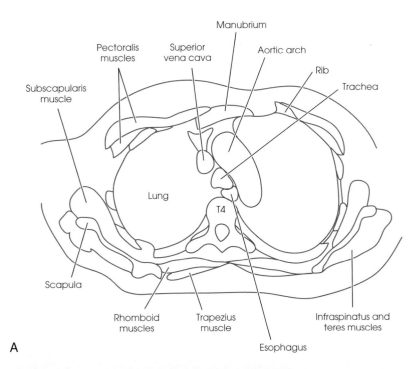

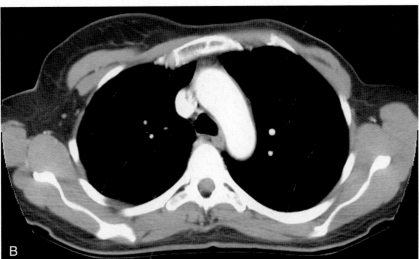

Fig. 28-31 A, Line drawing of CT section. **B,** CT image corresponding to level *D* in Fig. 28-27 through aortic arch.

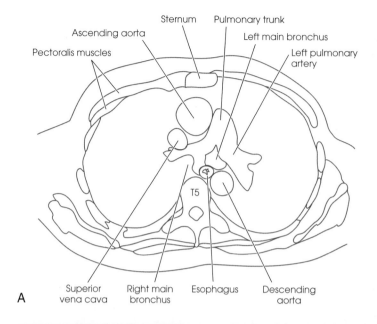

A

Pectoralis muscles

Ascending aorta

Sternum

Pulmonary trunk

Left main bronchus

Left pulmonary artery

Superior vena cava

Right main bronchus

Esophagus

Descending aorta

T5

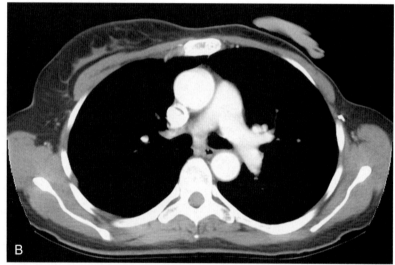

B

Fig. 28-32 A, Line drawing of CT section. **B,** CT image corresponding to level *E* in Fig. 28-27 through pulmonary trunk.

abdomen.) Note the normal difference in caliber between the ascending and descending aorta. The superior vena cava is located to the right of the ascending aorta, and the pulmonary trunk and left and right pulmonary arteries are located to the left of the ascending aorta at this level. The *pulmonary trunk* originates from the right ventricle of the heart and divides into the right and left *pulmonary arteries,* which carry deoxygenated blood to the lungs. The left pulmonary artery is seen bifurcating into the two lobar branches at the hilum of the left lung. Near the T5 level the trachea divides into the left and right *primary bronchi.* The esophagus (in which a small amount of air is seen) is found just posterior to the left main bronchus. Fig. 28-33 is an MR image that corresponds in position to the previous CT image. The main pulmonary artery and the left pulmonary artery are seen on this image, although the right pulmonary artery is not visible. Muscular structures are easily differentiated. The spinal cord is seen within the vertebral canal, where it is surrounded by CSF.

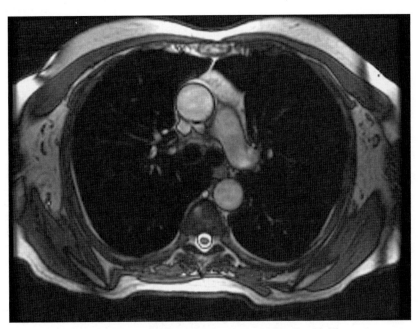

Fig. 28-33 MRI corresponding to level *E* in Fig. 28-27.

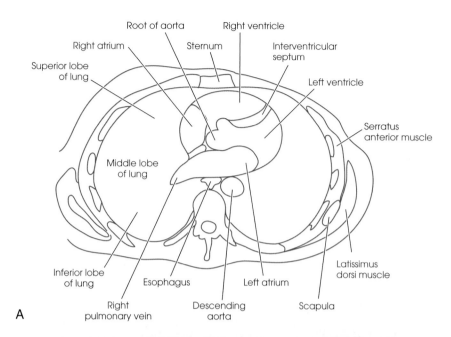

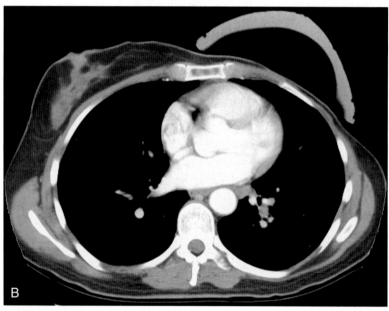

Fig. 28-34 A, Line drawing of CT section. **B,** CT image corresponding to level *F* in Fig. 28-27 through base of the heart.

The CT image depicted in Fig. 28-34 shows the *lungs* and the base of the *heart.* Generally, when the heart is imaged in cross section, the *left atrium* is the superiormost structure encountered, and the *pulmonary veins* are seen emptying into it (one of the right pulmonary veins can be seen here). The *right atrium* is seen lying the farthest toward the right side of the body, anterior and inferior to the left atrium. The superior vena cava may be seen at this level as it enters the right atrium. The *right ventricle* lies to the left of the right atrium and anterior to the more muscular *left ventricle.* Contrast-enhanced blood is seen here as blood exits the left ventricle to enter the root of the aorta. The *interventricular septum* can be seen between the ventricles.

The lungs are divided into superior and inferior lobes by the diagonally oriented *oblique fissure.* The *superior lobes* lie superior and anterior to the inferior lobes. The *superior lobe* of the right lung is divided further by the *horizontal fissure,* with the lower portion termed the *middle lobe.* The left lung has no horizontal fissure. The inferior and anterior portion of the left lung (corresponding to the right middle lobe) is termed the *lingula.* Although the fissures are not seen, the approximate locations of these lobes are identified here.

Muscular structures that can be seen at this level include the inferior insertions of the trapezius, the *latissimus dorsi,* and the *serratus anterior muscles.* The esophagus lies between the left atrium and the vertebral column at this level.

Fig. 28-35 lies at approximately T9 and shows the lower sternum and ribs. The descending aorta normally lies along the left anterolateral surface of the vertebral column, and the *azygos vein* is normally on the right anterolateral surface. Because this scan is inferior to the right ventricle, the *inferior vena cava* is seen between the heart and the liver. The superior portion of the liver is bulging against the base of the right lung, and the superiormost portion of the left hemidiaphragm is seen at the base of the left lung. The right and left ventricles of the heart and the interventricular septum can be seen surrounded by pericardium. The major muscle structures that are visible the serratus anterior, latissimus dorsi, and the deep back muscles.

Fig. 28-36 is a frontal CT localizer image representing the sagittal levels of the thorax presented here. Fig. 28-37 is located near the median sagittal plane of the chest. In this image, the central portion of the manubrium can be seen in the anterior thorax. The sternal angle is represented as a dark line separating the manubrium and the body of the sternum. Thoracic vertebral bodies, spinous processes, zygapophyseal joints, and intervertebral foramina border the posterior thorax. Because everyone has a slight degree of curvature in the spine, different structures are seen in the spinal column at different levels. Within the upper thorax, the cartilage rings of the trachea can be observed. The soft tissue structure posterior to the trachea is the esophagus. The heart and great vessels lie near the center of the thorax. In this image, the superiormost vascular structure is the arch of the aorta. At this level, the origin of the left common carotid artery is present. The left ventricle is the largest chamber of the heart and is seen here filled with contrast medium. It also empties into the aorta. The origin and ascending aorta can be seen just superior to the left ventricle. The left pulmonary artery lies immediately inferior to the aortic arch. This vessel is a branch of the pulmonary artery and originates from the right ventricle of the heart, which is anterior to the left ventricle. The left atrium of the heart is the posteriormost chamber and is seen here posterior to the pulmonary trunk and left ventricle. The diaphragm is located inferior to the heart and separates the thoracic cavity from the abdomen.

Fig. 28-38 is a CT image that passes just medial to the left sternoclavicular joint. In this image, the entire aorta is present, from the root, through the arch, and continuing as the descending portion. The origins of the left common carotid and the left subclavian arteries are seen at the superior border of the arch. The left common carotid artery courses from its origin superiorly into the neck near the trachea. The upper portion of the esophagus is posterior to the trachea. The left pulmonary artery is visible just inferior to the arch, and the air-filled structure posterior to this vessel is the left main bronchus.

Fig. 28-39 represents a sagittal section through the left sternoclavicular joint. Anteriorly, the bony structures include the clavicle, the upper-outer corner of the manubrium, and the costosternal articulations. The posterior bony anatomy includes the thoracic spine and the upper ribs. Within the thorax, the arch and

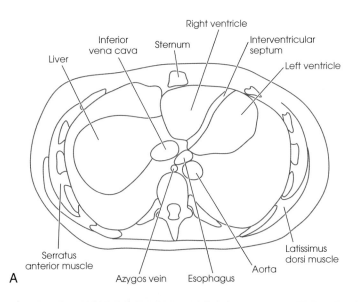

A

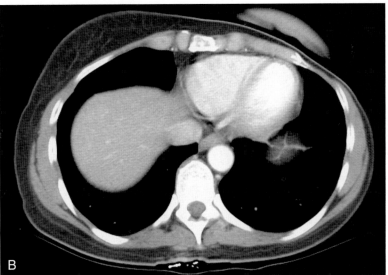

B

Fig. 28-35 A, Line drawing of CT section. **B,** CT image corresponding to level G in Fig. 28-27 through right hemidiaphragm.

ABC

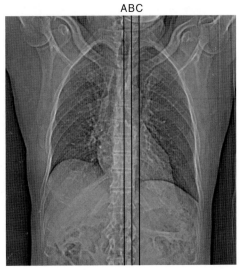

Fig. 28-36 CT localizer image representing levels of sagittal sections through thorax.

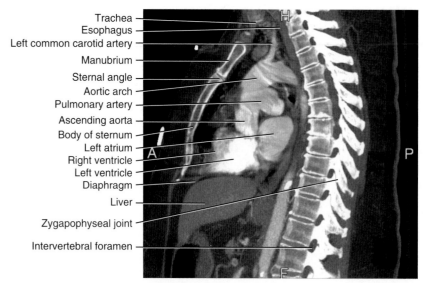

Trachea
Esophagus
Left common carotid artery
Manubrium
Sternal angle
Aortic arch
Pulmonary artery
Ascending aorta
Body of sternum
Left atrium
Right ventricle
Left ventricle
Diaphragm
Liver
Zygapophyseal joint
Intervertebral foramen

Fig. 28-37 Sagittal CT image of thorax corresponding to level *A* in Fig. 28-36.

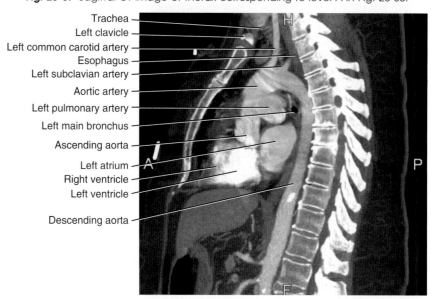

Trachea
Left clavicle
Left common carotid artery
Esophagus
Left subclavian artery
Aortic artery
Left pulmonary artery
Left main bronchus
Ascending aorta
Left atrium
Right ventricle
Left ventricle
Descending aorta

Fig. 28-38 Sagittal CT image of thorax corresponding to level *B* in Fig. 28-36.

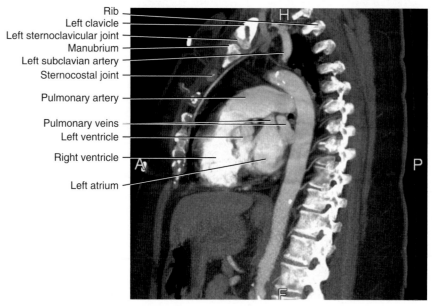

Rib
Left clavicle
Left sternoclavicular joint
Manubrium
Left subclavian artery
Sternocostal joint
Pulmonary artery
Pulmonary veins
Left ventricle
Right ventricle
Left atrium

Fig. 28-39 Sagittal CT image of thorax corresponding to level *C* in Fig. 28-36.

descending aorta are present. The left sub-clavian artery is the third branch from the aortic arch. This vessel passes superiorly to arch over the apex of the left lung. In this image, the proximal portion of this vessel is seen just superior to the aortic arch. In the anterior mediastinum, the contrast-filled right ventricle is pumping blood into the main pulmonary artery. The left pulmonary veins return blood from the lungs to the left atrium. The left ventricle lies between the right ventricle and the left atrium in this image.

Fig. 28-40 is a lateral chest x-ray to be used to localize the coronal sections of the thorax presented here. Fig. 28-41 is a coronal image passing through the anterior mediastinum. The clavicles, manubrium, and sternoclavicular joints are visible at the entrance into the thorax. Sections through the ribs line both lateral walls of the thoracic cavity. The setting for this image shows the lungs as black structures with a few vascular shadows visible within each. The mediastinum in the center of the thoracic cavity is occupied by the heart and great vessels. This scan passes through the anterior mediastinum, so the ascending portion of the aorta is visible. It lies between the pulmonary artery and the superior vena cava. In this slice, the superior vena cava is discernible at its entrance into the right atrium. The right ventricle is the anteriormost chamber of the heart and is seen here lateral to the right atrium.

The coronal thoracic section seen in Fig. 28-42 passes through a plane near the median coronal plane of the thorax. Clav-icles and ribs can be seen surrounding the superior and lateral thorax. The cartilage rings of the trachea lie in the median sagit-tal plane at the superior end of the thorax. The left lung is specked with several light gray vascular structures. The right lung shows infiltrates and central scar tissue from an old resection. This scan was per-formed with contrast enhancement, and the right axillary vein and superior vena cava are visible as bright white. The aortic arch gives rise to the vessels that supply the head and neck. In this image, the bra-chiocephalic artery and the origin of the left common carotid artery can be seen. The brachiocephalic veins are formed by the internal jugular and subclavian veins. The left brachiocephalic vein is located just to the left of the brachioce-phalic artery and superior to the origin of the common carotid artery in this image.

The main pulmonary artery is visible inferior to the aorta. A small portion of the left atrium and the right atrium and ventricle can be seen.

Fig. 28-43 shows anatomy in a posterior plane through the mediastinum. Because of the curve of the spine, the lower cervical and thoracic vertebrae are visible, but most of the thoracic spine is posterior to this imaging plane. Near the level of the fourth or fifth thoracic vertebrae, the trachea bifurcates into the right and left main bronchi. In this image, the lower trachea, its bifurcation, and the main bronchi are visible. On the right, the main bronchus is dividing into lobar bronchi. The soft tissue structure detectable near the top of the visible portion of the trachea is the esophagus. On the left side of the esophagus, the left subclavian artery, filled with contrast medium, is seen as it starts its arch over the apex of the lung. The round contrast-filled vessels that lie on the left side of the trachea are the aortic arch (superior) and the left pulmonary artery (inferior). Inferior to the trachea, the left atrium is detectable, filled with contrast medium. One of the four pulmonary veins is visible, filled with contrast medium and to the right of the left atrium. Because this image is relatively posterior in the mediastinum, no other chambers of the heart can be seen; however, a section of the descending aorta, filled with contrast medium, lies inferior to the left atrium.

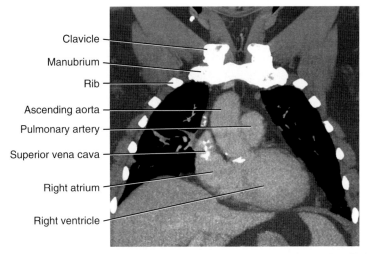

Fig. 28-41 Coronal CT image of thorax corresponding to level *A* in Fig. 28-40.

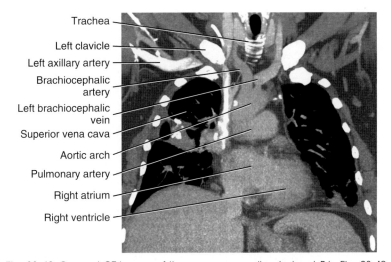

Fig. 28-42 Coronal CT image of thorax corresponding to level *B* in Fig. 28-40.

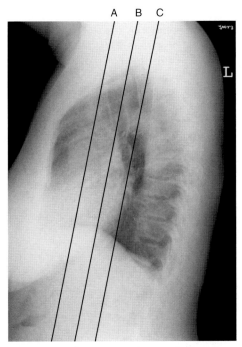

Fig. 28-40 Lateral chest x-ray representing levels of coronal sections through thorax.

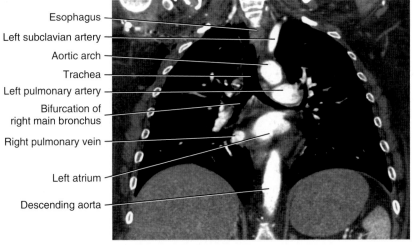

Fig. 28-43 Coronal CT image of thorax corresponding to level *C* in Fig. 28-40.

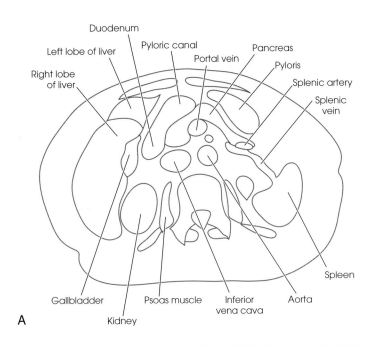

Duodenum
Left lobe of liver
Pyloric canal
Portal vein
Pancreas
Pyloris
Right lobe of liver
Splenic artery
Splenic vein
Spleen
Gallbladder
Kidney
Psoas muscle
Inferior vena cava
Aorta

A

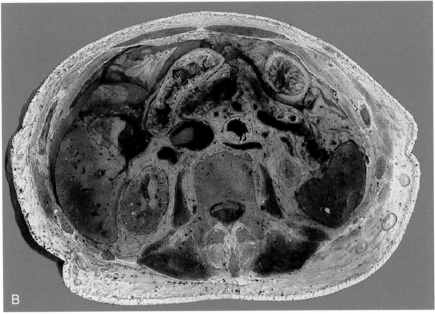

B

Fig. 28-44 A, Line drawing of gross anatomic section. **B,** Cadaveric section through central abdomen at the level of L2.

Abdominopelvic Region

The abdominopelvic region includes the diaphragm and everything inferior to it. Fig. 28-44 is a cadaveric image at the level of the second lumbar vertebra. Major abdominal organs and vascular structures can be identified in this image. In the abdomen, five lumbar vertebrae are visible. Although these vertebrae are slightly larger than the vertebrae in the thorax, the anatomic components are roughly the same. In the pelvis, the lower spine and hip bones (os coxae or innominate) form an attachment for the lower limbs and support for the trunk. The lower spine comprises the sacrum and coccyx. These are triangular bones with their broad bases oriented superiorly. Each os coxae lies obliquely situated in the pelvis, articulating with the sacrum (sacroiliac joint) posteriorly and with the opposite os coxae anteriorly (symphysis pubis). At birth, this bone consists of three components: the ilium, ischium, and pubis. These three ultimately fuse at the acetabulum. The superior, wing-shaped portion of the os coxae is the ilium. The superior edge is the crest, which lies at the level of the lower fourth lumbar vertebra. The anterior superior and anterior inferior iliac spines lie along the anterior surface of the ilium. At the posterior ilium, posterior superior and posterior inferior iliac spines are found at the top and bottom of the sacral articular surface. Below the posterior inferior iliac spine, the greater sciatic notch curves sharply toward the front of the bone. The inferior and anterior os coxae are composed of the pubis. The pubic bone extends from the acetabulum toward the midline, then curves inferiorly. The pubic bones articulate with each other at the symphysis pubis. The posterior inferior os coxae is formed by the ischium. This portion extends inferiorly from the acetabulum, then curls forward to meet the lower part of the pubis. The obturator foramen is a circular opening formed by the junction of the pubis and ischium.

The abdominal cavity is lined by a double-walled membrane called the *peritoneum*. Some organs develop posterior to the peritoneum and are referred to as *retroperitoneal*. Others invaginate into the peritoneum and are referred to as *intraperitoneal*. Several large folds of the peritoneum are identifiable on sectional images because of the large amount of fat found within it. The greater omentum extends from the greater curvature of the stomach and the transverse colon to blanket the anterior surface of the abdominal organs, especially the digestive organs. The small intestines invaginate into the peritoneum as they develop, and a large flap of peritoneum—the mesentery—anchors this part of the digestive system to the posterior abdominal wall.

The spleen is an organ belonging to the lymphatic system. It lies inferior to the left hemidiaphragm and posterior to the fundus of the stomach. On the medial surface of the spleen, blood vessels enter and exit at the hilum.

The organs of the alimentary tract include the esophagus, stomach, small intestine, and large intestine. The esophagus lies anterior to the spine and passes through the diaphragm to enter the abdomen at about the level of T10. In the abdomen, it passes toward the left to enter the stomach. The opening into the stomach is the cardiac orifice, and the junction is the esophagogastric junction. The stomach is a J-shaped pouch in the left upper quadrant. The region above the level of the esophagogastric junction is the fundus, the central region is the body, and the distal part is the pyloric antrum. This last portion normally lies at about the level of the second lumbar vertebra. The medial and lateral borders are referred to as the *lesser and greater curvatures*. Internally, the stomach is thrown into multiple folds termed *rugae*. Food passes from the distal stomach through the pyloric canal into the small intestine. A muscle called the *pyloric sphincter* controls passage through the canal. The small intestine consists of the duodenum, jejunum, and ileum. The first portion or duodenum extends from the stomach laterally to the liver, where the remainder curls inferiorly and medially to form a C-shaped loop around the head of the pancreas. The duodenum is approximately 10 to 12 inches (24 to 30 cm) long, and at the ligament of Treitz it continues as the jejunum. The jejunum is approximately 8 ft (2.4 m) long and mainly occu-

pies the left upper abdomen. It continues as the ileum. This distalmost part of the small bowel is about 10 ft (3 m) long and occupies the right inferior abdominal cavity and the pelvis. The large intestine is about 6 ft (1.8 m) long. It frames the periphery of the abdominal cavity and comprises the cecum, colon (ascending, transverse, descending, and sigmoid portions), rectum, and anus. The ileum empties into the saclike cecum in the right lower quadrant via the ileocecal valve. The vermiform appendix frequently can be seen projecting off the cecum. From the cecum, the ascending portion of the colon passes superiorly. Just below the liver, this portion curves anteriorly and medially at the hepatic (right colic) flexure. The transverse portion passes from here across the anterior abdomen. This portion dips inferiorly into the abdomen to a variable degree depending on the body habitus of the patient. As the colon reaches the spleen, it turns posteriorly and inferiorly at the splenic (left colic) flexure to become the descending colon. This portion passes down the posterior aspect of the left side of the abdomen toward the pelvis, where it continues as the sigmoid colon. The sigmoid colon curls medially and posteriorly in the pelvis, and at the mid-sacrum it curves inferiorly as the rectum. The rectum lies anterior to and follows the curve of the sacrum to become the anal canal as the large intestine exits the pelvis.

Several accessory organs of the digestive system are located in the upper abdomen. The liver occupies most of the right upper quadrant. This triangular organ is divided anatomically into a large right lobe and a much smaller left lobe. The falciform ligament is located along the division between these lobes on the anterior surface, and the ligamentum venosum and ligamentum teres are found along the division on the posterior surface of the liver. On the posteroinferior surface of the right lobe are two smaller lobes: the caudate (superior) and the quadrate (inferior). These two lobes are separated by the porta hepatis (hilum) of the liver. The hepatic artery, portal vein, and hepatic bile ducts enter and exit the liver here. The gallbladder rests against the undersurface of the liver. This organ functions as a storage vessel for bile, which is produced in the liver. Bile drains from the liver through the right and left hepatic ducts. These ducts unite to form the common hepatic duct, which meets the cystic duct

from the gallbladder. Distal to this junction, the continuation of this duct is known as the *common bile duct*. Bile passes through this duct to empty into the second part of the duodenum at the hepatopancreatic ampulla (ampulla of Vater). The pancreas, which functions as an endocrine and exocrine gland, lies transversely across the abdomen near the level of the second lumbar vertebra. The divisions of this retroperitoneal organ, from right to left, are the head, neck, body, and tail. The head is the inferiormost portion and is encircled by the duodenum. The tail is located near the hilum of the spleen. The pancreatic duct traverses the length of the organ and enters the second part of the duodenum at or near the common bile duct.

The urinary system includes the two kidneys and ureters, the bladder, and the urethra. The kidneys are retroperitoneal and lie between the 12th thoracic and 3rd lumbar vertebrae. The center or hilar region is normally near the interspace between L1 and L2. Suprarenal (adrenal) glands are perched on the upper surface of each kidney. The right adrenal gland can be seen between the liver and the right diaphragmatic crus, and the left lies between the left crus and the pancreatic tail and spleen. Each kidney is surrounded by a dense membrane, the renal fasciae, and a layer of fat, the perirenal fat. Urine is formed in the parenchyma of the kidney and collects in the calyceal system. The calyces unite to form the renal pelvis, which is continuous with the ureter. The ureters are musculomembranous tubes that extend down the posterior abdomen resting along the anterior surface of the psoas muscles. They are difficult to visualize unless filled with radiopaque contrast medium. In the pelvis, the ureters empty into the posteroinferior region of the bladder. The bladder is a collapsible muscular sac, which serves as a reservoir for urine until it is expelled from the body. The bladder rests on or near the pelvic floor, posterior to the symphysis pubis and anterior to the rectum in males or the vagina in females. The urethra is the muscular passageway that originates from the apex (inferior surface) of the bladder and by which urine is expelled. The urethra is relatively short in females, passing through the floor of the pelvis. The urethra is much longer in males because it passes through the prostate gland and the membranous and cavernous portions of the penis.

The internal organs of the male reproductive system include the ductus deferens, seminal vesicles, and prostate. Internal and external reproductive structures are connected by the spermatic cord, which includes the ductus deferens, testicular vessels, nerves, and lymphatic structures. The spermatic cord is seen anterior and medial to the femoral artery and vein and anterior and lateral to the pubis. The ductus deferens enters the pelvis through the spermatic cord and then arches over the anterior and lateral aspect of the bladder. It passes down the posterior surface of the bladder and enters the superior prostate. The seminal vesicles are found on the posterior and inferior surface of the bladder near the insertion of the ureters. The prostate gland lies inferior to the bladder, between the symphysis pubis and the rectum. The prostatic portion of the urethra passes through the prostate.

The organs of the female reproductive system include the uterus, uterine (fallopian) tubes, ovaries, and vagina. The uterus, which normally lays superior and posterior to the urinary bladder, is divided into a fundus, body, isthmus, and cervix. The fundus is the upper, rounded portion of the organ, superior to the orifices of the uterine tubes. The central portion is the body, which narrows at its lower end to become the isthmus. The narrowed lower ¾ inch (2 cm) of the uterus is the cervix, which is continuous with the vagina. The uterus is suspended in the pelvis by folds of peritoneum called the *broad ligaments.* The ovaries lie lateral to the body of the uterus within the broad ligament. They are normally found near the lateral pelvic wall at or slightly below the level of the anterior superior iliac spine. Extending between the ovaries and uterus, in the superior rim of the broad ligament, are the uterine tubes. The medial ends open into the upper body of the uterus. The lateral end of each tube, the infundibulum, is expanded and terminates in multiple fingerlike projections called *fimbriae.* This end of the tube is superior to the ovary but not attached. The inferiormost part of the internal female reproductive system is the vagina. This muscular tube lies between the rectum and the bladder and opens to the external body surface posterior to the urethral meatus.

Three vascular systems can be described in the abdomen: arterial, venous, and portal. The descending, or abdominal, aorta is the main conduit for arterial blood and passes through the diaphragm at approximately the level of T11 and extends to the pelvis along the left anterolateral surface of the vertebral bodies. Just below the diaphragm, at approximately the level of the 12th thoracic vertebra, the celiac artery originates from the anterior aorta. This fairly short vessel divides into the splenic, common hepatic, and left gastric arteries. The splenic artery passes toward the left to enter the hilum of the spleen. The common hepatic artery extends to the right to the porta hepatis. The superior mesenteric artery arises from the left anterior aorta near the first lumbar vertebra. The origin of this vessel is posterior to the neck of the pancreas. It extends anteriorly for a short distance and then turns inferiorly as it sends its branches to supply the small intestine and the proximal half of the large intestine. Near the level of the second lumbar vertebra, the renal arteries arise from the lateral surface of the aorta. The renal arteries pass laterally to enter the hila of the kidneys. The right renal artery is longer than the left because it must cross the spine to reach the right kidney. The inferior mesenteric artery arises from the abdominal aorta at L3 and supplies the distal half of the large bowel. At the fourth lumbar vertebra, the abdominal aorta bifurcates to form the right and left common iliac arteries. Each common iliac artery divides into internal and external iliac arteries near the top of the sacrum.

Internal iliac arteries divide rapidly as branches are sent to various structures within the pelvis. The external iliac arteries pass anteriorly and inferiorly through the pelvis. These vessels pass deep to the inguinal ligaments and become the femoral arteries.

The femoral veins carry venous blood from the lower limbs toward the pelvis. The femoral vein becomes the external iliac vein as it passes deep to the inguinal ligament. It is joined within the pelvis by the internal iliac vein to form the common iliac vein. The two common iliac veins unite at the level of the fifth lumbar vertebra to form the inferior vena cava. The inferior vena cava passes up the right anterolateral surface of the vertebral bodies, pierces the diaphragm, and empties into the inferior surface of the right atrium. The major tributaries of the inferior vena cava are the renal veins and the hepatic veins. The renal veins enter the lateral inferior vena cava near L2; the three hepatic veins enter near the top of the liver.

The vessels that drain the spleen and digestive system form the portal venous system. The major tributaries of this system are the superior and inferior mesenteric veins and the splenic vein. The inferior mesenteric vein empties into the splenic vein, which meets the superior mesenteric vein just posterior to the head of the pancreas. The junction of these two

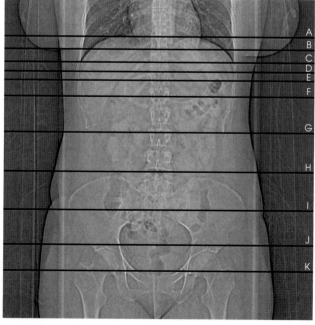

Fig. 28-45 CT localizer (scout) image of abdominopelvic region.

vessels forms the portal vein. These vessels extend superiorly to enter the porta hepatis of the liver.

Fig. 28-45 is a CT localizer, or scout, image representing an AP projection of the abdominopelvic region. Fig. 28-45 has 11 identifying lines showing the levels for each of the labeled images for this region.

Fig. 28-46 represents structures seen at the T9 level. The tip of the xiphoid process and lower ribs are seen. The image shows the *right hemidiaphragm* surrounding the superior portion of the *liver* and the *left hemidiaphragm* encircling the pericardial fat surrounding the apex of the heart and the *fundus* of the stomach. A small amount of oral contrast agent can be seen in the dependent portion of the stomach in this image. The *esophagus,* posterior to the liver, has migrated toward the patient's left as it nears its entrance into the stomach. The lower lobes of each lung are seen external to the diaphragm. The *aorta* is in its normal position, anterior and slightly left of the vertebral body; the azygos vein lies to the right of the aorta. The inferior vena cava appears embedded within the liver. Three *hepatic veins* drain into the inferior vena cava at this level. Serratus anterior muscles are seen external to the lateral aspects of the ribs; latissimus dorsi muscles extend superficially across the posterior abdomen.

Fig. 28-47 is a CT image at the level of the 10th thoracic vertebra. It shows the aorta and inferior vena cava and contrast-enhanced vessels within the liver. These represent branches of the hepatic and portal venous circulation. The right, left, and *caudate lobes* of the liver are visible. On the patient's left, the contrast-filled body of the stomach and the *spleen* can be identified. This is normally the level at which the esophagus enters the cardiac portion of the stomach. The *greater omentum* (a large fold of peritoneum) lies along the greater curvature of the stomach. Fig. 28-47 shows the greater omentum anterior and lateral to the stomach. The inferior lobes of the lungs are seen posterior to the liver and the spleen. The *crura of the diaphragm* are the lower tendinous insertions of this muscle. They can be seen extending around the anterior aorta and the posterior liver and spleen. This scan shows the latissimus dorsi and the lower reaches of the serratus anterior. The upper portions of the anterior abdominal muscles (rectus abdominis, external oblique) can also be seen.

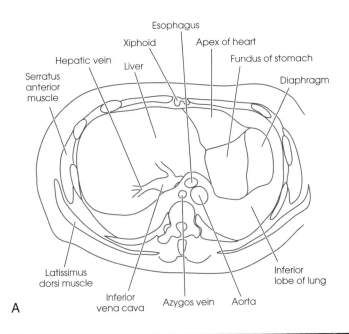

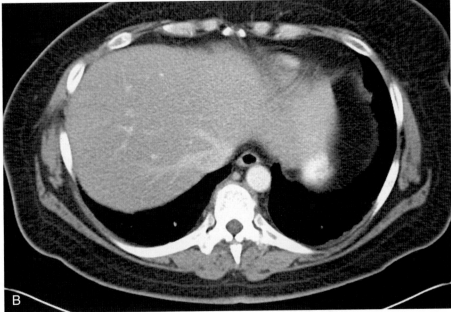

Fig. 28-46 A, Line drawing of CT section. **B,** CT image corresponding to level *A* in Fig. 28-45.

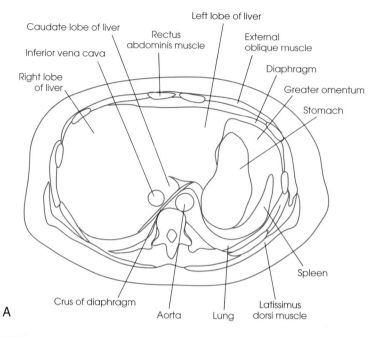

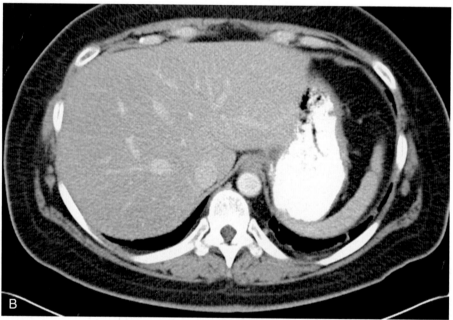

Fig. 28-47 A, Line drawing of CT section. **B,** CT image corresponding to level *B* in Fig. 28-45.

A CT image at the level of T11 (Fig. 28-48) shows the relationships among the liver, stomach, and spleen. The cardiac portion of the stomach is located at approximately the T10-11 level in the anterior aspect of the left upper quadrant, and the *pyloric portion* normally lies anterior to L2. This scan passes through the center or body of the stomach. An air-fluid level exists between the gas in the anterior stomach and the contrast medium in the posterior stomach. The spleen, located between the levels of T12 and L1, is in the posterolateral aspect of the left upper quadrant posterior to the fundus and body of the stomach. Contrast medium in the patient's colon is seen at the *splenic flexure,* seen here between the body of the stomach and the spleen. The liver is generally found between T11 and L3 and occupies the entire right upper quadrant. The right lobe of the liver has two small subdivisions, the caudate and *quadrate lobes,* which are bounded by the *gallbladder,* *ligamentum teres,* and inferior vena cava. The left lobe of the liver stretches across the midline and into the left upper quadrant. The *porta hepatis,* or hilum of the liver, is visible between the right and left lobes at this level. The inferior vena cava is found between the right and caudate lobes of the liver. In this image, it is nearly isodense with liver tissue. Large branches of the portal vein are seen at the porta hepatis.

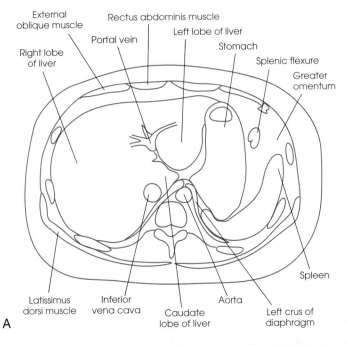

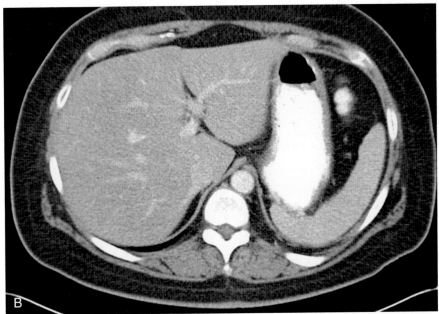

Fig. 28-48 A, Line drawing of CT section. **B,** CT image corresponding to level *C* in Fig. 28-45.

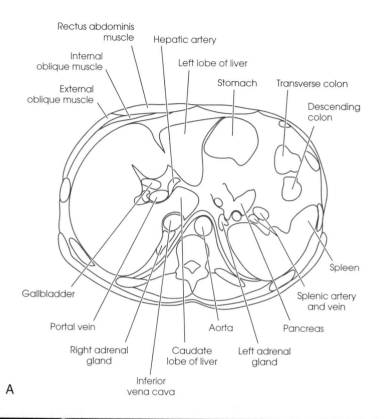

Rectus abdominis muscle
Internal oblique muscle
External oblique muscle
Hepatic artery
Left lobe of liver
Stomach
Transverse colon
Descending colon
Spleen
Splenic artery and vein
Pancreas
Left adrenal gland
Gallbladder
Portal vein
Aorta
Right adrenal gland
Caudate lobe of liver
Inferior vena cava

A

Fig. 28-49 lies at the inferior edge of T11. It shows the right, left, and caudate lobes of the liver and the porta hepatis. Anteriorly, the falciform ligament lies near the fissure between the right and left lobes (not seen on this image). The pyloric antrum of the stomach lies near the left lobe of the liver. This scan is inferior to the splenic flexure, so the *transverse and descending portions of the colon* can be differentiated. The spleen lies along the left posterior abdominal wall. This scan lies near the hilum, and vascular structures are seen in this region. The tail of the pancreas normally lies near the spleen and can be seen here between the stomach and spleen. The *suprarenal glands* are normally located superior to the kidney. The right suprarenal gland is found at this level between the liver and the right diaphragmatic crus. The left suprarenal gland is medial to the pancreas and spleen. The abdominal aorta is positioned anterior and to the left of the vertebral column; the inferior vena cava is between the right and caudate lobes of the liver. The portal vein is seen within the porta hepatis along with branches of the hepatic artery. The splenic artery is normally tortuous and not seen in its entirety. At this level, the bright circles along the posterior pancreas most likely represent portions of the contrast-filled *splenic artery*.

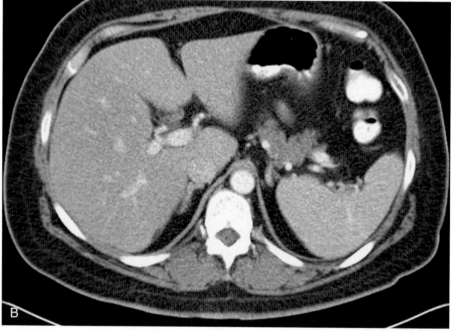

B

Fig. 28-49 A, Line drawing of CT section. B, CT image corresponding to level *D* in Fig. 28-45.

The CT scan in Fig. 28-50 passes through the upper portion of T12. The difference in density between the liver tissue and the bile-filled *gallbladder* makes these organs easy to differentiate. The antrum of the stomach, pyloric canal, and bulb (first portion) of the *duodenum* are seen in the anterior abdomen. The neck of the pancreas is posterior to the pyloric canal of the stomach in this image. The transverse and descending colon lie in the anterior left abdomen. The spleen is posterior to the descending colon. Loops of *jejunum,* the second part of the small bowel, are posterior to the antrum of the stomach. The left adrenal gland is lateral to the aorta and left diaphragmatic crus. The right adrenal gland is posterior to the IVC. The three branches of the *celiac trunk* (hepatic, splenic, left gastric arteries) supply the liver, spleen, pancreas, and stomach with oxygen-rich blood. In this image, the celiac trunk is seen as it divides into the *common hepatic artery* and the splenic artery. The left gastric artery is not seen. The splenic artery runs a tortuous course and normally cannot be visualized in its entirety in axial sections. Here, branches of the splenic artery and vein lie in close proximity and are difficult to differentiate. The inferior vena cava can be seen in its normal position anterior and to the right of the vertebral column. The main portion of the portal vein is just posterior to the duodenal bulb.

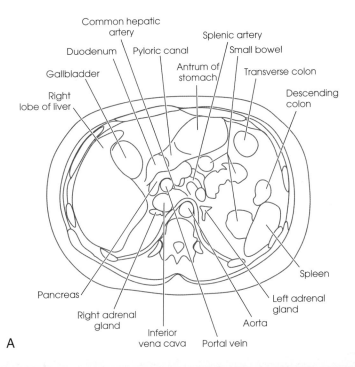

A

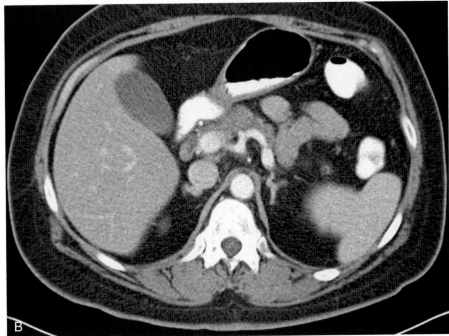

B

Fig. 28-50 A, Line drawing of CT section. **B,** CT image corresponding to level *E* in Fig. 28-45.

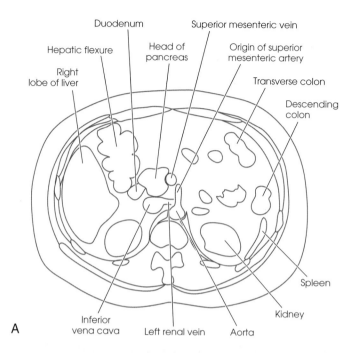

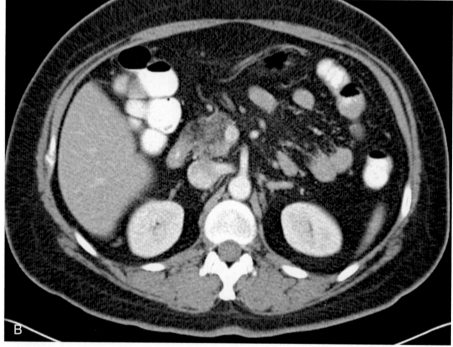

Fig. 28-51 A, Line drawing of CT section. **B,** CT image corresponding to level *F* in Fig. 28-45.

The muscles of the abdomen are located between the lower rib cage and the iliac crests. This group of muscles includes the *external oblique, internal oblique,* and *transverse abdominal muscles.* The two *rectus abdominis muscles* are located on the anterior aspect of the abdomen on either side of the midline and extend from the *pubic symphysis* to the xiphoid process.

The CT image in Fig. 28-51 is through the level of the first lumbar vertebra. The lower right lobe of the liver lies along the right side of the abdomen. The hepatic (right colic) flexure lies just medial to the liver. The duodenum forms a C-shaped loop around the head of the pancreas. In this scan, the head of the pancreas is seen between the duodenum (second portion) and the superior mesenteric vein. On the left side of the abdomen, loops of small bowel and the transverse and descending colon are seen. Folds of *mesentery* can be seen connecting some of the small bowel loops. The inferiormost edge of the spleen lies along the left posterior abdomen. The upper poles of the kidneys appear on either side of the vertebral body. At this level, the *superior mesenteric artery* is seen as it originates from the anterior aorta. The *left renal vein* can also be seen as it empties into the lateral aspect of the inferior vena cava.

Fig. 28-52 is a CT scan through the third lumbar vertebra. The ascending colon is found on the right side of the abdomen. In this image, most of the transverse colon can be seen across the anterior abdomen. The descending colon lies along the posterior left abdomen. Loops of small bowel are found in the central portion of the abdomen. Ileal loops are filled with contrast medium that has refluxed through the ileocecal valve from the colon. This level is just below the hila of the kidneys, and some of the central collecting system can be observed. The inferior vena cava and contrast-filled aorta lie anterior to the vertebral body. The rectus abdominis muscles lie on either side of the midline in the anterior abdomen. The three layers of the lateral abdominal muscles (external oblique, internal oblique, and transverse abdominis) are separated by fat and can plainly be seen in this scan. The *psoas muscles* originate from the body of T12 and the transverse processes of the lumbar vertebrae and descend the abdomen lateral to the vertebral bodies. The *quadratus lumborum muscles* are located posterolateral to the psoas muscles through the abdomen. These muscles can be seen on either side of the vertebra. The *spinal cord* normally terminates at the level of L1. Inferior to L1 the *spinal nerves,* known as *cauda equina,* are seen within the spinal canal.

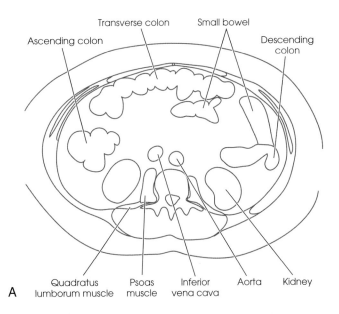

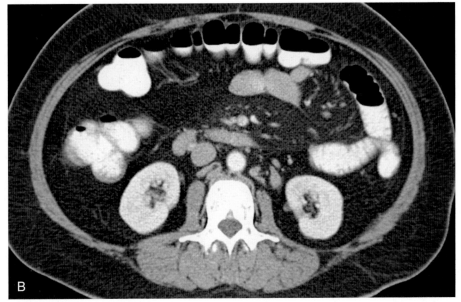

Fig. 28-52 A, Line drawing of CT section. **B,** CT image corresponding to level *G* in Fig. 28-45.

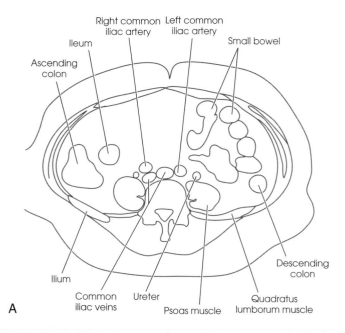

A

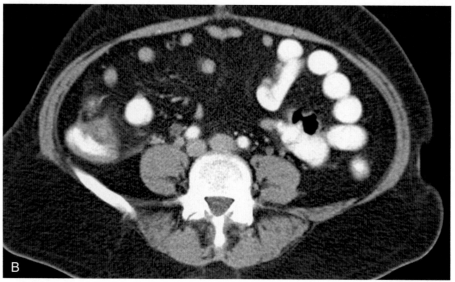

B

Fig. 28-53 A, Line drawing of CT section. **B,** CT image corresponding to level *H* in Fig. 28-45.

The CT scan in Fig. 28-53 lies near the interspace between the fourth and fifth lumbar vertebrae. The superior edge of the right *iliac crest* is visible in this image. The inferior portion of the cecum and the descending colon lie in the posterior abdomen on the right and left sides. Loops of small bowel are seen more anteriorly in the abdomen. The ureters normally lie just anterior to the psoas muscles. Because of peristalsis, no contrast medium is seen in the ureters on this image. At this level, the aorta has bifurcated to form the right and left *common iliac vessels.* The common iliac veins are fairly close to each other, indicating this scan is just inferior to their junction (which forms the inferior vena cava).

The CT image seen in Fig. 28-54 is of a female patient and was obtained at the upper sacral level. It shows the *wings* of the *ilia,* the right *anterior superior iliac spine,* and the *sacroiliac joints.* The descending colon is seen at the left lateral aspect of the pelvis, and multiple loops of *small intestine* are found throughout this level in the images. Three muscles lie posterior to the wings of the ilia: the gluteus minimus, gluteus medius, and gluteus maximus. The gluteus medius normally extends the farthest superiorly and is the first muscle visible as scans progress down through the pelvis. At the posterolateral aspect of the right ilium, two of the three *gluteal muscles* are visible—the gluteus medius and a small amount of the gluteus maximus—whereas on the left, only the gluteus medius is visible. The *iliacus muscle* is seen lining the internal aspect of the iliac wings near the psoas muscles. The two rectus abdominis muscles are found in the anterior abdomen on both sides of the midline. The external oblique, internal oblique, and transverse abdominis are seen extending anteriorly from the ilium on each side. The abdominal aorta bifurcates at L4 into the *common iliac arteries.* Each common iliac artery divides at the level of the anterior superior iliac spine into *internal* and *external iliac arteries.* The *internal iliac arteries* tend to be located in the posterior pelvis and branch to feed the pelvic structures. The *external iliac vessels* are found progressively anterior in succeeding inferior sections to become the femoral vessels at the superior aspect of the thigh. The internal and external iliac veins unite inferior to the anterior superior iliac spine to form the common iliac veins, and the inferior vena cava is formed anterior to L5 by the junction of the common iliac veins. This scan shows the internal and external iliac arteries. At this level, the internal and external iliac veins have joined to form the common iliac veins. The common iliac veins are positioned at the anterior aspects of the sacrum with the internal and external iliac arteries anterior and medial to the veins in these images.

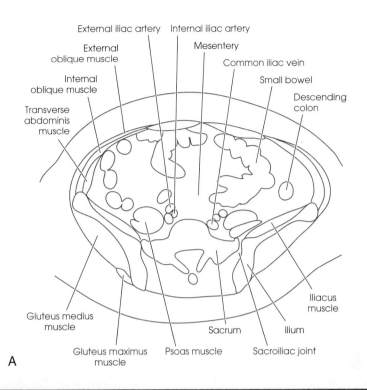

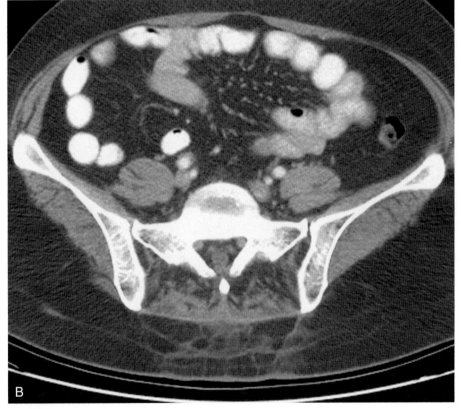

Fig. 28-54 A, Line drawing of CT section. **B,** CT image corresponding to level *I* in Fig. 28-45.

Abdominopelvic Region

293

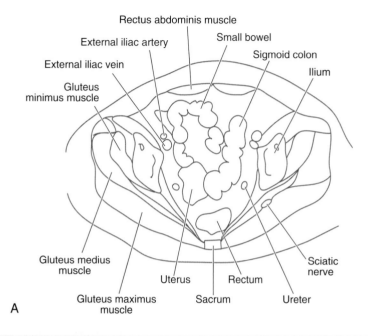

A

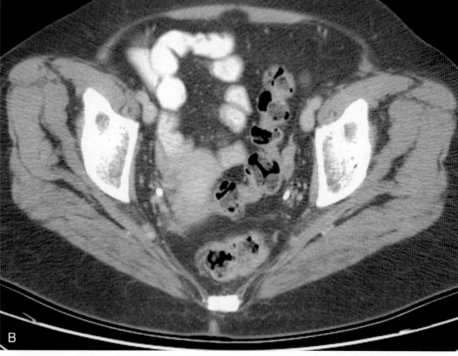

B

Fig. 28-55 A, Line drawing of CT section. **B,** CT image of female pelvis corresponding to level *J* in Fig. 28-45.

Fig. 28-55 is a CT image obtained just superior to the level of the *acetabulum*. In this image, the inferior sacrum is visible, and the junction of the *ilium, ischium,* and *pubis* lies near the upper part of the acetabulum. Loops of ileum, filled with contrast medium, are seen in the anterior right pelvis. The *haustral folds* of the *sigmoid colon* are found in the center of the pelvis as this part of the large intestine curls toward the sacrum. A portion of the rectum is seen just anterior to the sacrum in this image. The fundus of the *uterus* lies medial to the right acetabulum and posterior to the ileal folds. The ureters are filled with contrast medium in this image and are easily identifiable in the posterior and lateral regions of the pelvic cavity. The external iliac arteries and veins run a diagonal course through the pelvis, lying near the sacrum in the upper part of the pelvis and passing anteriorly as they pass down through the pelvis toward the lower extremities. In this scan the external iliac vessels are seen just medial to the anterior edges of the acetabula. Multiple muscular structures are found at this level. The rectus abdominis muscles lie on either side of the midline in the anterior abdomen. The gluteal muscles (maximus, medius, and minimus) lie along the external surface of the posterior pelvis. Other muscles of the lower limbs are found just anterior to the acetabula. The large sciatic nerve can be plainly seen on the left between the gluteus maximus and medius muscles.

The CT scan in Fig. 28-56 is of a female patient and is at a level just superior to the pubic symphysis. The pubic bones, *ischia, acetabula, femoral heads,* and *greater trochanters* are visualized. The relationship between the *rectum, cervix,* and wall of the *bladder* is shown from posterior to anterior in the pelvic region. The ureters entered the bladder just superior to this scan and so are no longer visible. The external iliac vessels are now referred to as the *femoral vessels,* with the name change occurring at the inguinal ligament, which is found between the pubic symphysis and the anterior superior iliac spine. The *iliopsoas muscles* (formed by the junction of the psoas and iliacus muscles) are found anterior to the femoral heads; the *obturator internus muscle,* with its characteristic right-angle bend, is found medial to the acetabulum.

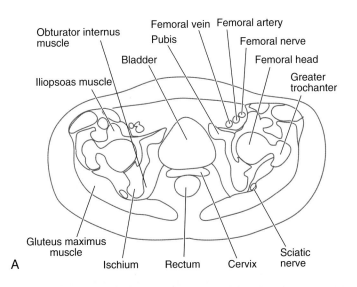

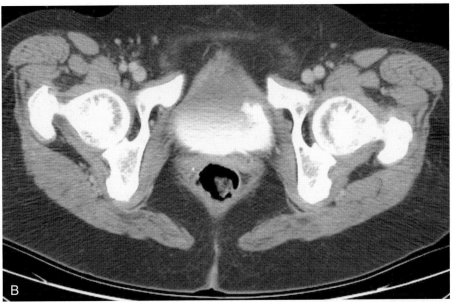

Fig. 28-56 A, Line drawing of CT section. **B,** CT image of female pelvis corresponding to level *K* in Fig. 28-45.

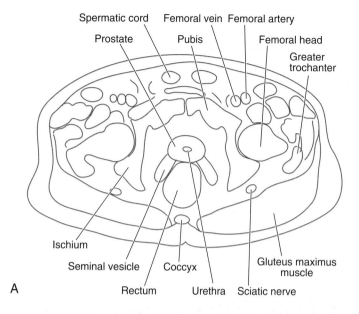

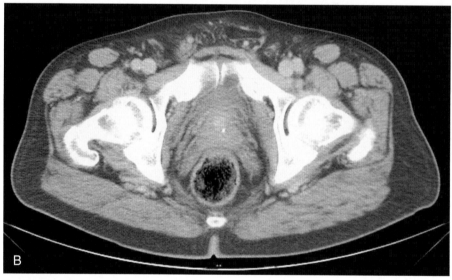

Fig. 28-57 A, Line drawing of CT section. **B,** CT image of male pelvis corresponding to level *K* in Fig. 28-45.

Fig. 28-57 is a CT scan through the lower pelvis of a male patient. This scan is at a slightly more inferior level than the previous scan. The symphysis pubis is seen here, along with the acetabula, *ischial spines,* and *femoral heads* and *greater trochanters.* The tip of the *coccyx* is visible in the posterior pelvis. In the male pelvis, the prostate gland lies inferior to the bladder and is traversed by the *urethra.* In this image, the prostate gland, seminal vesicles, and rectum occupy the pelvic cavity from anterior to posterior. The bright spot within the prostate gland is the contrast-filled urethra. The *spermatic cords* transmit the ductus deferens and vascular structures between the pelvis and the testicular structures and are found on either side of the midline just anterior to the symphysis pubis.

Fig. 28-58 is a sagittal MR image of the female pelvis near the midline. The fourth and fifth lumbar vertebrae, the sacrum, and the coccyx are visualized. The cauda equina is seen descending the spinal canal. The areas of signal void anterior to the sacrum represent the rectum. The musculature and cavity of the uterus are visible anterior to the rectum. In the anterior pelvis, the bladder is seen posterior and superior to the symphysis pubis. Multiple loops of small bowel fill the upper anterior region of the pelvis but are blurry owing to peristaltic motion. The rectus abdominis muscle extends superiorly from the pubis in the anterior abdominal wall. Fig. 28-59 is a sagittal MR image of a male patient. Note the prostate gland lying inferior to the bladder. A portion of the urethra can be seen passing through the prostate in this image.

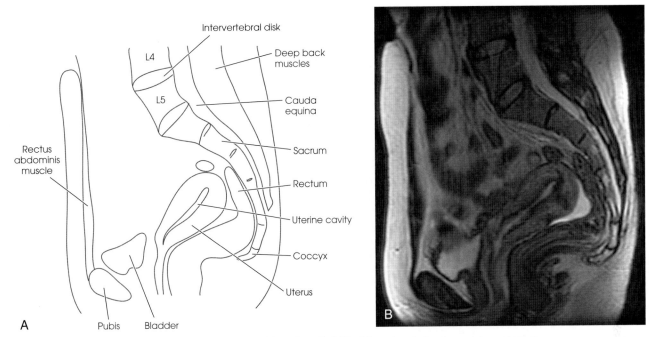

Fig. 28-58 A, Line drawing of MRI section. **B,** MRI of female abdominopelvic region at midsagittal plane.

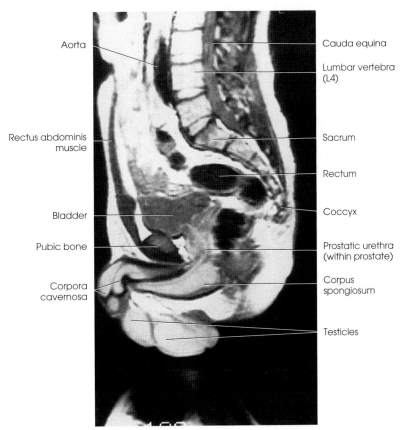

Fig. 28-59 MRI of male abdominopelvic region at midsagittal plane.

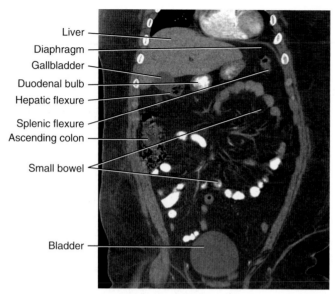

Liver
Diaphragm
Gallbladder
Duodenal bulb
Hepatic flexure
Splenic flexure
Ascending colon

Small bowel

Bladder

Fig. 28-60 Coronal CT image through anterior abdomen.

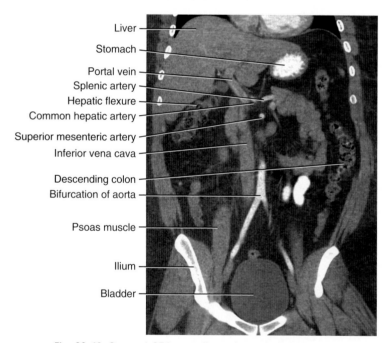

Liver
Stomach
Portal vein
Splenic artery
Hepatic flexure
Common hepatic artery
Superior mesenteric artery
Inferior vena cava
Descending colon
Bifurcation of aorta
Psoas muscle
Ilium
Bladder

Fig. 28-61 Coronal CT image through central abdomen.

Fig. 28-60 is a coronal CT image through the abdomen and pelvis. The only bony structures visible are the lower ribs. At the top of the abdomen, the diaphragm separates the heart and lungs from the liver and gastrointestinal structures. The right lobe of the liver occupies most of the right upper quadrant. On the inferolateral surface of the liver is a fluid-filled circle, which represents the gallbladder. Several structures of the gastrointestinal system are visible in this image. Near the midline, inferior to the liver, are contrast-filled structures, which represent the proximal duodenum and the stomach. The right (hepatic) and left (splenic) flexures of the large intestine are visible. The hepatic flexure is just inferior to the liver and gallbladder; the splenic flexure is just inferior to the left hemidiaphragm. The ascending colon lies along the right lateral abdominal wall, and multiple loops of small bowel with and without contrast enhancement can be seen within the central portion of the abdomen. The urinary bladder occupies the center of the pelvis.

Fig. 28-61 lies near the median coronal plane. At this level, the right and left lobes of the liver and a small portion of the gallbladder are apparent. The porta hepatis is the region of the liver where vascular structures enter and leave the organ. It is sometimes referred to as the hilum of the liver and is seen here on the inferior surface near the center. The contrast-filled body of the stomach lies near the left lobe of the liver. Several loops of small bowel are visible in the central abdomen, and the hepatic flexure and descending portion of the colon are along the lateral walls. The aorta and inferior vena cava are found anterior to the vertebral column within the abdomen. The aorta lies on the left, and the vena cava lies on the right. Major visceral branches of the abdominal aorta are (from superior to inferior) the celiac artery (sometimes called the celiac trunk), which originates from the anterior aorta near the level of T12; the superior mesenteric artery, which originates from the anterior aorta near the level of L1; the right and left renal arteries, which originate from the lateral aorta near the level of L2; the inferior mesenteric artery, which originates between the lateral and anterior surface of the aorta near the level of L3; and the common iliac arteries, which result when the aorta bifurcates near the level of L4. In this image, the aorta is bright because of contrast enhancement. The celiac trunk is a short vessel that almost immediately bifurcates into the common hepatic, splenic, and left gastric arteries. This image shows the common hepatic artery, which passes right to supply the liver, and the splenic artery, which branches toward the left to supply the spleen. Just below these vessels, the origin of the superior mesenteric artery is also apparent. The image clearly shows the lower abdominal aorta, its bifurcation, and the common iliac arteries. The portal system drains blood from the digestive system and carries nutrients to the liver. The portal vein is formed by the junction of the superior mesenteric vein and the splenic vein and can be seen within the porta hepatis.

Fig. 28-62 is a coronal CT image that represents a plane just posterior to the median coronal plane. Ribs are seen on the superior lateral aspect of the lower thorax and upper abdomen. Several lumbar vertebral bodies are visible in the center of the abdomen, and the iliac wings, acetabuli, femoral heads, and symphysis pubis are discernible in the pelvis. The right lobe of the liver lies in the right upper quadrant, and the spleen is found in the left upper quadrant where it is positioned lateral to the stomach and inferior to the diaphragm. The pancreas is a long, thin organ that lies horizontally across the center of the abdomen. In this scan, the tail of the pancreas can be found near the hilum of the spleen. The stomach, filled with contrast medium, rests inferior to the left hemidiaphragm, superior to the pancreatic tail, and between the liver and spleen. The right and left kidneys are retroperitoneal organs. Most of the right kidney is visible on this image; the anterior surface of the left kidney can also be seen. The central abdominal portions of the aorta and inferior vena cava are present in the center of the abdomen. The aorta is brighter owing to contrast enhancement. The left renal artery is visible at its origin from the aorta, and a small segment of the right renal artery is seen near the hilum of the right kidney.

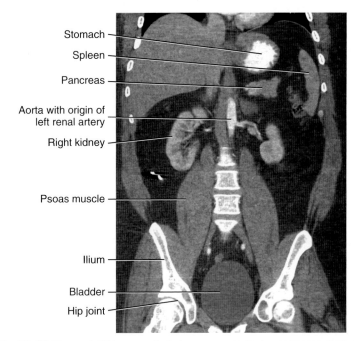

Stomach

Spleen

Pancreas

Aorta with origin of left renal artery

Right kidney

Psoas muscle

Ilium

Bladder

Hip joint

Fig. 28-62 Coronal CT image of abdomen posterior to midcoronal plane.

Selected bibliography

Applegate E: *The sectional anatomy learning system*, ed 3, Philadelphia, 2010, Saunders.

Bo WJ et al: *Basic atlas of sectional anatomy*, ed 4, Philadelphia, 2007, Saunders.

El-Khoury GY et al: *Sectional anatomy by MRI and CT*, ed 3, New York, 2007, Churchill Livingstone.

Ellis H et al: *Human cross-sectional anatomy: atlas of body sections and CT images*, ed 3, London, 2009, Hodder Arnold.

Kelley LL, Petersen CM: *Sectional anatomy for imaging professionals*, ed 3, St Louis, 2012, Mosby.

Madden, ME: *Introduction to Sectional Anatomy*, ed. 2, Philadelphia, 2008, Lippincott Williams & Wilkins.

National Institutes of Health: *The visible human project,* Available at: www.nlm.nih.gov/research/visible/visible_human.html. Accessed September 1, 2013.

Weber E et al: *Netter's concise radiologic anatomy*, Philadelphia, 2009, Saunders.

Weir J, Abrahams PH: *Imaging atlas of human anatomy*, ed 4, London, 2011, Mosby.

Sectional Anatomy for Radiographers

29
COMPUTED TOMOGRAPHY

GAYLE K. WRIGHT
NANCY M. JOHNSON

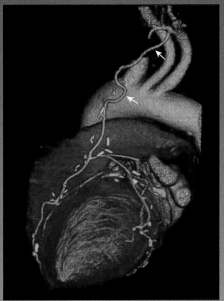

OUTLINE

Fundamentals of Computed
  Tomography, 302
Computed Tomography and
  Conventional Radiography, 302
Historical Development, 305
Computed Tomography Scanner
  Generation Classifications, 305
Technical Aspects, 308
System Components, 309
Diagnostic Applications, 313
Contrast Media, 316
Factors Affecting Image Quality, 318
Special Features, 321
Computed Tomography and
  Radiation Dose, 329
Comparison of Computed
  Tomography and Magnetic
  Resonance Imaging, 333
Future Considerations, 333
Basic Computed Tomography
  Examination Protocols, 336

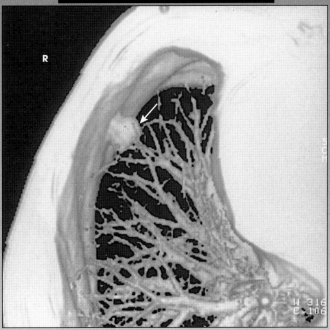

Fundamentals of Computed Tomography

*Computed tomography (CT)** is the process of creating a cross-sectional tomographic plane of any part of the body (Fig. 29-1). For CT, a patient is scanned by an x-ray tube rotating around the body part being examined. A detector assembly measures the radiation exiting the patient and feeds back the information, referred to as primary data, to the host computer. After the computer has compiled and calculated the data according to a preselected *algorithm,* it assembles the data in a *matrix* to form an *axial* image. Each image, or *slice,* is displayed in a cross-sectional format.

In the early 1970s, CT scanning was used clinically only for imaging of the brain. The first CT scanners were capable of producing only axial images and were called *CAT (computed axial tomography)*

*Almost all italicized words on the succeeding pages are defined at the end of this chapter.

units by the public; this term is no longer accurate because images can now be created in multiple planes. Dramatic technical advancements have led to the development of CT scanners that can be used to image virtually every structure within the human body. Improvements in scanner design and computer science have produced CT units with new imaging capabilities and reconstruction techniques. Three-dimensional reconstructions of images of the internal structures are used for surgical planning, CT angiography (CTA), radiation therapy planning, and virtual reality imaging.

Interventional procedures such as CT-guided biopsies and fluid drainage offer an alternative to surgery for some patients. Although these procedures are considered invasive, they offer shorter recovery periods, no exposure to anesthesia, and less risk of infection.

Computed Tomography and Conventional Radiography

When a conventional x-ray exposure is made, the radiation passes through the patient and produces an image of the body part. Frequently, body structures are superimposed (Fig. 29-2). Visualizing specific structures requires the use of contrast media, varied positions, and usually more than one exposure. Localization of masses or foreign bodies requires at least two exposures and a ruler calibrated for magnification.

During the CT examination, a tightly collimated x-ray beam is directed through the patient from many different angles, resulting in an image that represents a cross section of the area scanned. This imaging technique essentially eliminates the superimposition of body structures. The CT technologist controls the method of acquisition, the slice thickness, the reconstruction algorithm, and other factors related to image quality.

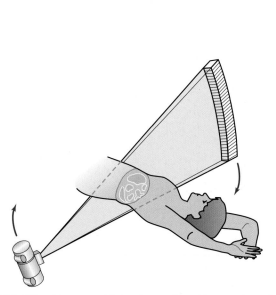

Fig. 29-1 CT scanner provides cross-sectional images by rotating around the patient.

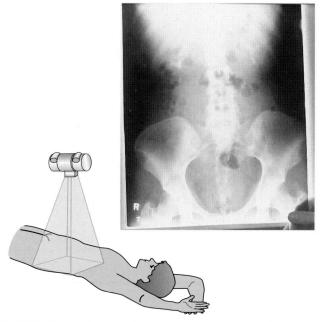

Fig. 29-2 Conventional radiograph superimposes anatomy and yields one diagnostic image with fixed density and contrast.

The digital radiograph of the abdomen illustrated in Fig. 29-3 shows high-density bone and low-density gas, but many soft tissue structures, such as the kidneys and intestines, are not clearly identified. A contrast medium is needed to visualize these structures. A CT examination of the abdomen would show all of the structures that lie within the slice. In Fig. 29-4, *A*, the liver, stomach, kidneys, spleen, and aorta can be identified. In addition to eliminating superimposition, CT is capable of differentiating among tissues with similar densities. This differentiation of densities is referred to as *contrast resolution*. The improved contrast resolution with CT compared with conventional radiography is due to a reduction in the amount of scattered radiation.

Fig. 29-4, *B*, is an axial image of the brain that differentiates the gray matter from the white matter and shows bony structures and cerebrospinal fluid within the ventricles. Because CT can show subtle differences in various tissues, radiologists are able to diagnose pathologic conditions more accurately than if they were to rely on radiographs alone. Because the image is digitized by the computer, numerous image manipulation techniques can be used to enhance and optimize the diagnostic information available to the physician (Fig. 29-5).

Computed Tomography and Conventional Radiography

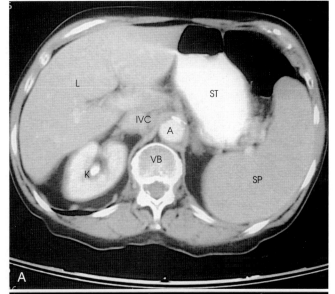
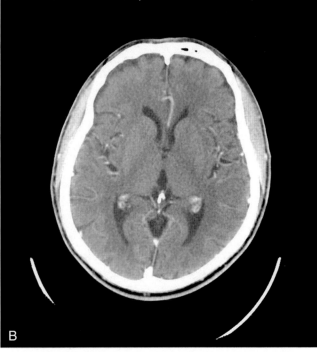

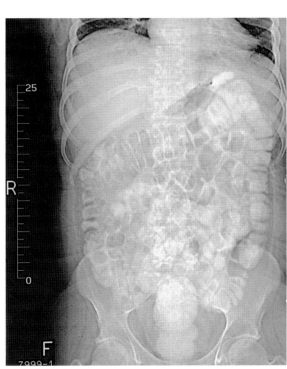

Fig. 29-3 Digital kidney, ureter, and bladder (KUB).

Fig. 29-4 A, Axial image of abdomen showing liver (*L*), stomach (*ST*), spleen (*SP*), aorta (*A*), inferior vena cava (*IVC*), vertebral body of thoracic spine (*VB*), and kidney (*K*). **B,** Axial CT scan of lateral ventricles–anterior horns (RightALV), posterior horns (LeftPLV), and third ventricle (3V).

(**B,** From Kelley LL, Petersen CM: *Sectional anatomy for imaging professionals*, ed 2, St Louis, 2007, Mosby.)

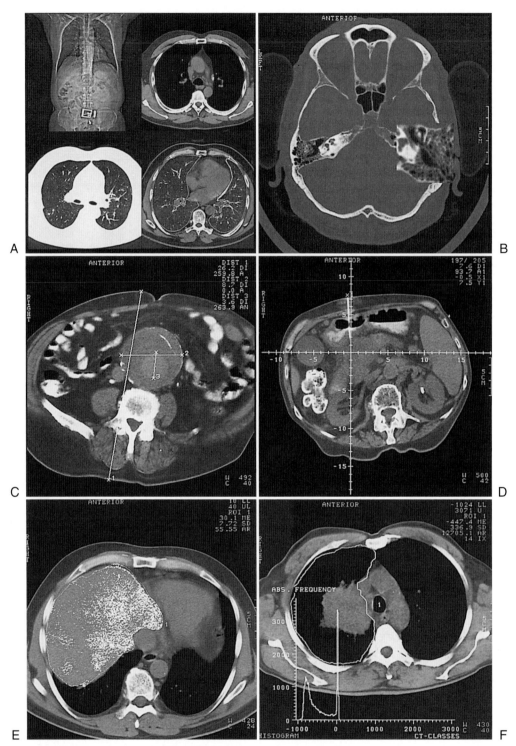

Fig. 29-5 Image manipulation techniques used to enhance diagnostic information in CT image. **A,** Multiple imaging windows. **B,** Image magnification. **C,** Measurement of distances. **D,** Superimposition of coordinates on the image. **E,** Highlighting. **F,** Histogram.

(Courtesy Siemens Medical Systems, Iselin, NJ.)

Historical Development

CT was first performed successfully in 1970 in England at the Central Research Laboratory of EMI, Ltd. Hounsfield, an engineer for EMI, and Cormack, a nuclear physicist from Johannesburg, South Africa, are generally given credit for the development of CT. For their research, they were awarded the Nobel Prize in medicine and physiology in 1979. After CT was shown to be a useful clinical imaging modality, the first full-scale commercial unit, referred to as a *brain tissue scanner,* was installed in Atkinson Morley's Hospital in 1971. An early dedicated head CT scanner is shown in Fig. 29-6. Physicians recognized its value for providing diagnostic neurologic information, and its use was accepted rapidly. The first CT scanners in the United States were installed in June 1973 at the Mayo Clinic, Rochester, Minnesota, and later that year at Massachusetts General Hospital, Boston. These early units were also dedicated head CT scanners. In 1974, Ledley at Georgetown University Medical Center, Washington, D.C., developed the first whole-body scanner, which greatly expanded the diagnostic capabilities of CT.

After physicians accepted CT as a diagnostic modality, numerous companies in addition to EMI began manufacturing scanners. Although the units differed in design, the basic principles of operation were the same.

Computed Tomography Scanner Generation Classifications

CT scanners have historically been categorized by *generation,* which is a reference to the level of technologic advancement of the tube and detector assembly. The original "generation" classification of scanners was a clear distinction of tube movement versus detector rotational path. As scanner technology has progressed, the tube movement and detector rotation relationship has remained relatively constant, but the tube power source and the detector configurations have changed. Some authors have used slip ring or detector advancements to assign a generation number. These varied opinions and discussions have led to some confusion concerning scanner generation classifications. The following discussion of scanner generations follows the original standards of tube movement versus detector rotation.

The early units, referred to as *first-generation scanners,* worked by a process known as *translate/rotate.* The tube produced a finely collimated beam, or pencil beam. Depending on the manufacturer, one to three *detectors* were placed

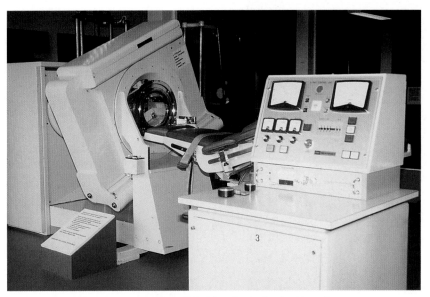

Fig. 29-6 First-generation EMI CT unit: dedicated head scanner.

(Photograph taken at Reöntgen Museum, Lennep, Germany.)

opposite the tube for radiation detection. The linear tube movement (translation) was followed by a rotation of 1 degree. Scan time was usually 3 to 5 minutes per scan, which required the patient to hold still for extended periods. Because of the slow scanning and reconstruction time, the use of CT was limited almost exclusively to neurologic examinations because of the aperture size and the water bag construction. A CT image from a first-generation scanner is shown in Fig. 29-7.

The *second-generation scanners* were considered a significant improvement over first-generation scanners. The x-ray tube emitted a fan-shaped beam that was measured by approximately 30 detectors placed closely together in a detector array. Tube and detector movement was still *translate/rotate;* however, the gantry rotated 10 degrees between each translation. These changes improved overall image quality and decreased scan time to about 20 seconds for a single slice. The time required to complete one CT examination remained relatively long, however.

The *third-generation scanners* introduced a *rotate/rotate movement,* in which the x-ray tube and detector array rotate simultaneously around the patient. An increase in the number of detectors (>750) and their arrangement in a "curved" detector array considerably improved image quality (Fig. 29-8). Scan times were decreased to 0.35 to 1 second per slice, which made the CT examination much easier for patients and helped decrease motion artifact. Advancements in computer technology also decreased image reconstruction time, substantially reducing examination time. Most current scanners are third-generation configurations with one of the following technical variations:

- *Helical CT, single-slice helical CT (SSHCT).* Slip-ring technology allows 360-degree continuous rotation of tube and detector. Reduces scan times to subsecond per slice.
- *Multislice detectors (MSHCT or MDCT).* Increase in number of detector rows allows multiple slices to be produced in one rotation. As detector rows increase, the fan beam geometry of the x-ray beam has been adapted, the beginning of cone-beam configuration. Began with two-slice scanners and quickly moved to four slices and more.
- *Volume CT (VCT).* Multislice scanners with 64 detector rows or more. The

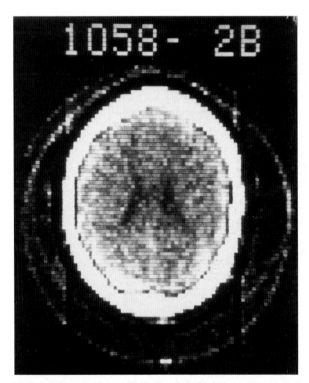

Fig. 29-7 Axial brain image from the first CT scanner in operation in the United States: Mayo Clinic, Rochester, Minnesota. The 80 × 80 matrix produced a noisy image. The examination was performed in July 1973.

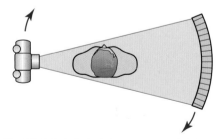

Fig. 29-8 Rotate/rotate movement: tube and detector movement of a third-generation scanner.

x-ray beam geometry must be a cone-beam configuration to accommodate the increased length of the scanning field.

- *Flat-panel CT (FP-CT or FD-CT).* A detector plate similar to plates used in digital radiography (DR) replaces the typical detector configuration. In dedicated breast units, the tube and detector travel a full 360 degrees. In other applications, interventional and intraoperative, the unit functions more like a C-arm fluoroscopy unit in which the tube and detector do not travel in a full 360 degrees. Scanners provide excellent spatial resolution but slightly lower contrast resolution.

The *fourth-generation scanners* introduced the *rotate-only movement* in which the tube rotates around the patient, but the detectors were in fixed positions, forming a complete circle within the gantry (Fig. 29-9). The use of stationary detectors required greater numbers of detectors to be installed in a scanner. Fourth-generation scanners tended to yield a higher patient dose per scan than previous generations of CT scanners because the CT tube is closer to the patient.

The *fifth-generation scanners* are classified as high-speed CT scanners because of millisecond acquisition times. These scanners are electron-beam scanners (EBCT) in which x-rays are produced from an electron beam in a fan beam configuration that strikes stationary tungsten target rings (Fig. 29-10). The detector rings are in a ±210-degree arc. These scanners were primarily used for cardiac studies because of the improved temporal resolution.

The *sixth-generation scanners* are dual-energy source (two x-ray tubes) (DSCT, DE-CT) that have two sets of detectors that are offset by 90 degrees. These DSCT scanners provide improved temporal resolution needed for imaging moving structures such as the heart (Fig. 29-11). The latest dual source/dual detector (DSDD) CT scanners offer dual-energy capabilities, typically 80kVp and 120kVp, between the two CT tubes. Using Flash Spiral scanning offered by Siemens, the dual source spiral scanning allows for gapless volume coverage using a pitch of 3.4, which increases the temporal resolution to one quarter of the rotation time. This technology allows a marked decrease in patient radiation dose as no overlapping scanning occurs.

Most scanners in use today are third-generation variations that have 4 to 320 rows of detectors in a single array. This increase in numbers of detector rows has increased the length of the scanning field, which requires the x-ray beam to be cone

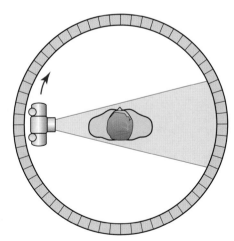

Fig. 29-9 Rotate-only movement: tube movement with stationary detectors of a fourth-generation scanner.

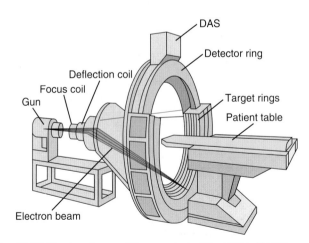

Fig. 29-10 Electron beam CT scanner configuration. X-rays, produced from electron beam, strike four target rings.

shaped to encompass the full detector array. This is a change from the original third-generation fan beam. The flat panel detector also requires cone-beam geometry. The increased detector size and the cone-beam geometry pose various challenges in maintaining image quality, but this discussion is too involved for this chapter.

Technical Aspects

The axial images acquired by CT scanning provide information about the positional relationships and tissue characteristics of structures within the section of interest. The computer performs a series of steps to generate one axial image. With the patient and gantry perpendicular to each other, the tube rotates around the patient, irradiating the area of interest. For every position of the x-ray tube, the detectors measure the transmitted x-ray values, convert them into an electrical signal, and relay the signal to the computer. The measured x-ray transmission values are called *projections (scan profiles)* or *raw data*. When collected, the electrical signals are digitized, a process that assigns a whole number to each signal. The value of each number is directly proportional to the strength of the signal.

The digital image is an array of numbers arranged in a grid of rows and columns called a *matrix*. A single square, or picture element, within the matrix is called a *pixel*. The slice thickness gives the pixel an added dimension called the *volume element*, or *voxel*. Each pixel in the image corresponds to the volume of tissue in the body section being imaged. The voxel volume is a product of the pixel area and slice thickness (Fig. 29-12). The *field of view* (FOV) determines the amount of data to be displayed on the monitor.

Each pixel within the matrix is assigned a number that is related to the linear attenuation coefficient of the tissue within each voxel. These numbers are called *CT numbers* or *Hounsfield units*. CT numbers are defined as a relative comparison of x-ray attenuation of a voxel of tissue with an equal volume of water. Water is used as reference material because it is abundant in the body and has a uniform density; water is assigned an arbitrary value of 0. Tissues that are denser than water are given positive CT numbers, and tissues with less density than water are assigned negative CT numbers. The scale of CT numbers ranges from −1000 (air/gas) to −3000 (dense bone). Average CT numbers for various tissues are listed in Table 29-1.

For displaying the digital image, each pixel within the image is assigned a level of gray. The gray level assigned to each pixel corresponds to the CT number for that pixel. The bit depth determines the number of shades of gray that can be assigned to a pixel. A bit depth of 8 would have 256 shades of gray available, whereas a bit depth of 12 would have 4096 shades.

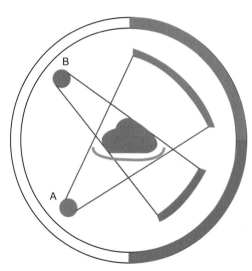

Fig. 29-11 Dual-source CT scanner (DSCT) configuration. This is considered a sixth-generation scanner.

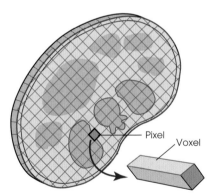

Fig. 29-12 CT image is composed of a matrix of pixels, with each pixel representing a volume of tissue (voxel).

TABLE 29-1

Average Hounsfield units (HU) for selected substances

Substance	HU
Air	−1000
Lungs	−250 to −850
Fat	−100
Orbit	−25
Water	0
Cyst	−5 to +10
Fluid	0 to +25
Tumor	+25 to +100
Blood (fluid)	+20 to +50
Blood (clotted)	+50 to +75
Blood (old)	+10 to +15
Brain	+20 to +40
Muscle	+35 to +50
Gallbladder	+5 to +30
Liver	+40 to +70
Aorta	+35 to +50
Bone	+150 to +1000
Metal	+2000 to +4000

System Components

The three major components of the CT scanner are shown in Fig. 29-13. Because each component has several subsystems, the following sections provide only a brief description of their main functions.

COMPUTER

The computer provides the link between the CT technologist and the other components of the imaging system. The computer system used in CT has four basic functions: control of data acquisition, image reconstruction, storage of image data, and image display.

Data acquisition is the method by which the patient is scanned. The technologist must select among numerous parameters, such as scanning in the conventional or helical mode, before the initiation of each scan. The *data acquisition system* (DAS) is involved in sequencing the generation of x-rays, turning the detectors on and off at appropriate intervals, transferring data, and monitoring the system operation.

The *reconstruction* of a CT image depends on the millions of mathematic operations required to digitize and recon-

struct the raw data. This image reconstruction is accomplished using an array processor that acts as a specialized computer to perform mathematic calculations rapidly and efficiently, freeing the host computer for other activities. Currently, CT units can acquire scans in less than 1 second and require only a few seconds more for image reconstruction.

The *host computer* in CT has limited storage capacity, so image data can be stored only temporarily. Other storage mechanisms are necessary to allow for long-term *data storage* and *retrieval*. After reconstruction, the CT image data can be transferred to another storage medium such as an optical disk. CT studies can be removed from the limited memory of the host computer and stored independently, a process termed *archiving*.

The reconstructed images are displayed on a monitor. At this point, the technologist or physician can communicate with the host computer to view specific images, post images on a scout, or implement image manipulation techniques such as zoom, control contrast and brightness, and image analysis techniques.

GANTRY AND TABLE

The *gantry* is a circular device that houses the x-ray tube, DAS, and detector array. Helical CT units also house the continuous *slip ring* and high-voltage generator in the gantry. The components housed in the gantry collect the necessary attenuation measurements to be sent to the computer for image reconstruction.

The x-ray tube used in CT is similar in design to the tubes used in conventional radiography, but it is specially designed to handle and dissipate excessive heat units created during a CT examination. The newest CT x-ray tubes use a rotating anode to increase heat dissipation, all metal larger anodes and a metal housing. Many CT x-ray tubes can handle around 8 million heat units (MHU), whereas advanced CT units can tolerate 20 MHU.

The detectors in CT function as image receptors. A detector measures the amount of radiation transmitted through the body and converts the measurement into an electrical signal proportional to the radiation intensity. Current detectors are gadolinium oxysulfide (GOS) ceramic scintillation (solid-state) detectors.

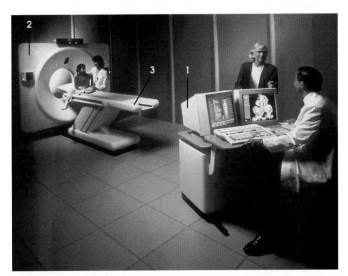

Fig. 29-13 Components of a CT scanner: *1*, Computer and operator's console; *2*, gantry; *3*, patient table.

(Courtesy GE Medical Systems, Waukesha, WI.)

The gantry can be tilted forward or backward up to 30 degrees to compensate for body part angulation. The opening within the center of the gantry is termed the *aperture*. Most apertures are about 28 inches (71.1 cm) wide to accommodate a variety of patient sizes as the patient table advances through it. To accommodate larger patients and for interventional applications, a 34-inch (85-cm) aperture is available.

For certain head studies, such as studies of facial bones, sinuses, or the sella turcica, a combination of patient positioning and gantry angulation results in a *direct coronal* image of the body part being scanned. Fig. 29-14 shows a typical direct coronal image of the paranasal sinuses.

The *table* is an automated device linked to the computer and gantry. It is designed to move in increments *(index)* according to the scan program. The table is an extremely important part of a CT scanner. Indexing must be accurate and reliable, especially when thin slices (1 or 2 mm) are taken through the area of interest. Most CT tables can be programmed to move in or out of the gantry, depending on the examination protocol and the patient.

CT tables are made of a low-density carbon fiber composite, both of which support the patient without causing image artifacts. The table must be very strong and rigid to handle patient weight and at the same time maintain consistent indexing. All CT tables have a maximum patient weight limit; this limit varies by manufacturer from 450 lb to 650 lb (204 kg to 295 kg). Exceeding the weight limit can cause inaccurate indexing, damage to the table motor, and even breakage of the tabletop, which could cause serious injury to the patient.

Accessory devices can be attached to the table for various uses. A special device called a *cradle* is used for head CT examinations. The head cradle helps hold the head still; because the device extends beyond the tabletop, it minimizes artifacts or attenuation from the table while the brain is being scanned. It can also be used in positioning the patient for direct coronal images.

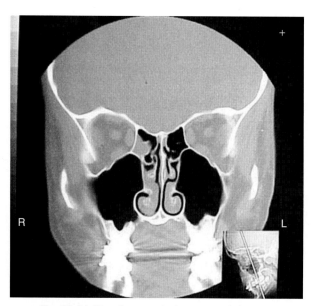

Fig. 29-14 Direct coronal of paranasal sinuses.

OPERATOR'S CONSOLE

The *operator's console* (Fig. 29-15) is the point from which the technologist controls the scanner. A typical console is equipped with a keyboard for entering patient data and a graphic monitor for viewing the images. Other input devices, such as a touch display screen and a computer mouse, may also be used. The operator's console allows the technologist to control and monitor numerous scan parameters. Imaging technique factors, slice thickness, table index, and reconstruction algorithm are some of the scan parameters that are selected at the operator's console.

Before starting an examination, the technologist must enter the patient infor-mation. A keyboard is still necessary for some functions. Usually the first scan program selected is the scout program from which the radiographer plans the sequence of axial scans. An example of a typical scout image is shown in Fig. 29-3. The operator's console is also the location of the monitor, where image manipulation takes place. Most scanners display the image on the monitor in a 1024 matrix interpolated by the computer from the 512 reconstructed images.

One of the most important functions of the operator's console is to initiate the process to store or archive the images for future viewing. Most modern imaging departments now have picture archiving and communications systems (PACS) that are used to store and retrieve soft copy (digital) images.

OTHER COMPONENTS
Display monitor

For the CT image to be displayed on a monitor in a recognizable form, the digital CT data must be converted into a *grayscale image*. This process is achieved by the conversion of each digital CT number in the matrix to an analog voltage. The brightness values of the grayscale image correspond to the pixels and CT numbers of the digital data they represent.

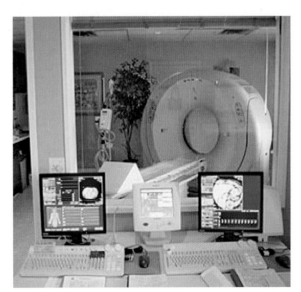

Fig. 29-15 CT operator's console, workstation for three-dimensional image manipulation, and power injector control panel.

Because of the digital nature of the CT image data, image manipulation can be performed to enhance the appearance of the image. One of the most common image processing techniques is called *windowing*, or *gray-level mapping*. This technique allows the technologist to alter the contrast of the displayed image by adjusting the window width (WW) and window level (WL). The *window width* is the range of CT numbers that are used to map signals into shades of gray. Basically, the window width determines the number of gray levels to be displayed in the image controlling contrast resolution. A narrow window width means that there are fewer shades of gray, resulting in higher contrast. Likewise, a wide window width results in more shades of gray in the image, or a longer gray scale. The *window level* determines the midpoint of the range of gray levels to be displayed on the monitor. It is used to set the center CT number within the range of gray levels being used to display the image and controls image brightness. The window level should be set to the CT number of the tissue of interest, and the window width should be set with a range of values that would optimize the contrast between the tissues in the image. Fig. 29-16 shows an axial image seen in two different windows: a standard abdomen window and a bone window adjusted for the spine.

The gray level of any image can be adjusted on the monitor to compensate for differences in patient size and tissue densities or to display the image as desired for the examination protocol. Examples of typical window width and level settings are listed in Table 29-2. These settings are averages and usually vary by vendor and radiologist's preference. The level, although an average, is approximately the same as the CT numbers expected for the tissue densities.

TABLE 29-2

Typical window settings

CT examination	Width	Center (level)
Brain	190	50
Skull	3500	500
Orbits	1200	50
Abdomen	400	35
Liver	175	45
Mediastinum	325	50
Lung	2000	−500
Spinal cord	400	50
Spine	2200	400

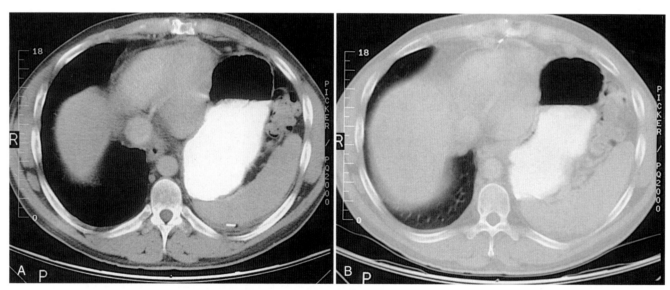

Fig. 29-16 A, Abdominal image, soft tissue window. **B,** Abdominal image, bone window.

Workstation for image manipulation and multiplanar reconstruction

Another advantage of the digital nature of the CT image is the ability to reformat the image data into coronal, sagittal, or oblique body planes without additional radiation to the patient. Image reformation in various planes is accomplished by stacking multiple contiguous axial images, creating a volume of data. Because the CT numbers of the image data within the volume are already known, a sectional image can be generated in any desired plane by selecting a particular plane of data. This postprocessing technique is termed *multiplanar reconstruction* (MPR). A coronal reformation from image data is shown in Figs. 29-17 and 29-18. Fig. 29-17 shows a coronal image of the abdomen (note the liver lesion), and Fig. 29-18 shows coronal images of the lungs displayed with a lung window width and window level. MPRs may also be performed in what is referred to as *curved planar reformations* to visualize structures better. Fig. 29-19 shows an axial image and oblique reformation of the mandible from the axial images. Other postprocessing techniques used today are three-dimensional imaging, surface rendering and volume rendering.

Diagnostic Applications

The original CT studies were used primarily for diagnosing neurologic disorders. As scanner technology advanced, the range of applications was extended to other areas of the body. The most commonly requested procedures involve the head, chest, abdomen, and pelvis. CT is the examination of choice for head trauma;

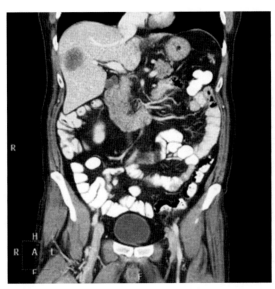

Fig. 29-17 Coronal reformatted image produced from axial images of abdomen and pelvis.

(Courtesy Philips Medical Systems.)

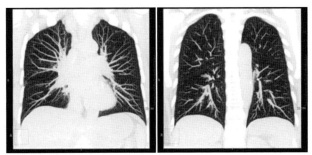

Fig. 29-18 Coronal reformatted images produced from axial low-dose lung nodule study of the chest. Scans produced with Philips Brilliance iCT.

(Courtesy Philips Medical Systems.)

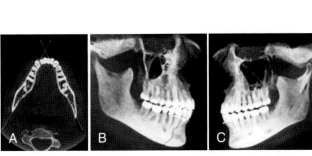

Fig. 29-19 A, Axial mandible showing reformatted planes. **B,** Oblique MPR left mandible (note fracture). **C,** Oblique MPR right mandible.

(Courtesy Philips Medical Systems.)

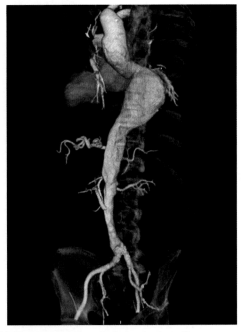

Fig. 29-20 Three-dimensional abdominal aortic aneurysm (*AAA*).

it clearly shows skull fractures and associated subdural hematomas. CT examinations of the head are one of the first exams performed on patients being evaluated for stroke or cerebrovascular accident where evidence of hemorrhage must be ruled out. CT imaging of the central nervous system can show infarctions, hemorrhage, disk herniations, craniofacial and spinal fractures, tumors, and cancers. CT imaging of the body excels at differentiating or distinguishing soft tissue structures within the chest, abdomen, and pelvis. Among the abnormalities shown in this region are metastatic lesions, aneurysms (Fig. 29-20), abscesses, and fluid collections from blunt trauma.

CT is also used for numerous interventional procedures, such as abscess drainage, tissue biopsy (Fig. 29-21), and cyst aspiration. In addition, CT is used during radiofrequency ablations and cryoabla-tions of tumors. Fig. 29-22 shows numerous structures and pathologic conditions identified by CT. Fig. 29-23 shows a liver lesion before radiofrequency ablation, during the procedure and after ablation.

For any procedure, a protocol is required to maximize the amount of diagnostic information available. Specific examination protocols vary according to the needs of different medical facilities and physicians.

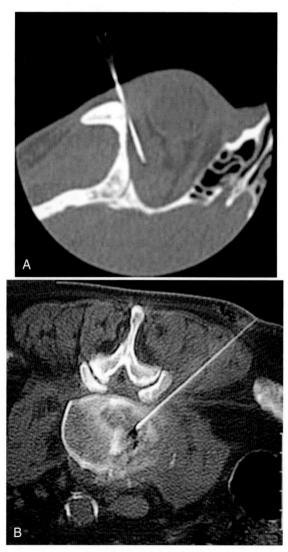

Fig. 29-21 A, Needle biopsy of orbital mass. **B,** Needle biopsy of infectious spondylitis of lumbar vertebral body.

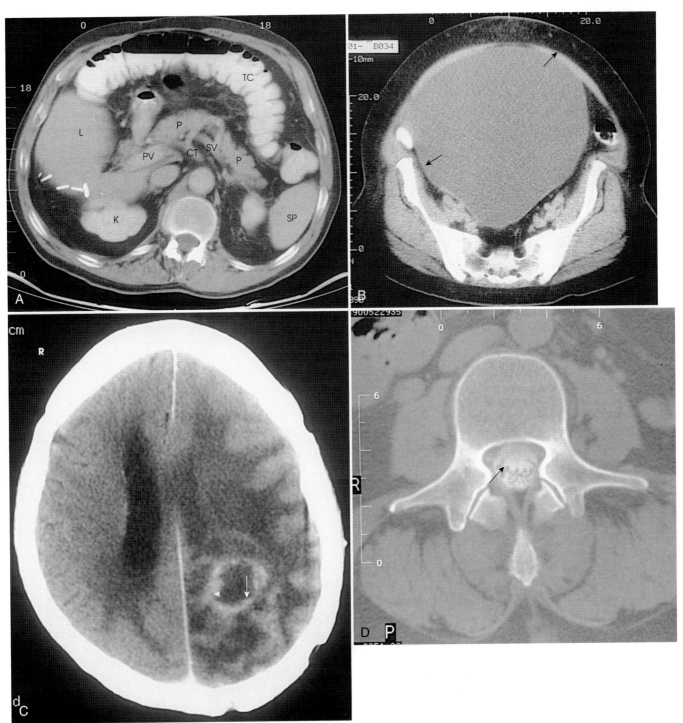

Fig. 29-22 A, Abdominal image showing transverse colon (*TC*) with air-fluid levels; liver (*L*), pancreas (*P*), spleen (*SP*), kidney (*K*), portal vein (*PV*), celiac trunk (*CT*), and splenic veins (*SV*) are shown with contrast medium. Surgical clips are seen in posterior liver. **B,** Abdominal image showing extremely large ovarian cyst (*arrows*). **C,** Brain image showing parietooccipital mass (*arrow*) with characteristic IV contrast ring enhancement (*arrowhead*). **D,** Image of L3 after myelography showing contrast material in thecal sac (*arrow*).

Contrast Media

A contrast medium is used in CT examinations to help distinguish normal anatomy from pathology and to make various disease processes more visible. A contrast agent can be administered intravenously, orally, or rectally. Generally, intravenous (IV) contrast media are the same as media used for excretory urograms. Most facilities use nonionic contrast material for these studies because of the low incidence of reaction and known safety factors associated with nonionic contrast material. IV contrast media are useful for demonstrating tumors within the head; Fig. 29-24 shows a brain scan with and without contrast media. The anterior lesion is evident in the unenhanced scan; in the enhanced scan, the tumor shows characteristic ring enhancement typical of specific tumors seen in CT scans. IV contrast media are also used to visualize vascular structures in the body.

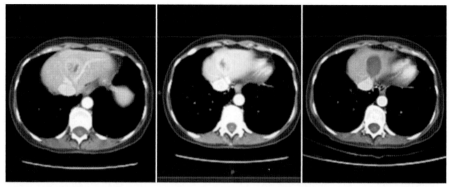

Fig. 29-23 Low-dose axial CT images from radiofrequency ablation study. Scans are before study (*left*), during study (*middle*), and after study (*right*).

(Courtesy Philips Medical Systems.)

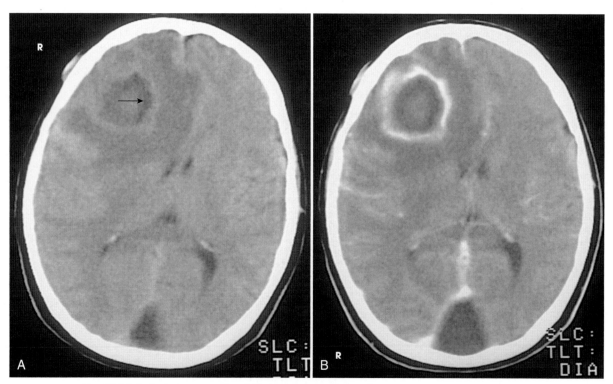

Fig. 29-24 A, Brain image without IV contrast agent showing a low-density lesion (*arrow*).
B, Brain image with IV contrast agent demonstrating ring enhancement.

IV contrast media should be used only with the radiologist's approval and after careful consideration of the patient's medical and allergy history. The patient's renal function must be evaluated before iodinated contrast material is given. Creatinine (CR) level and glomerular filtration rate (GFR) are the most common laboratory values used to determine renal function. Many CT examinations can be performed without IV contrast material if necessary; however, the amount of diagnostic information available may be limited.

Oral contrast media must be used for imaging the abdomen. When given orally, the contrast material in the gastrointestinal tract helps differentiate between loops of bowel and other structures within the abdomen. An oral contrast medium is generally a 2% barium mixture. The low concentration prevents contrast artifacts but allows good visualization of the stomach and intestinal tract. An iodinated contrast material such as oral Hypaque can be used, but it must be mixed at low concentrations to prevent contrast artifacts. A rectal contrast medium is often requested as part of an abdominal or a pelvic protocol. Usually mixed in the same concentration as the oral contrast medium, the rectal contrast material is useful for showing the distal colon relative to the bladder and other structures of the pelvic cavity. Tap water may also be used as a contrast medium depending on the area of interest and pathologic indications.

POWER INJECTOR USE FOR ADMINISTERING INTRAVENOUS CONTRAST MEDIA

Power injector use in CT examinations became mandatory when the first helical CT scanners were introduced. Faster delivery of IV contrast media became necessary with the reduced scan times used in helical CT. The advantage of power injector use is that a bolus injection of contrast medium can be delivered quickly, which provides for better contrast enhancement of structures and better opacification of the blood vessels. The use of power injectors also provides a means to reproduce examination parameters and allows for different vascular phases to be captured.

EQUIPMENT

Power injector equipment includes an injector assembly that is ceiling mounted next to the scanner or on a movable stand. The injector head typically has two syringes; however, some models may have only a single-syringe delivery system. If the injector head is a double-syringe system, each of the syringe controls is color coded. The same color-coding system is shown on the injector control module that is next to the CT scan console. The injector must be programmed at the control module, but operational buttons are located on the injector head as well.

The control module for the system is typically placed on or near the operator console of the scanner. Each injector system has controls for flow rate of the injection, pounds per square inch (psi) of pressure used for the injection, amount of contrast medium to be delivered, and time delays. Dual-head systems have dual sets of controls for each syringe. Dual-head systems are used when the radiologist requests a saline flush to follow the contrast injection.

Special pressure syringes and pressure tubing must be used when injecting. The pressure injections must be closely monitored, and care must be taken that no air is in the syringe or tubing. The pressure syringes have oval etchings on the side of the syringe as a safety feature. If the syringe is full of contrast material, the oval etchings appear round when viewed through the syringe owing to light refraction. If no fluid is present, the etchings remain oval in shape (Fig. 29-25).

Correct IV catheter size and placement is vital to the success of the CT examination. Catheters are typically placed in the arm veins in the antecubital fossa; however, veins lower in the forearm can also be used. Small veins should be avoided because of the pressures used

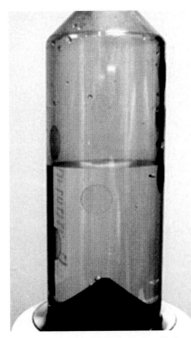

Fig. 29-25 CT pressure syringe partially filled with contrast material. Note oval etching above fluid level and round etching below fluid level.

when injecting. Catheter size depends on the type of CT examination being performed. A routine, non-CTA examination typically uses a 22-gauge Angiocath with an injection rate of 2 mL/sec. A CTA study requires a larger bore 18-gauge to 20-gauge Angiocath with an injection rate of 4 to 7 mL/sec.

PATIENT CARE AND INJECTION SAFETY

Patient positioning should be considered when placing the IV line. For many CT examinations, the patients must keep their arms resting above the head on a pillow or sponge during the examination. Care should be taken to make the patients as comfortable as possible while keeping their arms as straight as possible. The angiocatheter should not be placed in a site that would be bent when the patient elevates the arms above the head.

Proper placement of the Angiocath should always be confirmed with a hand test injection of saline that mimics the injection rate of the examination. The ease of injection and the injection site should be observed and palpated during the test injection to confirm patency of the vein. Patients should be instructed to notify the CT technologist immediately if they experience any pain or discomfort at the injection site during the procedure.

All connections between the Angiocath, injector tubing, and syringe should be checked and tightened to prevent air from entering the IV line. The pressure syringe should be checked for air bubbles, and the etchings on the side of the syringe should be confirmed as round. The injected head and syringe should be pointed down to ensure that any potential air bubble rises back into the syringe base and away from the IV line.

The patient should be instructed about the timing of the scan, the injection, and sensations of warmth and an odd taste caused by the dilation of the blood vessels. These sensations should be discussed with the patient, and the patient should be reassured that these are normal and fade quickly. The intensity of warmth and taste intensify as the injection amount and rate increase, so these are more intense for a patient having a CTA study.

If the patient complains of discomfort at or near the injection site, the injection should be terminated, and the patient should be checked for a contrast extravasation (contrast material leaking out of the vein). If there is any change in the appearance of the patient's arm (swelling, discoloration), the radiologist should be notified immediately. The CT technologist should be familiar with the department policy for the treatment of extravasation, which typically includes cold or hot compresses and elevation of the arm.

Factors Affecting Image Quality

In CT, the technologist has access to numerous scan parameters that can have a dramatic effect on image quality. The four main factors contributing to image quality are spatial resolution, contrast resolution, noise, and artifacts.

SPATIAL RESOLUTION

Spatial resolution is determined by the degree of blur or the ability to see the difference between two objects that are close together. The method most commonly used to evaluate spatial resolution is the number of line pairs per centimeter (lp/cm). The scan parameters that affect spatial resolution include scanning section thickness, display FOV, matrix, and reconstruction slice thickness and algorithm/kernel. The detector aperture width is the most significant geometric factor that contributes to spatial resolution.

CONTRAST RESOLUTION

Contrast resolution is the ability to differentiate between small differences in density within the image. Currently, tissues with density differences of less than 0.5% can be distinguished with CT. The scan parameters that affect contrast resolution are slice thickness, reconstruction algorithm, image display (window width), and x-ray beam energy. The size of the patient and the detector sensitivity also have a direct effect on contrast resolution.

TEMPORAL RESOLUTION

Temporal resolution is the ability of the CT system to freeze any motion of a scanned object. It is the shortest amount of time needed to acquire a complete data set. The use of CT in cardiac imaging requires high (shortest time) temporal resolution to decrease heart motion. Factors that improve temporal resolution include multidetector CT (i.e., 64-, 128-, 256-, 320-slice), tube/gantry rotation time, and the development of dual-source CT.

NOISE

The most common cause of *noise* in CT is *quantum noise*. This type of noise arises from the random variation in photon detection. Noise in a CT image primarily affects contrast resolution. As noise increases in an image, contrast resolution decreases. Noise gives an image a grainy quality or a mottled appearance. Among the scan parameters that influence noise are matrix size, slice thickness, x-ray beam energy, and reconstruction algorithm. Scattered radiation and patient size also contribute to the noise of an image. New technology is available to prevent scatter radiation from hitting the detector. Fig. 29-26 shows the ClearRay Anti-Scatter Collimator (Philips Medical Systems), which greatly reduces noise and increases contrast resolution.

ARTIFACTS

Metallic objects, such as dental fillings, pacemakers, and artificial joints, can cause starburst or *streak artifacts,* which can obscure diagnostic information. Dense residual barium from fluoroscopy examinations can cause *artifacts* similar to those caused by metallic objects. Many CT departments do not perform a CT examination in a patient until several days after barium studies to allow the body to eliminate the residual barium from the area of interest. Large differences in tissue densities of adjoining structures can cause artifacts that detract from image quality. Bone-soft tissue interfaces, such as occur with the skull and brain, often cause streak or shadow artifacts on CT images; these artifacts are referred to as *beam hardening* (Fig. 29-27).

New software developments have greatly improved image quality and reduced artifacts. Interactive reconstruction methods like Philips Medical's iDose4 and orthopedic metal artifact reduction (OMAR) (Fig. 29-28).

OTHER FACTORS
Patient factors

Patient factors also contribute to the quality of an image. If a patient cannot or will not hold still, the scan is likely to be nondiagnostic. Body size also can have an effect on image quality. Large patients attenuate more radiation than small patients; this can increase image noise, detracting from overall image quality. An increase in milliampere-seconds (mAs) is usually required to compensate for large body size. This increase results in a higher radiation dose to the patient. Image quality factors under technologist control include slice thickness, *scan time, scan diameter,* and patient instructions. Slice thickness is usually dictated by image *protocol.* As in

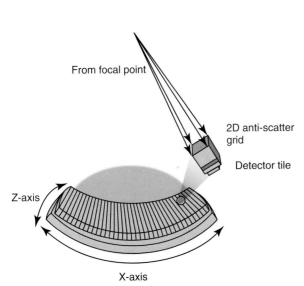

Fig. 29-26 Philips Medical Systems 2D Anti-scatter Grid, which can be focused for true three-dimensional cone-beam geometry. Scatter reduction improves low contrast resolution.

(Courtesy Philips Medical Systems.)

From focal point

2D anti-scatter grid

Detector tile

Z-axis

X-axis

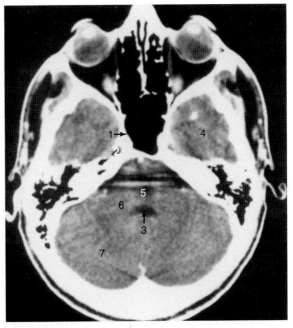

Fig. 29-27 Streaking through the posterior fossa represents beam-hardening artifact. Normal appearance of the brain. *1,* Sphenoid sinus; *2,* trigeminal ganglion; *3,* fourth ventricle; *4,* temporal lobe; *5,* pons; *6,* middle cerebellar peduncle; *7,* cerebellar hemisphere.

tomography, the thinner the slice thickness, the better the image-recorded detail. Thin-section CT scans, often referred to as *high-resolution scans,* are used to show structures better (Fig. 29-29). However, thinner slices require more mA increasing the dose to the patient.

As in conventional radiography, patient instructions are a crucial part of a diagnostic examination. Explaining the procedure fully in terms that the patient can understand increases the level of compliance from almost any patient.

Scan times

Scan times are usually preselected by the computer as part of the scan protocol, but they can be altered by the technologist.

When selecting a scan time, the technologist must take into account possible patient motion such as inadvertent body movements, breathing, or peristalsis. A good guideline is to choose a scan time that would minimize patient motion while providing a quality diagnostic image. When it is necessary to scan an uncooperative patient quickly, using the shortest scan time possible may allow the technologist to complete the examination, although the quality of the images obtained is likely to be compromised.

Scan diameter

The amount of the detector utilized for imaging is referred to as the scan FOV (SFOV). When imaging a pediatric

patient, the entire detector does not have to be active for such a small patient. The image that appears on the monitor depends on the *display FOV (DFOV).* The technologist can adjust the DFOV to include the entire cross section of the body part being scanned or to include only a specified region within the part. For most head, chest, and abdomen examinations, the selected scan diameter includes all anatomy of the body part to just outside the skin borders. Certain examinations may require the DFOV to be reduced to include specific anatomy, such as the sella turcica, sinuses, one lung, mediastinal vessels, suprarenal glands, one kidney, or the prostate.

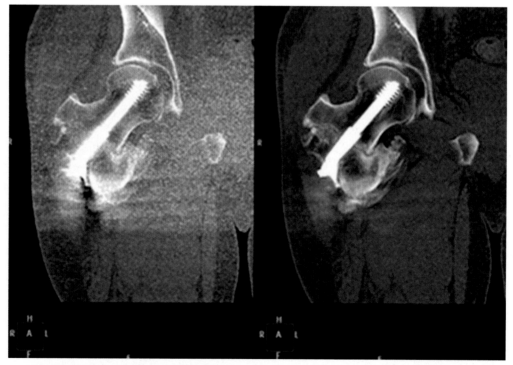

Fig. 29-28 Philips Medical Systems iDos4 and OMAR techniques to reduce noise and artifacts on patient with a hip pinning.

(Courtesy Philips Medical Systems.)

Special Features
DYNAMIC SCANNING

One advantage of CT is that data can be obtained for image reconstruction by the computer at a later time. The scanner can be programmed to scan through an area rapidly. In this situation, raw data are saved, but image reconstruction after each scan is bypassed to shorten scan time.

Dynamic scanning is based on the principle that after contrast agent administration, different structures enhance at different rates. Dynamic scanning can consist of rapid sequential scanning at the same level to observe contrast material filling within a structure, such as is performed when evaluating enhancement within a tumor. Another form is incremental dynamic scanning, which consists of rapid serial scanning at consecutive levels during the bolus injection of a contrast medium such as is performed when evaluating the patient for aortic aneurysm or perfusion imaging on stroke patients.

SINGLE SLICE SPIRAL OR HELICAL COMPUTED TOMOGRAPHY

Single slice *spiral CT* (SSCT) and *helical CT* are terms used to describe a method of data acquisition in CT. During spiral CT, the gantry is rotating continuously while the table moves through the gantry aperture. The continuous gantry rotation combined with the continuous table movement forms the spiral path from which raw data are obtained one slice per revolution (Fig. 29-30). Slip-ring technology has made continuous rotation of the x-ray tube possible by eliminating the large high-voltage cables between the x-ray tube and the generators.

One of the unique features of spiral CT is that it scans a volume of tissue rather than a group of individual slices. This method makes it extremely useful for the detection of small lesions because an arbitrary slice can be reconstructed along any position within the volume of raw data. In addition, because a volume of tissue is scanned in a single breath, respiratory motion can be minimized. For a volume scan of the chest, such as shown in Fig. 29-31, the patient is instructed to hold the breath, and a tissue volume of 24 mm is obtained in a 5-second spiral scan.

Two of the resultant images show a small lung nodule without breathing interference of *image misregistration;* a three-dimensional reconstruction of the lung clearly shows the pathologic condition. Spiral CT is especially useful when scanning uncooperative or combative patients; patients who cannot tolerate lying down for long periods; and patients who cannot hold still, such as pediatric patients or trauma patients. The use of spiral CT may

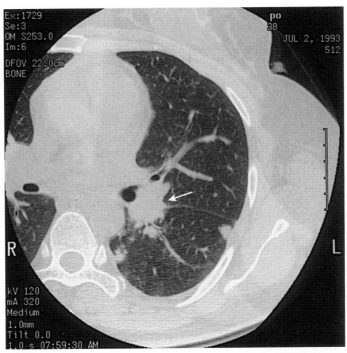

Fig. 29-29 High-resolution 1-mm slice using edge enhancement algorithm, showing nodule in left lung (*arrow*).

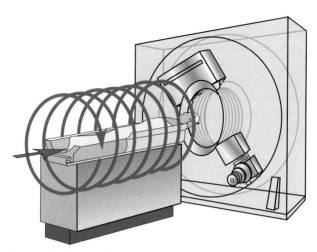

Fig. 29-30 Continuous gantry rotation combined with continuous table rotation, forming a spiral path of data.

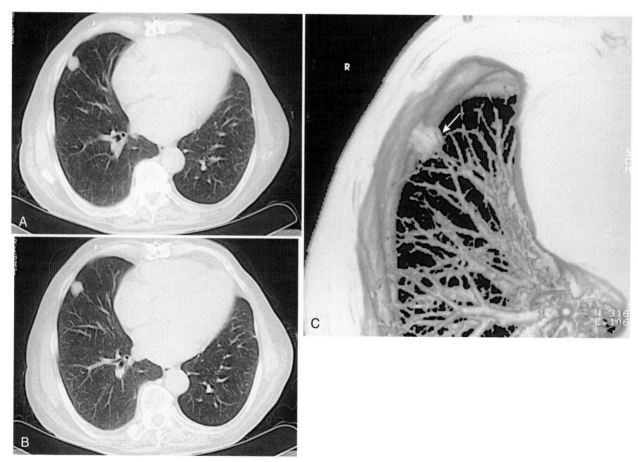

Fig. 29-31 A and **B,** Spiral images of lung showing lung nodule and associated vasculature. **C,** Three-dimensional reconstruction of lung nodule (*arrow*) after spiral scan.

(Courtesy Siemens Medical Systems, Iselin, NJ.)

decrease the amount of contrast medium necessary to visualize structures; this makes the examination safer and more cost-effective.

MULTISLICE SPIRAL OR HELICAL COMPUTED TOMOGRAPHY

Multislice helical CT (MSHCT) or *multidetector CT (MDCT)* systems incorporate a detector array that contains multiple rows of detector (channels) along the *z* axis compared with the single row of detectors in conventional spiral CT (SSCT). Each channel comprises numerous elements. In a "four-row" scanner, the detector array is connected to four data acquisition systems that generate four channels of data (Fig. 29-32). This type of detector array would allow a scan four times faster than the conventional single row spiral/helical scanner. Current technology detector arrays have 4, 8, 16, 32, 64, 128, 256, and 320 rows or channels. The increased width of the detector now requires the x-ray beam to be a cone-beam configuration compared with the fan beam used for SSCT. The 64-, 128-, 256-, and 320-row scanners are referred to as *volume CT (VCT)* systems because the amount of body section coverage in a single tube rotation. Figs. 29-33 and 29-34 were acquired on the Toshiba 320 row scanner in a single revolution. Fig. 29-33 is a three-dimensional volume rendering (VR) pediatric chest image acquired in 0.035 second. Fig. 29-34 shows a 16-cm volume coverage that allows for whole-brain perfusion imaging for evaluation of stroke.

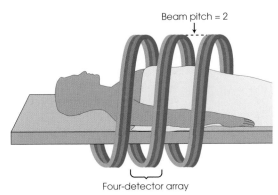

Fig. 29-32 Four-detector array with a beam pitch of 2 covers eight times the tissue volume of a single-slice spiral CT scan.

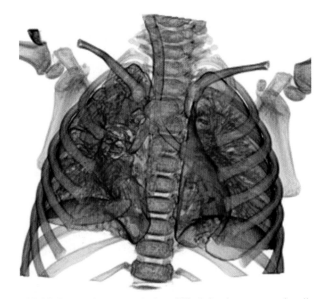

Fig. 29-33 Technology employing 320 detector rows makes it possible to scan an infant's chest with fine detail, low radiation dose, and fast acquisition times. This image is a three-dimensional VR acquired in a single rotation completed in 0.035 second.

(Courtesy Toshiba America Medical Systems.)

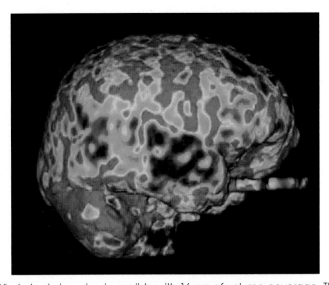

Fig. 29-34 Whole-brain imaging is possible with 16 cm of volume coverage. This three-dimensional VR whole-brain perfusion study shows evidence of acute stroke.

(Courtesy Toshiba America Medical Systems.)

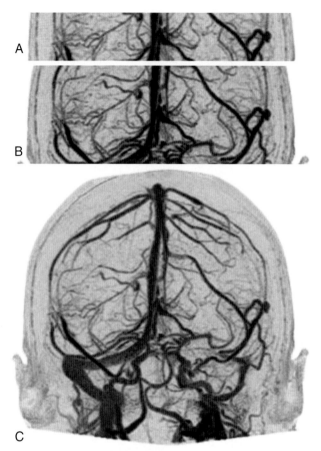

A

B

C

Fig. 29-35 Images show scan range for various row scanners. **A,** 64-row scanner. **B,** 128-row scanner. **C,** 320-row scanner. The 320-row scanner allows complete imaging of the cranial vessels with one table location.

(Courtesy Toshiba America Medical Systems.)

Cardiac imaging using VCT is a rapidly growing component of CT imaging. The advantages of MSHCT/MDCT include isotropic imaging and postprocessing, greater anatomic coverage, multiphase studies, faster examination times, and improved spatial resolution. The advancement of VCT, with increasing larger detector arrays, has provided unique clinical opportunities in diagnostic medicine. Fig. 29-35 compares the z-axis coverage of 64-, 128-, and 320-row detectors.

COMPUTED TOMOGRAPHY ANGIOGRAPHY

CTA is an application of spiral CT that uses three-dimensional imaging techniques. With CTA, the vascular system can be viewed in three dimensions. The three basic steps required to generate CTA images are as follows:

1. Choice of parameters for IV administration of the *bolus* of contrast medium (i.e., injection rate, injection duration, and delay between bolus initiation and the start of the scan sequence)
2. Choice of spiral parameters to maximize the contrast medium in the target vessel (i.e., *scan duration,* collimation, and *table speed*)
3. Reconstruction of two-dimensional image data into three-dimensional image data

CTA has several advantages over conventional angiography. CTA uses spiral technology; an arbitrary image within the volume of data can be retrospectively reconstructed without exposing the patient to additional IV contrast medium or radiation. During postprocessing of the image data, overlying structures can be eliminated so that only the vascular anatomy is reconstructed. Finally, because CTA is an IV procedure that does not require arterial puncture, only minimal postprocedure observation is necessary.

Currently, CTA is replacing angiography as a diagnostic tool for some studies. This is especially true in departments using multirow detectors that allow significantly faster scanning. Fig. 29-36 shows the vessels of the brain, whereas Fig. 29-37 shows the renal vessels in a three-dimensional format. The heart and coronary vessels are shown in Fig. 29-38,

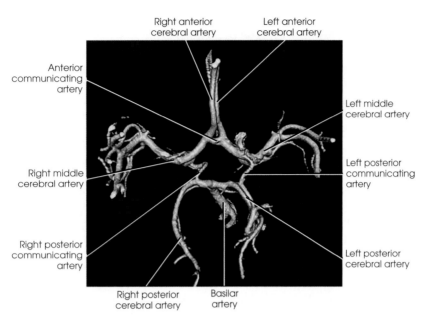

Right anterior
cerebral artery

Left anterior
cerebral artery

Anterior
communicating
artery

Left middle
cerebral artery

Right middle
cerebral artery

Left posterior
communicating
artery

Right posterior
communicating
artery

Left posterior
cerebral artery

Right posterior
cerebral artery

Basilar
artery

Fig. 29-36 Color CT angiography of circle of Willis.

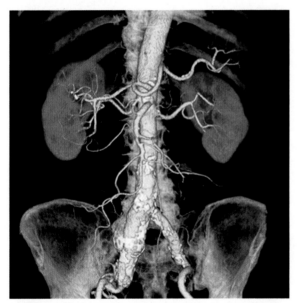

Fig. 29-37 Color CT angiography in three-dimensional format.

(Courtesy Toshiba America Medical Systems.)

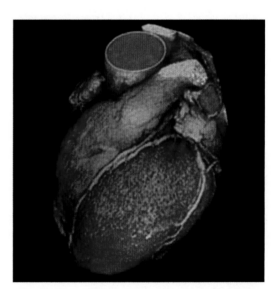

Fig. 29-38 Color three-dimensional cardiac CTA.

and a graft is shown in Fig. 29-39. Fig. 29-40 shows multiple reformations from a cardiac gated dose reduction method performed on a Philips Medical 256-row scanner. Fig. 29-41 is a brain perfusion study showing significant vascular changes on a patient with an acute stroke.

THREE-DIMENSIONAL IMAGING

A rapidly expanding area of CT is three-dimensional imaging. This is a *post-processing* technique that is applied to raw data to create realistic images of the surface anatomy to be visualized. The introduction of advanced computers and faster software programs has dramatically increased the applications of three-dimensional imaging. The common techniques used in creating three-dimensional images include *maximum intensity projection* (MIP), *shaded surface display* (SSD), and *volume rendering* (VR). All techniques use three initial steps to create the three-dimensional images from the original CT data:

1. *Construction* of a volume of three-dimensional data from the original two-dimensional CT image data. This same process is used in MPR.
2. *Segmentation* to crop or edit the target objects from the reconstructed data. This step eliminates unwanted information from the CT data.
3. *Rendering* or *shading* to provide depth perception to the final image.

Maximum intensity projection

MIP consists of reconstructing the brightest pixels from a stack of two-dimensional or three-dimensional image data into a three-dimensional image. The data are rotated on an arbitrary axis, and an imaginary ray is passed through the data in specific increments. The brightest pixel found along each ray is *mapped* into a grayscale image. MIP is commonly used for CTA.

Shaded surface display

SSD provides a three-dimensional image of the surface of a particular structure. After the original two-dimensional data are reconstructed into three-dimensional data, the different tissue types within the image need to be separated. This process, called *segmentation,* can be performed by drawing a line around the tissue of interest or, more commonly, by setting *threshold values.* A threshold value can be set for a particular CT number; the result is that any pixel that has an equal or greater CT number than the threshold value would be selected for the three-dimensional image. When the threshold value is set and the data are reconstructed into a three-dimensional image, a shading technique is applied. The shading or rendering technique provides depth perception in the reconstructed image.

Volume rendering

VR techniques incorporate the entire volume of data into a three-dimensional image by summing the contributions of each voxel along a line from the viewer's eye through the data set. This results in a three-dimensional image in which the dynamic range throughout the image is preserved. Rather than being limited to surface data, a VR image can display a wide range of tissues that accurately depict the anatomic relationships between vasculature and viscera. Because VR incorporates and processes the entire data set, much more powerful computers are required to reconstruct three-dimensional VR images at a reasonable speed.

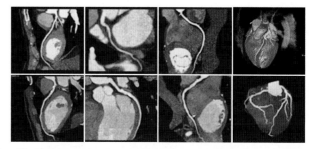

Fig. 29-40 Prospectively gated CT angiograms. Low-dose studies performed with Philips Step and Shoot Cardiac software that has arrhythmia detection that stops scans until ECG stabilizes.

(Courtesy Philips Medical Systems.)

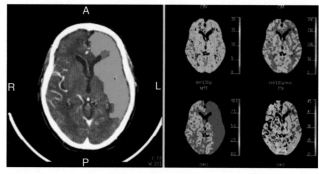

Fig. 29-41 CT brain perfusion study with brain perfusion parameter maps (*right four images*) and summary map overlays (*left*) showing areas of ischemic penumbra (*green*) and infarct (*red*). Images were acquired using a lower dose protocol on a Philips Brilliance CT scanner.

(Courtesy Philips Medical Systems.)

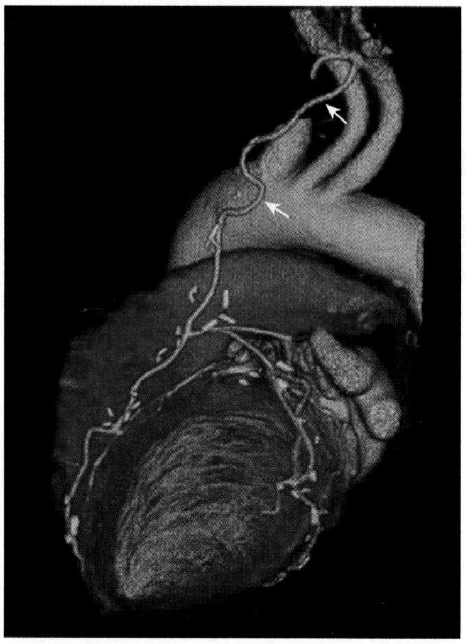

Fig. 29-39 Color three-dimensional cardiac CTA with graft (*arrows*).

Referring physicians and surgeons use three-dimensional images to correlate CT images clinically to the actual anatomic contours of their patients (Fig. 29-42). These reconstructions are especially useful in surgical procedures. Three-dimensional reconstructions are often requested as part of patient evaluation after trauma and for presurgical planning. Fig. 29-43 shows examples of the three common three-dimensional rendering techniques.

RADIATION TREATMENT PLANNING

Radiation therapy has been used for nearly as long as radiology has been in existence. The introduction of CT has had a major impact on radiation treatment planning. The use of spiral CT in conjunction with MPR provides a three-dimensional approach to radiation treatment planning. This method helps the dosimetrist plan treatment so that the radiation dose to the target is maximized and the dose to normal tissue is minimized. The three-dimensional simulation software offers the following: volumetric, high-precision localization; calculation of the geometric center of the defined target; patient marking systems; and virtual simulators capable of producing digitally reconstructed radiographs in *real time*. With the new, specially designed software, a single CT simulation procedure can replace a total of three procedures (one conventional CT scan and two conventional simulations) for radiation treatment planning (Fig. 29-44).

If the CT system is being used for radiation treatment planning, the standard curved couch cannot be used. Instead, a flat, firm board should be placed on the couch. Most radiation therapy departments have their own CT units today. A flat patient couch is substituted on the dedicated therapy units. In this way, the actual therapy delivery can be simulated more accurately. Fig. 29-45 shows the external skin markers and structures that would be in the beam's path.

PET/CT SCANNERS

When a CT scanner is coupled with a positron emission tomography (PET)

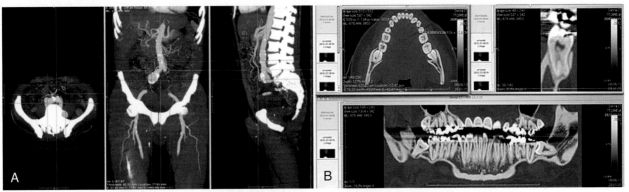

Fig. 29-42 A, MPR reconstruction of abdominal aorta. **B,** Curved MPR of mandible.

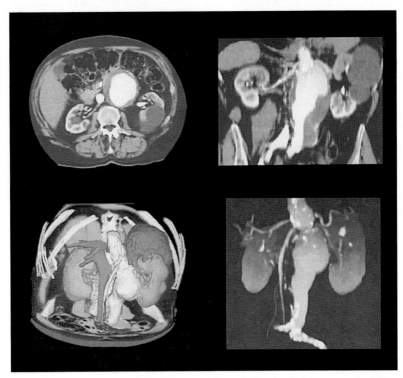

Fig. 29-43 Common three-dimensional rendering techniques used in CT.

(Courtesy Elicit, Hackensack, NJ.)

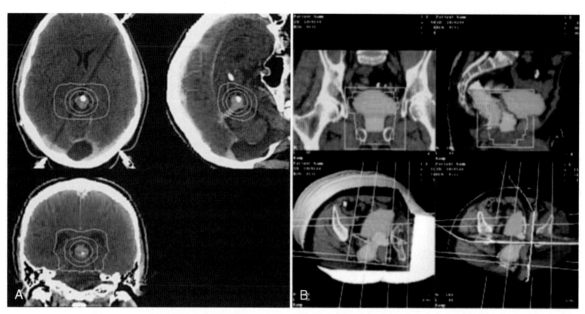

Fig. 29-44 A, Brain localization in three planes. **B,** Three-dimensional prostate therapy localization.

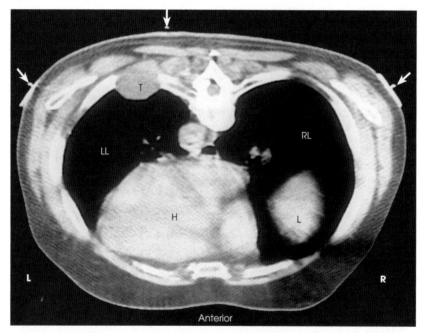

Fig. 29-45 Patient in prone position for radiation treatment planning. Radiopaque markers (*arrows*) show location of treatment field skin marks: tumor (*T*), heart (*H*), liver (*L*), right lung (*RL*), and left lung (*LL*).

scanner, it is referred to as a PET/CT scanner. The PET/CT scanner comprises two scanners in close proximity to each other with a single patient couch that travels between the two scanners. In some scanner configurations, there is a small gap between the scanner housings; in other configurations, the scanner appears to be a single unit. Current PET/CT scanners are typically third-generation scanners and incorporate the latest in detector technology. Most modern PET/CT scanners incorporate 8-, 16-, and 64-row detectors. PET/CT is discussed in more detail in Chapter 32; the scanners are typically housed in the nuclear medicine department instead of the CT department. The CT scanner is used for attenuation correction and anatomic correlation for the functional PET scans. Many patients require a more detailed diagnostic CT examination as well, however, which has required nuclear medicine technologists to obtain additional education and certification in CT to be able to perform the diagnostic CT exams. Fig. 29-46 shows sagittal reconstructed CT spine images and the corresponding PET images and PET/CT fusion image.

QUALITY CONTROL

The goal of any quality assurance program in CT is to ensure that the system is producing the best possible image quality with the minimum radiation dose to the patient. A CT system is a complex combination of sensitive and expensive equipment that requires systematic monitoring for performance and image quality. Most CT systems require weekly or biweekly preventive maintenance to ensure proper operation.

Preventive maintenance is usually performed by a service engineer from the manufacturer or a private company. Increasingly, the technologist is being assigned the responsibility of performing and documenting routine quality assurance tests. Many technologists routinely perform daily test scans on a water phantom to measure the consistency of the CT numbers and to record the standard deviation. As data are recorded over time, the CT scanner's current operating condition and its performance over longer time periods can be evaluated. Many units are also capable of *air calibrations,* which do not require the water phantom and can be performed between patients for unit self-calibration.

A CT phantom is typically multisectioned and is constructed from plastic cylinders, with each section filled with test objects designed to measure the performance of specific parameters. Some phantoms are designed to allow numerous parameters to be evaluated with a single scan. The recommended quality assurance tests for evaluating routine performance include contrast scale and mean CT number of water, high-contrast resolution, low-contrast resolution, laser light accuracy, noise and uniformity, slice thickness, and patient dose.

Computed Tomography and Radiation Dose

Calculating the radiation dose received during CT examinations presents a unique set of circumstances. Typically, radiation received during radiologic examinations comes from a fixed source with delivery to the patient in one or two planes (e.g., anteroposterior [AP] and lateral projections). These exposure parameters typically produce a much higher entrance skin dose than the exit skin dose, which creates a large dose gradient across the patient. In contrast, CT exposures (helical/spiral) originate from an essentially continuous source that rotates 360 degrees around the patient. This results in a radially symmetric radiation dose gradient within the patient.

Equipment manufacturers are developing new hardware to reduce patient dose to include off-focal radiation suppression devices, beam shaping filters, *z*-axis

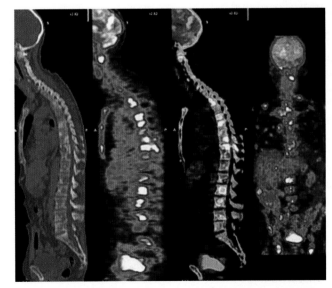

Fig. 29-46 Sagittal reformatted CT scan (*far left*), sagittal PET (*second from left*), PET/CT fusion image (*second from right*) and coronal PET (*far right*).

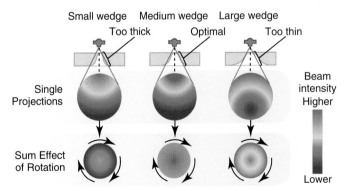

Fig. 29-47 Diagram represents selectable bowtie filters that reduce patient dose and improve image quality. These are referred to as SmartShape wedges on the Philips Brilliance iCT scanner. Note how correct wedge selection affects patient dose. Wedges are typically small (infants 0 to 18 months), medium (cardiac), and large (adult head and body). Wedge selection is built into scan protocols.

(Courtesy Philips Medical Systems.)

efficiency with increased collimation, and improved data acquisition systems (DAS). Fig. 29-47 demonstrates the SmartShape wedge from Philips Medical Systems, which is an example of a beam-shaping filter. Note the dose reduction shown on the center image when the appropriate filter is applied. Z-axis efficiency reduces dose effects related to "overscanning," which occurs in helical or spiral scanning systems. CT data acquisition systems are utilizing higher efficiency detector material to minimize electronic noise. Also software development has allowed optimization of image quality based on interative reconstruction. Using iterative reconstruction allows for a reduction in dose to the patient while maintaining image quality, reducing noise, which improves spatial resolution and low contrast detectability. For the pediatric population, dedicated protocols have been developed and included in the CT purchase.

Measurements of CT dose are typically performed using a circular CT dosimetry phantom that is made of polymethyl

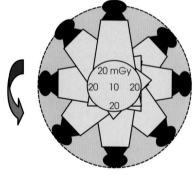

Fig. 29-48 CT dose profile for body.

(Data from McNitt-Gray MF: AAPM/RSNA physics tutorial for residents: topics in CT. Radiation dose in CT, *RadioGraphics* 22:1541, 2002.)

methacrylate (PMMA) with implanted thermoluminescent dosimeters (TLDs). The TLDs are positioned 1 cm below the surface around the periphery of the phantom and at the center (isocenter). The typical phantom sizes are 32 cm for body calculations and 16 cm for head calculations. For a single axial scan location (one full rotation of the tube, no table movement), the typical dose for the body phantom is 20 mGy at the periphery and 10 mGy at the isocenter. The typical dose for the head phantom is higher at 40 mGy at the periphery and 40 mGy at the isocenter. See Fig. 29-48 for the body and Fig. 29-49 for the head. Dose is size dependent (e.g., dose differs depending on head scan or body scan and whether the patient is a child or an adult).

Another component of dose to the patient is distribution of absorbed dose along the length of the patient from one single scan (full rotation at one table location). The radiation dose profile (Fig. 29-50) is not limited just to the slice location; the "tails" of the dose profile contribute to the absorbed dose outside of the primary beam. The size of the contribution to dose from the adjacent sections is directly related to the spacing of the slices and the width and shape of the radiation profile. The first method used to describe dose as a result of multiple scan locations was the *multiple scan average dose* (MSAD). MSAD described average dose resulting from scans over an interval length on the patient. Next was the *computed tomography dose index* (CTDI), which was calculated using a normalized beam width and a standard of 14 contiguous axial slices. This method required a dose profile measured with TLDs or film,

neither of which was convenient. To overcome the measurement limitations, another dose index, the $CTDI_{100}$, was developed. This dose index allowed profile calculations along the full length (100 mm) of a pencil ionization chamber and did not require nominal section widths. To provide a weighted average of the center and peripheral contributions, $CTDI_w$ was created. The final descriptor is $CTDI_{vol}$, which accounts for the helical pitch or axial scan spacing that is used for a specific protocol. The most common reporting method of dose reporting on the present scanners is the *dose-length product* (DLP). This is the $CTDI_{vol}$ multiplied by the length of the scan (cm). It is reported in mGy/cm.

Patient dose must be a part of the permanent record for each examination. Each manufacturer displays dose parameters in various ways. Fig. 29-51 is an example of how Philips Medical Systems displays dose information (note parameters within blue box just above the "go" button). To assist in preventing excessive exposure to patients, the American Association of Physicists in Medicine (AAPM) published a "Notifications Levels Statement" with preestablished *notification values* for individual scans using CTDI$_{vol}$ (mGy). Notification values (NV) are predetermined and set-up within the exam protocol, the technologist is notified when any scan series within the complete exam protocol exceeds the preset value. The alert value (AV) notifies the technologist when the cumulative dose index value exceeds the preset value. The dose checking systems will track and report all instances when established diagnostic reference levels (DRLs) have been exceeded.

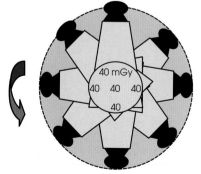

Fig. 29-49 CT dose profile for head.

(Data from McNitt-Gray MF: AAPM/RSNA physics tutorial for residents: topics in CT. Radiation dose in CT, *RadioGraphics* 22:1541, 2002.)

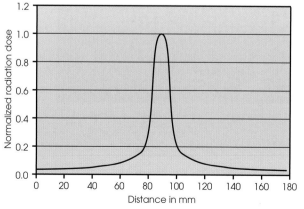

Fig. 29-50 Single-slice CT dose profile.

ESTIMATING EFFECTIVE DOSE

Effective dose takes into account where the radiation dose is being absorbed (e.g., which tissue or organ has absorbed the radiation). The International Commission on Radiological Protection (ICRP) sets the weighting factors for each radiosensitive organ (available at www.ICRP.org). Effective dose is measured in sieverts (Sv) or rems (100 rem = 1 Sv). The effective dose is determined by multiplying the DLP by a region-specific conversion factor. The conversion factors are 0.017 mSv/mGy/cm for chest imaging, 0.019 mSv/mGy/cm for pelvis imaging, and 0.0023 mSv/mGy/cm for head imaging. The conversion factor for head scans is considerably less because fewer radiosensitive organs are irradiated. (The DLP for a given chest examination is 375 mGy; the resulting estimated effective dose is 375 multiplied by 0.017, which equals 6.4 mSv.)

Factors That Affect Dose

The factors that directly influence the radiation dose to the patient are beam energy (kVp), tube current (mA), rotation or exposure time (seconds), section or slice thickness (beam collimation), object thickness and attenuation (size of the patient, pediatric versus adult), pitch or section spacing (table distance traveled in one 360-degree rotation), dose reduction techniques (mA modulation), and distance from the tube to isocenter. Patient shielding in the scan area is now possible with bismuth-filled shields, which yield little image artifact but provide 50% to 60% dose reduction. Adult breast shields, various sized pediatric breast shields, thyroid shields, and eye shields are presently available.

Each vendor has optimized the ability to use automatic exposure control in CT, developing a product for automatic tube current modulation (ATCM) and calculating or using patient attenuation measurements in one or more planes. Fig. 29-52 shows a technique of mA modulation that uses an AP and lateral scout image to calculate patient thickness, which results in automatic mA adjustments during the scan (see *red line*). New "selectable" filters (Fig. 29-53) have been developed that allow different filter applications based on body section or patient age or size. These filters can reduce dose by nearly 30% when using 120 kVp and 45% when using 80 kVp. Equipment manufactures include an automated dose-optimized selection of the tube voltage, as in some instances a lower kVp may provide better images with a lower dose.

Beam collimation (slice thickness) varies in single-detector scanners and multidetector scanners. Beam collimation for single-detector systems has minimal effect on dose; however, this is not the case for multidetector scanners. These

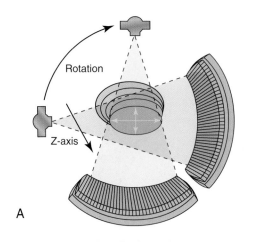

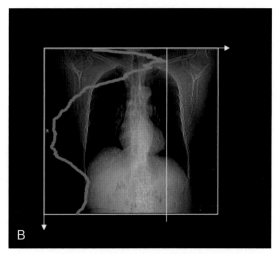

Fig. 29-51 Dose amounts must be reported for every series and protocol performed. Each manufacturer displays information differently. Note CTDI and DLP displayed inside the blue box.

(Courtesy Philips Medical Systems.)

Fig. 29-52 A, AP and lateral scout images performed for mA modulation calculations. Note thickness difference A/P versus R/L. **B,** Philips DoseRight automated tube current selection (ACS). *Red line* shows z-axis dose modulation. Note technique increase in shoulder and abdomen region and technique decrease in lung region.

(Courtesy Philips Medical Systems.)

scanners have multiple ways to scan and reconstruct images. A multidetector scanner can perform axial scans of 4 × 1.25 mm (5-mm beam width, 1.25-mm slice reconstruction), 4 × 2.5 mm (10-mm beam width, 2.25-mm slice reconstruction), and 4 × 5 mm (20-mm beam width, 5-mm slice reconstruction). When all other parameters are kept constant, there are significant differences in dose. Beam collimation, not reconstruction thickness, results in a difference in some cases of 55% in the head phantom and 65% in the body phantom when comparing single-detector to multidetector scanners. See Table 29-3 for single-detector imaging dose chart, Table 29-4 for multidetector imaging dose chart, and Table 29-5 for multidetector imaging with new dose reduction techniques.

Patient size must be considered carefully when setting up scan parameters. A small adult or pediatric patient absorbs less of the entrance radiation than a larger patient. This results in the exit radiation dose of higher intensity.

TABLE 29-3
Single-detector doses

Collimation (mm)	CTDI$_W$ head phantom (mGy)	CTDI$_W$ body phantom (mGy)
1	46	20
3	42	19
5	40	18
7	40	18
10	40	18

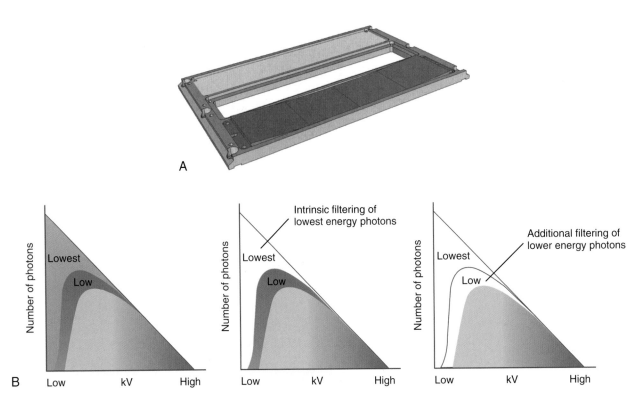

Fig. 29-53 A, IntelliBeam adjustable filter that controls beam hardness (quality). Filters are used in conjunction with wedges to reduce patient dose. **B,** Graph showing decrease in dose owing to elimination of low-energy photons (*far right diagram*).

(Courtesy Philips Medical Systems.)

Comparison of Computed Tomography and Magnetic Resonance Imaging

As CT was developing and advancing into a significant diagnostic modality, magnetic resonance imaging (MRI) was also progressing. Similar to CT, MRI was first used to image the brain; whole-body scans were developed shortly afterward. As MRI advanced and the quality of the images improved, it became apparent that MRI images exhibited better low-contrast resolution than CT images. Brain soft tissue detail is not shown as well with CT as with MRI performed at approximately the same level (Fig. 29-54).

The initial introduction of MRI raised concerns that CT scanners would become obsolete. Each modality has been found to have unique capabilities, however. CT and MRI are useful for different clinical applications. As previously mentioned, CT does not show soft tissue as well as MRI; however, CT shows bony structures better than MRI.

Patients often have ferrous metal within their bodies. MRI cannot always be used to scan such patients. CT is one option for these patients. The CT scanner does not affect metal in a patient, but metal can cause artifacts on CT images when the metal lies within the scan plane.

Many patients (especially pediatric and trauma patients) are extremely claustrophobic, combative, or uncooperative. CT is useful for scanning these patients quickly and easily because of the short gantry length, relatively large aperture, and short scan times.

Because equipment costs are less and a greater number of procedures can be accomplished per day, CT often is a less costly examination than MRI. Physicians have found that CT and MRI can be complementary examinations. In many situations, both examinations are ordered to provide as much diagnostic information as possible.

Future Considerations

Since 2010, the diagnostic capabilities of CT have increased significantly, and the dose used is lower than that previously required. The development of iterative reconstruction methods was central to the advancement of CT as a discipline. With the rapid advancements in technology, the CT technologist has an increased responsibility to understand contrast dynamics and the spiral scan parameters of pitch, collimation, scan timing, and table speed.

Advancements in dose reduction, improvement in spatial resolution, and temporal resolution will continue. Manufacturers are working hard to improve as low as reasonably achievable (ALARA) practices and to meet or exceed the standards published by Image Gently, The Alliance for Radiation Safety in Pediatric Imaging (imagegently.org) and Image Wisely, Radiation Safety in Adult Medical Imaging (imagewisely.org).

TABLE 29-4
Multidetector doses

Collimation (mm)	Total beam width (mm)	CTDI$_w$ head phantom (mGy)	CTDI$_w$ body phantom (mGy)
4 × 1.25	5	63	34
2 × 2.5	5	63	34
1 × 5	5	63	34
4 × 2.5	10	47	25
2 × 5	10	47	25
4 × 5	10	47	21

TABLE 29-5
Low-dose protocols (Philips Brilliance iCT)

Examination type	Scan mode	kVp	mAs	CTDIvol (mGy)
Adult abdomen and pelvis	Helical	120	160	11.4
Adult chest	Helical	140	20	2
Pediatric head	Helical	120	200	16.3

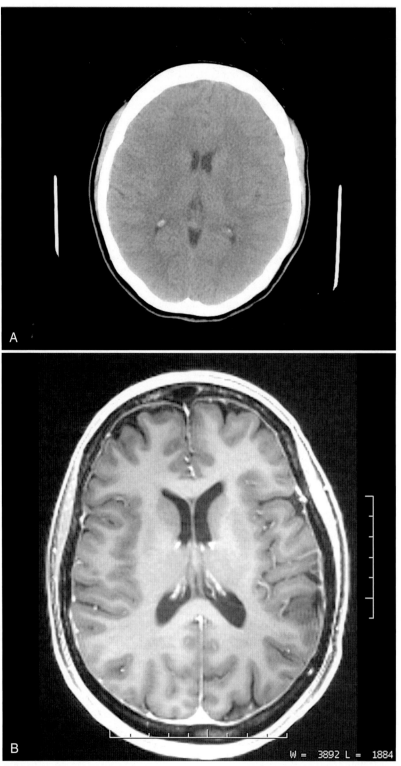

Fig. 29-54 A, Axial CT scan of lateral ventricles: anterior horns (ALV) and posterior horns (PLV), and third ventricle (3V). **B,** Axial MRI scan of the corpus callosum, anteriorly genu (G) and posteriorly splenium (S), and head of the caudate nucleus (CN).

(From Kelley LL, Petersen CM: *Sectional anatomy for imaging professionals,* St Louis, ed 2, 2007, Mosby.)

Advances in computing power and design have provided workstations that can generate three-dimensional models, rotate the models along any axis, and display the models with varying parameters (Figs. 29-55 and 29-56). Digital subtraction CT, multimodality image superimposition, and translucent shading of soft tissue structures are some newer applications. Virtual colonoscopy (Fig. 29-57), virtual bronchoscopy, virtual cholangiopancreatography, and virtual labyrinthoscopy (inner ear) continue to evolve. As higher-quality images increase the accuracy of diagnosis and treatment, patient care will improve. Because of the superb diagnostic information and cost-effectiveness that CT provides, this imaging modality will continue to be a highly respected diagnostic tool.

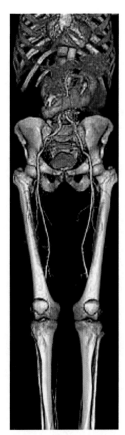

Fig. 29-55 Full-body three-dimensional reconstruction from 64-row CT scanner.

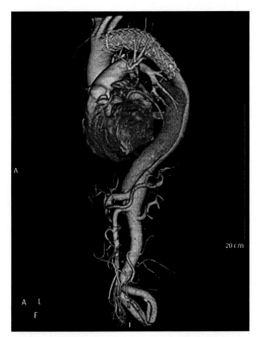

Fig. 29-56 Aortic arch stent shown on 500-mm three-dimensional reconstruction.

(Courtesy Philips Medical Systems.)

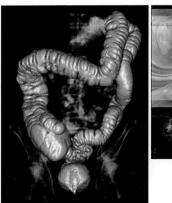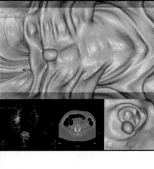

Fig. 29-57 CT colonography.

(Courtesy Philips Medical Systems.)

Basic Computed Tomography Examination Protocols

Because of the numerous scanner types, parameters, tube rotation speeds, and detector types that are used in CT imaging, it is impossible to list exact examination protocols. Technical factors are directly related to the detector configuration that is used: number of detector rows and fixed array versus adaptive array. Many scans are performed using auto tube current modulation as opposed to fixed mA. This is an overview of basic CT scan protocols using an adaptive array, 16-row scanner. The values listed are close approximations of what can be used for the various examinations.

BASIC HEAD

Anatomical scan range	Scan type	Localizer scans	kVp	mAs	FOV	Scan slice thickness	Recon slice thickness	Gantry tilt	Recon kernel	IV contrast	Oral contrast
Skull base thru vertex of head	Axial sequential	AP, LAT	120	250 auto	22cm	5mm	2.5mm	Match skull base	Medium average	No	No

Place patient in supine position with head in head holder. Assure that patient is not rotated or tilted. Elevate table to bring coronal alignment light to the center of the skull. Landmark per equipment requirements (table movement for scout images). Perform scout images. Prescribe scan locations from skull base to vertex of head. Angle gantry to match skull base (occipital bone) (foramen magnum) and frontal bone (roof of orbit).

CORONAL SINUSES

Anatomical scan range	Scan type	Localizer scans	kVp	mAs	FOV	Scan slice thickness	Recon slice thickness	Gantry tilt	Recon kernel	IV contrast	Oral contrast
Entire sphenoid sinus thru entire frontal sinus	Axial sequential	AP, LAT	120	200 auto	16cm	5mm 3mm	2.5mm 1.5mm	90° to max. sinus	Sharp bone	No	No

OPTION 1: Direct coronals - Place patient in prone position with extended chin resting in head holder (see diagram).
OPTION 2: Place patient in supine position with head in head holder (basic head positioning). Assure that patient is not rotated or tilted. Elevated table to bring coronal alignment light to the center of the skull. Landmark per equipment requirements (table movement for scout images). Perform scout images. Prescribe scan locations to include entire sphenoid sinus thru entire frontal sinus Angle gantry to 90° orientation to floor of maxillary sinus. Volume scans can be performed with either positioning option with MPR's in opposite planes. Direct coronal positioning provides better information about maxillary meatus.

SOFT TISSUE NECK

Anatomical scan range	Scan type	Localizer scans	kVp	mAs	FOV	Scan slice thickness	Recon slice thickness	Gantry tilt	Recon kernel	IV contrast	Oral contrast
Above floor of frontal fossa to mid aortic arch	Helical	AP, LAT	120	150 auto	20cm	5mm	2.5mm	Usually none	Medium average	Yes 15s delay	No

Place patient supine on table with head resting on radiolucent sponge. Assure that patient's head and neck is within table scan range. Assure that patient's head and shoulders are not rotated or tilted. Elevate table to bring coronal alignment light to the center of the neck. Landmark per equipment requirements (table movement for scout images). Tip chin up to bring plane of teeth perpendicular to tabletop. Perform scout images. Prescribe scan locations from above floor of frontal fossa to mid aortic arch. Usually no gantry tilt needed - however, scans should be perpendicular to midcoronal plane. Scans typically performed with IV contrast and a scan delay of 15 seconds.

CERVICAL SPINE

Anatomical scan range	Scan type	Localizer scans	kVp	mAs	FOV	Scan slice thickness	Recon slice thickness	Gantry tilt	Recon kernel	IV contrast	Oral contrast
Occipital condyles to below T2	Helical	AP, LAT	120	250 auto	16cm	3mm	1.5mm	Usually none	Sharp bone	No	No

Place patient supine on table with head resting on radiolucent sponge. Assure that patient's head and neck is within table scan range. Assure that patient's head and shoulders are not rotated or tilted. Elevate table to bring coronal alignment light to the center of the neck. Landmark per equipment requirements (table movement for scout images). Perform scout images. Prescribe scan locations from skull base/occipital condyles to below T1. Usually no gantry angle when scanning the entire C-Spine. If individual vertebral bodies are of interest - gantry can be angled to match vertebral bodies/disc spaces. Volume scans performed with MPR's in sagittal and coronal planes.

ROUTINE CHEST

	Anatomical scan range	Scan type	Localizer scans	kVp	mAs	FOV	Scan slice thickness	Recon slice thickness	Gantry tilt	Recon kernel	IV contrast	Oral contrast
	Above lung apices to below adrenal glands	Helical	AP, LAT	120	100 auto	Thorax margin	5mm	2.5mm	None	Medium average	Yes 25s delay	No

Place 22g needle in antecubital space - assure patency. Place patient in supine position with head on pillow, cushion under patient's knees for comfort. Assure that patient is not rotated or tilted. Elevate table to bring coronal alignment light to the center of the chest. Landmark per equipment requirements (table movement for scout images). Bring patient's arms above their head and support with sponges/pillows for comfort and to protect IV site. Perform scout images. Prescribe scan locations from above lung apices to below adrenal glands. Define FOV to include lateral margins of chest and use lateral scout to center FOV to include anterior and posterior margins of the chest. Scans typically performed with IV contrast and a scan delay of 25 seconds.

ROUTINE ABDOMEN

	Anatomical scan range	Scan type	Localizer scans	kVp	mAs	FOV	Scan slice thickness	Recon slice thickness	Gantry tilt	Recon kernel	IV contrast	Oral contrast
	Above hemidiaphragms to iliac crest	Helical	AP, LAT	120	200 auto	Body margin	5mm	2.5mm	None	Medium average	Yes 60s delay	Yes 24 hr/ 1 hr

Exams typically performed with oral contrast - give contrast 24 hours and 1 hour before exam or timing as requested by Radiologist. Place 22g needle in antecubital space - assure patency. Place patient in supine position with head on pillow, cushion under patient's knees for comfort. Assure that patient is not rotated or tilted. Elevate table to bring coronal alignment light to the center of the abdomen. Landmark per equipment requirements (table movement for scout images). Bring patient's arms above their head and support with sponges/pillows for comfort and to protect IV site. Perform scout images. Prescribe scan locations from above hemidiaphragms to iliac crest (scan area must include all of liver). Define FOV to include lateral margins of abdomen and use lateral scout to center FOV to include anterior and posterior margins of the abdomen. Scans typically performed with IV contrast and a scan delay of 60 seconds.

ROUTINE PELVIS

	Anatomical scan range	Scan type	Localizer scans	kVp	mAs	FOV	Scan slice thickness	Recon slice thickness	Gantry tilt	Recon kernel	IV contrast	Oral contrast
	Above Iliac crest to mid symphysis pubis	Helical	AP, LAT	120	200 auto	Body margin	5mm	2.5mm	Usually none	Medium average	Yes 120s delay	Yes 24 hr/ 1 hr

Exams typically performed with oral contrast - give contrast 24 hours and 1 hour before exam or timing as requested by Radiologist. Place 22g needle in antecubital space - assure patency. Place patient in supine position with head on pillow, cushion under patient's knees for comfort. Assure that patient is not rotated or tilted. Elevate table to bring coronal alignment light to the center of the pelvis. Landmark per equipment requirements (table movement for scout images). Bring patient's arms above their head and support with sponges/pillows for comfort and to protect IV site. Perform scout images. Prescribe scan locations from above iliac crest to mid symphysis or below symphysis. Define FOV to include lateral margins of pelvis and use lateral scout to center FOV to include anterior and posterior margins of the pelvis. Scans typically performed with IV contrast and a scan delay of 120-180 seconds.

Basic Computed Tomography Examination Protocols

EXTREMITY - KNEE

Anatomical scan range	Scan type	Localizer scans	kVp	mAs	FOV	Scan slice thickness	Recon slice thickness	Gantry tilt	Recon kernel	IV contrast	Oral contrast
Approx 2"-3" above to 2"-3" below joint or area of trauma	Helical	AP, LAT	120	140 200 auto	Knee margin	3mm	1.5mm	Usually none	Sharp bone	Depends on pathology	No

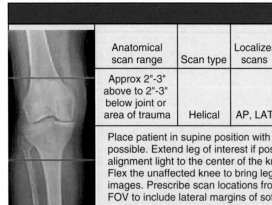

Place patient in supine position with head on pillow. Shift patient so extremity of interest is in midline of table if possible. Extend leg of interest if possible. Assure that patient is not rotated or tilted. Elevate table to bring coronal alignment light to the center of the knee. Landmark per equipment requirements (table movement for scout images). Flex the unaffected knee to bring leg and foot away from scan plane through affected knee if possible. Perform scout images. Prescribe scan locations from approximately 2"-3" above joint to 2"-3" below joint or area of interest. Define FOV to include lateral margins of soft tissues and use lateral scout to center FOV to include anterior and posterior margins of the knee. Volume scans performed followed by MPR's.

PEDIATRIC IMAGING

The following five points should be considered for pediatric imaging: (1) "Child size" the radiation dose, (2) scan only when necessary, (3) scan only indicated areas, (4) multiphase scanning usually not indicated, (5) utilize shielding whenever possible. Most protocols are adjusted based on patient weight as opposed to patient age, with 55kg being the top of the scale for pediatric adjustments. Note: kVp and mAs values listed are typical low/high ranges for imaging based on patient weight.

PEDIATRIC PROTOCOLS

Anatomical region	Pediatric considerations	Scan type	Localizer scans	kVp	mAs	FOV	Scan slice thickness	Recon slice thickness	Gantry tilt	Recon kernel	IV contrast	Oral contrast
Head	Avoid eyes with scan plane	Helical	AP, LAT	80 120	100 200 auto	16-20 cm	5mm 3mm	2.5mm 1.5mm	Match skull base	Medium average	No	No
Soft tissue neck	Typically same coverage as adults	Helical	AP, LAT	80 120	20 80 auto	10-14 cm	5mm 3mm	2.5mm 1.5mm	Usually none	Medium average	Typically yes	No
C-spine	Typically entire C-spine, avoid eyes	Helical	AP, LAT	80 120	40 100 auto	10-14 cm	3mm	1.5mm	Usually none	Sharp bone	No	No
Chest	Restrict to area of interest, typically single phase for peds	Helical	AP, LAT	80 120	20 70 auto	Edge of anatomy	5mm 3mm	2.5mm 1.5mm	Usually none	Medium average	Yes	No
Abdomen	Restrict to area of interest, typically single phase for peds	Helical	AP, LAT	80 120	40 100 auto	Edge of anatomy	5mm 3mm	2.5mm 1.5mm	Usually none	Sharp bone	Yes	Yes
Pelvis	Restrict to area of interest, typically single phase for peds	Helical	AP, LAT	80 120	40 100 auto	Edge of anatomy	5mm 3mm	2.5mm 1.5mm	Usually none	Sharp bone	Yes	Yes
Extremities	Typically same coverage as adults	Helical	AP, LAT	80 120	50 150 auto	Edge of anatomy	3mm	1.5mm	Usually none	Sharp bone	Depends on pathology	No

Definition of Terms

air calibration Scan of air in gantry; based on a known value of –1000 for air, the scanner calibrates itself according to this density value relative to actual density value measured.

algorithm Mathematic formula designed for computers to carry out complex calculations required for image reconstruction; designed for enhancement of soft tissue, bone, and edge resolution. Also referred to as *kernel*.

anisotropic spatial resolution Spatial resolution of a voxel in which all three axes of the volume element are not equal. Slice thickness is not equal to pixel size.

aperture Opening of the gantry through which patient passes during scan.

archiving Storage of CT images on long-term storage device such as cassette tape, magnetic tape, or optical disk.

artifact Distortion or error in image that is unrelated to subject being studied.

attenuation Coefficient CT number assigned to measured remnant radiation intensity after attenuation by tissue density.

axial Describes plane of image as presented by CT scan; same as *transverse*.

bolus Preset amount of radiopaque contrast medium injected rapidly per IV administration to visualize high-flow vascular structures, usually in conjunction with dynamic scan; most often injected using a pressure injector.

channel In multidetector CT, multiple rows of detectors (channels) are arranged along the longitudinal (z) axis of the patient. Each detector row (channel) consists of numerous elements.

computed tomography (CT) X-ray tube and detector assembly rotating 360 degrees around a specified area of the body; also called CAT (computed axial tomography) scan.

computed tomography dose index (CTDI) Radiation dose descriptor calculated with normalized beam widths for 14 contiguous sections or slices.

computed tomography dose index₁₀₀ (CTDI₁₀₀) Radiation dose descriptor calculated with the full length of a 100-mm pencil ionization chamber. Measures larger scan distances than CTDI, but only one location is calculated.

computed tomography dose indexvol (CTDIvol) Radiation dose descriptor that takes into account the parameters that are related to a specific imaging protocol. Considers helical pitch or axial scan spacing in its calculation. More accurate measure of dose per protocol.

computed tomography dose indexw (CTDIw) Radiation dose descriptor that provides a weighted average of the center and peripheral contributions to dose within the scan plane. More accurate than CTDI₁₀₀ owing to calculations from more than one location.

CT angiography Use of volumetric CT scanning with spiral technique to acquire image data that are reconstructed into three-dimensional CT angiograms.

CT number Arbitrary number assigned by computer to indicate relative density of a given tissue; CT number varies proportionately with tissue density; high CT numbers indicate dense tissue, and low CT numbers indicate less dense tissue. All CT numbers are based on the density of water, which is assigned a CT number of 0. Also referred to as a *Hounsfield unit*.

contrast resolution Ability to differentiate between small variations in density within the image.

curved planar reformations Postprocessing technique applied to stacks of axial image data that can be reconstructed into irregular or oblique planes.

data acquisition system (DAS) Part of detector assembly that converts analog signals to digital signals that can be used by the CT computer.

detector Electronic component used for radiation detection; made of either high-density photo reactive crystals or pressurized stable gases.

detector assembly Electronic component of CT scanner that measures remnant radiation exiting the patient, converting the radiation to an analog signal proportionate to the radiation intensity measured.

direct coronal Describes position used to obtain images in coronal plane; used for head scans to provide images at right angles to axial images; patient is positioned prone for direct coronal images and supine for reverse coronal images.

dose length product (DLP) Commonly reported dose descriptor on CT scanners. Calculated by multiplying the CTDIvol by the length of the scan (cm). DLP = CTDIvol × scan length.

dynamic scanning Process by which raw data are obtained by continuous scanning; images are not reconstructed but are saved for later reconstruction; most often used for visualization of high-flow vascular structures; can be used to scan an uncooperative patient rapidly.

field of view (FOV) Area of anatomy displayed on the monitor; can be adjusted to include entire body section or a specific part of the patient anatomy being scanned.

gantry Part of CT scanner that houses x-ray tube, cooling system, detector assembly, and DAS; often referred to as the "doughnut" by patients.

generation Description of significant levels of technologic development of CT scanners; specifically related to tube/detector movement.

grayscale image Analog image whereby each pixel in the image corresponds to a particular shade of gray.

helical CT Data acquisition method that combines continuous gantry rotation with continuous table movement to form a helical path of scan data; also called *spiral CT*.

high-resolution scans Use of scanning parameters that enhance contrast resolution of an image, such as thin slices, high matrices, high-spatial frequency algorithms, and small-display FOV.

host computer Primary link between system operator and other components of imaging system.

Hounsfield unit (HU) Number used to describe average density of tissue; term is used interchangeably with *CT number;* named in honor of Hounsfield, who is generally given credit for development of the first clinically viable CT scanner.

image misregistration Image distortion caused by combination of table indexing and respiration; table moves in specified increments, but patient movement during respiration may cause anatomy to be scanned more than once or not at all.

index Table movement; also referred to as *table increments*.

isotropic spatial resolution Spatial resolution of a voxel in which all three axes of the volume element are equal. Slice thickness is equal to pixel size.

mapping Assignment of appropriate gray level to each pixel in an image.

matrix Mathematical formula for calculation made up of individual cells for number assignment; CT matrix stores a CT number relative to the tissue density at that location; each cell or "address" stores one CT number for image reconstruction.

maximum intensity projection (MIP) Reconstruction of brightest pixels from stack of image data into a three-dimensional image.

multiplanar reconstruction (MPR) Postprocessing technique applied to stacks of axial image data that can be reconstructed into other orientations or imaging planes.

multiple scan average dose (MSAD) Dose descriptor that calculates average dose resulting from a series of scans over an interval length of scans.

noise Random variation of CT numbers around some mean value within a uniform object; noise produces a grainy appearance in the image.

partial volume averaging Calculated linear attenuation coefficient for a pixel that is a weighted average of all densities in the pixel; the assigned CT number and ultimately the pixel appearance are affected by the average of the different densities measured within that pixel.

pixel (picture element) One individual cell surface within an image matrix used for image display.

postprocessing techniques Specialized reconstruction techniques that are applied to CT images to display the anatomic structures from different perspectives.

primary data CT number assigned to the matrix by the computer; the information required to reconstruct an image.

protocol Instructions for CT examination specifying slice thickness, table increments, contrast administration, scan diameter, and any other requirements specified by the radiologist.

quantum noise Any noise in the image that is a result of random variation in the number of x-ray photons detected.

real time Ability to process or reconstruct incoming data in milliseconds.

reconstruction Process of creating a digital image from raw data.

region of interest (ROI) Measurement of CT numbers within a specified area for evaluation of average tissue density.

rendering Process of changing the shading of a three-dimensional image; commonly used to increase depth perception of an image.

retrieval Reconstruction of images stored on long-term device; can be done for extra film copies or when films are lost.

scan Actual rotation of x-ray tube around the patient; used as a generic reference to one slice or an entire examination.

scan diameter Also referred to as the zoom or focal plane of a CT scan; predetermined by the radiographer to include the anatomic area of interest; determines FOV.

scan duration Amount of time used to scan an entire volume during a single spiral scan.

scan time X-ray exposure time in seconds.

segmentation Method of cropping or editing target objects from image data.

shaded surface display (SSD) Process used to generate three-dimensional images that show the surface of a three-dimensional object.

shading Postprocessing technique used in three-dimensional reconstructions to separate tissues of interest by applying a threshold value to isolate the structure of interest.

slice One scan through a selected body part; also referred to as a *cut;* slice thickness can vary from 0.35 mm to 1 cm, depending on the examination.

slip ring Low-voltage electrical contacts within the gantry designed to allow continuous rotation of an x-ray tube without the use of cables connecting internal and external components.

spatial resolution Ability to identify visibly anatomic structures and small objects of high contrast.

spiral CT Scanning method that combines a continuous gantry rotation with a continuous table movement to form a spiral path of scan data; also called *helical CT.*

streak artifact Artifact created by high-density objects that result in an arc of straight lines projecting across the FOV from a common point.

system noise Inherent property of a CT scanner; the difference between the measured CT number of a given tissue and the known value for that tissue; most often evaluated through the use of water phantom scans.

table increments Specific amount of table travel between scans; can be varied to move at any specified increment; most protocols specify from 1 mm to 20 cm, depending on type of examination; also referred to as *indexing.*

table speed Longitudinal distance traveled by the table during one revolution of the x-ray tube.

temporal resolution Ability of CT system to freeze motions of the scanned object; the shortest amount of time needed to acquire a complete data set.

threshold value CT number used in defining the corresponding anatomy that comprises a three-dimensional object; any pixels within a three-dimensional volume having the threshold value (CT number) or higher would be selected for the three-dimensional model.

useful patient dose Radiation dose received by the patient that is actually and converted into an image.

voxel (volume element) Individual pixel with the associated volume of tissue based on the slice thickness.

window Arbitrary numbers used for image display based on various shades of gray; *window width* controls the overall gray level and affects image contrast; *window level* (center) controls subtle gray images within a certain width range and ultimately affects the brightness and overall density of an image.

Selected bibliography

American Association of Physicists in Medicine (AAPM), *AAPM guidelines of ruse of NEMA XR 25 CT dose check standard,* 2011, Available at: http://www.aapm.org/pubs/CTProtocols.

Bushong SC: *Radiologic science for technologists: physics, biology, and protection,* ed 9, St Louis, 2009, Mosby.

Griffey RT, Sodickson A: Cumulative radiation exposure and cancer risk estimates in emergency department patients undergoing repeat or multiple CT, *AJR Am J Roentgenol* 192:887, 2009.

Guide to Low Dose 2013, Siemens Healthcare, available at: www.siemens.com/low-dose.

Haaga JR et al: *CT and MRI of the whole body,* ed 5, vols I and II, St Louis, 2009, Mosby.

Image Gently, The Alliance for Radiation Safety in Pediatric Imaging Standards, available at: imagegently.org.

Image Wisely, Radiation Safety in Adult Medical Imaging, Available at: imagewisely.org.

Joemai RM et al: Assessment of patient and occupational dose in established and new applications of MDCT fluoroscopy, *AJR Am J Roentgenol* 192:881, 2009.

Seeram E: *Computed tomography: physical principles, clinical applications, and quality control,* ed 3, St Louis, 2009, Saunders.

30

MAGNETIC RESONANCE IMAGING

BARTRAM J. PIERCE
CHERYL DUBOSE

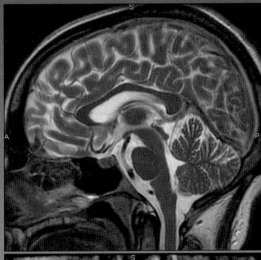

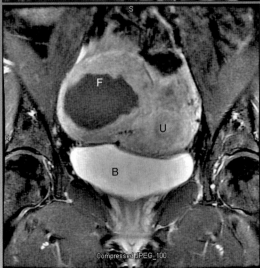

OUTLINE

Principles of Magnetic Resonance
  Imaging, 342
Comparison of Magnetic Resonance
  Imaging and Conventional
  Radiography, 342
Historical Development, 342
Physical Principles, 343
Equipment, 345
Safety of Magnetic Resonance
  Imaging, 348
Examination Protocols, 351
Clinical Applications, 357
Spectroscopy, 365
Functional Magnetic Resonance
  Imaging, 366
Conclusion, 367

Principles of Magnetic Resonance Imaging

*Magnetic resonance imaging** (MRI) is a noninvasive examination technique that provides anatomic and physiologic information. Similar to computed tomography (CT) (see Chapter 29), MRI is a computer-based cross-sectional imaging modality. The physical principles of MRI are totally different from those of CT and conventional radiography. MRI creates images of structures through the interactions of magnetic fields and radio waves with tissues without the use of ionizing radiation.

MRI was originally called *nuclear magnetic resonance* (NMR) imaging, with the word *nuclear* indicating that the non-radioactive atomic nucleus played an important role in the technique. This term was dropped because of public apprehension about nuclear energy and nuclear weapons—neither of which is associated with MRI in any way.

---

*Almost all italicized words on the succeeding pages are defined at the end of this chapter.

Comparison of Magnetic Resonance Imaging and Conventional Radiography

MRI provides cross-sectional images and serves as a useful addition to conventional x-ray techniques. On a radiograph, all body structures exposed to the x-ray beam are superimposed into one "flat" image. In many instances, multiple projections or contrast agents are required to distinguish one anatomic structure or organ clearly from another. Cross-sectional imaging techniques such as ultrasonography, CT, and MRI more easily separate the various organs because there is no superimposition of structures. Multiple slices (cross sections) or three-dimensional volumes are typically required to cover a single area of the body.

In addition to problems with overlapping structures, conventional radiography is limited in its ability to distinguish types of tissue. In radiographic techniques, *contrast* (the ability to discriminate between two different tissue densities) depends on differences in x-ray *attenuation* within the object and the ability of the recording medium (e.g., film or digital detectors) to detect these differences. It is difficult for radiographs to detect small attenuation changes. Typically conventional radiographs can distinguish only tissues with large differences in attenuation of the x-ray beam (air, fat, bone, and metal). Soft tissue structures such as the liver and kidneys cannot be separated by differences in x-ray attenuation alone. For these structures, differences are magnified through the use of contrast agents.

However, multislice helical CT, with its superior resolving power, is much more sensitive to these small changes in x-ray attenuation and is able to distinguish the liver from the kidneys on the basis of their differing x-ray attenuation and by position.

By manipulating completely different physical principles (interactions of matter with magnetic fields and radio waves), MRI is able to distinguish very small contrast differences among tissues.

Historical Development

In the mid-1940s, Felix Bloch, working at Stanford University, and Edward Purcell, working at Harvard University, discovered the principles of nuclear magnetic resonance. Their work led to the use of nuclear magnetic spectroscopy for the analysis of complex molecular structures and dynamic chemical processes. This process is still in use today for the nondestructive testing of chemical compounds. In 1952, Bloch and Purcell were jointly awarded the Nobel Prize in physics for their development of new ways and methods for nuclear magnetic precision measurements.

In 1969, Raymond Damadian proposed the first MRI body scanner. He discovered that the relaxation times* of tumors differed from the relaxation times of normal tissue. This finding suggested that images of the body might be obtained by producing maps of relaxation rates. In 1973, Paul Lauterbur published the first cross-sectional images of objects obtained with MRI techniques. These first images were crude, and only large objects could be distinguished. Mansfield further showed how the signals could be mathematically analyzed, which made it possible to develop useful imaging techniques. Mansfield also showed how extremely fast imaging could be achieved. Since that time, MRI technology has advanced rapidly. Very small structures are commonly imaged quickly and with increased resolution and contrast. In 2003, the Nobel Prize in physiology or medicine was jointly awarded to Lauterbur and Mansfield for their discoveries in MRI.

---

*This topic will be discussed later in the chapter.

Physical Principles
SIGNAL PRODUCTION

The structure of an atom is often compared with the structure of the solar system, with the sun representing the central atomic *nucleus* and the planets representing the orbiting electrons. MRI uses properties of the nucleus to generate the signal that contains the information used to construct the image. Clinical MRI scanners "image" hydrogen because it is the most abundant element in the body and is the strongest nuclear magnet on a per-nucleus basis.

Elements with odd atomic numbers, such as hydrogen, have magnetic properties causing them to act like tiny bar magnets (Fig. 30-1). Ordinarily, in the absence of a strong magnetic field, these protons point in random directions, as shown in Fig. 30-2, creating no net magnetization. At this point they are not useful for imaging. If the body is placed within a strong uniform magnetic field, the protons will attempt to align themselves in one of two orientations, with the field (parallel) or against the field (antiparallel). A slight majority will align with, or parallel to, the main magnetic field, also called the longitudinal plane, causing the tissues to be magnetized or have a slight net magnetization.

The protons do not line up precisely with the external field but at an angle to the field causing them to rotate around the direction of the magnetic field in a manner similar to the wobbling of a spinning top. This wobbling motion, depicted in Fig. 30-3, is called *precession* and occurs at a specific *frequency* (rate) for a given atom's nucleus in a magnetic field of a specific strength. These precessing protons can only absorb energy if that energy is presented at same frequency they are wobbling. In MRI, *radiofrequency* (RF) pulses at that specific precessional frequency are used. The absorption of energy by the precessing protons is referred to as *resonance*. This resonant frequency, called the Larmor frequency, varies depending on the field strength of the MRI scanner. At a field strength of 1.5 *tesla,* the frequency is approximately 63 MHz; at 1 tesla, the frequency is approximately 42 MHz; at 0.5 tesla, the frequency is approximately 21 MHz; and at 0.2 tesla, the frequency is approximately 8 MHz.

When the RF pulse, at the Larmor frequency, is applied, the protons absorb the energy resulting in a reorientation of the net tissue magnetization into a plane perpendicular to the main field. This is known as the *transverse plane.* The protons in the transverse plane also precess at the same resonant frequency. The precessing protons (a moving magnet) in the tissues create an electrical current, the MRI signal, in the receiving coil or *antenna.*

This follows Faraday's law of induction, in which a moving magnetic field (hydrogen protons) induces electrical current in a coil of wire (RF antenna or RF coil).

The MRI signal is picked up by this sensitive antenna or coil, amplified, and processed by a computer to produce a sectional image of the body. This image, similar to the image produced by a CT scanner, is a digital image that is viewed on a computer monitor. Because this is a digital image, it can be manipulated, or postprocessed, to produce the most acceptable image. Additional processing can be performed on a three-dimensional workstation if applicable, and hard copies can be produced if necessary.

Many other odd-numbered nuclei in the body are being used in MRI. Nuclei from elements such as phosphorus and sodium may provide useful or differing diagnostic information than hydrogen nuclei, particularly in efforts to understand the metabolism of normal and abnormal tissues. Metabolic changes may prove to be more sensitive and specific in detecting abnormalities than the more physical and structural changes recognized by hydrogen-imaging MRI. Nonhydrogen nuclei may also be used for combined imaging and spectroscopy, in which small volumes of tissue may be analyzed for chemical content.

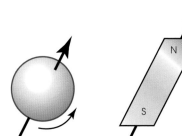

Fig. 30-1 A proton with magnetic properties can be compared with a tiny bar magnet. *Curved arrow* indicates that a proton spins on its own axis; this motion is different from that of precession.

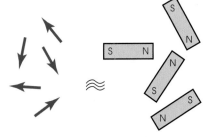

Fig. 30-2 In the absence of a strong magnetic field, the protons (*arrows*) point in random directions and cannot be used for imaging.

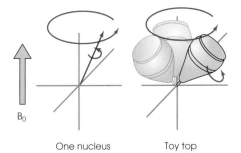

One nucleus   Toy top

Fig. 30-3 Precession. The protons (*arrow*) and the toy top spin on their own axes. Both also rotate (*curved arrows*) around the direction of an external force in a wobbling motion called *precession.* Precessing protons can absorb energy through resonance. B_0 represents the external magnetic field acting on the nucleus. The toy top precesses under the influence of gravity.

SIGNIFICANCE OF THE SIGNAL

Conventional radiographic techniques, including CT, produce images based on a single property of tissue: x-ray attenuation or density. MR images are more complex because they contain information about differing properties of tissue—proton density, relaxation rates, and flow phenomena. Each property contributes to the overall strength of the MRI signal. Computer processing converts signal strength to shades of gray on the image. Strong signals are represented by white in the image, and weak signals are represented by black.

One determinant of signal strength is the number of precessing protons in a given volume of tissue. Signal strength that depends on the concentration of protons is termed *proton density*. Most soft tissues, including fat, have a similar number of protons per unit volume; therefore, the use of proton density characteristics alone poorly separates these tissues. Some tissues have few hydrogen nuclei per unit of volume; examples include the cortex of bone and air in the lungs. These tissues have a weak signal as a result of low proton density and can be easily distinguished from other tissues.

MRI signal intensity also depends on the relaxation times of the nuclei. *Relaxation* is the release of energy by the excited protons. Excited nuclei relax through two processes. The process of nuclei releasing their excess energy to the general environment or lattice (the arrangement of atoms in a substance) is called *spin-lattice relaxation*. The rate of this relaxation process is measured in milliseconds and is labeled as T1. *Spin-spin relaxation* is the release of energy by excited nuclei through interaction among themselves. The rate of this process is also measured in milliseconds but is labeled as T2.

The rates of relaxation (T1 and T2) occur at different rates in different tissues. The environment of a hydrogen nucleus in the spleen differs from that of one in the liver; therefore, their relaxation rates differ, and the MRI signals created by these nuclei differ. The different relaxation rates in the liver and spleen result in different signal intensities and appearances on the image, enabling the viewer to discriminate between the two organs. Similarly, fat can be separated from muscle, and many tissues can be distinguished from others, based on the relaxation rates of their nuclei. The most important factor in tissue discrimination is the relaxation time.

The signals produced by MRI techniques contain a combination of proton density, T1, and T2 information. It is possible, however, to obtain images "weighted" toward any one of these three parameters by stimulating the nuclei with certain specific radio-wave *pulse sequences.* In most imaging sequences, a short T1 (fast spin-lattice relaxation rate) produces a high MRI signal on T1-weighted images. Conversely, a long T2 (slow spin-spin relaxation rate) generates a high signal on T2-weighted images.

The final property that influences image appearance is flow. For complex physical reasons, moving substances usually have weak MRI signals. (With some specialized pulse sequences, the reverse may be true; see the discussion of magnetic resonance angiography [MRA] later in the chapter.) With standard pulse sequences, flowing blood in vessels produces a low signal and is easily discriminated from surrounding stationary tissues without the need for the contrast agents required by regular radiographic techniques. Stagnant blood, such as an acute blood clot, typically has a high MRI signal in most imaging schemes as a result of its short T1 and long T2. The flow sequences of MRI may facilitate the assessment of vessel patency or the determination of the rate of blood flow through vessels (Fig. 30-4).

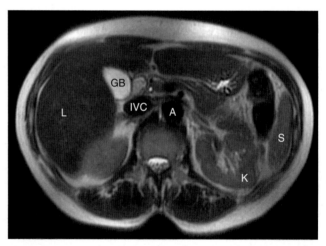

Fig. 30-4 T2-weighted image of an abdomen showing the flow void produced by flowing blood. *A,* Aorta; *GB,* gallbladder; *IVC,* inferior vena cava; *K,* kidney; *L,* liver; *S,* spleen.

Equipment

MRI requires a patient area (magnet room), an equipment room, and an operator's console. A separate diagnostic workstation is optional.

CONSOLE

The operator's console is used to control the imaging process (Fig. 30-5). Sitting at the console allows the operator to interact with the system's computers and electronics to manipulate all necessary examination parameters and perform the appropriate examination. Images are viewed on a computer monitor to ensure that the examination is of appropriate diagnostic quality. Images can be manipulated here, and hard copies of the exam can be produced if necessary. An independent or three-dimensional workstation may be used to perform additional imaging manipulation or post processing when required.

EQUIPMENT ROOM

The equipment room houses all the electronics and computers necessary to complete the imaging process. The RF cabinet controls the transmission of the radio-wave pulse sequences. The gradient cabinet controls the additional time-varying magnetic fields necessary to localize the MRI signal. The array processors and computers receive and process the large amount of *raw data* received from the patient and constructs the images the operator sees on the operator's console.

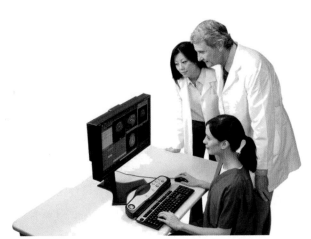

Fig. 30-5 Operator's console. This device controls the imaging process and allows visualization of images.

(Courtesy General Electric Healthcare.)

Equipment

MAGNET ROOM

The magnet is the major component of the MRI system in the scanning room. This magnet must be large enough to surround the patient and any antennas (coils) that are required for radio-wave transmission and reception. Antennas are typically wound in the shape of a positioning device for a particular body part. These are commonly referred to as *coils, or RF antennas.* As the patient lies on the table, coils are either placed on, under, or around the part to be imaged. Once positioned the patient is advanced into the center of the magnet (isocenter) (Fig. 30-6).

Various magnet types may be used to provide the strong uniform magnetic field required for imaging, as follows:

• *Resistive magnets* are simple but large electromagnets consisting of coils of wire. A magnetic field is produced by passing an electrical current through the wire coils. High magnetic fields are produced by passing a large amount of current through numerous coils. The electrical resistance of the wire produces heat and limits the maximum magnetic field strength of resistive magnets. The heat produced is conducted away from the magnet by a cooling system.

• *Superconductive (cryogenic) magnets* are also electromagnets. Their wire loops are cooled to very low temperatures with liquid helium to reduce electrical resistance. This permits higher magnetic field strengths than produced by resistive magnets.

• *Permanent magnets* are a third source for producing the magnetic field. A permanent magnet has a constant field that does not require additional electricity or cooling. The early permanent magnets were extremely heavy even compared with the massive superconductive and resistive units. Because of their weight, these magnets were difficult to place for clinical use. With improvements in technology, permanent magnets have become more competitive with the other magnet types. The magnetic field of permanent magnets does not extend as far away from the magnet (*fringe field*) as do the magnetic fields of other types of magnets. Fringe fields are a problem because of their effect on nearby electronic equipment.

Various MRI systems operate at different magnetic field strengths. Magnetic field strength is measured in tesla (T) or *gauss* (G). Most MRI examinations are performed with field strengths ranging from 0.2 to 3 tesla. Resistive systems generally do not exceed 0.6 tesla, and permanent magnet systems do not exceed 0.3 tesla. Higher field strengths require superconductive technology, with popular field strengths of 1.5 tesla and 3 tesla. Most research has concluded that field strengths used for diagnostic clinical imaging do not produce any substantial harmful effects.

Regardless of magnet type, MRI units are a challenge to install in hospitals. Current units are quite heavy—up to 10 tons for resistive and superconductive magnets and approximately 100 tons for some permanent magnets. Some institutional structures cannot support these weights without reinforcement. In addition, choosing a location for the MRI unit can be difficult because of magnetic fringe fields. With resistive and superconductive magnets, the fringe field extends in all directions and may interfere with nearby electronic or computer equipment, such as television monitors and other electronic devices. In addition, metal objects moving near the magnetic fringe field, such as automobiles or elevators, may cause ripples in the field, similar to the ripples caused by a pebble thrown into a pond. These ripples can be carried into the center of the magnet, where they distort the field and ruin the images. Efforts are made to shield the magnetic fringe field to prevent its extension beyond the MRI suite. Shielding will limit the effects of the magnetic field on metal objects or electronic devices and their effect on the magnetic field.

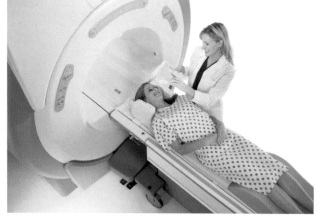

Fig. 30-6 Patient prepared for MRI.

(Courtesy General Electric Healthcare.)

Stray radio waves present another difficulty in the placement of MRI units. The radio waves used in MRI may be the same as the radio waves used for other nearby radio applications. Stray radio waves can be picked up by the MRI antenna coils and interfere with normal image production. MRI facilities require specially constructed rooms to shield the receiving antennas from outside radio interference, adding to the cost of the installation.

Specialty units have become available for limited applications. One example is an extremity MRI scanner (Fig. 30-7). This unit is designed so that the patient can sit comfortably in a chair while having an extremity or musculoskeletal joint imaged. These units are lightweight (approximately 1500 lb) and take up less space than conventional MRI scanners, and they produce good image quality (Fig. 30-8).

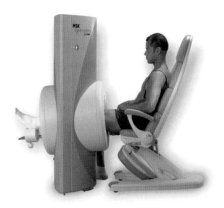

Fig. 30-7 Extremity MRI scanner, 1 tesla.

(Courtesy ONI Medical Systems, Inc, Wilmington, MA.)

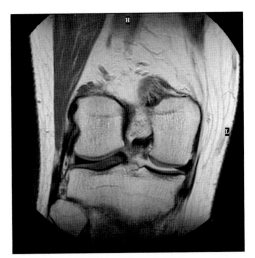

Fig. 30-8 Coronal MRI of the knee obtained with extremity MRI scanner.

(Courtesy ONI Medical Systems, Inc, Wilmington, MA.)

Infection Control

Because of the inherent dangers found within the MRI suite (projectiles, torque effects), developing and maintaining a strict infection control protocol can be a challenge. Although it may be expected that all technologists practice standard precautions, some may not realize that cleanliness of the magnet room is typically the responsibility of the technologist. In many institutions, housekeeping is not allowed in the magnet room. It is important for technologists to be aware of the infection control policies for their institution. Research has shown that various pathogens, including methicillin-resistant *Staphylococcus aureus* (MRSA), will grow within the bore of the magnet. For this reason technologists must be diligent in their practice of infection control.

Safety of Magnetic Resonance Imaging

MRI is generally considered safe. It is often preferred over CT for imaging of children because it does not use ionizing radiation, which has known potential adverse health effects. A growing child's body is thought to be more susceptible to the effects of ionizing radiation. Nevertheless, many potential safety issues concerning MRI must be raised—some related to potential direct effects on the patient from the imaging environment and others related to indirect hazards.

Opinions differ about the safety of the varying magnetic and RF fields to which the patient is directly exposed. Many studies in which experimental animal and cell culture systems were exposed to these fields over long periods have reported no adverse effects, whereas others have reported changes in cell cultures and embryos. RF energy is deposited in the patient during imaging and is dissipated in the body as heat. The resulting changes seem to be less than the levels considered clinically significant, even in areas of the body with poor heat dissipation, such as the lens of the eye. The significance of direct short-term exposure (i.e., exposure of a patient) and long-term exposure (i.e., exposure of an employee who works with MRI) is unclear. No clear association of MRI with adverse effects in humans has been proven, but research is continuing.

Hazards related to MRI have been well documented. Objects containing ferromagnetic metals (e.g., iron, nickel, cobalt) may be attracted to the imaging magnet with sufficient force to injure patients or personnel who may be interposed between them. Scissors, oxygen tanks, and patient gurneys are among the many items that have been drawn into the magnetic field at MRI sites. Metallic implants within patients or personnel may become displaced or dislodged and cause injury if they are in delicate locations. Examples include intracranial aneurysm clips, auditory implants, and metallic foreign bodies in the eye. Surgical clips, metal hardware and artificial joints do not pose problems. Electromechanical implants such as pacemakers or internal cardiac defibrillators can malfunction when exposed to strong magnetic fields or RF energy. These patients should not be allowed near the magnet. Fortunately, manufacturers continue to develop *MRI safe and conditional* implants, allowing these patients to be scanned safety. Anyone entering the magnet room (patients, visitors, and personnel) should be screened to ensure that they do not carry metallic objects into the magnet room or have objects in their bodies that could be adversely affected by exposure to strong magnetic fields.

Patients have received local burns from wires, such as electrocardiogram (ECG) leads, and other monitoring devices touching their skin during MRI examinations. These injuries have resulted from electrical burns caused by currents induced in the wires or thermal burns caused by heating of the wires. Such burns can be prevented by checking wires for frayed insulation, ensuring that no wire loops are within the magnetic field, and placing additional insulation between the patient and any wires exiting the MRI system.

The varying magnetic forces (gradients) in an MRI unit act on the machine itself, causing knocking or banging sounds. These noises can be loud enough to produce temporary or permanent hearing damage. The use of earplugs or other-sound damping devices is required to prevent auditory complications. Claustrophobia can be a significant impediment to MRI in up to 20% of patients (Fig. 30-9). Patient education is perhaps most important in preventing this problem, but tranquilizers, appropriate lighting, air movement, and mirrors or prisms that enable a patient to look out of the imager may be helpful. Claustrophobia can also be prevented by having a family member or friend accompany the patient and be present in the room during the scan.

In superconductive magnet systems, rapid venting (quench) of the super cooled liquid gases (helium) from the magnet or its storage containers into the surrounding room space is a rare but potential hazard. As the helium fills the magnet room, it replaces the oxygen resulting in unsafe levels which can lead to unconsciousness or asphyxiation. Oxygen monitoring devices in the magnet or cryogen storage room can signal personnel when the oxygen concentration becomes too low. Personnel may then evacuate the area and activate ventilation systems to exchange the escaped gas for fresh air.

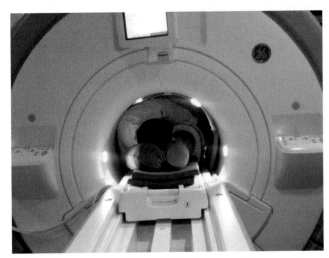

Fig. 30-9 Patient inside a superconducting 1.5-tesla magnet. Some patients cannot be scanned because of claustrophobia.

(Courtesy General Electric Healthcare.)

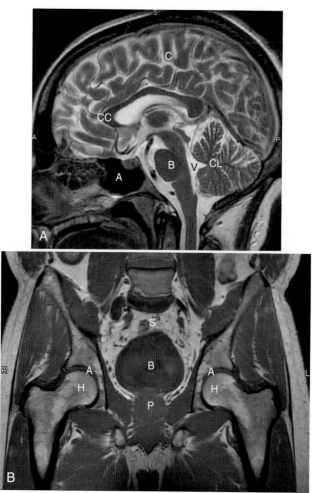

Fig. 30-10 Two images (different patients) from a 3-tesla superconductive MRI scanner, showing excellent resolution of images. **A,** This image shows remarkable anatomic detail in a midsagittal image of the head. *A,* air in sinuses; *B,* brain stem; *C,* cerebrum; *CC,* corpus callosum; *CL,* cerebellum; *V,* ventricle. **B,** This coronal image of the pelvis shows anatomic relationships of the prostate (*P*), which is enlarged and elevating the bladder (*B*). Hips (*H*) and acetabula (*A*) are also shown. A loop of the sigmoid (*S*) colon is on top of the bladder. This degree of resolution in coronal or sagittal images would be difficult to obtain by reformatting a series of transverse CT slices.

Examination Protocols

IMAGING PARAMETERS

The availability of many adjustable parameters makes MRI a complex imaging technique. Knowledge of the patient's clinical condition or disease is important in choosing the proper technique.

The operator may choose to obtain MR images in sagittal, coronal, transverse, or oblique planes. These are independently and directly acquired images with equal resolution in any plane (Fig. 30-10). In contrast, data can be obtained only in the transverse plane with CT. Sagittal and coronal CT images are generated by reformatting the data. Another MRI technique, especially when numerous thin slices or multiple imaging planes are desired, is three-dimensional imaging. In this technique, MRI data are collected simultaneously from a three-dimensional block of tissue rather than from a series of slices. Special data collection techniques and subsequent computer analysis allow the images from the single imaging sequence to be displayed in any plane (Fig. 30-11).

Slice thickness is important in the visualization of pathology. More MRI signal is available from a thicker slice than a thinner slice, so thicker slices may provide images that are less grainy. The surrounding tissues in the thicker slices may hide

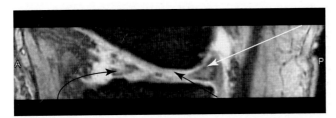

Fig. 30-11 Single slice from three-dimensional acquisition of the knee on a 3-tesla MRI unit. Data from an entire volume within the imaging coil are obtained concurrently. The data may be reconstructed into thin slices in any plane, such as the sagittal image shown here. This imaging sequence shows hyaline cartilage (*black arrow*) as a fairly high signal intensity rim overlying the bone. Meniscal fibrocartilage (*white arrow*) has low signal intensity. High signal intensity from joint fluid in a tear (*curved arrow*) within the anterior horn of the meniscus is visualized.

small pathologic lesions, however. Slice thickness may need to be adjusted based on the type of lesion under investigation.

Another important MRI parameter is overall imaging time. As imaging time (per slice) is lengthened, more MRI signal is available for analysis. Image quality improves with increased signal. Fewer patients can be imaged, however, when extended data acquisitions are performed. In addition, patient motion increases with prolonged imaging times, which in turn reduces image quality.

The set of imaging parameters used in MRI are called *pulse sequences*. A pulse sequence is a combination of gradients and RF pulses chosen to favor a particular tissue (contrast) as quickly as possible (speed) while minimizing artifacts and maximizing SNR. Depending on the choice of pulse sequence and imaging parameters, the resulting images may be more strongly weighted toward proton density, T1, or T2 information. Depending on the relative emphasis given to these factors, normal anatomy (Fig. 30-12) or a pathologic lesion (Fig. 30-13) may be more easily recognized. It is not unusual for a lesion to stand out dramatically when one pulse sequence is used yet be nearly invisible (same MRI signal as surrounding normal tissue) with a different pulse sequence.

Pulse sequences are classed depending on the timing of the gradient and RF pulses. Although the discussion of pulse sequences is outside the scope of this chapter, they can be divided into three categories. *Spin echo* sequences yield true T1-, T2-, or proton density–weighted images and are the standard pulse sequences used for all routine imaging. Classic spin echo sequences tend to have long scan times, so researchers have developed fast or turbo spin echo, which

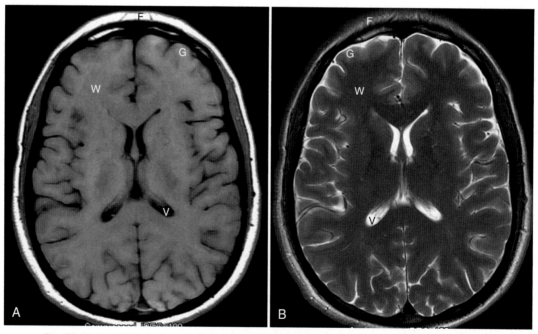

Fig. 30-12 Axial 3-tesla images through a normal brain. **A,** T1-weighted image shows relatively low differentiation of gray matter (*G*) and white matter (*W*) within the brain. **B,** Heavily T2-weighted image shows improved differentiation between gray and white matter. Cerebrospinal fluid within the ventricles (*V*) also changes in appearance with change in pulse sequence (low signal on T1-weighted image); fat (*F*) normally shows high signal intensity, whereas on the T2-weighted image, the signal intensity of fat is less than cerebrospinal fluid.

can dramatically shorten the scan time. *Gradient echo* sequences are used where the scan time must be short, such as breath hold abdominal scans. They generate T1- and T2-* weighted images and are also used in imaging flowing blood (see the discussion of MRA later in this chapter). *Echo planar* imaging is another extremely rapid imaging sequence used where motion is an issue. *Inversion recovery* is a sequence that can minimize or null signal intensity of a particular tissue. Most common are short tau inversion recovery (STIR), which nulls fat signal, and fluid attenuated inversion recovery (FLAIR), which nulls out signal from cerebrospinal fluid (CSF) in brain imaging. Researchers are continually developing new pulse sequences for specific applications.

POSITIONING

Patient positioning for MRI is usually straightforward. Generally, the patient lies supine on a table that is subsequently advanced into the magnetic field. As previously discussed, it is important to ensure that the patient has no contraindications to MRI, such as a cardiac pacemaker or intracranial aneurysm clips. Claustrophobia may be a problem for some patients as previously noted because the imaging area is tunnel shaped in most MRI system configurations (see Fig. 30-9).

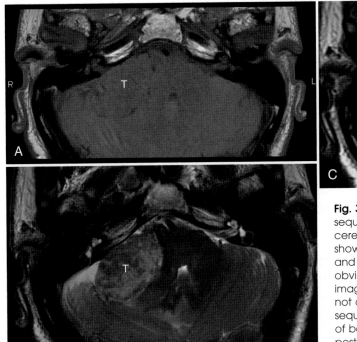

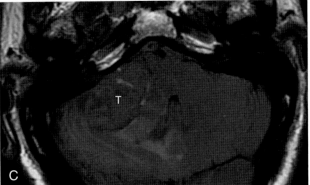

Fig. 30-13 Axial MRI showing the use of different pulse sequences and their effect on the visualization of the cerebellopontine angle tumor. **A,** T1-weighted image shows that limited contrast exists between the tumor (*T*) and normal brain. **B,** Lesion becomes dramatically more obvious using the pulse sequence of the T2-weighted image. **C,** Lesion is still visible on FLAIR pulse sequence but not as well as the T2-weighted image. Choice of pulse sequence is critical. These images also show how the lack of bone artifact makes MRI superior to CT for imaging of posterior fossa lesions.

COILS

The *coils* used for MRI are necessary for transmitting the RF pulse or receiving the MRI signal (as described earlier in the section on signal production). Some coils can transmit and receive (transmit/receive coils), whereas others may only receive the signal (receive only coils).

The body part to be examined determines the placement and shape of the antenna coil that is used for imaging (Fig. 30-14). Most coils are round or oval, and the body part to be examined is inserted into the coil's open center. Some coils, rather than encircling the body part, are placed directly on the patient over the area of interest. These surface coils are best when used for the imaging of thin body parts, such as the limbs, or superficial portions of a larger body structure, such as the orbit within the head or the spine within the torso. Another form of receiver coil is the endocavity coil, which is designed to fit within a body cavity such as the rectum. This enables a receiver coil to be placed close to some internal organs that may be distant from surface coils applied to the exterior body. Endocavity coils also may be used to image the wall of the cavity itself (Fig. 30-15).

PATIENT MONITORING

Although most MRI sites are constructed so that the operator can see the patient during imaging, the visibility is often limited, and the patient is relatively isolated within the MRI room (see Fig. 30-9). At most sites, intercoms are used for verbal communication with the patient, and all units have "panic buttons" with which the patient may summon assistance. These devices may be insufficient, however, to monitor the health status of a sedated, anesthetized, or unresponsive patient. MRI—safe/conditional devices are available to monitor multiple physiologic parameters such as heart rate, respiratory rate, blood pressure, and oxygen concentration in the blood. The technologist should always monitor the patient visually and verbally at all times.

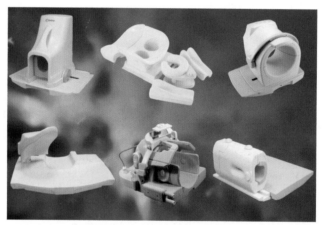

Fig. 30-14 Examples of coils used for MRI. *Upper row, left to right,* Foot/ankle coil, breast coil, and knee coil. *Lower row, left to right,* Shoulder coil, functional head coil, and wrist coil.

(Courtesy Invivo Corporation.)

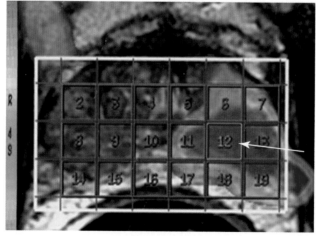

Fig. 30-15 Axial image of prostate obtained with an endorectal coil. The increased resolution allowed by the endorectal coil makes it possible to perform MRS (*PROSE*). The spectroscopy map shows an elevated citrate level (*arrow*) consistent with tumor.

(Courtesy GE Healthcare.)

CONTRAST MEDIA

Contrast agents widen the signal differences in MR images between various normal and abnormal structures. In CT scanning, the use of high-attenuation, orally administered contrast medium allows clear differentiation of the bowel from surrounding lower attenuation structures. In MRI scans, the bowel may lie adjacent to normal or pathologic structures of low, medium, and high signal intensity, and these intensities may change as images of varying T1 and T2 weighting are obtained. Air, water, fatty liquids (e.g., mineral oil), dilute iron solutions (e.g., Geritol), gadolinium compounds designed for intravenous (IV) use, barium sulfate, kaolin (a clay), and various miscellaneous agents have been used.

MRI contrast agents most commonly used in the United States for routine clinical use in the whole body are gadolinium-containing compounds. Gadolinium is a metal with *paramagnetic* effects. Pharmacologically, an intravenously administered gadolinium compound acts similarly to radiographic iodinated IV agents: It is distributed through the vascular system, its major route of excretion is the urine, and it respects the blood-brain barrier (i.e., it does not leak out from the blood vessels into the brain substance unless the barrier has been damaged by a pathologic process).

New contrast agents used for MRA examinations are known as blood pool agents and contain a gadolinium base. By binding to albumin found in the body, these blood pool agents produce shorter T1 relaxation times than regular gadolinium compounds, resulting in a brighter signal on the final image. These agents also prolong retention in the bloodstream, allowing for longer imaging times. Imaging using these agents may allow estimates of tissue perfusion and ischemia. Enhancement of heart muscle could assist in differentiating healthy, ischemic, or infarcted myocardial tissue.

Gadolinium compounds are used most commonly in evaluation of the central nervous system. The most important clinical action of gadolinium compounds is the shortening of T1. In T1-weighted images, this provides a high-signal, high-contrast focus in areas where gadolinium has accumulated by leaking through the broken blood-brain barrier into the brain substance (Fig. 30-16). In gadolinium-enhanced T1-weighted images, brain tumors or metastases are better distinguished from their surrounding edema than in routine T2-weighted images. Gadolinium improves the visualization of small tumors or tumors that have a signal intensity similar to that of a normal brain, such as meningiomas. Rapid intravenous

(IV) injections of gadolinium are routinely used in dynamic imaging studies of body organs such as the liver and kidneys, similar to techniques using standard radiographic iodinated agents in CT. Contrast-enhanced MRA is routinely performed to image the blood vessels in the neck (carotid) and body.

In general, gadolinium agents are nonspecific; however, organ specific agents have been developed primarily for imaging the liver. Iron oxide mixtures known as *superparamagnetic* contrast agents are available but not widely used. These agents are referred to as T2 contrast agents because they shorten the T2 relaxation times of normal tissue. Research and development of novel contrast agents to improve the specificity of MRI imaging continues.

Despite the fact the gadolinium is a toxic substance, gadolinium containing contrast agents (GBCAs) are well tolerated and typically have fewer side effects and are less nephrotoxic than iodine-based contrast agents. Nevertheless, patients with severe kidney disease and reduced renal function are susceptible to developing a life-threatening condition known as nephrogenic systemic fibrosis (NSF). Care should be taken when using GBCAs in this patient population.

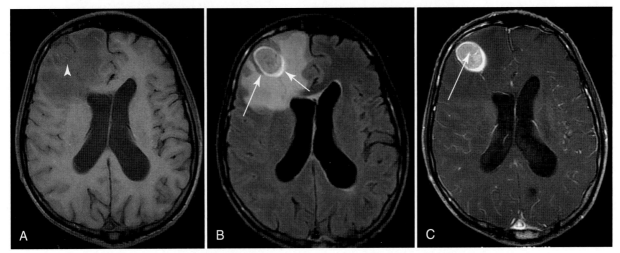

Fig. 30-16 Use of IV gadolinium contrast medium for lesion enhancement in axial images of the brain. **A,** T1-weighted sequence. A single brain lesion (*arrowhead*) is seen as a focal area of low signal intensity in a large area of edema. The borders of the lesion are difficult to delineate. **B,** FLAIR image. High signal areas (*arrows*) represent tumor and surrounding edema. **C,** T1-weighted image obtained using similar parameters after IV administration of gadolinium. Lesion borders and size (*arrow*) are much more conspicuous.

GATING

Gated imaging is another technique for improving image quality in areas of the body in which involuntary patient motion is a problem. A patient can hold his or her head still for prolonged data acquisition, but heartbeat and breathing cannot be suspended for the several minutes required for standard MRI studies. Even fast pulse sequences are susceptible to motion *artifact* from the beating heart; this is a problem when images of the chest or upper abdomen are desired. If special techniques are not used, part of the MRI signal may be obtained when the heart is contracted (systole) and part when the heart is relaxed (diastole). When information is combined into one image, the heart appears blurred. This problem is analogous to photographing a moving subject with a long shutter speed. Similar problems in MRI occur with the different phases of respiration.

Gating techniques are used to organize the signal so that only the signal received during a specific part of the cardiac or respiratory cycle is used for image production (Fig. 30-17). Gated images may be obtained in one of two ways. In one technique of cardiac gating, the imaging pulse sequence is initiated by the heartbeat (usually monitored by an ECG). The data collection phase of the pulse sequence occurs at the same point in the cardiac cycle. Another method is to obtain data throughout the cardiac cycle but record the point in the cycle at which each group of data was obtained. After enough data are collected, the data are reorganized so that all data recorded within a certain portion of the cardiac cycle are collated together: data collected during the first eighth of the cycle, second eighth of the cycle, and so on. Each grouping of data can be combined into a single image, producing multiple images at different times in the cycle.

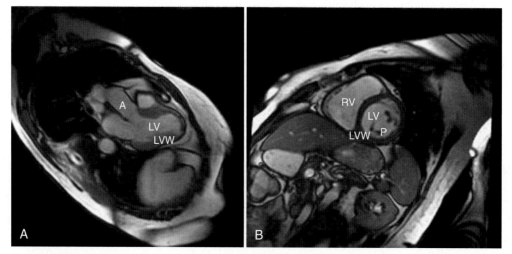

Fig. 30-17 ECG gated images of the heart. **A,** Left ventricular outflow tract (*LVOT*). **B,** Short-axis images. *A,* aorta; *LV,* left ventricle; *LVW,* left ventricular wall; *P,* papillary muscles; *RV,* right ventricle.

OTHER CONSIDERATIONS

When MRI was introduced, long imaging times were required to obtain enough information to reconstruct the sectional images, and this remains the standard for most routine imaging. With advances in technology, it has become possible to obtain enough data quickly (within seconds) to reconstruct an image by using special fast-imaging pulse sequences. These fast-imaging pulse sequences are becoming more popular for specialized applications, such as obtaining a dynamic series of images after IV administration of contrast agents. In many such sequences, fluid has a high signal intensity. This high signal intensity can produce a myelogram-like effect in studies of the spine or an arthrogram-like effect in evaluation of joint fluid (see Fig. 30-11). Quality assurance is important in a complex technology such as MRI. Calibration of the unit is generally performed by service personnel. Routine scanning of phantoms by the technologist can be useful for detecting any problems that may develop.

Clinical Applications
CENTRAL NERVOUS SYSTEM

MRI is the modality of choice for imaging of the central nervous system. It is routinely used in almost all examinations of the brain with the exception of acute trauma. MRI is superior in the brain because of its inherent ability to differentiate the natural contrast among tissues such as gray and white matter (see Fig. 30-12). This ability allows MRI to be more sensitive than CT in detecting changes in white matter disease such as multiple sclerosis. The development of specialized pulse sequences such as fluid attenuation inversion recovery (FLAIR) helps visualize lesions in the periventricular area that were previously difficult to detect. MRI is also superior at imaging the posterior fossa (cerebellum and brain stem) because cortical bone does not produce any signal in MRI (see Fig. 30-13). This area is often obscured on CT because of the beam-hardening artifact. Almost all brain lesions—such as primary and metastatic tumors, pituitary tumors, acoustic neuromas (tumors of the eighth cranial nerve), and meningiomas—are better shown by MRI. The additional use of IV gadolinium–based contrast materials has allowed better differentiation and increased sensitivity in detecting these lesions (Fig. 30-18). Cerebral infarction is identified sooner using diffusion-weighted imaging compared with CT. Diffusion-weighted imaging also gives MRI the ability to determine the age of lesions or differentiate acute from chronic ischemic changes.

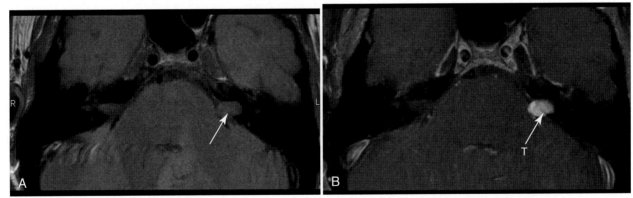

Fig. 30-18 Axial MRI of the brain in a patient with acoustic nerve tumor arising from the seventh and eighth cranial nerve complex. **A,** Precontrast T1-weighted image shows inhomogeneous area of abnormality (*white arrows*), with mass effect expanding the area of the nerve complex. **B,** Image obtained at the same level after gadolinium enhancement. Active tumor (*T*) shows high signal intensity.

MRI is also routinely used to image the spinal canal and its contents. The ability of MRI to image directly in the sagittal plane allows for the screening of a large area in a single examination. T2-weighted pulse sequences permit the separation of cerebrospinal fluid and the spinal cord similar to myelography without the use of contrast media (Fig. 30-19). Because of its inherent ability to differentiate slight changes in soft tissue contrast, MRI is exquisitely sensitive at detecting spinal cord tumor and cystic changes within the cord. The visualization of bony marrow is useful in the detection and diagnosis of metastatic disease and pathologic and nonpathologic vertebral fractures and diskitis (infection). The most prolific use of MRI in the spine is the imaging of disk disease. Direct visualization of the posterior longitudinal ligament in the sagittal plane and vertebral disks in the oblique plane shows the severity of herniated disks (Fig. 30-20). The use of IV gadolinium contrast material helps differentiate between disk herniation and postoperative scar tissue, which is a crucial clinical distinction.

CHEST

MRI is extremely sensitive to physiologic motion, so imaging within the chest is difficult. Advances in multislice/helical CT and the technical challenges of imaging moving anatomy have limited the use of MRI for examining the chest. Cardiac gating (imaging only during a certain part of the cardiac cycle), respiratory gating or triggering, breath-hold scans, and ultrafast imaging sequences have enabled MRI to excel at cardiac imaging, MRI is able to show anatomy and produce functional (ejection fractions, chamber volume) data similar to nuclear medicine and echocardiography. The study of congenital heart disease, imaging of masses, and evaluation of heart muscle viability are now routine (Fig. 30-21). MRI may also be used to image the chest wall, thoracic outlet, and brachial plexus region.

Since its approval in 1991 by the U.S. Food and Drug Administration (FDA) as a supplemental imaging tool, MR mammography or breast MRI has become an essential part of breast imaging. The FDA lists breast MRI in its screening criteria. Breast imaging is routinely used to screen high-risk patients. Surgeons also use it preoperatively to define the extent of the lesion, look for additional lesions, and image the contralateral breast. In addition, it is being used to monitor adjuvant therapy (chemotherapy and radiation therapy) (Fig. 30-22) and diagnose/verify breast implant rupture.

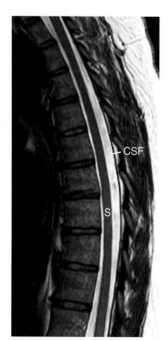

Fig. 30-19 Sagittal T2-weighted MRI through thoracic spine. High signal from CSF outlines the normal spinal cord (*S*), giving a myelogram-like effect without the use of contrast agents.

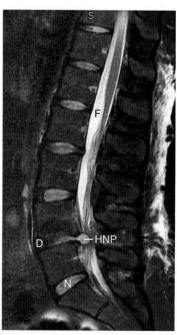

Fig. 30-20 Sagittal T2-weighted image of lumbar spine. Spinal canal is filled with high signal intensity cerebrospinal fluid (*F*) except for low signal intensity linear nerve roots running within the spinal canal. Normal vertebral disks have a high signal intensity nucleus pulposus (*N*). Desiccated disks (*D*) show low signal intensity. At L4-5, note the herniated nucleus pulposus (*HNP*) protruding into the spinal canal and compressing the nerve roots.

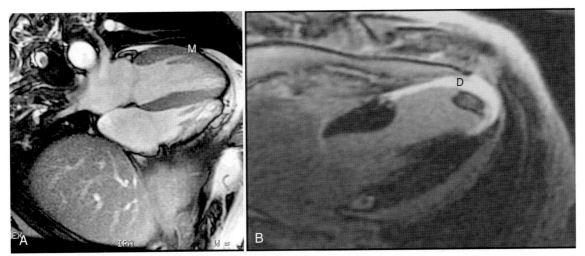

Fig. 30-21 Cardiac MRI: four-chamber view from two different patients. **A,** T2-weighted image showing normal myocardium in the wall of the left ventricle (*M*) before the administration of contrast medium. **B,** Delayed enhancement image (inversion recovery) showing bright signal in the wall of the left ventricle represented infarcted or dead myocardium (*D*).

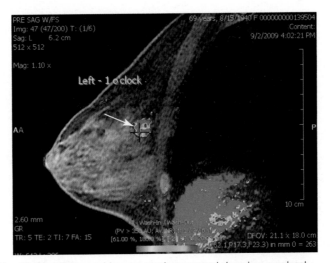

Fig. 30-22 MRI breast image postprocessed showing contrast washin and washout. The patient is a 68-year-old woman with an enhancing mass in the left breast at 1 o'clock position (*arrow*).

ABDOMEN

Although abdominal imaging is also affected by respiratory motion, the use of ultrafast scanning techniques with the ability to acquire two-dimensional and three-dimensional volumes in a breath-hold has made MRI extremely useful in the abdomen as a problem-solving tool. Typically not used as a primary diagnostic tool, MRI is used to follow-up questionable results from other modalities such as CT and ultrasound. One exception is liver imaging, in which MRI may be more sensitive in detecting primary and metastatic tumors. The use of liver-specific IV contrast agents has improved the sensitivity and specificity of liver lesions. MRI has the ability to predict the histologic diagnosis of certain abnormalities such as hepatic hemangiomas, which have a distinctive appearance. The use of in-phase and out-of-phase images can distinguish between benign and malignant adrenal tumors (Figs. 30-23 and 30-24).

PELVIS

Respiratory motion has little effect on the structures in the pelvis. As a result, these structures can be better visualized than structures in the upper abdomen. The ability of MRI to image in the coronal and sagittal planes is helpful in examining the curved surfaces in the pelvis. Bladder tumors are shown well, including tumors at the dome and base of the bladder that can be difficult to evaluate in the transverse dimension. In the prostate (see Fig. 30-15), MRI is useful in detecting neoplasm and its spread. In the female pelvis, MRI can be used to image benign and malignant conditions (Fig. 30-25).

MUSCULOSKELETAL SYSTEM

MRI produces excellent images of the limbs because involuntary motion is not a problem, and MRI contrast among the soft tissues is excellent. The lack of bone artifact on MRI permits excellent visualization of the bone marrow. On plain film radiography and occasionally on CT, dense cortical bone is often hidden in the marrow space. As previously stated, calcium within tumors is better visualized with CT, however, because of the lower MRI signal from calcium.

Overall, the ability to image in multiple planes, along with excellent visualization of soft tissues and bone marrow, has rapidly expanded the role of MRI in musculoskeletal imaging. MRI is particularly valuable for the study of joints, and it is replacing arthrography and, to a lesser extent, arthroscopy in the evaluation of injured knees (see Fig. 30-11), ankles, and shoulders. Small joints are also well evaluated with MRI. Local staging of soft tissue and bone tumors is best accomplished with MRI. Early detection of ischemic necrosis of bone is a strength of MRI.

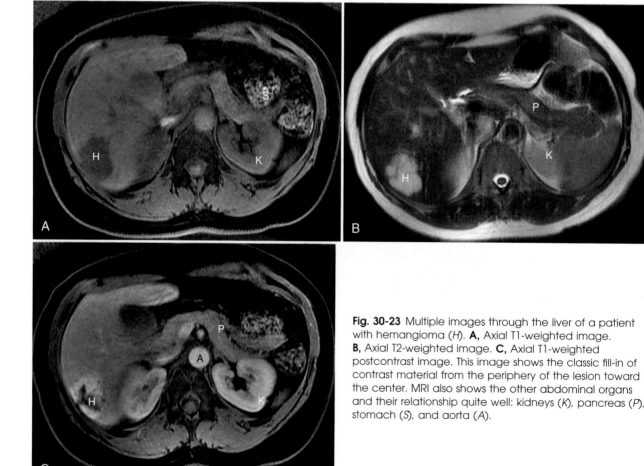

Fig. 30-23 Multiple images through the liver of a patient with hemangioma (*H*). **A,** Axial T1-weighted image. **B,** Axial T2-weighted image. **C,** Axial T1-weighted postcontrast image. This image shows the classic fill-in of contrast material from the periphery of the lesion toward the center. MRI also shows the other abdominal organs and their relationship quite well: kidneys (*K*), pancreas (*P*), stomach (*S*), and aorta (*A*).

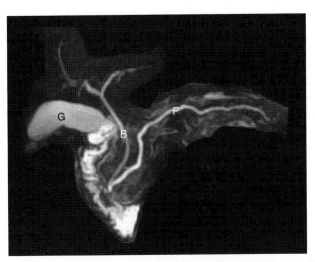

Fig. 30-24 Magnetic resonance cholangiopancreatography (MRCP): heavily T2-weighted images specially designed to image the gallbladder (*G*), biliary (*B*), and pancreatic ducts (*P*).

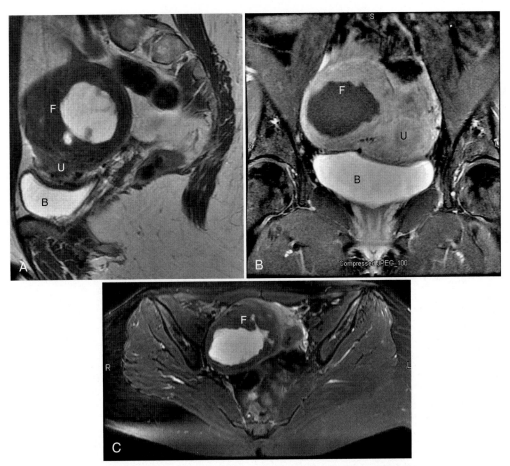

Fig. 30-25 Multiple images through a female pelvis. **A,** Sagittal T2-weighted image. **B,** Coronal T1-weighted image after contrast agent administration. **C,** Axial T1-weighted image after contrast agent administration with fat saturation. All images show the different components of a uterine fibroid (*F*). The relationship between the uterus (*U*) and bladder (*B*) is shown well using multiple imaging planes.

The ability to image in multiple planes, along with excellent visualization of soft tissues and bone marrow and the lack of physiologic motion, has rapidly expanded the role of MRI in musculoskeletal imaging. The lack of bone artifact in MRI permits excellent visualization of the bone marrow (Fig. 30-26) and helps in the more effective diagnosis of pathologic conditions such as stress fractures and avascular necrosis (Fig. 30-27). MRI has become the imaging choice for joints. It has replaced radiographic arthrography in all joints, although magnetic resonance arthrography is now routinely performed. The ability to quantify cartilage loss is very helpful in treating osteoarthritis. Staging of soft tissue and bone tumors is best accomplished with MRI (Fig. 30-28).

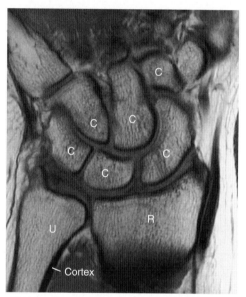

Fig. 30-26 T1-weighted coronal MRI of the wrist using a surface coil to improve visualization of superficial structures. Marrow within the carpal bones (*C*), radius (*R*), and ulna (*U*) has high signal as a result of its fat content. A thin black line of low signal cortex surrounds the marrow cavity of each bone, and trabecular bone can be seen as low signal detail interspersed within marrow.

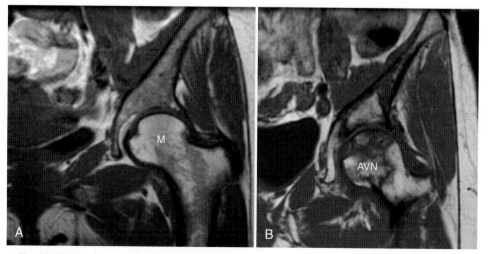

Fig. 30-27 Two T1-weighted images of the left hip from different patients. **A,** Normal bone marrow signal (*M*). **B,** Abnormal bone marrow signal consistent with avascular necrosis (*AVN*).

VESSELS

MRA is the imaging of vascular structures by magnetic resonance. Two techniques used to obtain images of flowing blood are time of flight (TOF) and phase contrast (PC). Using either of these techniques, MR angiograms can be obtained in two-dimensional or three-dimensional volumes. In TOF imaging, a special pulse sequence is used that suppresses the MRI signal from the anatomic area surrounding the vessels of interest. Consequently, an MRI signal is given only by material that is outside the area of study when the signal-suppressing pulse occurs. Incoming blood makes vessels appear bright, whereas stationary tissue signal is suppressed (Fig. 30-29). PC imaging takes advantage of the shifts in phase, or orientation, experienced by magnetic nuclei moving through the MRI field. Special pulse sequences enhance these effects in flowing blood, producing a bright signal in vessels when the unchanging signal from stationary tissue is subtracted. PC imaging is used when data about velocity and direction of blood are needed.

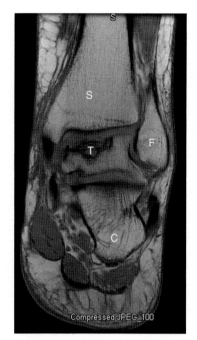

Fig. 30-28 Coronal T1-weighted image of the ankle. Bone marrow shows high signal intensity because of fat. Osteochondral defect seen in dome of the talus (*T*) shows low signal intensity. *C,* calcaneus; *F,* fibula; *S,* tibia.

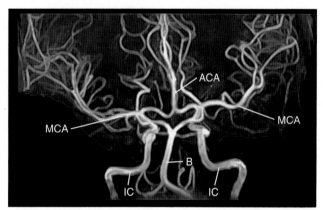

Fig. 30-29 MRA shows intracranial arterial vessels in AP view. *ACA,* anterior cerebral arteries; *B,* basilar artery; *IC,* internal carotids; *MCA,* middle cerebral artery. In the center is the circle of Willis.

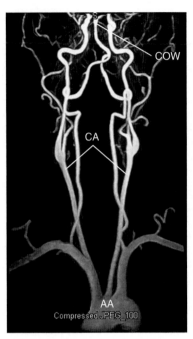

Fig. 30-30 Contrast-enhanced MRA shows carotid arteries (*CA*) from the aortic arch (*AA*) to the circle of Willis (*COW*).

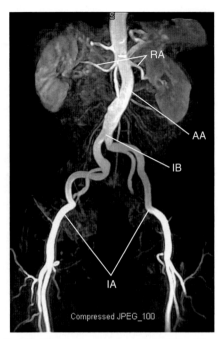

Fig. 30-31 Contrast-enhanced MRA of the abdominal aorta (*AA*), shows the renal arteries (*RA*), iliac bifurcation (*IB*), and iliac arteries (*IA*).

TOF imaging can be used with the injection of gadolinium-containing IV contrast material. Gadolinium shortens the T1 relaxation time of blood, increasing its signal intensity and allowing a decrease in imaging time (breath-hold sequences) and three-dimensional volume imaging in the long axis of the vessel. Imaging of the carotid (Fig. 30-30), thoracic, abdominal, and pelvic arteries (Fig. 30-31) is possible. With the use of a moving table, the aorta can be imaged from the heart to the feet. This is routinely performed to screen for vascular lesions in the peripheral vasculature. Vascular imaging can be used to look for dissections, aneurysms, arteriovenous malformations, plaques, stenosis, and occlusions.

In routine MRI, fast flowing blood typically has a signal void. This signal void is helpful in determining whether flow is normal or visualizing thrombus within the vessel.

DIFFUSION AND PERFUSION

The sensitivity of MRI to motion can be a handicap and a potential source of information. Motion artifacts interfere with upper abdominal images that are affected by heart and diaphragmatic motion, yet flow-sensitive pulse sequences can image flowing blood in blood vessels.

Specialized techniques have been developed that can image the *diffusion* and *perfusion* of molecules within matter. Molecules of water undergo random motion within tissues, but the cellular membranes (or lack thereof) affect the rate of this diffusion. Tissues have structure, and this structure affects the rates of diffusion and perfusion and their direction; in other words, diffusion and perfusion are not entirely random in a structured tissue. These microscopic motions can be detected by specialized MRI pulse sequences that can image their rate and direction. Diffusion and perfusion motion differ among tissue types. Diffusion patterns of gray matter in the brain differ from the diffusion patterns in more directionally oriented fiber tracts of white matter. This concept is currently used in diffusion tensor imaging.

Diffusion and perfusion imaging is most often used in the brain to visualize ischemic changes such as stroke. Recovery from acute stroke can be predicted by viewing the mismatch between the diffusion and perfusion images. Diffusion and perfusion imaging can produce clinically significant images that may help in the understanding of white matter degenerative diseases (e.g., multiple sclerosis, ischemia, infarction) (Fig. 30-32); the development of possible therapies to return blood flow to under perfused brain tissue; and the characterization of brain tumors. Similar applications for the rest of the body may be developed if technical difficulties, particularly difficulties related to patient motion such as breathing, can be overcome.

Spectroscopy

In routine MRI, the purpose is to produce detailed pictures of the anatomy being imaged. This is accomplished by spatially localizing the MRI signal in a volume of tissue. In magnetic resonance spectroscopy (MRS), the result is a graph, or spectra, of the chemical composition of the volume of tissue being "imaged." This graph not only denotes the chemical compounds present but also the relationship between the amount of each compound. In pathologic conditions in which the imaging characteristics are similar or difficult to interpret, MRS can add vital information leading to a more accurate interpretation.

MRS is most commonly used in the brain. It can be helpful in diagnosing metabolic conditions, tumor recurrence versus necrosis, and pathologic processes (Fig. 30-33). The use of MRS is becoming more widespread in breast and prostate imaging to differentiate between normal and abnormal tissue. It has also been used to study normal physiologic changes such as seen in muscle contraction (Fig. 30-34).

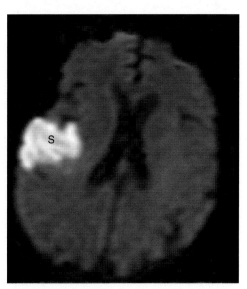

Fig. 30-32 Diffusion-weighted image shows acute ischemic infarct (stroke) (*S*) in the right middle cerebral artery territory. Lack of diffusion in this area turns this area bright on this heavily T2-weighted image.

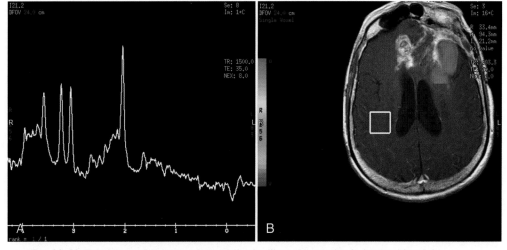

Fig. 30-33 Routine spectroscopy in a patient with a primary brain tumor. Voxel shows normal brain spectra in an area unaffected by the brain tumor.

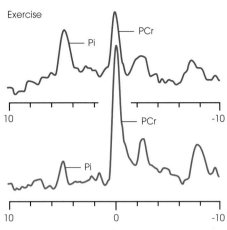

Fig. 30-34 Spectra from human muscle before (*red line*) and during (*blue line*) exercise. Thin horizontal lines represent separate baselines for each spectrum. Each peak represents a different chemical species, and the area under the peak down to the baseline indicates the amount of substance present. The inorganic phosphate (*Pi*) peak increases with exercise as energy-rich phosphocreatine (*PCr*) is used to provide energy for muscle contraction.

Functional Magnetic Resonance Imaging

Functional MRI (fMRI) records active areas of the brain during certain activities or after the introduction of stimuli, such as visual or auditory stimuli. Typically, fMRI uses the differences in the magnetic properties of oxygenated and deoxygenated blood to visualize active areas of the brain. The use of oxygenated and deoxygenated blood as a contrast agent is known as blood oxygen level dependent (BOLD) imaging. The human body is composed of approximately 50% oxygenated and 50% deoxygenated blood. Oxygenated blood displays diamagnetic properties; that is, it does not affect molecules in the surrounding area. Deoxygenated blood is a paramagnetic substance, which increases T2* decay and decreases the availability of signal in the area immediately surrounding it (magnetic susceptibility artifact). Because of this increase in magnetic susceptibility artifact, it is possible for MRI to measure the difference between oxygenated and deoxygenated blood. As blood flow increases to areas of activation, the MRI scanner is able to distinguish the subtle differences in signal and register the area of brain activity.

Currently, fMRI is used for many areas of research in an effort to increase understanding of human brain anatomy and function. Studies involving the visual cortex, memory, Alzheimer's disease, schizophrenia, and many others have been performed. fMRI may prove useful in areas of lie detection and mind reading. fMRI displays promise for the future of MRI not only as a diagnostic tool but also as a predictor of future behaviors and disease processes.

Conclusion

Since its inception in the 1970s, MRI has evolved into a sophisticated tool useful in the diagnosis and staging of disease processes. At present, MRI is the imaging modality of choice for the central nervous system and musculoskeletal system, and it is expanding to play a vital role in the areas of breast, cardiac, and abdominal imaging. MRI remains a complementary tool for other imaging modalities and is becoming a vital tool of its own with the addition of fMRI.

Although it remains an expensive technology, MRI applications continue to increase because of its inherent flexibility and hardware and software advances. New organ-specific and blood pool contrast agents allow imaging techniques that may increase available information regarding normal anatomy and pathology. These advances will help MRI maintain its place in the imaging world.

Definition of Terms

antenna Device for transmitting or receiving radio waves.

artifact Spurious finding in or distortion of an image.

attenuation Reduction in energy or amount of a beam of radiation when it passes through tissue or other substances.

coil Single or multiple loops of wire (or another electrical conductor such as tubing) designed to produce a magnetic field from current flowing through the wire or to detect a changing magnetic field by voltage induced in the wire.

contrast Degree of difference between two substances in some parameter, with the parameter varying depending on the technique used (e.g., attenuation in radiographic techniques or signal strength in MRI).

cryogenic Relating to extremely low temperature (see *superconductive magnet*).

diffusion Spontaneous random motion of molecules in a medium; a natural and continuous process.

echo planar imaging Fast pulse sequence that can be used to create MR images within a few seconds.

fat-suppressed images Images in which the fat tissue in the image is made to be of a lower, darker signal intensity than the surrounding structures.

frequency Number of times that a process repeats itself in a given period (e.g., the frequency of a radio wave is the number of complete waves per second).

fringe field Portion of the magnetic field extending away from the confines of the magnet that cannot be used for imaging but can affect nearby equipment or personnel.

gating Organizing data so that the information used to construct the image comes from the same point in the cycle of a repeating motion, such as a heartbeat. The moving object is "frozen" at that phase of its motion, reducing image blurring.

gauss (G) Unit of magnetic field strength (see *tesla*).

gradient echo Fast pulse sequence that is often used with three-dimensional imaging to generate T2-weighted images.

inversion recovery Standard pulse sequence available on most MRI imagers; the name indicates that the direction of longitudinal magnetization is reversed (inverted) before relaxation (recovery) occurs.

longitudinal plane Plane that extends along the long axis of the body, dividing the body into either right and left portions or anterior and posterior portions. This plane corresponds to the direction of the main magnetic field in superconducting magnets and is the location of protons awaiting excitation by the RF coil.

magnetic resonance (MR) Process by which certain nuclei, when placed in a magnetic field, can absorb and release energy in the form of radio waves. This technique can be used for chemical analysis or for the production of cross-sectional images of body parts. Computer analysis of the radio-wave data is required.

MRI conditional An item that has been demonstrated to pose no known hazards in a specified MRI environment with specified conditions of use.

MRI safe An item that poses no known hazards in all MRI environments.

noise Random contributions to the total signal that arise from stray external radio waves or imperfect electronic apparatus or other interference. Noise cannot be eliminated, but it can be minimized; it tends to degrade the image by interfering with accurate measurement of the true MRI signal, similar to the difficulty in maintaining a clear conversation in a noisy room.

nuclear magnetic resonance (NMR) Another name for magnetic resonance; this term is not commonly used.

nucleus Central portion of an atom, composed of protons and neutrons.

paramagnetic Referring to materials that alter the magnetic field of nearby nuclei. Paramagnetic substances are not themselves directly imaged by MRI but instead change the signal intensity of the tissue where they localize, acting as MRI contrast agents. Paramagnetic agents shorten the T1 and the T2 of the tissues they affect, actions that tend to have opposing effects on signal intensity. In clinical practice, agents are administered in a concentration in which either T1 or T2 shortening predominates (usually the former) to provide high signal on T1-weighted images.

perfusion Flow of blood through the vessels of an organ or anatomic structure; usually refers to blood flow in the small vessels (e.g., capillary perfusion).

permanent magnet Object that produces a magnetic field without requiring an external electricity supply.

precession Rotation of an object around the direction of a force acting on that object. This should not be confused with the axis of rotation of the object itself (e.g., a spinning top rotates on its own axis, but it may also precess [wobble] around the direction of the force of gravity that is acting on it).

proton density Measure of proton (i.e., hydrogen, because its nucleus is a single proton) concentration (number of nuclei per given volume); one of the major determinants of MRI signal strength in hydrogen imaging.

pulse See *radiofrequency (RF) pulse.*

pulse sequence Series of radio-wave pulses designed to excite nuclei in such a way that their energy release has varying contributions from proton density, T1, or T2 processes.

radiofrequency (RF) pulse A short burst of radio waves. If the radio waves are of the appropriate frequency, they can give energy to nuclei that are within a magnetic field by the process of magnetic resonance. Length of the pulse determines amount of energy given to the nuclei.

rapid acquisition recalled echo Commonly known as fast, or turbo, spin echo; a fast pulse sequence used to create spin echo–like T2-weighted images rapidly.

raw data Information obtained by radio reception of the MRI signal as stored by a computer. Specific computer manipulation of these data is required to construct an image from them.

relaxation Return of excited nuclei to their normal, unexcited state by the release of energy.

relaxation time Measure of the rate at which nuclei, after stimulation, release their extra energy.

resistive magnet Simple electromagnet in which electricity passing through coils of wire produces a magnetic field.

resonance Process of energy absorption by an object that is tuned to absorb energy of a specific frequency only. All other frequencies would not affect the object (e.g., if one tuning fork is struck in a room full of tuning forks, only the forks tuned to that identical frequency would vibrate [resonate]).

signal In MRI, induction of current into a receiver coil by precessing magnetization.

slice Cross-sectional image; can also refer to the thin section of the body from which data are acquired to produce the image.

spectroscopy Science of analyzing the components of an electromagnetic wave, usually after its interaction with some substance (to obtain information about that substance).

spin echo Standard MRI pulse sequence that can provide T1-weighted, T2-weighted, or proton density–weighted images. The name indicates that a declining MRI signal is refocused to gain strength (similar to an echo) before it is recorded as raw data.

spin-lattice relaxation Release of energy by excited nuclei to their general environment; one of the major determinants of MRI signal strength. T1 is a rate constant measuring spin-lattice relaxation.

spin-spin relaxation Release of energy by excited nuclei as a result of interaction among themselves; one of the major determinants of MRI signal strength. T2 is a rate constant measuring spin-spin relaxation.

superconductive magnet Electromagnet in which the coils of wire are cooled to an extremely low temperature so that the resistance to the conduction of electricity is nearly eliminated (superconductive).

superparamagnetic Material that has a greater effect with a magnetic field; it can dramatically decrease the T2 of tissues, causing a total loss of signal by the absorbing structures.

T1 Rate constant measuring spin-lattice relaxation.

T2 Rate constant measuring spin-spin relaxation.

tesla (T) Unit of magnetic field strength; 1 tesla equals 10,000 gauss or 10 kilogauss (other units of magnetic field strength). The earth's magnetic field approximates 0.5 gauss.

transverse plane Plane that extends across the axis of the body from side to side, dividing the body part into upper and lower portions.

Selected bibliography

Bloch F: Nuclear induction, *Physiol Rev* 70:460, 1946.

Burghart G, Finn CA: *Handbook of MRI scanning*, St Louis, 2010, Mosby

Bushong SC: *MRI physical and biological principles*, ed 3, St Louis, 2003, Mosby.

Damadian R: Tumor detection by nuclear magnetic resonance, *Science* 171:1151, 1971.

Kelley LL, Petersen CM: *Sectional anatomy for imaging professionals*, ed 2, St Louis, 2007, Mosby.

Purcell EM et al: Resonance absorption by nuclear magnetic moments in a solid, *Physiol Rev* 69:37, 1946.

Shellock FG: *Magnetic resonance procedures: health effects and safety*, Boca Raton, FL, 2001, CRC Press.

Shellock FG: *Reference manual for magnetic resonance safety, implants, and devices*, Los Angeles, 2005, Biomedical Research Publishing Group.

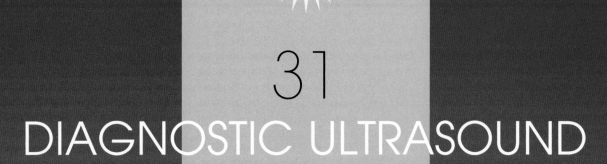

31

DIAGNOSTIC ULTRASOUND

SUSANNA L. OVEL

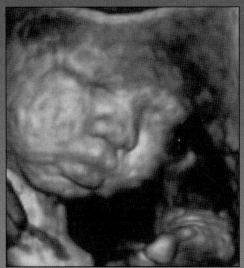

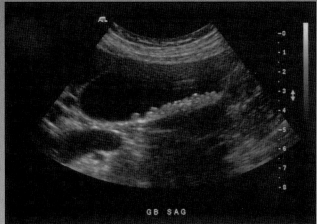

GB SAG

OUTLINE

Principles of Diagnostic
  Ultrasound, 370
Historical Development, 371
Physical Principles, 372
Anatomic Relationships and
  Landmarks, 373
Clinical Applications, 374
Cardiologic Applications, 393
Conclusion, 396

Principles of Diagnostic Ultrasound

Diagnostic medical sonography is a general term used to encompass abdominal, breast, cardiac, gynecologic, obstetric, and vascular sonography. *Registered diagnostic medical sonographers* (RDMSs) specialize in abdominal sonography, obstetrics/gynecology imaging, breast sonography, musculoskeletal imaging, or neonatal neurosonography. *Registered diagnostic cardiac sonographers* (RDCSs) specialize in fetal, pediatric, or adult echocardiography. *Registered vascular technologists* (RVTs) specialize in abdominal vasculature imaging, imaging of arteries and veins of the upper and lower extremities, imaging of extracranial arteries and veins, transcranial duplex sonography, and physiologic vascular testing in pediatric and adult patients. One overall physics examination, encompassing sonographic principles, hemodynamics, and instrumentation, is required for all these specialties.

Diagnostic medical sonography employs high-frequency transducers ranging from 2 to 30 MHz. The transducer emits short pulses of ultrasound (pulse waves) into the human body. The transducer receives real-time reflections or frequency shifts from structures or vessels along the sound waves path, and they are displayed as a grayscale, color Doppler, spectral, or duplex image. Velocity of the red blood cells can be calculated using the Doppler technique. Pulse wave, continuous wave, and color Doppler techniques show blood flow direction, flow resistance and turbulence within the vessel, and regurgitation of the cardiac chamber.

Diagnostic medical sonography has evolved into a unique imaging tool. Sonography was previously thought to be a completely noninvasive technique; however, with the introduction of intracavity and intraluminal transducers, collection of diagnostic data of the pelvic and cardiovascular regions has been shown to improve patient management and care.

CHARACTERISTICS OF DIAGNOSTIC MEDICAL SONOGRAPHERS

The diagnostic medical sonographer uses complicated equipment, independent judgment, and systematic problem-solving skills to acquire quality images and technical data for assistance in a patient's diagnosis, management, and care. Integrity and honesty are important qualities in all medical professionals. In sonography, these character traits are crucial because almost 90% of observed data is discarded.

After each examination, the sonographer provides the reading physician with a technical report detailing the size and description of normal and abnormal anatomy or hemodynamics along with possible differential diagnostic considerations.

Similar to radiography, diagnostic medical sonography has national standardized protocols for each examination. The sonographer has the ability to expand on basic examination protocols when additional information is needed without fear of ionizing radiation. In-depth knowledge of pathophysiology, laboratory values, and other medical imaging modalities (i.e., computed tomography [CT], magnetic resonance imaging [MRI]) is an important part of sonography education.

Physical requirements play an additional role in sonography. Sonographers must be able to aid in moving patients and medical equipment. Attention to the use of proper body mechanics is essential (Fig. 31-1). Repetitive usage injury or syndrome of the neck, shoulder, elbow, wrist, and back has been documented. The sonographer should be in good physical, emotional, and nutritional health and possess a dedication to continual learning. The career can be exciting and rewarding as well as stressful, demanding, frustrating, and occasionally depressing.

RESOURCE ORGANIZATIONS

Resource organizations devoted exclusively to ultrasound include the American Society of Echocardiography (ASE), the Society of Diagnostic Medical Sonography (SDMS), the American Institute of Ultrasound in Medicine (AIUM), the Society of Radiologists in Ultrasound (SRU), and the Society of Vascular Ultrasound (SVU). International Foundation for Sonography Education and Research (IFSER) is a unique organization devoted to the educators of ultrasound.

Historical Development

The development of *sonar** was the precursor to the development of medical ultrasound. Sonar equipment was initially constructed for defense efforts during World War II to detect the presence of submarines. Various investigators later proved that ultrasound had a valid contribution to make to medicine.

In 1947, Dussick positioned two transducers on opposite sides of the head to

---

*Almost all italicized words on the succeeding pages are defined at the end of this chapter.

measure ultrasound transmission profiles. He also discovered that this technique could detect tumors and other intracranial lesions. In the early 1950s, Dussick with Heuter, Bolt, and Ballantyne continued to use *through-transmission* techniques and computer analysis to aid in the diagnosis of brain lesions in the intact skull. They discontinued their studies, however, after concluding that the technique was too complicated for routine clinical use.

In the late 1940s, Howry (a radiologist), Wild (a diagnostician interested in tissue characterization), and Ludwig (interested in reflections from gallstones) independently showed that when ultrasound waves generated by a piezoelectric crystal transducer were transmitted into the human body, these waves would be returned to the transducer from tissue interfaces of different *acoustic impedances*. At this time, research efforts were directed toward transforming naval sonar equipment into a clinically useful diagnostic tool. In 1948, Howry developed the first ultrasound scanner, consisting of a cattle watering tank with a wooden rail anchored along the side. The transducer carriage moved along the rail in a horizon-

tal plane, and the object to be scanned and the transducer were positioned inside the water tank.

Hertz and Edler developed echocardiographic techniques in 1954 in Sweden. These investigators were able to distinguish normal heart valve motion from the thickened, calcified valve motion seen in patients with rheumatic heart disease. In 1957 in Scotland, Brown and Donald built an early obstetric contact-compound scanner. This scanner was used primarily to evaluate the location of the placenta and to determine the gestational age of the fetus.

Further developments resulted in real-time ultrasound instrumentation. High-frequency transducers with improved *resolution* allow the sonographer to accumulate several images per second at a rate of up to 30 frames per second. Today's ultrasound systems include color Doppler, spectral analysis, and three- and four-dimensional imaging in addition to real-time imaging. Diagnostic ultrasound as used in clinical medicine has not been associated with any harmful biologic effects and is generally accepted as a safe modality.

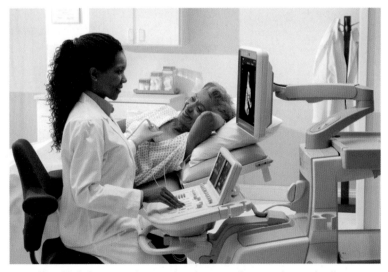

Fig. 31-1 Sonographer performing an ultrasound examination.

(Courtesy Philips Medical Systems.)

Physical Principles
PROPERTIES OF SOUND WAVES

Sound waves are traveling variations of pressure, density, and particle motion. Matter must be present for sound to travel; it cannot travel through a vacuum. Sound carries energy, not matter, from one place to another. Vibrations from one molecule carry to the next molecule along the same axis. These oscillations continue until friction causes the vibrations to cease.

Ultrasound refers to sound waves beyond the audible range (>20 kHz). Diagnostic medical sonography can use frequencies of 2 to 30 MHz.

Acoustic impedance

Sound travels through tissues at different speeds depending on the density and stiffness of the medium. Acoustic impedance of a medium determines how much of the wave transmits to the next medium (Fig. 31-2).

Velocity of sound

Propagation speed is the speed with which a sound wave travels through a medium. It is determined by the density and stiffness of a medium. In soft tissue, the propagation speed of sound is 1540 m/sec. Bone shows a very high propagation speed (4080 m/sec), whereas air shows the lowest propagation speed (330 m/sec).

TRANSDUCER SELECTION

Diagnostic ultrasound transducers operate on the principle of piezoelectricity. The *piezoelectric effect* states that some materials produce a voltage when deformed by an applied pressure. Diagnostic ultrasound transducers convert electrical energy into acoustic energy during transmission and acoustic energy into electrical energy for reception. Diagnostic imaging transducers routinely operate in a frequency range of 2 to 15 MHz. Transducers may be linear, convex, sector, or vector in construction (Fig. 31-3). Higher frequencies are used in intracavity and intraluminal transducers and for visualizing the extremities or superficial structures. Lower frequencies are needed for deeper structures of the thoracic cavity, abdomen, and pelvis. Lower frequencies provide necessary penetration depth at the expense of *detail resolution*.

Pulse wave transducers transmit pulses of sound and receive returning echoes producing a grayscale ultrasound image. A continuous wave transducer produces a continuous wave of sound and is composed of a separate transmit and receiver element within a single transducer assembly. Continuous wave transducers do not produce an image.

VOLUME SCANNING AND THREE-DIMENSIONAL AND FOUR-DIMENSIONAL IMAGING

Volume scanning allows for quick "sweeps" of specific areas of the body or fetus. These sweeps give volume data that can be rendered even after the patient has left the ultrasound department. Three-dimensional imaging systems allow the sonographer to acquire volume data. The sonographer can reconstruct these data into a three-dimensional image on the ultrasound machine or at a workstation. With four-dimensional imaging, the

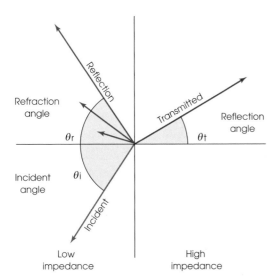

Fig. 31-2 Relationship among incident, reflected, and transmitted waves.

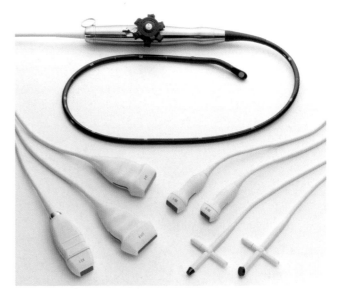

Fig. 31-3 Various ultrasound transducers.

(Courtesy Philips Medical Systems.)

ultrasound system is able to acquire and display three-dimensional images in real time.

Anatomic Relationships and Landmarks

The use of anatomic landmarks to define specific areas of the human body is an important part of the imaging and orientation skills of the sonographer. The middle hepatic vein is a sonographic landmark used to locate the division between the left and right hepatic lobes (Fig. 31-4, A). The main lobar fissure is used to locate the gallbladder fossa (Fig. 31-4, B). The ovaries are located medial and anterior to the iliac vessels (Fig. 31-4, C). The use of anatomic landmarks is a routine part of many sonographic examinations.

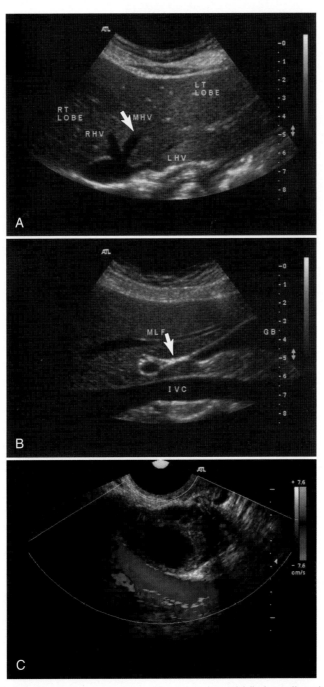

Fig. 31-4 A, Transverse sonogram of liver showing middle hepatic vein (*MHV*) dividing left and right hepatic lobes. *LHV,* left hepatic vein; *RHV,* right hepatic vein. **B,** Sagittal image of main lobar fissure (*MLF*) and its relationship to gallbladder (*GB*). **C,** Sagittal color Doppler image of right ovary lying anterior and medial to iliac vessels.

(Courtesy Paul Aks, BS, RDMS, RVT.)

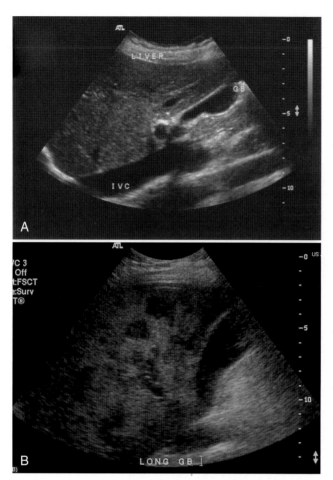

Fig. 31-5 A, Sagittal sonogram of normal homogeneous liver. **B,** Longitudinal sonogram of heterogeneous hepatic lobe in a patient with a history of breast carcinoma.

Clinical Applications
CHARACTERISTICS OF THE SONOGRAPHIC IMAGE

The sonographer uses specific terms to characterize the sonographic image. If the echo pattern is similar throughout a structure or mass, it is termed *homogeneous* (Fig. 31-5, *A*). If the echo pattern is dissimilar throughout a structure or mass, it is termed *heterogeneous* (Fig. 31-5, *B*). Internal composition of a structure or mass is described using the terms *anechoic* (without internal echoes), *echogenic* (with internal echoes), and *complex* (containing anechoic and echogenic regions) (Fig. 31-6). The sonographer also uses descriptive terms to describe the borders of a mass. Are the borders smooth or irregular, thin or thick, calcified or dilated?

Imaging artifacts are an additional concern for the sonographer. Acoustic artifacts include reflections that are missing; not real; improperly positioned; or of improper brightness, number, shape, or size (Fig. 31-7). Understanding the assumptions of the ultrasound system and the physical principles of sound waves, the sonographer is better able to comprehend the real-time images.

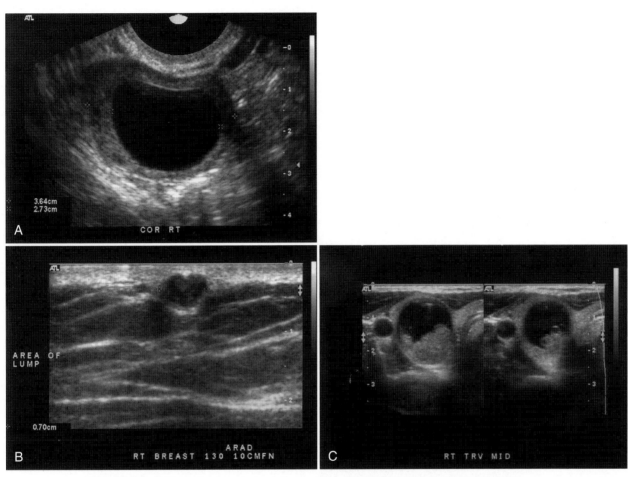

Fig. 31-6 A, Endovaginal sonogram of anechoic ovarian cyst. **B,** Echogenic mass is measured in upper inner quadrant of right breast. **C,** Transverse sonogram of complex thyroid mass.

(Courtesy Paul Aks, BS, RDMS, RVT.)

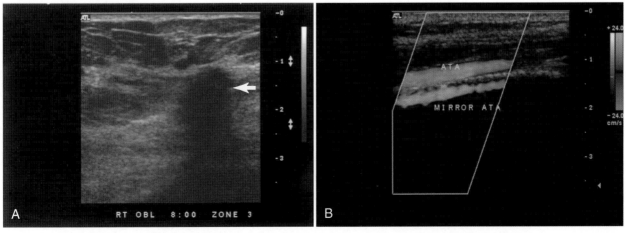

Fig. 31-7 A, Breast carcinoma showing posterior acoustic shadowing (*arrow*). **B,** Mirror image of anterior tibial artery.

ABDOMEN AND RETROPERITONEUM

The abdominal ultrasound examination generally includes a survey of the liver, pancreas, gallbladder, spleen, great vessels, and kidneys in the sagittal and transverse planes (Figs. 31-8 and 31-9). Specific protocols are followed to image size, shape, and echogenicity of the organ *parenchyma* and anatomic relationships of the surrounding structures. Doppler flow patterns of the upper abdominal blood vessels may be included. Patients are examined in two different body positions (i.e., supine and decubitus). The use of two positions shows mobility of gallstones and repositions interfering bowel gas. Air reflects most of the sound wave, making visualization of the abdominal and retroperitoneal structures difficult. Abdominal examinations are typically scheduled in the morning with the patient fasting 6 to 8 hours before the sonogram.

The retroperitoneal ultrasound examination includes a survey of the great vessels, kidneys, and bladder in the sagittal and transverse planes before and after voiding. Specific protocols are followed to image the size, shape, cortical thickness, and echogenicity of the renal parenchyma. Anterior-posterior diameters of the inferior vena cava, aorta, and common iliac arteries are measured and documented. Doppler flow patterns of the great vessels and kidneys may be included. Retroperitoneum examinations can be scheduled in the morning or afternoon with the patient drinking 8 to 16 oz. of water 1 hour before the sonogram.

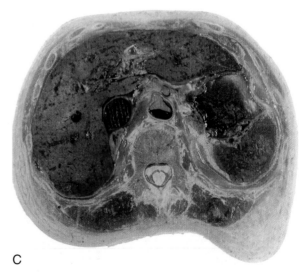

A

B

Aorta and
trunk of superior
Round ligament mesenteric artery
Splenic artery

Liver,
caudate
process

Left
lobe
of liver

Porta
hepatis

Stomach

Inferior
vena
cava

Left
adrenal
gland

Right
adrenal
gland

Spleen

Right
lobe
of liver

Spine   Spinal cord

C

Fig. 31-8 A, Transverse sonogram of right upper quadrant over right lobe of liver. **B,** Line drawing of gross anatomic section. **C,** Gross anatomic section at approximately same level as **A.**

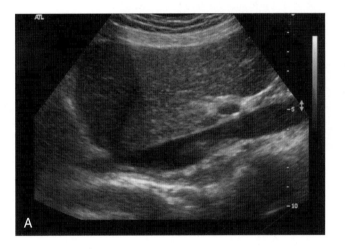

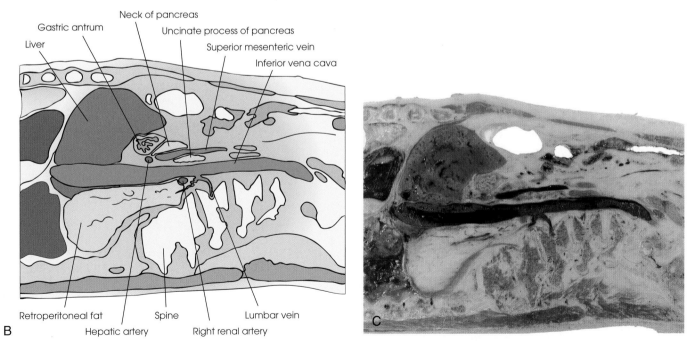

Fig. 31-9 A, Sagittal sonogram of right upper quadrant over medial segment of left lobe of the liver, hepatic vein, and inferior vena cava. **B,** Line drawing of gross anatomic section. **C,** Gross anatomic section at approximately same level as **A.**

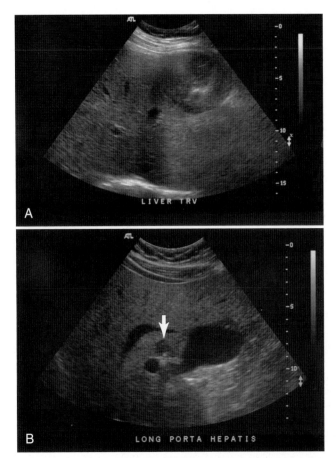

Fig. 31-10 A, Transverse sonogram of liver shows a complex mass in the left lobe.
B, Sonogram of liver shows fatty infiltration with small area of normal liver parenchyma anterior to porta hepatis (*arrow*).

(**A,** Courtesy Paul Aks, BS, RDMS, RVT.)

To produce an adequate survey of the abdominal and retroperitoneal cavities, the sonographer must have an understanding of the patient's clinical history. Although ultrasound cannot diagnose the specific pathology of a lesion or condition, a complete clinical picture may lead to more specific differential diagnostic considerations.

Liver and biliary tree

Sonographic examinations of the liver and biliary tree are generally requested in patients with right upper quadrant pain or elevations in liver function laboratory tests. The liver is assessed for size and echogenicity of the parenchyma. Under normal circumstances, the liver parenchyma appears moderately echogenic and homogeneous. Some types of liver pathologies shown on ultrasound include fatty infiltration, cirrhosis, cavernous hemangioma, and hepatoma (Fig. 31-10). Doppler evaluation of the hepatic artery, hepatic veins, and portal veins is included with a patient history or suspicion of cirrhosis, portal hypertension, portal vein thrombosis, and Budd-Chiari syndrome.

The biliary tree includes the gallbladder and the intrahepatic and extrahepatic bile ducts. The gallbladder is evaluated for size, wall thickness, and absence of internal echoes. Under normal circumstances, the gallbladder is a pear-shaped anechoic structure located in the gallbladder fossa on the posterior surface of the liver (Fig. 31-11). The intrahepatic biliary ducts converge near the *porta hepatis* forming the common hepatic duct. The cystic duct joins the common hepatic duct to form the extrahepatic common bile duct. The biliary tree is evaluated for size and evidence of intraductal stones or masses. Some abnormalities of the biliary tree shown on ultrasound include intrahepatic and extrahepatic biliary obstruction, cholelithiasis, and cholecystitis (Fig. 31-12).

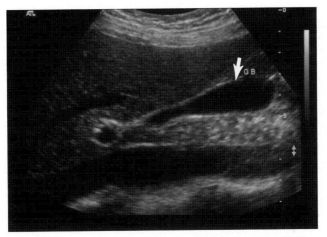

Fig. 31-11 Sagittal sonogram of normal gallbladder (*GB*).

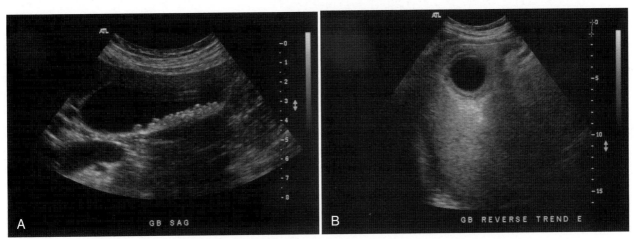

Fig. 31-12 A, Sagittal sonogram of gallbladder showing multiple small gallstones with posterior acoustic shadowing. **B,** Transverse sonogram of acute cholecystitis.

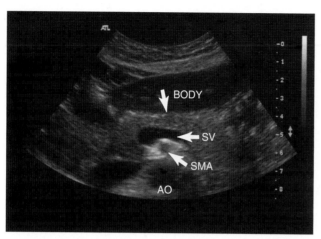

Fig. 31-13 Transverse sonogram of normal pancreas. The body of the pancreas lies anterior to splenic vein (*SV*), superior mesenteric artery (*SMA*), and aorta (*AO*).

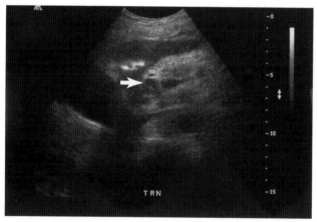

Fig. 31-14 Transverse sonogram shows hypoechoic mass in head of the pancreas (*arrow*).

Pancreas

The pancreas is an elongated organ oriented in a *transverse oblique plane* in the epigastric and left hypochondriac regions of the retroperitoneal cavity. The head of the pancreas lies in the descending portion of the duodenum and lateral to the superior mesenteric artery. The body is the largest portion, lying anterior to the superior mesenteric artery and splenic vein (Fig. 31-13). The tail is the superiormost portion lying posterior to the antrum of the stomach and generally extends toward the splenic hilum. The echogenicity of the pancreas varies depending on the amount of fat but should appear homogeneous throughout the organ. Ultrasound examinations of the pancreas are requested in patients with a history of unexplained weight loss, epigastric pain, and elevation in pancreatic enzymes or liver function laboratory tests. The pancreas is evaluated for size and echogenicity of the parenchyma. The distal common bile duct is routinely measured in the posterior lateral portion of the head of the pancreas. Some abnormalities of the pancreas shown on ultrasound include inflammation, calcifications, tumor, or abscess formation (Fig. 31-14).

Spleen

The spleen is the predominant organ in the left upper quadrant located inferior to the diaphragm and anterior to the left kidney. Ultrasound examinations of the spleen are requested in patients with a history of abdominal trauma, chronic liver disease, and leukocytosis. Increase in hepatic pressures from liver disease may cause an abnormal increase in the size of the spleen (Fig. 31-15). The normal spleen appears moderately echogenic, similar to the normal liver parenchyma. The spleen is evaluated for size and echogenicity of the parenchyma. Some abnormalities of the spleen shown on ultrasound include splenomegaly, splenic rupture, calcifications, or abscess formation. Doppler evaluation of the splenic artery and vein is included with a patient history or suspicion of portal hypertension.

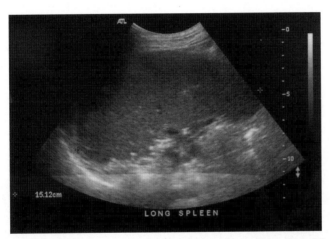

Fig. 31-15 Sagittal sonogram of enlarged spleen measuring greater than 15 cm in length (splenomegaly).

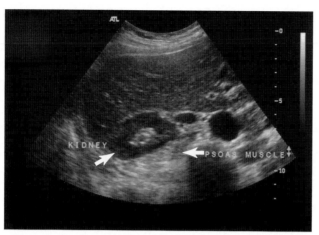

Fig. 31-16 Transverse sonogram of right kidney lying posterior to the liver and lateral to the psoas muscle.

Kidneys and bladder

The kidneys are bean-shaped structures lying in a *sagittal* oblique plane lateral to the psoas muscles in the retroperitoneal cavity (Fig. 31-16). Ultrasound examinations of the kidneys and bladder are requested in patients with a history of urinary tract infection, flank pain, hematuria, and increase in creatinine levels. The normal adult renal cortex shows a moderate- to low-level echo pattern, *hypoechoic,* to the liver and spleen. The renal sinus is the most echogenic portion of the kidney and considered *hyperechoic* to the surrounding structures. The kidneys are evaluated for contour, size, cortical thickness, dilation of calyces (hydronephrosis), and echogenicity of the renal parenchyma. Ultrasound guidance is used to localize the kidney during renal biopsy procedures and to evaluate for any postbiopsy complications.

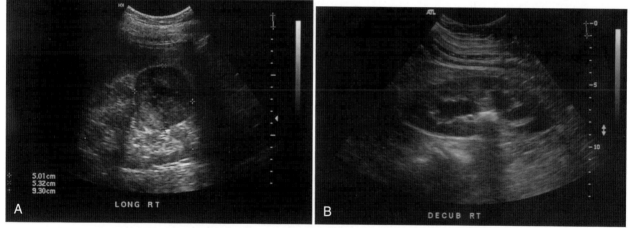

Fig. 31-17 A, Sagittal sonogram shows hypoechoic mass in anterior right kidney.
B, Sagittal sonogram of right kidney shows mild hydronephrosis and hyperechoic kidney stone.

Ultrasound is a useful imaging tool to monitor a renal transplant. The transplant is typically placed superficially in the right iliac fossa. Sonograms of the transplant include grayscale images to evaluate size, contour, echogenicity, and cortical thickness. The renal artery and vein are evaluated with Doppler checking for intimal thickening, stenosis, and thrombosis.

A partially distended urinary bladder is evaluated for wall thickness, contour, and evidence of neoplasm. Postvoid imaging is included to evaluate the amount of residual urine and competence of the ureteral valves. Abnormalities of the kidneys and bladder shown on ultrasound include urinary obstruction, nephrolithiasis, abscess formation, cortical thinning, and benign and malignant neoplasms (Fig. 31-17).

MUSCULOSKELETAL STRUCTURES

The musculoskeletal system provides movement of the body parts and organs. Ultrasound examinations of the musculoskeletal structures are requested in patients with a history of trauma, palpable mass, and chronic pain. On ultrasound, normal muscles show a low to medium shade of gray echo pattern with hyperechoic striations throughout. Tendons appear homogeneous with hyperechoic linear bands. Some abnormalities of the musculoskeletal system shown on ultrasound include muscle or tendon tears, inflammation, hematoma, and edema (Fig. 31-18).

SUPERFICIAL STRUCTURES

Superficial structures image well with ultrasound and include soft tissues, thyroid glands, breast, scrotum, and abdominal wall. The echogenicity of the thyroid glands and testes is similar showing a moderately echogenic parenchymal pattern. Breast tissue varies depending on the amount of fat content. In sonography, all breast tissues are compared with the medium level echo pattern of normal breast fat. Abdominal wall ultrasound examinations may be requested to rule out evidence of herniation or hematoma. Soft tissue ultrasound examinations are generally requested to evaluate a specific mass. Abnormalities of the superficial structures shown on ultrasound include inflammation, herniation, hematomas, and benign and malignant neoplasms (Figs. 31-19 and 31-20).

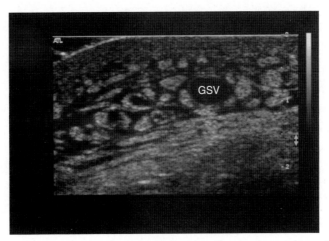

Fig. 31-18 Transverse sonogram of medial thigh shows tissue edema surrounding great saphenous vein (*GSV*).

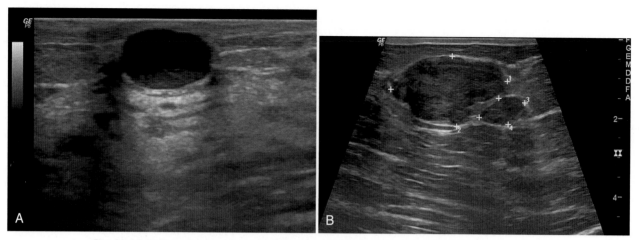

Fig. 31-19 A, Breast cyst with debris is shown demonstrating well-defined borders, fluid-fluid level and increased through transmission. **B,** Fibroadenomas (*calipers*) demonstrate well-defined borders and may have some increased transmission; however, the internal echo pattern is solid and homogeneous. Benign lesions typically demonstrate a mass wider than tall.

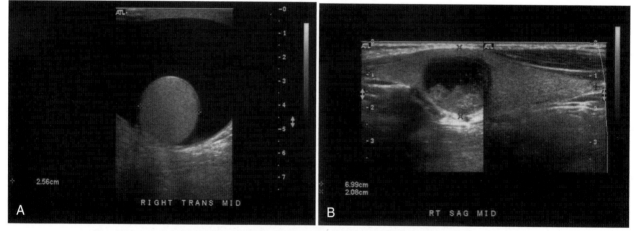

Fig. 31-20 A, Transverse sonogram of right testis surrounded by anechoic fluid (hydrocele). **B,** Sagittal image of complex thyroid mass.

(Courtesy Paul Aks, BS, RDMS, RVT.)

NEONATAL NEUROSONOGRAPHY

Premature infants are susceptible to intracranial hemorrhage resulting from stress on the immature ventricular walls and vascular circulation. The anatomy of the neonatal brain and ventricular system is easily visualized through the small opening of the anterior fontanelle. Portability of ultrasound equipment allows performance of the sonogram in the neonatal intensive care unit. The neonatal brain is evaluated for ventricular dilation and intracranial hemorrhage. Abnormalities of the neonatal brain shown on ultra-sound include intracranial hemorrhage, ventriculomegaly, agenesis of the corpus callosum, and arteriovenous malformation (Fig. 31-21).

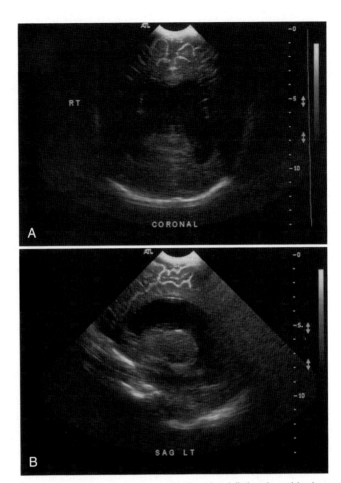

Fig. 31-21 A, Coronal sonogram in a neonate showing bilateral ventriculomegaly. **B,** Sagittal sonogram of left lateral ventricle showing ventriculomegaly.

GYNECOLOGIC APPLICATIONS
Anatomic features of the pelvis

The pelvis is divided into the true and false pelvis by the *iliopectineal line*. The *false pelvis* contains loops of bowel and is bound by the abdominal wall, ala of the iliac bones, and base of the sacrum. The *true pelvis* contains the female reproductive organs, urinary bladder, distal ureters, and bowel (Fig. 31-22). It is bound by the symphysis pubis, sacrum, and coccyx. The pelvic floor is formed by ligaments and the levator ani, piriformis, and coccygeus muscles.

The *retrouterine pouch or pouch of Douglas* lies between the uterus and the rectum. Free fluid routinely accumulates in this area. All pelvic recesses should be imaged on all transabdominal and endovaginal sonograms.

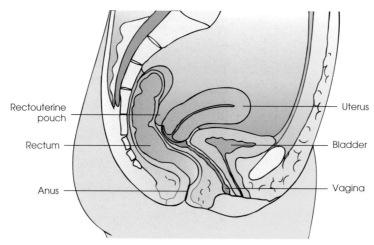

Rectouterine pouch

Rectum

Anus

Uterus

Bladder

Vagina

Fig. 31-22 Sagittal line drawing of female pelvis.

Sonography of the female pelvis

Sonography of the female pelvis is clinically useful in the premenarche, menarche, and postmenopausal periods. Pelvic ultrasound examinations are requested for assessment of a pelvic mass, pelvic pain, or abnormal uterine bleeding; infertility monitoring; and localization of an intrauterine device.

A complete transabdominal examination of the female pelvis includes evaluation and documentation of the distended urinary bladder, uterus, cervix, endometrial canal, vagina, ovaries, adnexal regions, pelvic recesses, and supporting pelvic musculature. The full bladder helps to reposition the intestines laterally into the false pelvis. The urinary bladder serves as an *acoustic window* and anechoic landmark in transabdominal imaging. Real-time imaging allows the sonographer to evaluate the entire pelvic area for pathology and peristalsis of the bowel (Fig. 31-23).

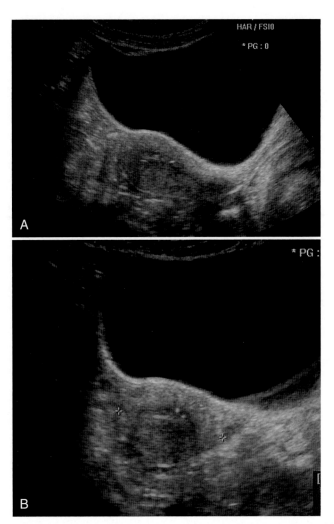

Fig. 31-23 A, Transabdominal sagittal sonogram of uterus. **B,** Transabdominal tranverse sonogram of uterus with measurements.

Endovaginal transducers show excellent detail resolution of the uterine endometrium at the expense of penetration depth and acoustic windows (Fig. 31-24). Endovaginal sonography should be used in conjunction with a transabdominal pelvic examination. A high-frequency transducer is inserted into the vaginal canal to evaluate the uterus, endometrium, ovaries, adnexal regions, and pelvic recesses in the sagittal and coronal planes (Fig. 31-25).

The normal adult uterine myometrium appears homogeneous and moderately echogenic on ultrasound. The echogenicity and thickness of the normal endometrium vary with the menstrual cycle but should not exceed 14 mm in anteroposterior diameter. Normal ovaries appear moderately echogenic with small functional cysts (follicles) of varying size and number. Monitoring the number and size of *follicular cysts* is a common practice in infertility treatment. Ultrasound is used to aid the gynecologist in determining when the ovum is ready for stimulation with high doses of human chorionic gonadotropin. Some abnormalities of the female pelvis shown on ultrasound include congenital malformation, leiomyoma, endometrial polyp, ovarian cyst, and tubal ovarian abscess (Fig. 31-26).

OBSTETRIC APPLICATIONS

Obstetric sonography is probably the most well known ultrasound examination. An obstetric sonogram allows the obstetrician to view and monitor the developing *embryo* and *fetus*. Routine screening examinations are requested between 16 and 24 *gestational weeks* to measure *gestational age*, evaluate fetal anatomy, localize placental placement, assess amniotic fluid, and evaluate cervical competence. Evaluation of the fetus is relatively easy because the fetus occupies a fluid-filled *gestational sac,* an excellent acoustic window for ultrasound.

In the first trimester, endovaginal imaging is more likely to image an early gestational sac, yolk sac, amniotic cavity, and embryo (Figs. 31-27 and 31-28). The number of viable embryos is easily diagnosed with a first-trimester sonogram. The gestational sac may be visualized at 4.5 gestational weeks, and embryo cardiac activity can be identified at 5.5 gestational weeks with endovaginal sonography. By the 9th gestational week, the cerebral hemispheres and limb buds are evident. By the 12th gestational week, the fetus has a skeletal body.

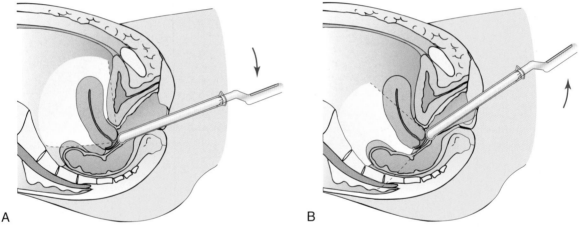

Fig. 31-24 A, Transvaginal sagittal scan with anterior angulation to visualize better the fundus of normal anteflexed uterus. **B,** Transvaginal sagittal scan with posterior angulation to visualize better cervix and rectouterine recess.

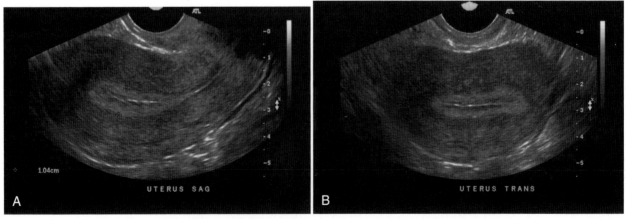

Fig. 31-25 A, Endovaginal sagittal sonogram of uterus. **B,** Coronal sonogram of uterus.

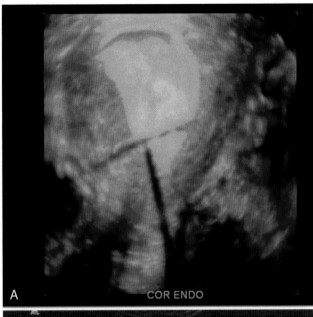

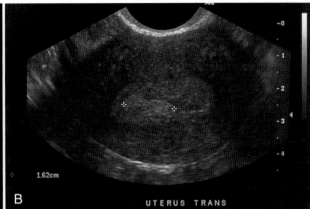

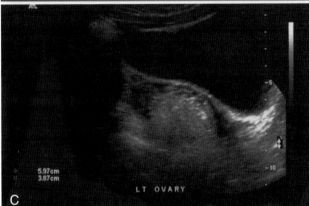

Fig. 31-26 A, Volumetric coronal sonogram of uterine cervix showing improper location of an intrauterine device. **B,** Coronal image of the endometrium showing a hyperechoic neoplasm (calipers). **C,** Sagittal image of complex left ovarian mass.

(**A** and **C,** Courtesy Paul Aks, BS, RDMS, RVT.)

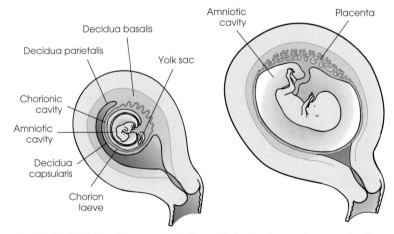

Fig. 31-27 First-trimester representations of developing embryo and yolk sac within amniotic and chorionic cavities of the uterus.

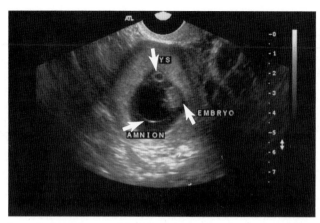

Fig. 31-28 Endovaginal sonogram of first-trimester pregnancy. Yolk sac (*YS*), embryo, and amnion are easily visualized within fluid-filled gestational sac.

(Courtesy Sharon Ballestero, RT, RDMS.)

During the second trimester (13 to 28 gestational weeks), detailed anatomy of the fetus is identified. Structures such as the brain, face, limbs, spine, abdominal wall, stomach, kidneys, bladder, and heart are evaluated and documented. Measurements of the biparietal diameter, circumference of the fetal head, abdominal circumference, and femur length are used to determine gestational age and are termed *biometric measurements* (Fig. 31-29). Documentation of the placenta, amniotic fluid, and fetal position is also included.

In the third trimester (29 to 40 gestational weeks), the fetus grows an additional 4 inches in length and gains 2000 to 2800 g in weight (4 to 6 lb). Third-trimester ultrasound examinations are

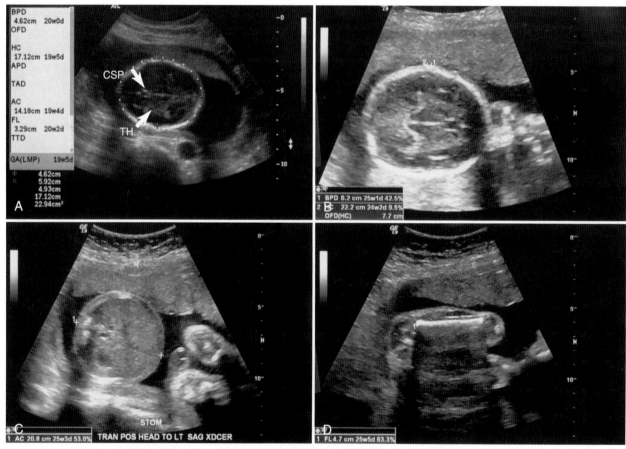

Fig. 31-29 A, Biparietal diameter (*BPD*) is measured perpendicular to falx cerebri in a plane that passes through the third ventricle and thalami. **B,** Fetal head circumference is measured in a plane that must include the cavum septi pellucidi (*CSP*) and tentorial hiatus. **C,** Abdominal circumference is a cross-sectional measurement slightly superior to cord insertion at junction of left and right portal veins and shows a short length of umbilical vein and left portal vein. **D,** Femur length (*FL*) is measured parallel to femoral shaft at level of femoral head cartilage and distal femoral condyle.

(Courtesy Sharon Ballestero, RT, RDMS.)

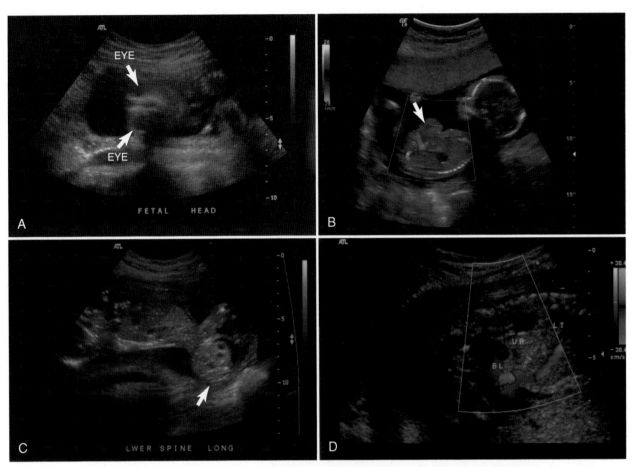

Fig. 31-30 A, Early second-trimester sonogram of the fetal face showing anencephaly (frog-face). **B,** Sagittal image of early second-trimester fetus showing gastroschisis. **C,** Sagittal image of second-trimester fetus showing sacral teratoma (*arrow*). **D,** Sagittal image of left kidney showing hydronephrosis.

(**B,** Courtesy Sharon Ballestero, RT, RDMS. **C,** Courtesy B. Alex Stewart, RT, RDMS.)

generally requested to evaluate fetal growth and position, amniotic fluid volume, and placental placement.

Obstetric sonography is a safe imaging modality for evaluating normal and abnormal development of embryologic and fetal anatomy. A detailed ultrasound examination can assess complications of pregnancy, such as ectopic pregnancy, fetal demise, neural tube defects, nuchal cord, skeletal or limb anomalies, cardiac defects, gastrointestinal and genitourinary defects, and head anomalies (Fig. 31-30). Evaluation of the fetus using three-dimensional and four-dimensional imaging is not presently a routine part of obstetric screening examinations (Fig. 31-31).

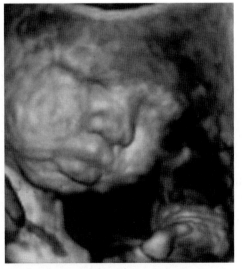

Fig. 31-31 Three-dimensional sonogram of second-trimester fetal face.

(Courtesy Kimberly Smith, BS, RDMS, RVT.)

VASCULAR APPLICATIONS

Sonography applications for evaluating the hemodynamics and anatomy of vascular structures continue to increase. Color Doppler imaging and spectral analysis can evaluate blood flow characteristics of the vascular structures in the neck, upper and lower extremities, abdomen, and pelvis. Registered vascular technologists have specialized education and training in arterial and venous anatomy, hemodynamics, arterial and venous abnormalities, and additional physiologic vascular testing (i.e., pulse volume recording).

Abdominal duplex examinations are requested in patients with a history or suspicion of portal hypertension, mesenteric ischemia, renal artery stenosis, and portal vein thrombosis. Spectral analysis of blood flow velocity and direction is evaluated and documented. Specific criteria are used to diagnose the degree of arterial narrowing shown on the spectral analysis.

The extracranial carotid arteries are evaluated using duplex sonography (Fig. 31-32). Arterial patency, blood flow velocity, resistance, direction, and evidence of turbulence are evaluated with color Doppler and spectral analysis. The highest flow velocities in the common carotid, internal carotid, external carotid, vertebral, and subclavian arteries are recorded. The velocity difference between the common and internal carotid arteries is used to diagnose the degree or percentage of stenosis (i.e., 50%) (Fig. 31-33).

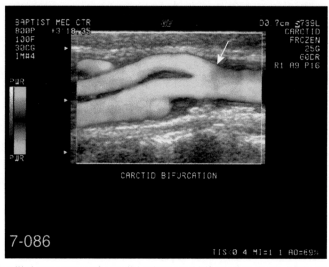

Fig. 31-32 Sagittal sonogram of carotid artery and bifurcation (*arrow*) into internal and external carotid arteries.

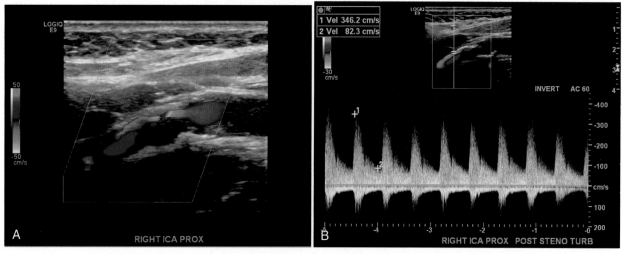

Fig. 31-33 A, Sagittal image of carotid artery with high-grade stenosis in proximal internal carotid artery. **B,** Color Doppler and spectral analysis show increases in flow velocity in stenotic internal carotid artery.

Duplex sonograms of the lower extremity arterial arteries are requested in patients with symptoms of claudication, rest pain, decrease in palpable pedal pulse, and bypass graft surveillance. Patients with a clinical history of hypertension, cigarette smoking, and diabetes mellitus have an increased risk of developing peripheral arterial disease. Duplex examination of the lower extremities begins at the distal aorta. The common and external iliac arteries are examined for any inflow abnormalities. The common femoral, deep femoral, femoral, popliteal, anterior tibial, posterior tibial, and peroneal arteries are evaluated in grayscale, with color Doppler and spectral analysis for patency, plaque formation, increases in flow velocity, and, when applicable, degree of stenosis. Upper extremity arterial duplex examinations are requested in patients with arm or hand pain, asymmetric blood pressures, and changes in skin pallor. Using duplex sonography, the subclavian, axillary, brachial, ulnar, and radial arteries are evaluated for patency, plaque formation, increase in flow velocities, and, when applicable, degree of stenosis.

Duplex sonographic examination of the lower extremity veins is an inexpensive imaging modality to evaluate for deep vein thrombosis and venous insufficiency. Lower extremity venous duplex sonograms are requested to map venous incompetence before an ablation procedure. Incompetence of the venous valves (venous insufficiency) is the most common cause of varicose vein development. Lower extremity venous duplex examinations are requested in patients with a history of acute or chronic leg pain, edema, changes in skin pigmentation, and varicose veins.

The deep venous system is evaluated for patency and valve competency. The small and great saphenous veins are measured and evaluated for patency, valve competency, and association with vari-

cosities. Visible perforator veins are also evaluated for patency and valve competency. The sonographer provides a technical report to the reading physician detailing the findings regarding evidence of lower extremity deep vein thrombosis, venous insufficiency, and possible source of varicosities (Fig. 31-34). Upper extremity venous examinations are requested in patients with indwelling catheters, arm or hand swelling, and arm pain. The internal jugular, subclavian, axillary, brachial, cephalic, and basilic veins are evaluated for patency and *phasic flow*.

Additional physiologic testing is used to evaluate peripheral arterial and venous flow. The ankle/brachial index (ABI), venous return time, and pulse volume recording are examples of nonimaging vascular testing.

Cardiologic Applications

Real-time echocardiography of the fetal, neonatal, pediatric, and adult heart has proven to be a tremendous diagnostic aid for the cardiologist and internist. Multiple imaging windows are used to image cardiac anatomy in detail, including the four chambers of the heart, four heart valves (mitral, tricuspid, aortic, and pulmonic), interventricular and interatrial septa, muscular wall of the ventricles, papillary muscles, and chordae tendineae cordis. Difficult cases can be imaged using a transesophageal technique in which the transducer is passed from the mouth, through the esophagus, to the orifice of the stomach.

PROCEDURE FOR ECHOCARDIOGRAPHY

The echocardiographic examination begins with the patient in a left lateral decubitus position. This position allows the heart to move away from the sternum and fall closer to the chest wall, providing a better cardiac "window," or open area, for the sonographer to image. The transducer is placed in the third, fourth, or fifth intercostal space to the left of the sternum. The protocol for a complete echocardiographic examination includes images in the long axis, short axis, apical, and suprasternal windows (Fig. 31-35). Contrast agents improve visualization of viable myocardial tissue.

CARDIAC PATHOLOGY

Echocardiography is used to evaluate many cardiac conditions. Atherosclerosis or previous rheumatic fever may lead to scarring, calcification, and thickening of the valve leaflets. With these conditions, valve tissue destruction continues, causing stenosis and regurgitation of the leaflets and subsequent chamber enlargement.

The effects of sub-bacterial endocarditis can also be evaluated with echocardiography. With this infectious process, multiple small vegetations form on the endocardial surface of the valve leaflets, causing the leaflets to tear or thicken, with resultant severe regurgitation into subsequent cardiac chambers. The echocardiogram of a patient with congestive cardiomyopathy shows generalized four-chamber enlargement, valve regurgitation, and the threat of thrombus formation along the nonfunctioning ventricular wall. The pericardial sac surrounds the ventricles and right atrium and may fill with fluid, impairing normal cardiac function.

Analysis of ventricular function and serial evaluation of patients after a myocardial infarction are accomplished with two-dimensional echocardiography and, in some cases, stress dobutamine echocardiography. Complications of myocardial infarction include rupture of the ventricular septum, development of a left ventricular aneurysm in the weakest area of the wall, and coagulation of thrombus in the akinetic or immobile apex of the left ventricle (Fig. 31-36).

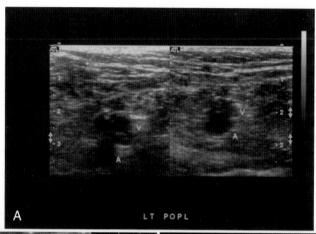

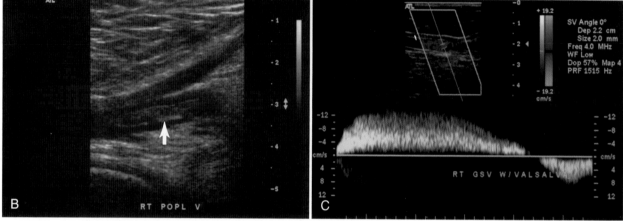

Fig. 31-34 A, Transverse sonograms of popliteal artery and vein without compression (*left image*) and with compression (*right image*) showing a deep vein thrombosis. **B,** Sagittal sonogram of popliteal vein showing echogenic thrombus (*arrow*). **C,** Spectral analysis of great saphenous vein shows venous reflux during Valsalva maneuver signifying venous incompetence at this level.

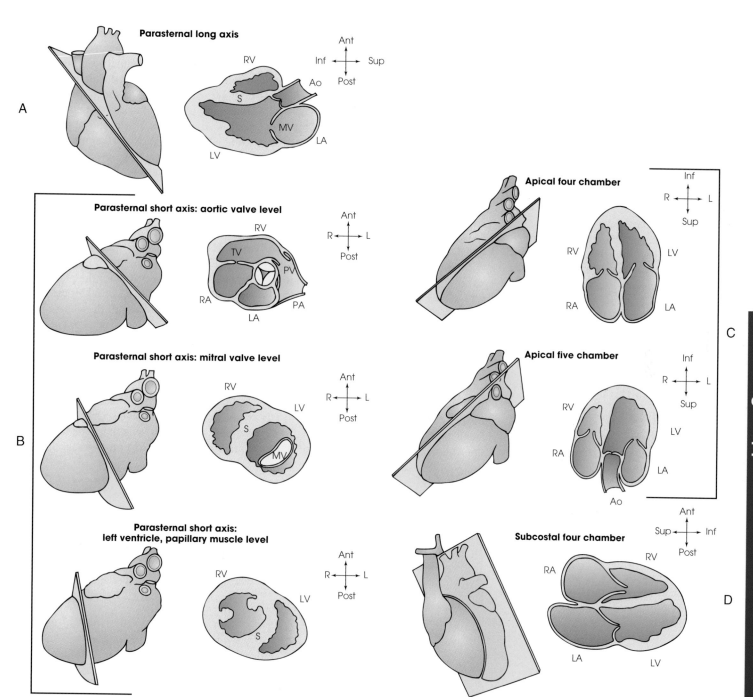

Fig. 31-35 A, Parasternal long-axis drawing. *Ao,* aorta; *LA,* left atrium; *LV,* left ventricle; *MV,* mitral valve; *RV,* right ventricle; *S,* septum. **B,** Parasternal short-axis drawings at various levels: aortic valve level; mitral valve level; and left ventricle, papillary muscle level. *LA,* left atrium; *LV,* left ventricle; *MV,* mitral valve; *PA,* pulmonary artery; *PV,* pulmonic valve; *RA,* right atrium; *RV,* right ventricle; *S,* septum; *TV,* tricuspid valve. **C,** Apical four-chamber image and apical five-chamber image. *Ao,* aorta; *LA,* left atrium; *LV,* left ventricle; *RA,* right atrium; *RV,* right ventricle. **D,** Subcostal four-chamber image. *LA,* left atrium; *LV,* left ventricle; *RA,* right atrium; *RV,* right ventricle.

Within the figure:

Parasternal long axis

RV, Ao, S, MV, LA, LV
Ant / Inf — Sup / Post

Parasternal short axis: aortic valve level

RV, TV, PV, RA, LA, PA
Ant / R — L / Post

Parasternal short axis: mitral valve level

RV, LV, S, MV
Ant / R — L / Post

Parasternal short axis: left ventricle, papillary muscle level

RV, LV, S
Ant / R — L / Post

Apical four chamber

RV, LV, RA, LA
Inf / R — L / Sup

Apical five chamber

RV, LV, RA, LA, Ao
Inf / R — L / Sup

Subcostal four chamber

RA, RV, LA, LV
Ant / Sup — Inf / Post

Congenital heart lesions

Echocardiography has been used to diagnose congenital lesions of the heart in fetuses, neonates, and young children. The cardiac sonographer is able to assess abnormalities of the four cardiac valves, determine the size of the cardiac chambers, assess the interatrial and interventricular septum for the presence of shunt flow, and identify the continuity of the aorta and pulmonary artery with the ventricular chambers to look for abnormal attachment relationships.

A premature infant has an improved chance of survival if the correct diagnosis is made early. If the neonate is cyanotic, congenital heart disease or respiratory failure may be rapidly diagnosed with echocardiography. Critical cyanotic disease in a premature infant may include hypoplastic left heart syndrome, transposition of the great vessels with pulmonary atresia, or severe tetralogy of Fallot.

Conclusion

The contribution of diagnostic ultrasound to clinical medicine has been assisted by technologic advances in instrumentation and transducer design, increased ability to process the returned echo information, and improved methodology for three-dimensional reconstruction of images. The development of high-frequency *endovaginal*, *endorectal*, and *transesophageal transducers* with endoscopic imaging has aided the visualization of previously difficult areas. Improved computer capabilities and advances in teleradiography have enabled the sonographer to obtain more information and process multiple data points to obtain a comprehensive report from the ultrasound study. Color-flow Doppler has made it possible for the sonographer to distinguish the direction and velocity of arterial and venous blood flow from vascular and other pathologic structures in the body. Doppler has allowed the sonographer to determine the exact area of obstruction or leakage present and to determine precisely the degree of turbulence within a vessel or cardiac chamber.

Modifications in transducer design have improved resolution in superficial structures, muscles, and tendons. Advancements in equipment and transducer design have also improved the results of ultrasound examinations in neonates and children. Increased sensitivity allows the sonographer to define the texture of organs and glands with more detail and greater tissue differentiation. Improvements in resolution have aided the visualization of small cleft palate defects, abnormal development of fingers and toes, and small spinal defects. The ability to image the detail of the fetal heart has assisted the early diagnosis of congenital heart disease.

Advanced research and development of computer analysis and tissue characterization of echo reflections should contribute further to the total diagnostic approach using ultrasound. Various abdominal contrast agents continue to be investigated to improve visualization of the stomach, pancreas, and small and large intestines. Cardiac contrast agents are already being used to improve the visualization of viable myocardial tissue within the heart. Saline and other contrast agents are being injected into the endometrial cavity to outline the lining of the endometrium for the purpose of distinguishing polyps and other lesions from the normal endometrium.

Ultrasound has rapidly emerged as a powerful, inexpensive, diagnostic imaging modality with various applications in patient management and care. Expected advancements include further developments in transducer design, image resolution, tissue characterization applications, color-flow sensitivity, and four-dimensional reconstruction of images.

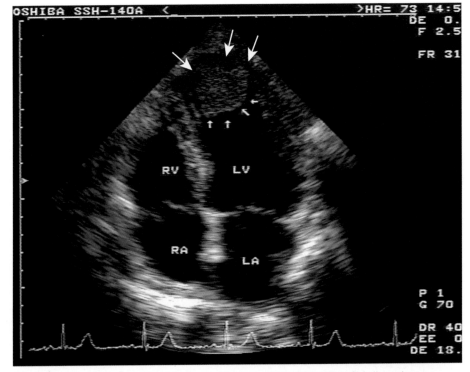

Fig. 31-36 Apical four-chamber image with large apical thrombus. This thrombus (*arrows*) is distinguished from an artifact because it is located in a region with abnormal wall motion, is attached to the apical endocardium, has well-defined borders, and moves in the same direction as the apex. *LA*, left atrium; *LV*, left ventricle; *RA*, right atrium; *RV*, right ventricle.

Definition of Terms

acoustic impedance Resistance of sound as it propagates through a medium.

acoustic window Ability of sonography to visualize a particular area. The full urinary bladder is a good acoustic window to image the uterus and ovaries in a transabdominal sonogram. The intercostal margins may be a good acoustic window to image the liver parenchyma.

anechoic Property of being free of echoes or without echoes.

angle of incidence Angle at which the ultrasound beam strikes an interface with respect to normal (perpendicular) incidence.

ankle/brachial index (ABI) Ratio of ankle pressure to brachial pressure to provide a general guide to help determine the degree of disability of the lower extremity.

attenuation Weakening of the sound wave as it propagates through a medium.

axial resolution Ability to distinguish two structures along a path parallel to the sound beam.

biparietal diameter (BPD) Largest dimension of the fetal head perpendicular to the midsagittal plane; measured by ultrasonic visualization and used to measure fetal development.

color-flow Doppler Velocity in each direction is quantified by allocating a pixel to each area; each velocity frequency change is allocated a color.

complex Containing anechoic and echogenic areas.

continuous wave ultrasound Wave in which cycles repeat indefinitely; consists of a separate transmit and receiver transducer housed within one assembly.

coronal image plane Anatomic term used to describe a plane perpendicular to the sagittal and transverse planes of the body.

detail resolution Includes axial and lateral resolution.

Doppler effect Shift in frequency or wavelength, depending on the conditions of observation; caused by relative motions among sources, receivers, and medium.

Doppler ultrasound Application of Doppler effect to ultrasound to detect movement of a reflecting boundary relative to the source, resulting in a change of the wavelength of the reflected wave.

duplex imaging Combination of grayscale real-time imaging and color or spectral Doppler.

echogenic Refers to a medium that contains echo-producing structures.

embryo Term used for a developing zygote through the 10th week of gestation.

endometrium Inner layer of the uterine canal.

endorectal transducer High-frequency transducer that can be inserted into the rectum to visualize the bladder and prostate gland.

endovaginal transducer High-frequency transducer (and decreased penetration) that can be inserted into the vagina to obtain high-resolution images of the pelvic structures.

false pelvis Region above the pelvic brim.

fetus Term used for the developing embryo from the 11th gestational week until birth.

follicular cyst Functional or physiologic ovulatory cyst consisting of an ovum surrounded by a layer of cells.

frequency Number of cycles per unit of time, usually expressed in Hertz (Hz) or megahertz (MHz) (a million cycles per second).

gestational age Length of time calculated from the first day of the last menstrual period; also known as gestational weeks.

gestational sac Fluid-filled structure normally found in the uterus containing the pregnancy.

grayscale Range of amplitudes (brightness) between white and black.

heterogeneous Having a mixed composition.

homogeneous Having a uniform composition.

hyperechoic Producing more echoes than normal.

hypoechoic Producing less echoes than normal.

iliopectineal line Bony ridge on the inner surface of the ileum and pubic bones that divides the true and false pelvis.

intima Inner layer of the vessel; the middle layer is the media and the outer layer is the adventitia.

ischemia Area of the cardiac myocardium that has been damaged by disruption of the blood supply by the coronary arteries.

isoechoic Having a texture nearly the same as that of the surrounding parenchyma.

lateral resolution Ability to distinguish two structures lying perpendicular to the sound beam.

leiomyoma Most common benign tumor of the uterine myometrium.

myometrium Thick middle layer of the uterine wall.

noninvasive technique Procedure that does not require the skin to be broken or an organ or cavity to be entered (e.g., taking the pulse).

oblique plane Slanting direction or any variation that is not starting at a right angle to any axis.

parenchyma Functional tissue or cells of an organ or gland.

phasic flow Normal venous respiratory variations.

piezoelectric effect Conversion of pressure to electrical voltage or conversion of electrical voltage to mechanical pressure.

porta hepatis Region in hepatic hilum containing common duct, proper hepatic artery, and main portal vein.

posterior acoustic enhancement Increase in reflection amplitude from structures that lie behind a weakly attenuating structure (i.e., cyst).

posterior acoustic shadowing Reduction in reflection amplitude from reflectors lying behind a strongly reflecting or attenuating structure.

pulse wave ultrasound A transducer emits short pulses of ultrasound into the human body and receives reflections from the body before emitting another pulse of sound.

real-time imaging Imaging with rapid frame rate visualizing moving structures or scan planes continuously.

reflection Redirection (return) of a portion of the sound beam back to the transducer.

refraction Phenomenon of bending wave fronts as the acoustic energy propagates from the medium of one acoustic velocity to a second medium of differing acoustic velocity.

regurgitation Occurs when blood leaks from one high-pressure chamber to a chamber of lower pressure.

resolution Measure of ability to display two closely spaced structures as discrete targets.

retroperitoneal cavity Area posterior to the peritoneal cavity that contains the aorta, inferior vena cava, pancreas, part of the duodenum and colon, kidneys, and adrenal glands.

retrouterine pouch Pelvic space located anterior to the rectum and posterior to the uterus; also known as pouch of Douglas.

sagittal Plane that travels vertically from the top to the bottom of the body along the *y* axis.

scattering Diffusion or redirection of sound in several directions on encountering a particle suspension or rough surface.

sonar Instrument used to discover objects under the water and to show their location.

sound wave Longitudinal waves of mechanical energy propagated through a medium.

transducer Device that converts energy from one form to another.

transverse Plane that passes through the width of the body in a horizontal direction.

ultrasound Sound with a frequency greater than 20 kHz.

velocity of sound Speed with direction of motion specified.

Selected bibliography

Callen PW: *Ultrasonography in obstetrics and gynecology,* ed 5, Philadelphia, 2008, Saunders.

Curry RA, Tempkin BB: *Ultrasonography: an introduction to normal structure and function,* ed 3, Philadelphia, 2011, Saunders.

Hagen-Ansert SL: *Textbook of diagnostic ultrasonography,* ed 7, vols I and II, St Louis, 2012, Elsevier Mosby.

Henningsen C: *Clinical guide to ultrasonography,* St Louis, 2005, Mosby.

Henningsen C, Kuntz, K, Youngs D: *Clinical guide to ultrasonography,* ed 2, St Louis, 2014, Mosby.

Kremkau FW: *Diagnostic ultrasound principles and instrumentation,* ed 8, St Louis, 2011, Saunders.

Ovel S: *Sonography exam review: physics, abdomen, obstetrics and gynecology,* ed 2, St Louis, 2014, Mosby.

Rumack CM et al: *Diagnostic ultrasound,* ed 4, St Louis, 2011, Elsevier Mosby.

Zweibel WJ, Pellerito J, editors: *Introduction to vascular ultrasonography,* ed 5, St Louis, 2005, Mosby.

32

NUCLEAR MEDICINE

KIM CHANDLER

OUTLINE

Principles of Nuclear Medicine, 400
Historical Development, 400
Comparison with Other
    Modalities, 401
Physical Principles of Nuclear
    Medicine, 403
Radiation Safety in Nuclear
    Medicine, 407
Instrumentation in Nuclear
    Medicine, 408
Imaging Methods, 410
Clinical Nuclear Medicine, 415
Principles and Facilities in Positron
    Emission Tomography, 421
Clinical Positron Emission
    Tomography, 432
Future of Nuclear Medicine, 435
Conclusion, 437

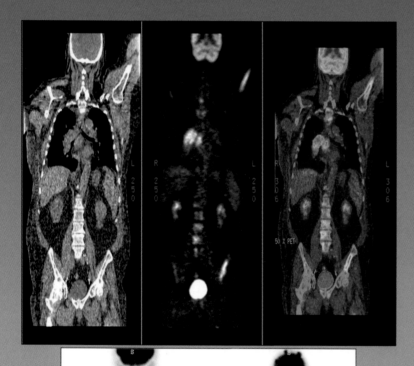

Principles of Nuclear Medicine

Nuclear medicine is a medical specialty that focuses on the use of radioactive materials called *radiopharmaceuticals** for diagnosis, therapy, and medical research. In contrast to radiographic procedures that determine the presence of disease based on structural appearance, nuclear medicine determines the cause of a medical problem based on the physiologic function of organs or tissues.

For a nuclear medicine procedure, the radioactive material, commonly referred to as a *radiopharmaceutical* or a *radiotracer,* is primarily introduced into the body by injection, ingestion, or inhalation. Different radiotracers are used to study different parts of the body. Specific tracers are selected based on their ability to localize in specific organs or tissues. Radiotracers undergo radioactive decay to produce gamma-ray emissions that allow for the detection of the tracer's presence. A special piece of equipment, known as a *gamma* or *scintillation camera,* is used to transform these emissions into images that provide information about the function (primarily) and anatomy of the organ or system being studied. The lowest amount of radiotracer that can be used to ensure a satisfactory examination or therapeutic goal is administered to reduce the radiation exposure to the patient.

Nuclear medicine procedures are performed by a team of specially educated professionals: a nuclear medicine physician, a specialist with extensive education in the basic and clinical science of medicine who is licensed to use radioactive materials; a nuclear medicine technologist who performs the tests and is educated in the theory and practice of nuclear medicine procedures; a physicist who is experienced in the technology of nuclear medicine and the care of the equipment, including computers; and a pharmacist or specially prepared technologist who is qualified to prepare the necessary radioactive pharmaceuticals.

Historical Development

Dalton is considered the father of the modern theory of *atoms* and molecules. In 1803, Dalton, an English schoolteacher,

---

*Almost all italicized words on the succeeding pages are defined at the end of this chapter.

stated that all atoms of a given element are chemically identical, are unchanged by chemical reaction, and combine in a ratio of simple numbers. Dalton measured atomic weights in reference to hydrogen, to which he assigned the value of 1 (the atomic number of this element).

The discovery of x-rays by Roentgen in 1895 was a great contribution to physics and the care of the sick. A few months later, another physicist, Becquerel, discovered naturally occurring radioactive substances. In 1898, Curie discovered two new elements in the uranium ore pitchblende. Curie named these trace elements *polonium* (after her homeland, Poland) and *radium.* Curie also coined the terms *radioactive* and *radioactivity.*

In 1923, de Hevesy, often called the "father of nuclear medicine," developed the tracer principle. He coined the term *radioindicator* and extended his studies from inorganic to organic chemistry. The first radioindicators were naturally occurring substances such as radium and radon. The invention of the *cyclotron* by Lawrence in 1931 made it possible for de Hevesy to expand his studies to a broader spectrum of biologic processes by using ^{32}P (phosphorus-32), ^{22}Na (sodium-22), and other cyclotron-produced (synthetic) radioactive tracers.

Radioactive elements began to be produced in *nuclear reactors* developed by Fermi and colleagues in 1946. The nuclear reactor greatly extended the ability of the cyclotron to produce radioactive tracers. A key development was the introduction of the *gamma camera* by Anger in 1958. In the early 1960s, Edwards and Kuhl made the next advance in nuclear medicine with the development of a crude single photon emission computed tomography (SPECT) camera known as the MARK IV. With this new technology, it was possible to create three-dimensional images of organ function instead of the two-dimensional images created previously. It was not until the early 1980s, when computers became fast enough to acquire and process all of the information successfully, that SPECT imaging could become standard practice.

With the development of more suitable *scintillators,* such as sodium iodide (NaI), and more sophisticated nuclear counting electronics, positron coincidence localization became possible. Wrenn demonstrated the use of positron-emitting radioisotopes for the localization of brain tumors in

1951. Brownell further developed instrumentation for similar studies. The next major advance came in 1967, when Hounsfield demonstrated the clinical use of computed tomography (CT). The mathematics of positron emission tomography (PET) image *reconstruction* is similar to that used for CT reconstruction techniques. Instead of x-rays from a point source traversing the body and being detected by a single or multiple detectors as in CT, PET imaging uses two opposing detectors to count pairs of 511-KeV photons simultaneously that originate from a single positron-electron annihilation event.

From 1967 to 1974, significant developments occurred in computer technology, scintillator materials, and *photomultiplier tube* (PMT) design. In 1975, the first closed-ring transverse positron tomograph was built for PET imaging by Ter-Pogossian and Phelps.

Developments now continue on two fronts that have accelerated the use of PET. First, scientists are approaching the theoretic limits (1 to 2 mm) of PET scanner resolution by employing smaller, more efficient scintillators and PMTs. Microprocessors tune and adjust the entire ring of *detectors* that surround the patient. Each ring in the PET tomograph may contain 1000 detectors. The tomograph may be composed of 30 to 60 rings of detectors. The second major area of development is in the design of new radiopharmaceuticals. Agents are being developed to measure blood flow, metabolism, protein synthesis, lipid content, receptor binding, and many other physiologic parameters and processes.

During the mid-1980s, PET was used predominantly as a research tool; however, by the early 1990s, clinical PET centers had been established, and PET was routinely used for diagnostic procedures on the brain, heart, and tumors. In the middle to late 1990s, three-dimensional PET systems that eliminated the use of interdetector *septa* were developed. This development allowed the injected dose of the radiopharmaceutical to be reduced by approximately 6-fold to 10-fold.

One of the first organs to be examined by nuclear medicine studies using *external radiation detectors* was the thyroid. In the 1940s, investigators found that the rate of incorporation of radioactive iodine by the thyroid gland was greatly increased in hyperthyroidism (overproduction of thyroid hormones) and greatly decreased in hypothyroidism (underproduction of thyroid hormones). Over the years, tracers and instruments were developed to allow almost every major organ of the body to be studied by application of the tracer principle. Images subsequently were made of structures such as the liver, spleen, brain, and kidneys. At the present time, the emphasis of nuclear medicine studies is more on function and chemistry than anatomic structure. In PET, new image reconstruction methods have been developed to characterize better the distribution of annihilation photons from these three-dimensional systems.

Beginning in 2000, major nuclear medicine camera manufacturers developed combined PET and CT systems that can simultaneously acquire PET functional images and CT anatomic images. Both modalities are coregistered or exactly matched in size and position. The success of these camera systems led to the development of combined SPECT and CT systems, as well. Significant benefits are expected for diagnosing metastatic disease because precise localization of tumor site and function can now be determined. In addition to anatomic registration, CT has allowed for improved attenuation correction in PET and SPECT. By more accurately mapping the different densities in the body, more accurate correction of the different gamma attenuators can be applied to PET and SPECT data. Rapid

enhancements and developments are anticipated to continue with this technology over the next several years.

In addition to the hybrid fusion of PET and CT, the first PET/magnetic resonance imaging (MRI) system was approved by the U.S. Food and Drug Administration (FDA) for customer purchase in 2011. The integration of PET and MRI is not straightforward and challenges the technical design of both systems. PET/MRI merges the metabolic ability of PET imaging with the morphologic imaging of MRI (see Chapter 30) to generate diagnostic images for oncologic, cardiologic, and neurologic purposes. With only a few PET/MRI systems installed throughout the United States, growth in this area is anxiously anticipated.

Comparison with Other Modalities

Nuclear medicine is predominantly used to measure human cellular, organ, or system function. A parameter that characterizes a particular aspect of human physiology is determined from the measurement of the radioactivity emitted by a radiopharmaceutical in a given volume of tissue. In contrast, conventional radiography measures the structure, size, and position of organs or human anatomy by determining x-ray transmission through a given volume of tissue. X-ray attenuation

by structures interposed between the x-ray source and the radiographic image receptor provides the contrast necessary to visualize an organ. CT creates cross-sectional images by computer reconstruction of multiple x-ray transmissions (see Chapter 29). The characteristics of radiologic imaging modalities are compared in Table 32-1.

Radionuclides used for conventional nuclear medicine include ^{99m}Tc (technetium), ^{123}I (iodine), ^{131}I (iodine), ^{111}In (indium), ^{201}Tl (thallium), and ^{67}Ga (gallium). Labeled compounds with these high atomic weight radionuclides often do not mimic the physiologic properties of natural substances because of their size, mass, and distinctly different chemical properties. Compounds labeled with conventional nuclear medicine radionuclides are poor radioactive *analogs* for natural substances. Imaging studies with these agents are qualitative and emphasize nonbiochemical properties. The elements hydrogen, carbon, nitrogen, and oxygen are the predominant constituents of natural compounds found in the body. They have low-atomic-weight radioactive counterparts including ^{11}C (carbon), ^{13}N (nitrogen), and ^{15}O (oxygen). Different from conventional radionuclides, these radionuclides emit positrons and can directly replace their stable isotopes in substrates, metabolites, drugs, and other biologically active compounds without disrupting

TABLE 32-1

Comparison of imaging modalities

Modality information	PET	SPECT	MRI	CT
Measures	Physiology	Physiology	Anatomy (physiology*)	Anatomy
Resolution	3-5 mm	8-10 mm	0.5-1 mm	1-1.5 mm
Technique	Positron annihilation	Gamma emission	Nuclear magnetic resonance	Absorption of x-rays
Harmful	Radiation exposure	Radiation exposure	None known	Radiation effects exposure
Use	Research and clinical	Clinical	Clinical (research*)	Clinical
No. examinations per day	4-12	5-10	10-15	15-20

*Secondary function.

normal biochemical properties. In addition, the most commonly used PET radionuclide, ^{18}F (fluorine), can replace hydrogen in many molecules, providing an even greater assortment of biologic analogs that are useful PET radiopharmaceuticals.

SPECT, or single-photon emission computed tomography, is a conventional nuclear imaging technique that is used to determine tissue function. Because SPECT employs collimators and lower energy photons, it is less sensitive (by 10^1 to 10^5) and less accurate than PET. Generally, PET resolution is better than SPECT resolution by a factor of 2 to 10. PET easily accounts for photon loss through attenuation by performing a *transmission scan.* This is difficult to achieve and not routinely done with SPECT imaging; however, newly designed SPECT instrumentation that couples a low-output x-ray CT to the gamma camera for the collection of attenuation information is now being used in selected sites to correct for gamma attenuation. Software approaches are also being investigated that assign known *attenuation coefficients* for specific tissues to *segmented regions* of images for analytic attenuation correction of SPECT data.

The differences between the various imaging modalities can be highlighted using a study of brain blood flow as an example. Without an intact circulatory system, an intravenously injected radiotracer cannot make its way into the brain for distribution throughout the brain's capillary network ultimately diffusing into cells that are well perfused. For radiographic procedures such as CT, structures within the brain may be intact, but there may be impaired or limited blood flow to and through major vessels within the brain. Under these circumstances, the CT scan may appear almost normal despite reduced blood flow to the brain. If the circulatory system at the level of the capillaries is not intact, a PET scan can be performed, but no perfusion information is obtained because the radioactive water used to measure blood flow is not transported through the capillaries and diffused into the brain cells.

The image-enhancing contrast agents used in many radiographic studies may cause a toxic reaction. The x-ray dose to the patient in these radiographic studies is greater than the radiation dose in nuclear imaging studies. The radiotracers used in PET studies are similar to the body's own biochemical constituents and are administered in very small amounts. Biochemical compatibility of the tracers within the body minimizes the risks to the patient because the tracers are not toxic. Trace amounts minimize alteration of the body's *homeostasis.*

An imaging technique that augments CT and PET is *magnetic resonance imaging* (MRI) (see Chapter 30). Images obtained with PET and MRI are shown in Fig. 32-1. MRI is used primarily to measure anatomy or morphology. In contrast to CT, which derives its greatest image contrast from varying tissue densities (bone from soft tissue), MRI better differentiates tissues by their proton content and the degree to which the protons are bound in lattice structures. The tightly bound protons of bone make it virtually transparent to MRI.

CT, MRI, and other anatomic imaging modalities provide complementary information to nuclear medicine imaging and PET. These imaging modalities benefit from *image coregistration* with CT and MRI by pinpointing physiologic function from precise anatomic locations. Greater emphasis is being placed on multimodality image coregistration between PET, CT, SPECT, and MRI for brain research and for tumor localization throughout the body (Fig. 32-2). All new PET imaging systems are fused with a CT scanner for attenuation and anatomic positioning information. Many SPECT imaging systems incorporate CT technology for the same purposes.

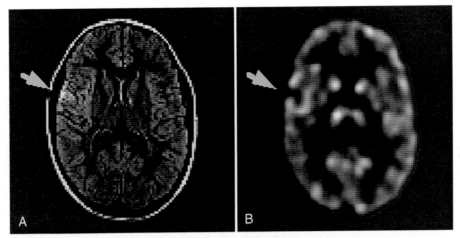

Fig. 32-1 Coregistered MRI and PET scans. *Arrows* indicate an abnormality on the anatomic image (**A,** MRI scan) and the functional image (**B,** PET scan). ^{18}F-FDG PET image depicts hypometabolic area of seizure focus (*arrow*) in a patient with a diagnosis of epilepsy.

Physical Principles of Nuclear Medicine

An understanding of radioactivity must precede an attempt to grasp the principles of nuclear medicine and how images are created using radioactive compounds. The term *radiation* is taken from the Latin word *radii,* which refers to the spokes of a wheel leading out from a central point. The term *radioactivity* is used to describe the radiation of energy in the form of high-speed *alpha* or *beta particles* or waves (gamma rays) from the nucleus of an atom.

BASIC NUCLEAR PHYSICS

The basic components of an atom include the nucleus, which is composed of varying numbers of *protons* and *neutrons,* and the orbiting *electrons,* which revolve around the nucleus in discrete energy levels. Protons have a positive electrical charge, electrons have a negative charge, and neutrons are electrically neutral. Protons and neutrons have masses nearly 2000 times the mass of the electron; the nucleus comprises most of the mass of an atom. The Bohr atomic model (Fig. 32-3) can describe this configuration. The total number of protons, neutrons, and electrons in an atom determines its characteristics, including its stability.

The term *nuclide* is used to describe an atomic species with a particular arrangement of protons and neutrons in the nucleus. Elements with the same number of protons but a different number of neutrons are referred to as *isotopes.* Isotopes have the same chemical properties as one another because the total number of protons and electrons is the same. They differ simply in the total number of neutrons contained in the nucleus. The neutron-to-proton ratio in the nucleus determines the stability of the atom. At certain ratios, atoms may be unstable, and a process known as spontaneous *decay* can occur as the atom attempts to regain stability. Energy is released in various ways during this decay, or return to *ground state.*

Radionuclides decay by the emission of alpha, beta, and gamma radiation. Most radionuclides reach ground state through various decay processes, including alpha, beta, or positron emission; *electron capture;* and several other methods. These decay methods determine the type of particles or gamma rays given off in the decay.

To explain this process better, investigators have created decay schemes to

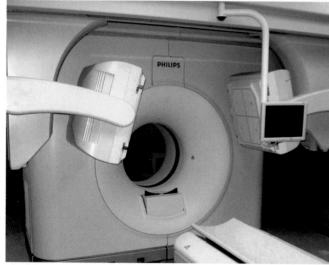

Fig. 32-2 Combined SPECT/CT camera for a blending of imaging function and form.

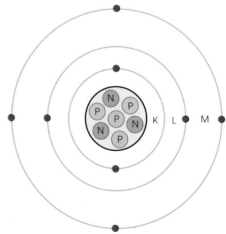

Fig. 32-3 Diagram of Bohr atom containing a single nucleus of protons (*P*) and neutrons (*N*) with surrounding orbital electrons of varying energy levels (e.g., *K, L, M*).

show the details of how a *parent* nuclide decays to its *daughter* or ground state (Fig. 32-4, *A*). Decay schemes are unique for each radionuclide and identify the type of decay, the energy associated with each process, the probability of a particular decay process, and the rate of change into the ground state element, commonly known as the *half-life* (T$\frac{1}{2}$) of the radionuclide.

Radioactive decay is considered a purely random and spontaneous process that can be mathematically defined by complex equations and represented by average decay rates. The term *half-life* is used to describe the time it takes for a quantity of a particular radionuclide to decay to one half of its original activity. This radioactive decay is a measure of the physical time it takes to reach one half of the original number of atoms through spontaneous disintegration. The rate of decay has an exponential function, which can be plotted on a linear scale (Fig. 32-4, *B*). If plotted on a semilogarithmic scale, the decay rate would be represented as a straight line. Radionuclide half-lives range from milliseconds to years. The half-lives of most radionuclides used in nuclear medicine range from several hours to several days.

NUCLEAR PHARMACY

The radionuclides used in nuclear medicine are produced in reactors, or *particle accelerators*. Naturally occurring radionuclides have very long half-lives (i.e., thousands of years). These natural radionuclides are unsuitable for nuclear medicine imaging because of limited availability and the high-absorbed dose the patient would receive. The radionuclides for nuclear medicine are produced in a particle accelerator through nuclear reactions created between a specific target chemical and high-speed charged particles. The number of protons in the target nuclei is changed when the nuclei are bombarded by the high-speed charged particles, and a new element or radionuclide is produced. Radionuclides can be created in nuclear reactors either by inserting a target element into the reactor core where it is irradiated or by separating and collecting the *fission* products.

The most commonly used radionuclide in nuclear medicine is ^{99m}Tc, which is produced in a generator system. This system makes available desirable short-lived radionuclides—the *daughters*—which are formed by the decay of relatively longer lived radionuclides—the *parents*. The generator system uses ^{99}Mo (molybdenum-99) as the parent; ^{99}Mo has a half-life of 66.7 hours and decays (86%) to a daughter product known as *metastable* ^{99m}Tc. Because ^{99m}Tc and ^{99}Mo are chemically different, they can easily be separated through an ion-exchange column. ^{99m}Tc exhibits nearly ideal characteristics for use in nuclear medicine examinations, including a relatively short physical half-life of 6.04 hours and a high-yield (98.6%), 140-keV, low-energy, gamma photon (see Fig. 32-4, *A*).

Because radiopharmaceuticals are administered to patients, they need to be sterile and *pyrogen-free*. They also need to undergo all of the quality control measures required of conventional drugs. A radiopharmaceutical generally has two components: a *radionuclide* and a *phar-*

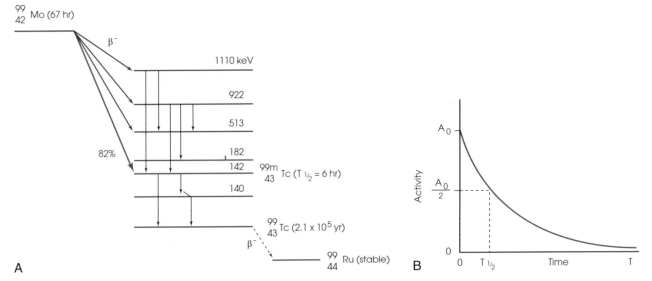

Fig. 32-4 A, Decay scheme illustrating the method by which radioactive molybdenum (*^{99}Mo*) decays to radioactive technetium (*^{99m}Tc*), one of the most commonly used radiopharmaceuticals in nuclear medicine. **B,** Graphic representation showing the rate of physical decay of a radionuclide. The *y* (vertical) axis represents the amount of radioactivity, and the *x* (horizontal) axis represents the time at which a specific amount of activity has decreased to one half of its initial value. Every radionuclide has an associated half-life that is representative of its rate of decay.

maceutical. The pharmaceutical is a biologically active compound chosen on the basis of its preferential localization or participation in the physiologic function of a given organ. A radionuclide is the radioactive material used to tag the pharmaceutical to allow for localization of the compound within the body (Fig. 32-5). After the radiopharmaceutical is administered, the target organ is localized by means of the physiologic pharmaceutical distribution, and the radiation emitted from it can be detected by imaging instruments, or gamma cameras.

The following characteristics are desirable in an imaging radiopharmaceutical:

- Ease of production and ready availability
- Low cost
- Lowest possible radiation dose to the patient
- Primary photon energy between 100 keV and 400 keV
- Physical half-life greater than the time required to prepare the material for injection
- Effective half-life longer than the examination time
- Suitable chemical forms for rapid localization
- Different uptake in the structure to be detected than in the surrounding tissue
- Low toxicity in the chemical form administered to the patient
- Stability or near-stability

A commonly used radiopharmaceutical is ^{99m}Tc tagged to a macroaggregated albumin (MAA). After intravenous injection, this substance follows the pathway of blood flow to the lungs, where it is distributed throughout and trapped in the small pulmonary capillaries (Fig. 32-6). Blood clots along the pathway prevent this radiopharmaceutical from distributing in the area beyond the clot. As a result, the image shows a void or clear area, often described as *photopenia* or a *cold spot.* More than 30 different radiopharmaceuticals are used in nuclear medicine (Table 32-2).

Radiopharmaceutical doses vary depending on the radionuclide used, the examination to be performed, and the size of the patient. The measure of radioactivity is expressed as either the *becquerel* (Bq), which corresponds to the decay rate, expressed as 1 disintegration per second (dps), or as the *curie* (Ci), which equals 3.73×10^{10} dps, relative to the number of decaying atoms in 1 g of radium.

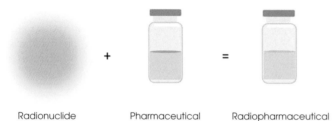

Radionuclide   Pharmaceutical   Radiopharmaceutical

Fig. 32-5 A radionuclide is chosen based on the characteristics of its gamma emission and ability to tag to a specific pharmaceutical; the pharmaceutical is chosen based on its ability to localize to a specific organ or function. When combined, a radiopharmaceutical, *or tracer*, is synthesized to visualize specific organs or functions in the body by detecting the radioactive emissions of the radiopharmaceutical that has been physiologically incorporated into the organ or function via pharmaceutical distribution.

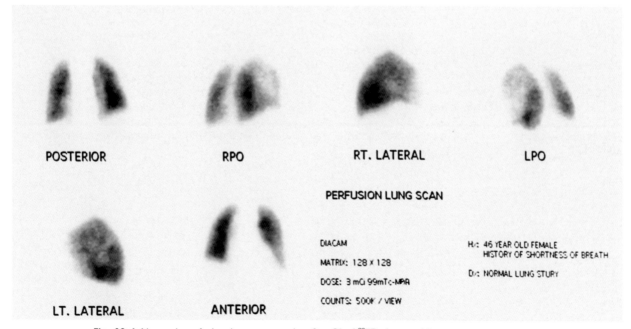

POSTERIOR   RPO   RT. LATERAL   LPO

PERFUSION LUNG SCAN

LT. LATERAL   ANTERIOR

DIACAM

MATRIX: 128 × 128

DOSE: 3 mCi 99mTc-MAA

COUNTS: 500K / VIEW

Hx: 46 YEAR OLD FEMALE
HISTORY OF SHORTNESS OF BREATH

Dx: NORMAL LUNG STUDY

Fig. 32-6 Normal perfusion lung scan using 3 mCi of ^{99m}Tc tagged to a macroaggregated albumin (^{99m}Tc MAA) on a large field-of-view gamma camera approximately 5 minutes after injection of the radiopharmaceutical. *LPO,* left posterior oblique; *LT,* left; *RPO,* right posterior oblique; *RT,* right.

(Courtesy Siemens Medical Systems, Iselin, NJ.)

TABLE 32-2

Radiopharmaceuticals used in nuclear medicine

Radionuclide	Symbol	Physical half-life	Chemical form	Diagnostic use
Chromium	^{51}Cr	27.8 days	Sodium chromate	Red blood cell volume and survival
			Albumin	Gastrointestinal protein loss
Cobalt	^{57}Co	270 days	Cyanocobalamin (vitamin B_{12})	Vitamin B_{12} absorption
Fluorine	^{18}F	110 min	Fluorodeoxyglucose	Oncology and myocardial hibernation
Gallium	^{67}Ga	77 hr	Gallium citrate	Inflammatory process and tumor imaging
Indium	^{111}In	67.4 hr	DTPA	Cerebrospinal fluid imaging
			Ibritumomab tiuxetan	Localization of tumor
			OctreoScan (pentetreotide)	Neuroendocrine tumors
			ProstaScint (capromab pendetide)	Prostate cancer
			Oxine	White blood cell/abscess imaging
Iodine	^{123}I	13.3 hr	Sodium iodide	Thyroid function and imaging
			Human serum albumin	Plasma volume
	^{131}I	8 days	Sodium iodide	Thyroid function, imaging, and therapy
			Hippurate	Renal function
Nitrogen	^{13}N	10 min	Ammonia	Myocardial perfusion
Rubidium	^{82}Rb	75 sec	Rubidium chloride	Cardiovascular imaging
Technetium	^{99m}Tc	6 hr	Sodium pertechnetate	Imaging of brain, thyroid, scrotum, salivary glands, renal perfusion, and pericardial effusion; evaluation of left-to-right cardiac shunts
			Sulfur colloid	Imaging of liver and spleen and renal transplants, lymphoscintigraphy
			Macroaggregated albumin	Lung imaging
			Sestamibi	Cardiovascular imaging, myocardial perfusion
			DTPA	Brain and renal imaging
			DMSA	Renal imaging
			MAG3	Renal imaging
			Diphosphonate	Bone imaging
			Pyrophosphate	Bone and myocardial imaging
			Red blood cells	Cardiac function imaging
			HMPAO	Functional brain imaging and white blood cell/abscess imaging
			Iminodiacetic derivations	Liver function imaging
			Neurolite (Bicisate)	Brain imaging
			Myoview (Tetrofosmin)	Myocardial perfusion
			CEA-scan (arcitumomab)	Gastrointestinal tract
			Cardiolite (Sestamibi)	Myocardial perfusion
			Apcitide (AcuTect)	Acute venous thrombosis
Thallium	^{201}Tl	73.5 hr	Thallous chloride	Myocardial imaging
Xenon	^{133}Xe	5.3 days	Xenon gas	Lung ventilation imaging

DMSA, dimercaptosuccinic acid; *DTPA,* diethylenetriamine pentaacetic acid; *HMPAO,* hexamethylpropyleneamine oxime; *MAG3,* mertiatide.

Radiation Safety in Nuclear Medicine

The radiation protection requirements in nuclear medicine differ from the general radiation safety measures used for diagnostic radiography. The radionuclides employed in nuclear medicine are in liquid, solid, or gaseous form. Because of the nature of radioactive decay, these radionuclides continuously emit radiation after administration (in contrast to diagnostic x-rays, which can be turned on and off mechanically). Special precautions are required.

Generally, the quantities of radioactive tracers used in nuclear medicine present no significant hazard. Nonetheless, care must be taken to reduce unnecessary exposure. The high concentrations or activities of the radionuclides used in a nuclear pharmacy necessitate the establishment of a designated preparation area that contains isolated ventilation, protective lead or glass shielding for vials and syringes, absorbent material, and gloves. The handling and administration of diagnostic doses to patients warrants the use of gloves and a lead or tungsten syringe shield, which is especially effective for reduction of exposure to hands and fingers during patient injection, at all times (Fig. 32-7). Any radioactive material that is spilled continues to emit radiation and must be cleaned up and contained immediately. Because radioactive material that contacts the skin can be absorbed and may not be easily washed off, it is very important to wear protective gloves when handling radiopharmaceuticals.

Technologists and nuclear pharmacists are required to wear appropriate radiation monitoring (dosimetry) devices, such as film badges and thermoluminescent dosimetry (TLD) rings, to monitor radiation exposure to the body and hands. The *ALARA* (as low as reasonably achievable) program applies to all nuclear medicine personnel.

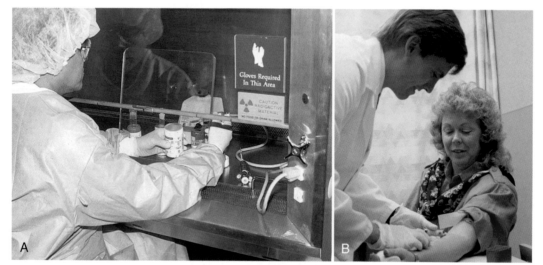

Fig. 32-7 A, Area in a radiopharmacy in which doses of radiopharmaceuticals are prepared in a clean and protected environment. **B,** Nuclear medicine technologist administering a radiopharmaceutical intravenously using appropriate radiation safety precautions, including gloves and a syringe shield.

Instrumentation in Nuclear Medicine
MODERN-DAY GAMMA CAMERA

The term *scintillate* means to emit light photons. Becquerel discovered that ionizing radiation caused certain materials to glow. A *scintillation detector* is a sensitive element used to detect ionizing radiation by observing the emission of light photons induced in a material. When a light-sensitive device is affixed to this material, the flash of light can be converted into small electrical impulses. The electrical impulses are amplified so that they may be sorted and counted to determine the amount and nature of radiation striking the scintillating materials. Scintillation detectors were used in the development of the first-generation nuclear medicine scanner, the *rectilinear scanner*, which was built in 1950.

Scanners have evolved into complex imaging systems known today as *gamma cameras* (because they detect gamma rays). These cameras are still scintillation detectors that use a thallium-activated sodium iodide crystal to detect and transform radioactive emissions into light photons. Through a complex process, these light photons are amplified, and their locations are electronically recorded to produce an image that is displayed on computer output systems. Scintillation cameras with single or multiple crystals are used today. The gamma camera has many components that work together to produce an image (Fig. 32-8).

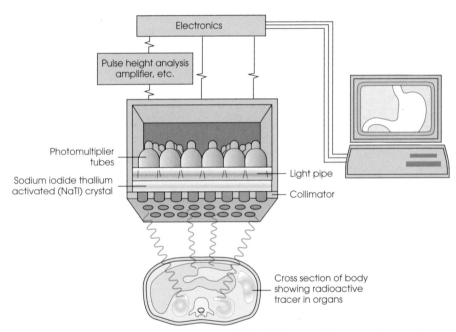

Fig. 32-8 Typical gamma camera system, which includes complex computers and electronic mechanical components for acquiring, processing, displaying, and analyzing nuclear medicine images.

Nuclear Medicine

Collimator

Located at the face of the detector, where photons from radioactive sources first enter the camera, is a *collimator*. The collimator is used to separate gamma rays and keep scattered rays from entering the scintillation crystal. *Resolution* and *sensitivity* are terms used to describe the physical characteristics of collimators. Collimator sensitivity is determined by the fraction of photons that are transmitted through the collimator and strike the face of the camera crystal. Spatial resolution refers to the system's ability to define detail in an image.

Collimators are usually made of a material with a high atomic number, such as lead, which absorbs scattered gamma rays. Different collimators are used for different types of examinations, depending on photon energy and the desired level of sensitivity and resolution.

Crystal and light pipe

The scintillation crystals commonly used in gamma cameras are made of sodium iodide with trace quantities of thallium added to increase light production. This crystal composition is effective for stopping most common gamma rays emitted from the radiopharmaceuticals used in nuclear medicine.

The thickness of the crystal varies from $\frac{1}{4}$ inch to $\frac{1}{2}$ inch (0.6 to 1.3 cm). Thicker crystals are better for imaging radiopharmaceuticals with higher energies (>180 keV) but have decreased resolution because of the decreased ability of the electronics to localize the exact location of the photon absorption within the thicker crystal. Thinner crystals provide improved resolution but cannot efficiently image photons with a higher kiloelectron voltage because of the inability of the thinner crystals to stop the higher-energy photons from passing through the crystal without being absorbed.

A *light pipe* may be used to attach the crystal to the PMTs. The light pipe is a disk of optically transparent material that helps direct photons from the crystal into the PMTs.

An array of PMTs is attached to the back of the crystal or light pipe. Inside the detector are PMTs used to detect and convert light photons emitted from the crystal into an electronic signal that amplifies the original photon signal by a factor of up to 10^7. A typical gamma camera detector head contains 80 to 100 PMTs.

The PMTs send the detected signal through a series of processing steps, which include determining the location *(x, y)* of the original photon and its amplitude or energy *(z)*. The *x* and *y* values are determined by where the photon strikes the crystal. Electronic circuitry known as a *pulse height analyzer* is used to eliminate the *z* signals that are not within a desired preset energy range for a particular radionuclide. This helps reduce scattered lower energy, unwanted photons ("noise") that generally would degrade resolution of the image. When the information has been processed, the signals are transmitted to the display system, which includes a cathode ray tube and a film imaging system or computer to record the image.

Multihead gamma camera systems

The original gamma camera was a single detector that could be moved in various positions around the patient. Today, gamma camera systems may include up to three detectors (heads). Dual-head gamma camera systems are the most common, allowing for simultaneous anterior and posterior planar imaging, and are ideal for SPECT. Triple-head systems are not as popular as dual-head systems and are generally used for brain and heart studies. Although the triple-head systems are primarily suited for SPECT, they can also provide multiplanar images (see the section on imaging methods presented later in this chapter).

Multi-crystal gamma camera

Multi-crystal gamma cameras utilize an array of crystals that are coupled to position sensitive photomultiplier tubes (PSPMTs) or photodiodes. PSPMTs work under the same principle as conventional PMTs but have the ability to retain spatial information that conventional PMTs lose. With a unique cathode configuration and the use of an array of anodes, the system is able to direct electrons generated at different locations on the photocathode toward a corresponding array of anodes. Silicon photodiodes are semiconductor (or solid state) devices used for the detection of light and are ideal because they can be manufactured in any geometry; they produce low noise, and they are small and fast. Semiconductor detectors eliminate the need for light output from the crystal and convert the absorbed gamma ray energy directly into an electric charge. The photodiodes generate a current when

the anode/cathode junction in the semiconductor is illuminated by light. Avalanche photodiodes (APDs) are similar to silicon photodiodes but utilize avalanche multiplication and can be used in MRI systems or hybrid PET/MRI systems because their performance is not altered by the strong magnetic field.

COMPUTERS

Computers have become an integral part of the nuclear medicine imaging system. Computer systems are used to acquire and process data from gamma cameras. They allow data to be collected over a specific time frame or to a specified number of counts; the data can be analyzed to determine functional changes occurring over time (Fig. 32-9, *A* and *B*). A common example is the renal study, in which the radiopharmaceutical that is administered is cleared by normally functioning kidneys in about 20 minutes. The computer can collect images of the kidney during this period and analyze the images to determine how effectively the kidneys clear the radiopharmaceutical (Fig. 32-9, *C* to *E*). The computer also allows the operator to enhance a particular structure by adjusting the contrast and brightness of the image.

Computerization of the nuclear pharmacy operation also has become an important means of record keeping and quality control. Radioactive dosages and dose volumes can be calculated more quickly by computer than by hand. The nuclear pharmacy computer system may be used to provide reminders and keep records as required by the Nuclear Regulatory Commission (NRC), the FDA, and individual state regulatory agencies. Computers also assist in the scheduling of patients, based on dose availability and department policies.

Computers are necessary to acquire and process SPECT images (see the next section). SPECT uses a scintillation camera that moves around the patient to obtain images from multiple angles for tomographic image reconstruction. SPECT studies are complex and, similar to MRI studies, require a great deal of computer processing to create images in transaxial, sagittal, or coronal planes. Rotating three-dimensional images can also be generated from SPECT data (Fig. 32-10).

Computer networks are an integral part of the way a department communicates información within and among institutions. In a network, several or many computers are connected so that they all have access to the same files, programs, and printers. Networking allows the movement of image-based and text-based data to any computer or printer in the network. Networking improves the efficiency of a nuclear medicine department. A computer network can serve as a vital component, reducing the time expended on menial tasks while allowing retrieval and transfer of information. Consolidation of all reporting functions in one area eliminates the need for the nuclear medicine physician to travel between departments to read studies. Centralized archiving, printing, and retrieval of most image-based and non–image-based data have increased the efficiency of data analysis, reduced the cost of image hard copy, and permitted more sophisticated analysis of image data than would routinely be possible.

Electronically stored records can decrease reporting turnaround time, physical image storage requirements, and use of personnel for record maintenance and retrieval. Long-term computerized records can also form the basis for statistical analysis to improve testing methods and predict disease courses. Most institutions now use some form of picture archiving and communication systems (PACS) to organize all of the imaging that is done. PACS are the foundation of a digital department, allowing for easy transfer, retrieval, and archiving of all imaging done in the nuclear medicine department.

QUANTITATIVE ANALYSIS

Many nuclear medicine procedures require some form of quantitative analysis to provide physicians with numeric results based on and depicting organ function. Specialized software allows computers to collect, process, and analyze functional information obtained from nuclear medicine imaging systems. Cardiac ejection fraction is a common quantitation study (Fig. 32-11). In this dynamic study of the heart's contractions and expansions, the computer accurately determines the ejection fraction, or the amount of blood pumped out of the left ventricle with each contraction.

Imaging Methods

A wide variety of diagnostic imaging examinations are performed in nuclear medicine. These examinations can be described on the basis of the imaging method used: static, whole-body, dynamic, SPECT, and PET.

STATIC IMAGING

Static imaging is the acquisition of a single image of a particular structure. This image can be thought of as a

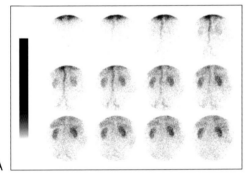
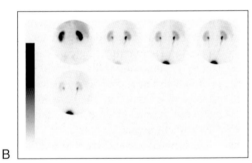
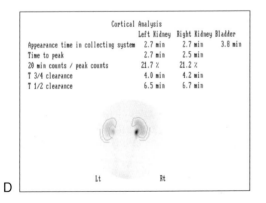
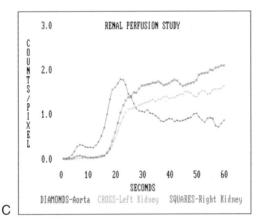
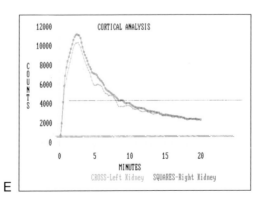

Fig. 32-9 A, Posterior renal blood flow in an adult patient using 10 mCi of ^{99m}Tc with DTPA imaged at 3 seconds per frame. The image in the *lower right corner* is a blood-pool image taken immediately after the initial flow sequence. Together the images show normal renal blood flow to both kidneys. B, Normal, sequential dynamic 20-minute ^{99m}Tc with mertiatide (MAG3) images. C, Renal arterial perfusion curves showing minor renal blood flow asymmetry. D, Renal cortical analysis curves showing rapid uptake and prompt parenchymal clearance. E, Quantitative renal cortical analysis indices showing normal values.

snapshot of the radiopharmaceutical distribution within a part of the body. Examples of static images include lung scans, spot bone scan images, and thyroid images. Static images are usually obtained in various orientations around a particular structure to show all aspects of that structure. Anterior, posterior, and oblique images are often obtained.

In static imaging, low radiopharmaceutical activity levels are used to minimize radiation exposure to the patients. Because of these low activity levels, images must be acquired for a preset time or a minimum number of counts or radioactive emissions. This time frame may vary from a few seconds to several minutes to acquire 100,000 to more than 1 million counts. Generally, it takes 30 seconds to 5 minutes to obtain a sufficient number of counts to produce a satisfactory image.

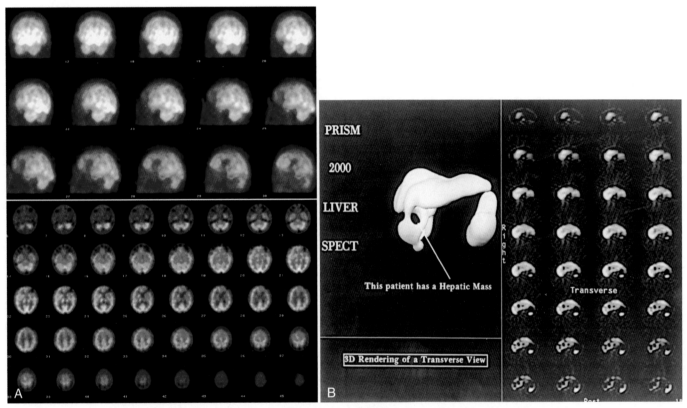

Fig. 32-10 A, Three-dimensional SPECT brain study using 20 mCi of ^{99m}Tc ECD showing a patient with a left frontal lobe brain infarct (*top*). Baseline and Diamox challenge transaxial, coronal, and sagittal images of the same patient, showing the left frontal lobe brain infarct (*bottom*). **B,** Three-dimensional SPECT liver study using 8 mCi of ^{99m}Tc sulfur colloid. A mass is seen on the three-dimensional image (*left*) and transaxial images (*right*).

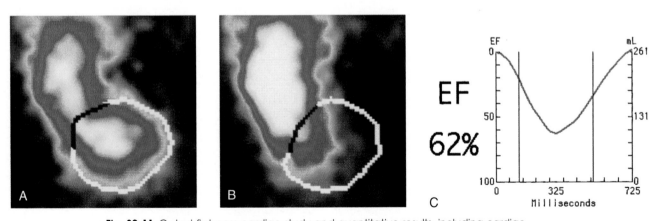

Fig. 32-11 Gated first-pass cardiac study and quantitative results, including cardiac ejection fraction, of a normal patient. **A,** Anterior image of the left ventricle at end-diastole (relaxed phase), with a region of interest drawn around the left ventricle. **B,** Same view showing end-systole (contracted phase). **C,** Curve representing the volume change in the left ventricle of the heart before, during, and after contraction. This volume change is referred to as the ejection fraction (*EF*); normal value is approximately 62%.

WHOLE-BODY IMAGING

Whole-body imaging uses a specially designed moving detector system to produce an image of the entire body or a large body section. In this type of imaging, the gamma camera collects data as it passes over the body. Earlier detector systems were smaller and required two or three incremental passes to encompass the entire width of the body.

Nearly all camera systems used for whole-body imaging incorporate a dual-head design for simultaneous anterior and posterior acquisition. Whole-body imaging systems are used primarily for whole-body bone or whole-body tumor imaging and other clinical and research applications (Fig. 32-12).

DYNAMIC IMAGING

Dynamic images display the distribution of a particular radiopharmaceutical over a specific period. A dynamic or "flow" study of a particular structure is generally used to evaluate blood perfusion to the tissue; this can be thought of as a sequential or time-lapse image. Images may be acquired and displayed in time sequences of one tenth of a second to longer than 10 minutes per image. Dynamic imaging is commonly used for first-pass cardiac studies, hepatobiliary studies, and renal studies.

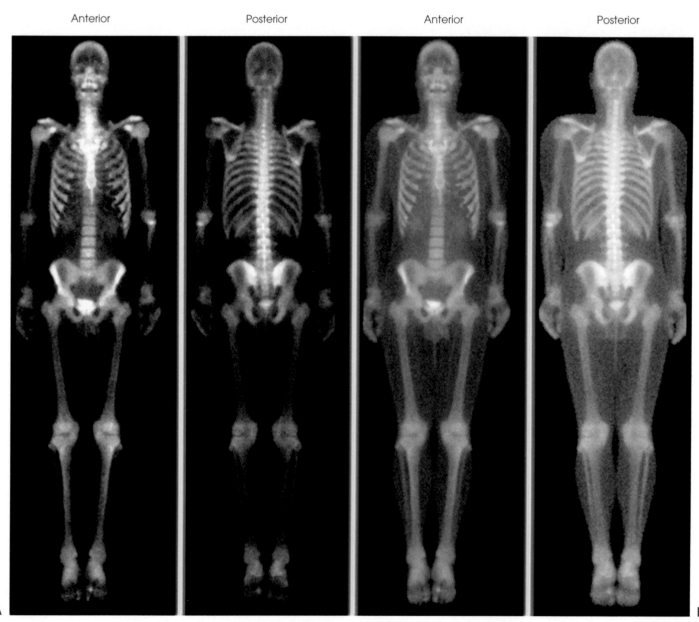

Anterior   Posterior   Anterior   Posterior

A   B

Fig. 32-12 Whole-body scan performed using 25 mCi ^{99m}Tc HDP in a 25-year-old man. Study was normal. **A,** Anterior and posterior whole-body view in linear gray scale. **B,** Anterior and posterior whole-body view in square-root gray scale, to enhance soft tissue.

(Courtesy General Electric.)

SPECT IMAGING

The reconstruction of SPECT data produces image projections similar to those obtained by CT or MRI. This reconstruction technique is used to create thin slices through a particular organ are different angles, or planes, to help delineate small lesions within tissues. These images can be created for virtually any structure or organ that is acquired using SPECT. Improved clinical results with SPECT are due to improved target-to-background ratios. Planar images record and show all radioactive emissions from the patient within the region of interest (ROI) as well as above and below the ROI, causing degradation of the image. In contrast, SPECT eliminates the unnecessary information.

With SPECT, typically, two gamma detectors are used to produce tomographic images (Fig. 32-13). Tomographic systems are designed to allow the detector heads to rotate 360 degrees around a patient's body to collect "projection" image data. The image data is reconstructed by a computer using reconstruction algorithms that populate all acquired projections to display the radiopharmaceutical distribution of the object into several formats include transaxial, sagittal, coronal, planar, and three-dimensional representations. These computer-generated images allow for the display of thin slices through

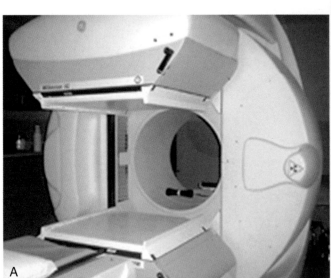
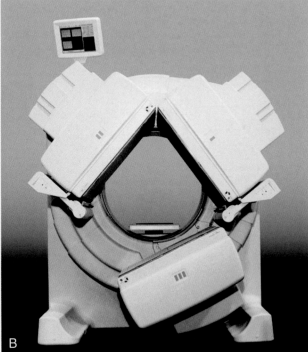

Fig. 32-13 SPECT camera systems. **A,** Dual-headed SPECT/CT system. **B,** Triple-headed system.

(**B,** Courtesy Marconi Medical Systems.)

different planes of an organ or structure, helping to identify small abnormalities.

The most common uses of SPECT include cardiac perfusion, brain, liver (see Fig. 32-10, *B*), tumor, and bone studies. An example of a SPECT study is the myocardial perfusion thallium study, which is used to identify perfusion defects in the left ventricular wall. The ^{201}Tl is injected intravenously while the patient is being physically stressed on a treadmill or is being infused with a vasodilator. The radiopharmaceutical distributes in the heart muscle in the same fashion as blood flowing to the tissue. An initial set of images is acquired immediately after the stress test. A second set is obtained several hours later when the patient is rested (when the ^{201}Tl has redistributed to viable tissue) to determine whether any blood perfusion defects that were seen on the initial images have resolved. By comparing the two image sets, the physician may be able to tell whether the patient has damaged heart tissue resulting from a myocardial infarction or myocardial ischemia (Fig. 32-14).

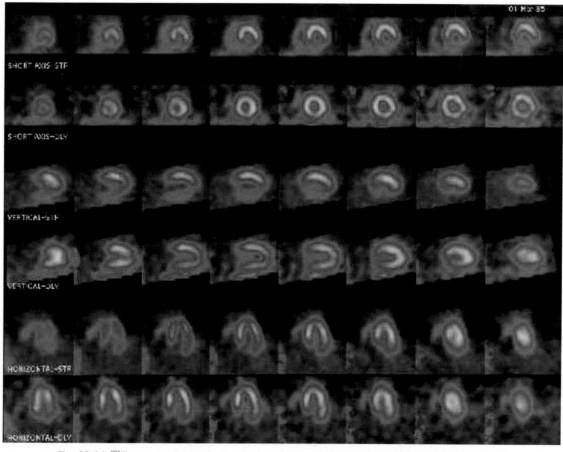

Fig. 32-14 ^{201}Tl myocardial perfusion study comparing stress and redistribution (resting) images in various planes of the heart (short axis and long axis). Perfusion defect is identified in stress images but not seen in redistribution (rest) images. This finding is indicative of ischemia.

COMBINED SPECT AND COMPUTED TOMOGRAPHY IMAGING

A blending of imaging function and form is available. By merging the functional imaging of SPECT with the anatomic landmarks of CT, more powerful diagnostic information is obtainable (Fig. 32-15). This combination has a significant impact on diagnosing and staging malignant disease and on identifying and localizing metastases. This new technology can be used for anatomic localization and attenuation correction. According to manufacturers, statistics show that adding CT (for attenuation correction and anatomic definition) changes the patient course of treatment 25% to 30% from what would have been done when interpreting the functional image alone.

Clinical Nuclear Medicine

The term *in vivo* means "within the living body." Because all diagnostic nuclear medicine imaging procedures are based on the distribution of radiopharmaceuticals within the body, they are classified as in vivo examinations.

Patient preparation for nuclear medicine procedures is minimal, with most tests requiring no special preparation. Patients usually remain in their own clothing. All metal objects outside or inside the clothing must be removed because they may attenuate anatomic or pathologic conditions on nuclear medicine imaging. The waiting time between dose administration and imaging varies with each study. After completion of a routine procedure, patients may resume all normal activities.

Technical summaries of commonly performed nuclear medicine procedures follow. After each procedure summary is a list, by organ or system, of many common studies that may be done in an average nuclear medicine department.

BONE SCINTIGRAPHY

Bone scintigraphy is generally a survey procedure to evaluate patients with malignancies, diffuse musculoskeletal symptoms, abnormal laboratory results, and hereditary or metabolic disorders. Tracer techniques have been used for many years to study the exchange between bone and blood. Radionuclides have played an important role in understanding normal

bone metabolism and the metabolic effects of pathologic involvement of bone. Radiopharmaceuticals used for bone imaging can localize in bone and in soft tissue structures. Skeletal areas of increased uptake are commonly a result of tumor, infection, or fracture.

Bone scan
Principle

It is unclear how ^{99m}Tc-labeled diphosphonates are incorporated into bone at the molecular level; however, regional blood flow, osteoblastic activity, and extraction efficiency seem to be the major factors that influence the uptake. In areas in which osteoblastic activity is increased, active hydroxyapatite crystals with large surface areas seem to be the most suitable sites for uptake of the diphosphonate portion of the radiopharmaceutical.

Radiopharmaceutical

The adult dose of 20 mCi (740 MBq) of ^{99m}Tc hydroxymethylene diphosphonate (HDP) or 20 mCi (740 MBq) of ^{99m}Tc methylene diphosphonate (MDP) is injected intravenously. The pediatric dose is adjusted according to the patient's weight.

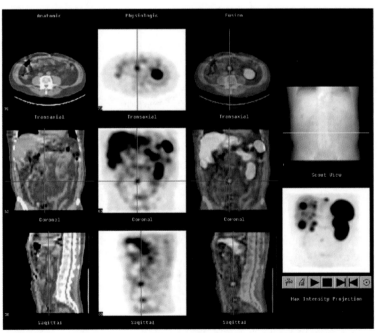

Fig. 32-15 ^{111}In-Octreotide SPECT/CT fusion images showing numerous foci of increased uptake within liver. This is consistent with the patient's known hepatic metastases. Very small focus of increased uptake is also seen in the inferior abdomen, near midline, anterior to the lumbar spine, and is consistent with nodal metastasis. These findings are indicative of somatostatin-avid hepatic and probable nodal metastases.

Scanning

A routine survey (whole-body, local views, or SPECT) begins about 3 hours after radiopharmaceutical injection and takes 30 to 60 minutes. A flow study would begin immediately after the injection; extremity imaging may be needed 4 to 5 hours later. The number of camera images acquired depends on the indication for the examination.

Bone (skeletal) studies

Skeletal studies include bone scan, bone marrow scan, and joint scan.

NUCLEAR CARDIOLOGY

Nuclear cardiology has experienced rapid growth in recent years and currently constitutes a significant portion of daily nuclear medicine procedures. These noninvasive studies assess cardiac performance, evaluate myocardial perfusion, and measure viability and metabolism. Advances in computers and scintillation camera technology have facilitated the development of a quantitative cardiac evaluation unequaled by any other noninvasive or invasive methods. The stress test is performed with the patient using a treadmill or pharmacologic agent. During the stress test, the patient's heart rate, electrocardiogram (ECG), blood pressure, and symptoms are continuously monitored. Some patients cannot exercise because of peripheral vascular disease, neurologic problems, or musculoskeletal abnormalities. In these patients, a pharmacologic intervention can be used in place of the exercise test to alter the blood flow to the heart in a way that simulates exercise, allowing the detection of myocardial ischemia.

Radionuclide angiography
Principle

Gated radionuclide angiography (RNA) can be used to measure left ventricular ejection fraction and evaluate left ventricular regional wall motion. RNA requires that the blood be labeled with an appropriate tracer such as ^{99m}Tc. The technique is based on imaging using a multigated acquisition (MUGA) format. During a gated acquisition, the cardiac cycle is divided into 16 to 20 frames. The R wave of each cycle resets the gate so that each count is added to each frame, until there are adequate count statistics for analysis. RNA requires simultaneous acquisition of

the patient's ECG and images of the left ventricle. The *ejection fraction* and wall motion analysis are measured at rest.

Radiopharmaceutical

The adult dose is 25 or 30 mCi (1110 MBq) of ^{99m}Tc-labeled red blood cells, depending on whether the test is an ejection fraction only or a rest MUGA based on the patient's body surface area (i.e., height and weight). The pediatric dose is adjusted according to the patient's weight.

Scanning

Imaging can begin immediately after the injection and takes about 1 hour. For a rest MUGA, imaging of the heart should be obtained in the anterior, left lateral, and left anterior oblique positions. For an ejection fraction–only MUGA, only the left anterior oblique is obtained.

Thallium-201 myocardial perfusion study
Principle

The stress ^{201}Tl study has high sensitivity (about 90%) and specificity (about 75%) for the diagnosis of coronary artery disease. This study also has been useful for assessing myocardial viability in patients with known coronary artery disease and for evaluating patients after revascularization. At rest, symptoms may not be apparent. ^{201}Tl is an analog of potassium and has a high rate of extraction by the myocardium over a wide range of metabolic and physiologic conditions. ^{201}Tl is distributed in the myocardium in proportion to regional blood flow and myocardial cell viability. Under stress, myocardial ^{201}Tl uptake peaks within 1 minute. ^{201}Tl uptake in the heart ranges from about 1% of the injected dose at rest to about 4% with maximum exercise. Regions of the heart that are infarcted or hypoperfused at the time of injection appear as areas of decreased activity (photopenia).

Radiopharmaceutical

The adult dose for a stress study is 3 mCi (111 MBq) of ^{201}Tl thallous chloride administered intravenously at peak stress; 1 mCi (37 MBq) of ^{201}Tl is administered intravenously before the delayed study, generally 3 to 4 hours after stress. The adult dose for a rest study is 4 mCi (148 MBq) of ^{201}Tl administered intrave-

nously before the rest study. The minimum dose recommended for pediatric patients is 300 µCi (11.1 MBq) of ^{201}Tl thallous chloride. Whenever possible, ^{99m}Tc sestamibi should be used in place of ^{201}Tl in obese patients so that a higher dose may be administered for clearer imaging results.

Scanning

Images obtained include the anterior planar image of the chest and heart, followed by a 180-degree SPECT study (45 degrees right anterior oblique to 45 degrees left posterior oblique).

Technetium-99m sestamibi myocardial perfusion study
Principle

Similar to ^{201}Tl, ^{99m}Tc sestamibi is a cation; however, it has a slightly lower fractional extraction than ^{201}Tl, particularly at high flow rates. ^{99m}Tc sestamibi has favorable biologic properties for myocardial perfusion imaging. It is used to assess myocardial salvage resulting from therapeutic intervention in acute infarction, to determine the myocardial blood flow during periods of spontaneous chest pain, and to diagnose coronary artery disease in obese patients. A first-pass flow study can be performed with a rest or stress ^{99m}Tc sestamibi myocardial perfusion scan. A first-pass study evaluates heart function (ejection fraction) during the short time (in seconds) that it takes the injected bolus to travel through the left ventricle.

Radiopharmaceutical

The adult dose for the stress study is 25 mCi (925 MBq) for a 2-day study and 40 mCi (1480 MBq) for a 1-day study of ^{99m}Tc sestamibi administered intravenously at peak stress. The adult dose for a rest study is 10 mCi (370 MBq) for a 1-day study and 34 mCi (1295 MBq) for a 2-day study of ^{99m}Tc sestamibi administered intravenously.

Scanning

SPECT imaging should normally be done 30 to 60 minutes after injection of the dose for stress and rest studies. When needed, more delayed images can be obtained for 4 to 6 hours after injection. A 2-day protocol provides optimal image quality, but the 1-day protocol is more convenient for patients, technologists, and physicians.

Cardiovascular studies

Cardiovascular studies include aortic/mitral regurgitant index, cardiac shunt study, dobutamine MUGA, rest MUGA, rest MUGA–ejection fraction only, exercise MUGA, stress testing (myocardial perfusion), ^{201}Tl myocardial perfusion scan, ^{99m}Tc sestamibi first-pass study, ^{99m}Tc sestamibi myocardial perfusion scan, ^{99m}Tc pyrophosphate (PYP) myocardial infarct scan, and rest ^{201}Tl scan with infarct quantitation.

CENTRAL NERVOUS SYSTEM IMAGING

The central nervous system consists of the brain and spinal cord. For patients with diseases of the central or peripheral nervous systems, nuclear medicine techniques can be used to assess the effectiveness of surgery or radiation therapy, document the extent of involvement of the brain by tumors, and determine progression or regression of lesions in response to different forms of treatment. Brain perfusion imaging is useful in the evaluation of patients with stroke; transient ischemia; and other neurologic disorders such as Alzheimer's disease, epilepsy, and Parkinson disease. Radionuclide cisternography is particularly useful in facilitating the diagnosis of cerebrospinal fluid leakage after trauma or surgery and normal-pressure hydrocephalus. More recent studies indicate that documented lack of cerebral blood flow should be the criterion of choice to confirm brain death when clinical criteria are equivocal, when a complete neurologic examination cannot be performed, or when patients are younger than 1 year.

Brain spect study

Principle

Some imaging agents are capable of penetrating the intact blood-brain barrier. After a radiopharmaceutical crosses the *blood-brain barrier*, it becomes trapped inside the brain. The regional uptake and retention of the tracer are related to the regional perfusion. Before the imaging agent is injected, the patient is placed in a quiet, darkened area and instructed to close the eyes. These measures are helpful in reducing uptake of the tracer in the visual cortex.

Radiopharmaceutical

The adult dose is 20 mCi (740 MBq) of ^{99m}Tc ethylcysteinate dimer (ECD) or ^{99m}Tc hexamethylpropyleneamine oxime (HMPAO). The pediatric dose is based on body surface area.

Scanning

Imaging begins 1 hour after ^{99m}Tc ECD injection or ^{99m}Tc HMPAO injection. Tomographic images of the brain are obtained.

Dopamine transporter study

Principle

A reduction of dopaminergic neurons in the striatal region of the brain is a characteristic of Parkinson's disease, parkinsonian syndromes, multiple system atrophy and progressive supranuclear palsy. ^{123}I ioflupane has a high binding affinity for presynaptic dopamine transporters in the striatal region of the brain and when introduced, as a radiopharmaceutical, will allow for quantitate measurement of the transporters.

Radiopharmaceutical

A thyroid blocker, such as Lugol's solution, should be given prior to ^{123}I ioflupane administration to protect the thyroid. The adult dose is a slow infusion of 3 to 5 mCi (111 to 185 MBq) of ^{123}I ioflupane.

Scanning

Imaging begins 3 to 6 hours after injection. Tomographic images of the brain are obtained.

Central nervous system studies

Central nervous system studies include brain perfusion imaging–SPECT study, brain imaging–acetazolamide challenge study, central nervous system shunt patency, cerebrospinal fluid imaging–cisternography/ventriculography, ^{201}Tl scan for recurrent brain tumor, and ^{99m}Tc HMPAO scan for determination of brain death.

IMAGING OF THE ENDOCRINE SYSTEM

The endocrine system organs, located throughout the body, secrete hormones into the bloodstream. Hormones have profound effects on overall body function and metabolism. The endocrine system consists of the thyroid, parathyroid, pituitary, and suprarenal glands; the islet cells of the pancreas; and the gonads. Nuclear medicine procedures have played a significant part in the current understanding of the function of the endocrine glands and their role in health and disease. These procedures are useful for monitoring treatment of endocrine disorders, especially in the thyroid gland. Thyroid imaging is performed to evaluate the size, shape, nodularity, and functional status of the thyroid gland. Imaging is used to screen for thyroid cancer and to differentiate hyperthyroidism, nodular goiter, solitary thyroid nodule, and thyroiditis.

Thyroid scan

Principle

^{99m}Tc pertechnetate or ^{123}I can be used to image the thyroid gland. ^{99m}Tc pertechnetate is trapped by the thyroid gland but, in contrast to ^{123}I, is not organified *into* the gland. It offers the advantages of low radiation dose to the patient, no particulate radiation (in contrast to ^{131}I), and well-resolved images. ^{123}I is organified into the gland. Imaging is used to determine the relative function in different regions within the thyroid, with special emphasis on the function of nodules compared with the rest of the gland. Scanning can also determine the presence and site of thyroid tissue in unusual areas of the body, such as the tongue and anterior chest (ectopic tissue).

Radiopharmaceutical

The adult dose is 5 mCi (185 MBq) of ^{99m}Tc pertechnetate administered intravenously, or 1 mCi ^{123}I administered orally. The pediatric dose is adjusted according to the patient's weight. Uptake may be affected by thyroid medication and by foods or drugs, including some iodine-containing contrast agents used for renal radiographic imaging and CT scanning.

Scanning

Scanning should start 20 minutes after the injection of ^{99m}Tc, or 4 to 24 hours after the administration of ^{123}I. A gamma camera with a pinhole collimator is used to obtain anterior, left anterior oblique, and right anterior oblique thyroid. The pinhole collimator is a thick, conical collimator that allows for magnification of the thyroid.

Iodine-131 thyroid uptake measurement

Principle

Radioiodine is concentrated by the thyroid gland in a manner that reflects the ability of the gland to handle stable dietary iodine. ^{131}I uptake is used to estimate the function of the thyroid gland by measuring its avidity for administered radioiodine. The higher the uptake of ^{131}I, the more active the thyroid; conversely, the lower the uptake, the less functional the gland. Uptake conventionally is expressed as the percentage of the dose in the thyroid gland at a given time after administration. Measurement of ^{131}I uptake is valuable in distinguishing between thyroiditis (reduced uptake) and Graves disease and toxic nodular goiter (Plummer disease), which have an increased uptake. It is also used to determine the appropriateness of a therapeutic dose of ^{131}I in patients with Graves disease, residual or recurrent thyroid carcinoma, or thyroid remnant after thyroidectomy.

Radiopharmaceutical

All doses of ^{131}I sodium iodide are administered orally. The adult dose for a standard uptake test is 3 to 5 μCi (148 to 222 kBq) of ^{131}I. The pediatric dose is adjusted according to the patient's weight. A standard dose is counted with the thyroid probe the morning of the uptake measurement and is used as the 100% uptake value. The patient's total count is compared with the standard count to obtain the patient percent uptake.

Measurements are obtained using an uptake probe consisting of a 2 × 2 inch (5 × 5 cm) sodium iodide/PMT assembly fitted with a flat-field lead collimator (Fig. 32-16). Uptake readings are generally acquired at 6 hours, at 24 hours, or both.

Total-body iodine-123 scan

Principle

A total-body ^{123}I (TBI) scan is recommended for locating residual thyroid tissue or recurrent thyroid cancer cells in patients with thyroid carcinoma. Most follicular or papillary thyroid cancers concentrate radioiodine; other types of thyroid cancer do not. A TBI scan is usually performed 1 to 3 months after a thyroidectomy to check for residual normal thyroid tissue and metastatic spread of the cancer before ^{131}I ablation therapy. After the residual thyroid tissue has been ablated

(destroyed), another ^{123}I TBI scan may be performed to check for residual disease.

Radiopharmaceutical

The adult dose for a TBI scan is generally 5 mCi (185 MBq) of ^{123}I sodium iodide administered orally. Thyrotropin alfa (Thyrogen) may be injected on each of 2 days before dose administration to allow the patient to remain on thyroid medication. The pediatric dose is adjusted according to the patient's weight.

Scanning

Total-body imaging begins 24 hours after dose administration. Images are obtained of the anterior and posterior whole body. SPECT imaging can also be performed to localize any specific areas of interest better.

Endocrine studies

Endocrine studies include the adrenal scan (^{131}I or ^{123}I-labeled MIBG), ectopic thyroid scan (^{131}I or ^{123}I), thyroid scan (^{123}I or ^{99m}Tc pertechnetate), thyroid uptake measurement (^{131}I or ^{123}I), thyroid uptake/scan (^{123}I), total body iodine scan (^{131}I or ^{123}I), parathyroid scan, and ^{111}In pentetreotide scan.

IMAGING OF THE GASTROINTESTINAL SYSTEM

The gastrointestinal system, or alimentary canal, consists of the mouth, oropharynx, esophagus, stomach, small bowel, colon, and several accessory organs (salivary glands, pancreas, liver, and gallbladder). The liver is the largest internal organ of the body. The portal venous system brings blood from the stomach, bowel, spleen, and pancreas to the liver.

Liver and spleen scan

Principle

Liver and spleen scanning is used to evaluate the liver for functional disease (e.g., cirrhosis, hepatitis, metastatic disease) and to look for residual splenic tissue after splenectomy. Imaging techniques such as ultrasonography, CT, and MRI provide excellent information about the anatomy of the liver, but nuclear medicine studies can assess the *functional* status of this organ. Liver and spleen scintigraphy is also useful for detecting hepatic lesions and evaluating hepatic morphology and function. It is also used to determine whether certain lesions found with other methods may be benign (e.g., focal nodular hyperplasia), obviating the need for biopsy. Uptake of a radiopharmaceutical in the liver, spleen, and bone marrow depends on blood flow and the functional capacity of the phagocytic cells. In normal patients, 80% to 90% of the radiopharmaceutical is localized in the liver, 5% to 10% is localized in the spleen, and the rest is localized in the bone marrow.

Radiopharmaceutical

Adults receive 6 mCi (222 MBq) of ^{99m}Tc sulfur colloid injected intravenously. The pediatric dose is adjusted according to the patient's weight.

Scanning

Images obtained may be planar (anterior, posterior, right and left anterior oblique, right and left lateral, right posterior oblique, and a marker view) or SPECT.

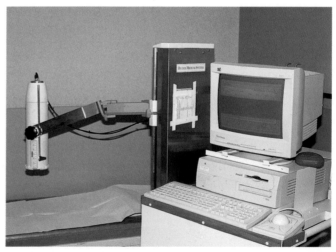

Fig. 32-16 Uptake probe used for thyroid uptake measurements over the extended neck area.

Gastrointestinal studies

Gastrointestinal studies include anorectal angle study, colonic transit study, colorectal/neorectal emptying study, esophageal scintigraphy, gastroesophageal reflux study, gastric emptying study, small-bowel transit study, hepatic artery perfusion scan, hepatobiliary scan, hepatobiliary scan with gallbladder ejection fraction, evaluation of human serum albumin for protein-losing gastroenteropathy, liver and spleen scan, liver hemangioma study, Meckel diverticulum study, and salivary gland study.

GENITOURINARY NUCLEAR MEDICINE

Genitourinary nuclear medicine studies are recognized as reliable, noninvasive procedures for evaluating the anatomy and function of the systems in nephrology, urology, and kidney transplantation. These studies can be accomplished with minimal risk of allergic reactions, unpleasant side effects, or excessive radiation exposure to the organs.

Dynamic renal scan
Principle

Renal imaging is used to assess renal perfusion and function, particularly in renal failure and renovascular hypertension and after renal transplantation. ^{99m}Tc mertiatide (MAG3) is secreted primarily by the proximal renal tubules and is not retained in the parenchyma of normal kidneys.

Radiopharmaceutical

The adult dose is 10 mCi (370 MBq) of ^{99m}Tc MAG3. The pediatric dose is adjusted according to the patient's weight.

Scanning

Imaging is initiated immediately after radiopharmaceutical injection. Because radiographic contrast media may interfere with kidney function, renal scanning should be delayed for 24 hours after contrast studies. Images are often taken over the posterior lower back, centered at the level of the 12th rib. Transplanted kidneys are imaged in the anterior pelvis. Patients need to be well hydrated, determined by a specific gravity test, before all renal studies.

Genitourinary studies

Genitourinary studies include dynamic renal scan, dynamic renal scan with furosemide, dynamic renal scan with captopril, pediatric furosemide renal scan, ^{99m}Tc dimercaptosuccinic acid (DMSA) renal scan, residual urine determination, testicular scan, and voiding cystography.

IN VITRO AND IN VIVO HEMATOLOGIC STUDIES

In vitro and in vivo hematologic studies have been performed in nuclear medicine for many years. Quantitative measurements are made after a radiopharmaceutical has been administered, often at predetermined intervals. The two types of nonimaging nuclear medicine procedures are as follows:

- *In vitro* radioimmunoassay for quantitating biologically important substances in the serum or other body fluids.
- *In vivo* evaluation of physiologic function by administering small tracer amounts of radioactive materials to the patient and subsequently counting specimens of urine, blood, feces, or breath. A wide variety of physiologic events may be measured, including vitamin B12 absorption (Schilling test), red blood cell survival and sequestration, red blood cell mass, and plasma volume.

Hematologic studies

Hematologic studies include plasma volume measurement, Schilling test, red blood cell mass, red blood cell survival, and red blood cell sequestration.

IMAGING FOR INFECTION

Imaging for infection is another useful nuclear medicine diagnostic tool. Inflammation, infection, and abscess may be found in any organ or tissue and at any location within the body. ^{67}Ga scans and ^{111}In-labeled white blood cell scans are useful for diagnosis and localization of infection and inflammation.

Infection studies

Infection studies include ^{67}Ga gallium scan, ^{111}In white blood cell scan, ^{99m}Tc HMPAO, and studies after total hip or knee replacement surgery.

RESPIRATORY IMAGING

Respiratory imaging commonly involves the demonstration of pulmonary perfusion using limited, transient capillary blockade and the assessment of ventilation using an inhaled radioactive gas or aerosol. Lung imaging is most commonly performed to evaluate pulmonary emboli, chronic obstructive pulmonary disease, chronic bronchitis, emphysema, asthma, and lung carcinoma. It is also used for lung transplant evaluation.

Xenon-133 lung ventilation scan
Principle

Lung ventilation scans are used in combination with lung perfusion scans. The gas used for a ventilation study must be absorbed significantly by the lungs and diffuse easily. ^{133}Xe has adequate imaging properties, and the body usually absorbs less than 15% of the gas.

Radiopharmaceutical

The adult dose is 15 to 30 mCi (555 to 1110 MBq) of ^{133}Xe gas administered by inhalation.

Scanning

Imaging starts immediately after inhalation of the ^{133}Xe gas begins in a closed system to which oxygen is added and carbon dioxide is withdrawn. When ^{133}Xe gas is used, the ventilation study must precede the ^{99m}Tc perfusion scan. Posterior and anterior images are obtained for the first breath equilibrium and *washout*. If possible, left and right posterior oblique images should be obtained between the first breath and equilibrium.

Technetium-99m macroaggregated albumin lung perfusion scan
Radiopharmaceutical

The adult dose is 4 mCi (148 MBq) of ^{99m}Tc MAA. The pediatric dose is adjusted according to the patient's weight.

Scanning

Imaging starts 5 minutes after radiopharmaceutical injection. Eight images should be obtained: anterior, posterior, right and left lateral, right and left anterior oblique, and right and left posterior oblique. The nuclear medicine physician may need additional images. All patients should have a chest radiograph within 24 hours of the lung scan. The chest radiograph is required for accurate interpretation of the lung scans so as to determine the probability for pulmonary embolism.

Respiratory studies

Respiratory studies include ^{99m}Tc diethylenetriamine pentaacetic acid (DTPA) lung aerosol scan, ^{99m}Tc MAA lung perfusion scan, and ^{133}Xe lung ventilation scan.

SENTINEL NODE IMAGING

Many tumors metastasize via lymphatic channels. Defining the anatomy of lymph nodes that drain a primary tumor site helps guide surgical and radiation treatment for certain tumor sites. Contrast lymphangiography, MRI, and CT are the standard methods to evaluate the status of the lymph nodes. Radionuclide lymphoscintigraphy has been useful in patients in whom the channels are relatively inaccessible. This method has been used primarily in patients with truncal melanomas and prostate and breast cancer to map the routes of lymphatic drainage and permit more effective surgical or radiation treatment of draining regional lymph nodes.

Principle

Colloidal particles injected intradermally or subcutaneously adjacent to a tumor site show a drainage pattern similar to that of the tumor. Colloidal particles in the 10- to 50-nm range seem to be the most effective for this application. The colloidal particles drain into the sentinel lymph node, where they are trapped by phagocytic activity; this aids in the identification of the lymph nodes most likely to be sites of metastatic deposits from the tumor.

Radiopharmaceutical

The adult dose is 100 μCi of ^{99m}Tc sulfur colloid in a volume of 0.1 mL per injection site.

Scanning

Patients with malignant melanoma should be positioned supine or prone on the imaging table. Images are acquired immediately after injection, then every few minutes for the first 15 minutes followed by every 5 minutes for 30 minutes. Additional lateral and oblique views are required after visualization of the sentinel node. Patients with breast cancer should be positioned supine on the imaging table with the arms extended over the head.

THERAPEUTIC NUCLEAR MEDICINE

The potential that radionuclides have for detecting and treating cancer has been recognized for decades. Radioiodine is a treatment in practically all adults with Graves disease except women who are pregnant or breastfeeding. High-dose ^{131}I therapy ($\geq$30 mCi) is used in patients with residual thyroid cancer or thyroid metastases. ^{32}P in the form of sodium phosphate can be used to treat polycythemia, a disease characterized by the increased production of red blood cells. ^{32}P chromic phosphate colloid administered into the peritoneal cavity is useful in the postoperative management of ovarian and endometrial cancers because of its effectiveness in destroying many of the malignant cells remaining in the peritoneum. Skeletal metastases occur in more than 50% of patients with breast, lung, or prostate cancer in the end stages of the disease. ^{99}Sr (strontium-99) is often useful for managing patients with bone pain from metastases when other treatments have failed.

Therapeutic procedures

Therapeutic procedures include ^{131}I therapy for hyperthyroidism and thyroid cancer, ^{32}P therapy for polycythemia, ^{32}P intraperitoneal therapy, ^{32}P intrapleural therapy, and ^{89}Sr bone therapy.

SPECIAL IMAGING PROCEDURES

Special imaging procedures include dacryoscintigraphy, the LeVeen shunt patency test, and lymphoscintigraphy of the limbs.

TUMOR IMAGING

Octreoscan

^{111}In pentetreotide (OctreoScan) is a radiolabeled analog of the neuroendocrine peptide somatostatin. It localizes in somatostatin receptor–rich tumors, primarily of neuroendocrine origin. It is currently indicated for the scintigraphic localization of the following tumors: carcinoid, islet cell carcinoma, gastrinoma, motilinoma, pheochromocytoma, small cell carcinoma, medullary thyroid carcinoma, neuroblastoma, paraganglioma, glucagonoma, pituitary adenoma, meningioma, VIPoma, and insulinoma.

Principle

Somatostatin is a neuroregulatory peptide known to localize on many cells of neuroendocrine origin. Cell membrane receptors with a high affinity for somatostatin have been shown to be present in most neuroendocrine tumors, including carcinoids, islet cell carcinomas, and gonadotropin hormone–producing pituitary adenomas. Tumors such as meningiomas, breast carcinomas, astrocytomas, and oat cell carcinomas of the lung have been reported to have numerous binding sites.

Radiopharmaceutical

The adult dose is 5 to 6 mCi (203.5 MBq) of ^{111}In pentetreotide administered intravenously. The pediatric dose is adjusted according to the patient's weight.

Scanning

The patient should be well hydrated before administration of OctreoScan. At 4 hours after injection, anterior and posterior whole-body images should be acquired. At 24 hours, anterior and posterior spot views of the chest and abdomen should be obtained. SPECT imaging is most helpful in the localization of intraabdominal tumors. SPECT/CT can assist in lesion localization.

Tumor studies

Tumor studies include ^{67}Ga tumor scan, ^{99m}Tc sestamibi breast scan, ^{111}In capromab pendetide (ProstaScint) scan, ^{99m}Tc nofetumomab merpentan (Verluma) for small cell lung cancer, and ^{111}In OctreoScan.

Principles and Facilities in Positron Emission Tomography

Positron emission tomography (PET) is a noninvasive nuclear imaging technique that involves the administration of a positron-emitting radioactive molecule and subsequent imaging of the distribution and kinetics of the radioactive material as it moves into and out of tissues. PET imaging of the heart, brain, lungs, or other organs is possible if an appropriate radiopharmaceutical, also called a *radiotracer* or *radiolabeled molecule,* can be synthesized and administered to the patient.

Three important factors distinguish PET from all radiologic procedures and from other nuclear imaging procedures. First, the results of the data acquisition and analysis techniques yield an image related to a particular physiologic parameter such as blood flow or metabolism. The ensuing image is aptly called a *functional* or *parametric image.* Second, the images are created by the simultaneous detection of a pair of *annihilation* radia-tion photons that result from *positron* decay (Fig. 32-17). The third factor that distinguishes PET is the chemical and biologic form of the radiopharmaceutical. The radiotracer is specifically chosen for its similarity to naturally occurring biochemical constituents of the human body. Because extremely small amounts of the radiopharmaceutical are administered, equilibrium conditions within the body are not altered. If the radiopharmaceutical is a form of sugar, it behaves much like the natural sugar used by the body. The kinetics or the movement of the radiotracer such as sugar within the body is followed by using the PET scanner to acquire many images that measure the distribution of the *radioactivity concentration* as a function of time. From this measurement, the local tissue metabolism of the sugar may be deduced by converting a temporal sequence of images into a single parametric image that indicates tissue glucose use or, more simply, tissue metabolism.

This discussion focuses on major concepts of *positrons,* PET, and the equipment used in this type of imaging. PET is a multidisciplinary technique that involves four major processes—radionuclide production, radiopharmaceutical production, data acquisition (PET scanner or tomograph), and a combination of image reconstruction and image processing—to create images that depict tissue function.

POSITRONS

Living organisms are composed primarily of compounds that contain the elements hydrogen, carbon, nitrogen, and oxygen. In PET, radiotracers are made by synthesizing compounds with radioactive isotopes of these elements. Chemically, the radioactive isotope is indistinguishable from its equivalent stable isotope. Neutron-rich (i.e., having more neutrons than protons) radionuclides emit electrons or beta particles. The effective range or distance traveled for a 1-MeV beta particle (β^-) in human tissue is only 4 mm. These radionuclides typically do not emit other types of radiation that can be easily measured externally with counters or scintillation detectors. The only radioisotopes of these elements that can be detected outside the body are positron-emitting

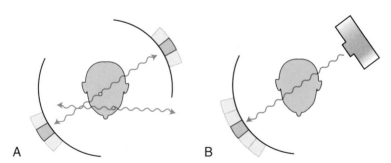

Fig. 32-17 A, PET relies on the simultaneous detection of a pair of annihilation radiations emitted from the body. **B,** In contrast, CT depends on the detection of x-rays transmitted through the body.

nuclides. The stable and radioactive nuclides of several elements are depicted in Fig. 32-18.

Positron-emitting radionuclides have a neutron-deficient nucleus (i.e., the *nucleus* contains more protons than neutrons and is also called a *proton-rich* nucleus). Positrons (β^+) are identical in mass to electrons, but they possess positive instead of negative charge. The characteristics of positrons are listed in Table 32-3. Positron decay occurs in unstable radioisotopes only if the nucleus possesses excess energy greater than the energy equivalent of two electron rest masses, or a total of 1.022 MeV. Positrons are emitted from the nucleus with high velocity and kinetic energy. They are rapidly slowed by interactions in the surrounding tissues until all of the positron kinetic energy is lost. At this point, the positron combines momentarily with an electron. The combination of particles totally annihilates or disintegrates, and the combined positron-electron mass of 1.022 MeV is transformed into two equal-energy photons of 0.511 MeV, which are emitted at 180 degrees from each other (Fig. 32-19).

These annihilation photons behave like gamma *rays,* have sufficient energy to

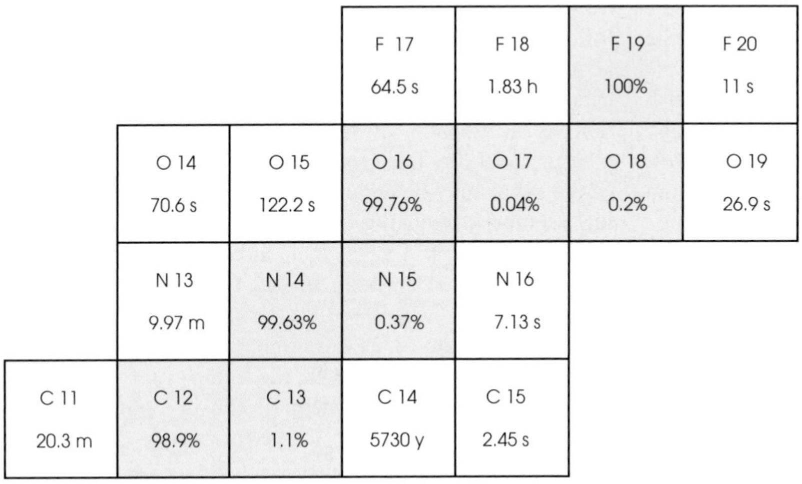

			F 17 64.5 s	F 18 1.83 h	F 19 100%	F 20 11 s
	O 14 70.6 s	O 15 122.2 s	O 16 99.76%	O 17 0.04%	O 18 0.2%	O 19 26.9 s
	N 13 9.97 m	N 14 99.63%	N 15 0.37%	N 16 7.13 s		
C 11 20.3 m	C 12 98.9%	C 13 1.1%	C 14 5730 y	C 15 2.45 s		

Fig. 32-18 Excerpt from *The Chart of the Nuclides* showing the stable elements (*shaded boxes*), positron emitters (*to the left of the stable elements*), and beta emitters (*to the right of the stable elements*). Isotopes farther from their stable counterparts have very short half-lives. The most commonly used PET nuclides are ^{11}C, ^{13}N, ^{15}O, and [18]F.

(From Walker FW et al: *The chart of the nuclides,* ed 13, San Jose, CA, 1984, General Electric Company.)

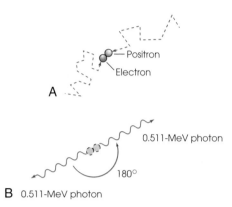

Fig. 32-19 Neutron-deficient nuclei decay by positron emission. A positron is ejected from the nucleus and loses kinetic energy by scattering (*erratic line in* **A**) until it comes to rest and interacts with a free electron. Two photons of 0.511 MeV ($E = mc^2$) result from the positron and electron annihilation (*wavy line in* **B**).

TABLE 32-3
Positron characteristics

Definition	Positively charged electron
Origin	Neutron-deficient nuclei
Production	Accelerators
Nuclide decay	$p = n + \beta^+$ neutrino
Positron decay	Annihilation to two 0.511-MeV photons
Number	About 240 known
Range	Proportional to kinetic energy of β^+
Routine PET nuclides	^{11}C, ^{13}N, ^{15}O, ^{18}F, ^{68}Ga, ^{82}Rb

traverse body tissues with only modest attenuation, and can be detected externally. Because two identical or isoenergetic photons are emitted at exactly 180 degrees from each other, the nearly simultaneous detection of both photons defines a line that passes through the body. The line is located precisely between the two scintillators that detected the photons. A simplified block diagram for a single coincidence circuit is shown in Fig. 32-20. The creation of images from coincidence detection is discussed in the section on data acquisition.

The positron annihilation photons from the positron-emitting radionuclides of carbon, nitrogen, and oxygen can be used for external detection. Table 32-4 depicts the positron ranges for three positron energies in tissue, air, and lead. Hydrogen has no positron-emitting radioisotope; however, ^{18}F is a positron (β^+) emitter that is used as a hydrogen substitute in many compounds. This substitution of ^{18}F for hydrogen is successfully accomplished because of its small size and strong bond with carbon.

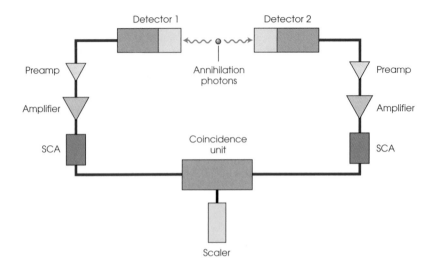

Fig. 32-20 Simplified coincidence electronics for one pair of detectors in a PET tomograph.

TABLE 32-4

Range (R) of positrons (β^+) in centimeters

E(MeV)*	R_{tissue}	R_{air}	R_{lead}
0.5	0.15	127	0.01
1.0	0.38	279	0.03
1.5	0.64	508	0.05

*The average positron energy is approximately one third the maximum energy (see Fig. 32-21).
From U.S. Department of Health, Education, and Welfare: *Radiological health handbook,* Rockville, MD, 1970, Bureau of Radiological Health.

RADIONUCLIDE PRODUCTION

Positron-emitting radionuclides are produced when a *nuclear particle accelerator* bombards appropriate nonradioactive *target* atoms with nuclei accelerated to high energies. The high energies are necessary to overcome the electrostatic and nuclear forces of the target nuclei so that a nuclear reaction can occur. An example is the production of ^{15}O. Deuterons, or heavy hydrogen ions (the deuterium atom is stripped of its electron, leaving only the nucleus with one proton and one neutron), are accelerated to approximately 7 MeV. The target material is stable nitrogen gas in the form of an N_2 molecule. The resultant nuclear reaction yields a neutron and an ^{15}O atom, which can be written in the following form: $^{14}N(d,n)^{15}O$. The ^{15}O atom quickly associates with a stable ^{16}O atom that has been intentionally added to the target gas to produce a radioactive ^{15}O-^{16}O molecule in the form of O_2.

The unstable or radioactive ^{15}O atom emits a positron when it decays. This radioactive decay process transforms a proton into a neutron. On decay, the ^{15}O atom becomes a stable ^{15}N atom, and the O_2 molecule breaks apart. This process is shown in Fig. 32-21, and the decay schemes for the four routinely produced PET radionuclides are depicted in Fig. 32-22. The common reactions used for the production of positron-emitting forms of carbon, nitrogen, oxygen, and fluorine are given in Table 32-5.

Because of the very short half-lives of the routinely used positron-emitting nuclides of oxygen, nitrogen, and carbon, nearby access to a nuclear particle accelerator is necessary to produce sufficient quantities of these radioactive materials. The most common device to achieve nuclide production within reasonable space (250 ft² [223 m²]) and energy (150 kW) constraints is a compact medical cyclotron (Fig. 32-23). This device is specifically designed for the following: (1) simple operation by the technologist staff, (2) reliable and routine operation with minimal downtime, and (3) computer-controlled automatic operation to reduce overall staffing needs.

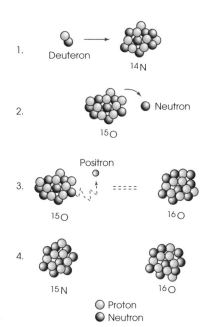

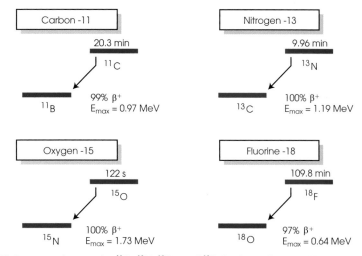

Fig. 32-21 Typical radionuclide production sequence. The $^{14}N(d,n)^{15}O$ reaction is used for making ^{15}O-^{16}O molecules. *1,* A deuteron ion is accelerated to high energy (7 MeV) by a cyclotron and impinges on a stable ^{14}N nucleus. *2,* As a result of the nuclear reaction, a neutron is emitted, leaving a radioactive nucleus of ^{15}O. *3,* ^{15}O atom quickly associates with ^{16}O atom to form O_2 molecule. Later, unstable ^{15}O atom emits a positron. *4,* As a result of positron decay (i.e., positron exits nucleus), ^{15}O atom is transformed into stable ^{15}N atom, and O_2 molecule breaks apart.

Fig. 32-22 Decay schemes for ^{11}C, ^{13}N, ^{15}O, and ^{18}F. Each positron emitter decays to a stable nuclide by ejecting a positron from the nucleus. E_{max} represents the maximum energy of the emitted positron. Electron capture is a competitive process with positron decay; positron decay is not always 100%.

TABLE 32-5
Most common production reactions and target materials for typical nuclides used in positron emission tomography

| Nuclide | Half-life (min) | Reaction(s) | | Target material |
		Proton	Deuteron	
^{11}C	20.4	$^{14}N(p,\alpha)^{11}C$		N_2 (gas)
^{13}N	9.97	$^{16}O(p,\alpha)^{13}N$		H_2O (liquid)
^{15}O	2.03	$^{15}N(p,n)^{15}O$	$^{14}N(d,n)^{15}O$	$N^2 + 1\% O_2$ (gas)
^{18}F	109.8	$^{18}O(p,n)^{18}F$		95% $^{18}O - H_2O$ (liquid)
			$^{20}Ne(d,\alpha)^{18}F$	Ne + 0.1% F_2 (gas)

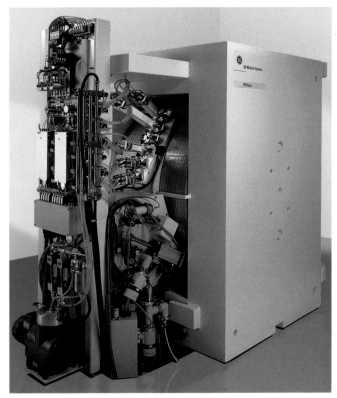

Fig. 32-23 Compact cyclotron (2.2 m high × 1.5 m wide × 1.5 m deep) used for routine production of PET isotopes. Cyclotron can be located in a concrete vault, or it can be self-shielded. Particles are accelerated in vertical orbits and impinge on targets located near the top center of the machine. This is an example of a negative-ion cyclotron.

(Courtesy GE Medical Systems, Milwaukee, WI.)

Nuclear Medicine

RADIOPHARMACEUTICAL PRODUCTION

Radiopharmaceuticals are synthesized from radionuclides derived from the target material. These agents may be simple, such as the ^{15}O-^{16}O molecules described earlier, or they may be complex. Regardless of the chemical complexity of the radioactive molecule, all radiopharmaceuticals must be synthesized rapidly. This entails specialized techniques not only to create the labeled substance but also to verify the purity (chemical, radiochemical, and radionuclide) of the radiotracer.

Two important radiopharmaceuticals are presently used in many PET studies. The simplest is ^{15}O-water (^{15}O-H_2O), which is produced continuously from the $^{14}N(d,n)^{15}O$ nuclear reaction or in batches from the $^{15}N(p,n)^{15}O$ nuclear reaction. As previously discussed, the radioactive oxygen quickly combines with a stable ^{16}O atom, which has been added to the stable N_2 target gas, to form an oxygen molecule (O_2). The ^{15}O-^{16}O molecule is reduced over a platinum catalyst with small amounts of stable H_2 and N_2 gas. Radioactive water vapor is produced and collected in sterile saline for injection. A typical bolus injection of ^{15}O-H_2O is approximately 30 to 50 mCi in a volume of 1 to 2 mL of saline for use in a PET scanner that acquires data in two-dimensional form and approximately 3 to 8 mCi in the same volume of saline for a PET tomograph of the newer three-dimensional design. A dose of radioactive water can be prepared every 2 to 5 minutes. Radioactive ^{15}O-H_2O is used primarily for the determination of *local cerebral blood flow* (LCBF). PET LCBF images from one subject using two different techniques are shown in Fig. 32-24. Blood flow to tumor, heart, kidney, or other tissues can also be measured using ^{15}O-H_2O.

The most widely used PET radiopharmaceutical for clinical PET imaging is more complex than labeled water and employs ^{18}F-labeled fluoride ions (F–) to form a sugar analog called [^{18}F]-2-fluoro-2-deoxy-D-glucose (^{18}F-FDG). This agent is used to determine the *local metabolic rate of glucose use* in tumor, brain, heart, or other tissues that use glucose as a metabolic substrate. The glucose obtained from food is metabolized by the brain to provide the adenosine triphosphate necessary for maintaining the membrane potential of neurons within the brain. The metabolism of glucose is proportional to the neural activity of the brain and brain metabolism. Radioactive ^{18}F-FDG and glucose enter the same biochemical pathways in the brain. In contrast to glucose, ^{18}F-FDG cannot be completely metabolized in the brain, however, because its metabolism is blocked at the level of fluorodeoxyglucose-6-phosphate ([^{18}F]-FDG-6-PO_4). Because ^{18}F-FDG follows the glucose pathway into the brain, the concentration of [^{18}F]-FDG-6-PO_4 within the brain cells is proportional to brain tissue metabolism. These pathways for glucose and ^{18}F-FDG are shown schematically in Fig. 32-25.

Injected doses of ^{18}F-FDG range from 5 to 20 mCi; a standard dose is 15 to 20 mCi. FDG is dissolved in a few milliliters of isotonic saline and is administered intravenously. The total time for FDG production, which includes target irradiation (1 hour to 90 minutes), radiochemical synthesis (30 minutes to 1 hour), and purity certification (15 minutes), is approximately 2 to 3 hours, depending on

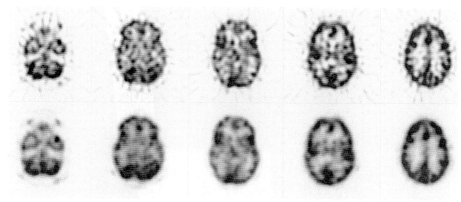

Fig. 32-24 PET LCBF images. Images in the *top row* were created using a standard filtered back-projection reconstruction technique. An iterative reconstructive method was used to create images in the *bottom row* from the same raw data that were used for upper images. In all images, dark areas correspond to high brain blood flow. There is about an 8-mm separation between each brain slice within a row.

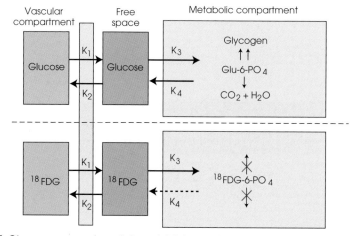

Fig. 32-25 Glucose compartmental model (*above dashed line*) compared with the ^{18}F-FDG model (*below dashed line*). ^{18}F-FDG does not go to complete storage (glycogen) or metabolism (CO_2 + H_2O) as does glucose. The constants (*K*) refer to reaction rates for moving substances from one compartment to another. *Dashed arrow* refers to extremely small K value that can usually be neglected.

the exact synthesis method used. Because of the short half-life of most positron-emitting radioisotopes, radiopharmaceutical production must be closely tied to the clinical patient schedule.

DATA ACQUISITION

The positron-electron annihilation photons are detected and counted with a PET scanner or tomograph (Fig. 32-26). The bore width of these scanners is approximately 70 cm, with newer scanners being slightly larger in diameter. The radial field of view (FOV) or the imaging dimension parallel to the detector rings for these scanners is approximately 10 inches (24 cm) and 22 inches (55 cm) (Fig. 32-27). The z axis or dimension perpendicular to the detector rings is 6 to 20 inches (15 to 50 cm). Typical new scanners have 800 to 1000 detectors per ring. A detector module consists of *scintillators* organized into a matrix (6×6, 7×8, or 8×8) of small rectangular boxes (3 to 6 mm long, 3 to 6 mm wide, and 10 to 30 mm deep), which are coupled to PMTs. Scintillators can be constructed from various different materials. Different materials have different characteristics that may improve or degrade the quality of the system. Characteristics such as short decay time, high light output, high-energy resolution, and high stopping power would create the most efficiency PET detector material. Characteristics of the commercial materials available are listed in Table 32-6. The most newest scintillator, lutetium orthosilicate ($Lu_2SiO_5:Ce$), has a higher light output (approximately

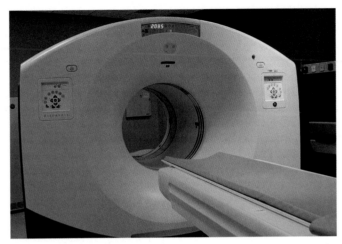

Fig. 32-26 Typical whole-body PET/CT scanner. The bed is capable of moving in and out of the scanner to measure the distribution of PET radiopharmaceuticals throughout the body, and it adjusts to a very low position for easy patient access. Sophisticated computer workstations are required to view and analyze data.

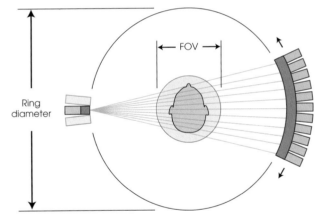

Fig. 32-27 Detector arrangement in neurologic PET ring (head-only scanner). Rays from opposed detector pairs (*lines* between detectors) depict possible coincidence events. The useful field of view (*FOV*) is delineated by the *central circle*.

TABLE 32-6
Properties of PET scintillator materials

Property	NaI sodium iodide	BGO bismuth germanium oxide $Bi_4Ge_3O_{12}$	GSO gadolinium oxyorthosilicate $Gd_2SiO_5(Ce)$	LSO lutetium oxyorthosilicate $Lu_2SiO_5(Ce)$	LYSO lutetium yttrium orthosilicate $Lu_{2(1-x)}Y_{2x}SiO_5(Ce)$
Z (atomic number) stopping power	50	74	58	66	65
Density (g/cm³)	3.7	7.1	6.7	7.4	7.1
Light yield	100	15	26	75	80
Decay constant (nsec)	230	300	65	40	41
Energy resolution @ 511 keV (%)	6.6	10.2	8.5	10	14
Attenuation length (mm) for 511 keV photons	28.8	10.5	14.3	11.6	12
Attenuation coefficient (cm⁻¹) @ 511 keV	0.34	0.94	0.67	0.87	0.83

four times that of bismuth germanate [BGO]) and faster photofluorescent decay (approximately 7.5 times that of BGO). Scintillator dimensions are being reduced to improve resolution. At the present time, the resolution within the image plane for PET scanners is between 3 mm and 5 mm full width at half maximum. An image of a point source of radioactivity appears to be 3 to 5 mm wide at half the maximum intensity of the source image. The concept of PET scanner resolution can be explained using a bicycle wheel as an example. In the case of PET, lines drawn between detectors or *rays* correspond to the bicycle spokes. The highest density of spokes is located at the hub. At the rim of the wheel, the density of spokes is reduced. The same is true for the density of rays between detectors. That is why the selected radial imaging FOV for these scanners is approx-

imately the middle third of the distance from one detector face to the opposite detector face. Adequate ray density for the best resolution for image reconstruction is achieved only within this FOV. The same holds for the axial or longitudinal dimension (*z* axis). Approximately two thirds of the axial FOV contains sufficient ray sampling. By acquiring several axial FOV, which is achieved by moving the bed through the PET scanner, the amount of data undersampled is significantly reduced. Each axial FOV is overlapped with the next. Sufficient axial sampling is achieved for all but the first and last bed position.

Coincidence counts are collected not only for detector pairs within each ring (direct-plane information), but also between adjacent rings (cross-plane information) as shown in Fig. 32-28. Not all

photons emitted from the patient can be detected, however. Some of the pairs of 0.511-MeV photons from the positron annihilation impinge on detectors in the tomograph ring and are detected; most do not. The photon pairs are emitted 180 degrees from each other. The emission process is *isotropic,* which means that the annihilation photons are emitted with equal probability in all directions so that only a small fraction of the total number of photons emitted from the patient actually strike the tomograph detectors (Fig. 32-29).

PET scanners originally used ray information only from the nearest adjacent planes. With improvements in software reconstruction techniques and the elimination of septa between detector rings, the second, third, fourth, and upward adjacent planes are used to produce

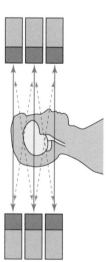

Fig. 32-28 Side-view schematic of a small portion of a multiring (three-ring) PET tomograph. *Darker green squares* indicate the scintillator-matrix, which is attached to multiple-photocathode PMTs. *Solid lines* indicate the direct planes, and *dashed lines* depict the cross planes. The determined by the pair of cross planes forms a data plane located between direct planes. Improvements in PET scanner instrumentation not only permit cross-plane information between adjacent rings to be acquired, but it also allows for expansion to the second, third, fourth, and fifth near neighbor rings. This significantly enhances overall scanner sensitivity.

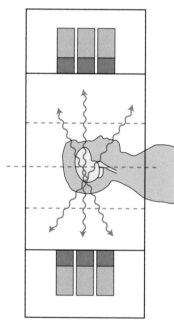

Fig. 32-29 Side view of PET scanner, illustrating possible photon directions. Only 15% of the total number of emitted photons from the patient can be detected in a whole-body tomograph (ring diameter 39 inches [100 cm]). This is increased to 25% for a head tomograph (ring diameter 24 inches [60 cm]). For these estimates, axis coverage was considered to be 6 inches (15 cm). The actual number of detected coincidences would be less than either the 15% or 25% estimate because the detector efficiency is not 100% (typical efficiency 30%).

three-dimensional PET images. With inclusion of the additional cross-plane information, PET scanner *sensitivity* is greatly increased. The injected doses of radiopharmaceutical are significantly reduced (50% to 90% less radioactivity given) to yield PET images with a quality equivalent to that of images obtained from the original dose levels used in two-dimensional PET scanners with septa.

When pairs of photons are detected, they are counted as valid events (i.e., true positron annihilation) only if they appear at the detectors within the resolving time for the coincidence electronics. For many PET tomographs, this is typically 8 to 12 nsec. If one photon is detected and no other photon is observed during that time window, the original event is discarded. This is defined as electronic collimation. No conventional lead collimators as needed with SPECT are used in PET scanners. Thick lead shields absorb annihilation photons created out of the axial FOV, however, before interacting with the PET detectors. These shields help reduce random events and high singles counting events. PET scanners must operate with high sensitivity, and as a result scanners must also be able to handle very high count rates with minimum *deadtime* losses.

For PET procedures, data acquisition is not limited to images of tomographic count rates. The creation of *quantitative* parametric images of glucose metabolism requires that the blood concentrations of the radiopharmaceutical be measured. This measurement is accomplished by discrete or continuous arterial sampling, discrete or continuous venous sampling, or *region of interest* (ROI) analysis of a sequential time series of major arterial vessels observed in reconstructed tomographic images. For arterial sampling, an indwelling catheter is placed in the radial artery. Arterial blood pressure forces blood out of the catheter for collection and radioactivity measurement. For venous sampling, blood is withdrawn through an indwelling venous catheter. For obtaining *arterialized venous blood*, the patient's hand is heated to 104°F to 108°F (40°C to 42.2°C). In this situation, arterial blood is shunted directly to the venous system. The arterial concentration of radioactivity can be assessed by measuring the venous radioactivity concentration.

If plasma radioactivity measurement is required in discrete samples, the red blood cells are separated from whole blood by centrifugation, and the radioactivity concentration within plasma is determined by discrete sample counting in a gamma well counter. Continuous counting is performed on whole blood by directing the blood through a radiation detector via small-bore tubing. A peristaltic pump, a syringe pump, or the subject's arterial blood pressure is used for continuous or discrete blood sampling. For ROI analysis, the arterial blood curve is generated directly from each image of a multiple-frame, time-series PET scan. ROI is placed around the arterial vessel visualized in the PET images. The average number of counts for the ROI from each frame is plotted against time. Actual blood sampling is not usually required for ROI analysis. A single venous (or arterial) blood sample may be taken, however, at times when tracer equilibrium has been established between arterial and venous blood to position the blood curve appropriately on an absolute scale.

A typical set of blood and tissue curves is given in Fig. 32-30. Curves created from plasma data and other information (e.g., nonradioactive plasma glucose level) are supplied to a mathematical model that appropriately describes the physiologic process being measured (i.e., metabolic rate of glucose use in tissue). Applying the model to the original PET image data creates parametric or functional images.

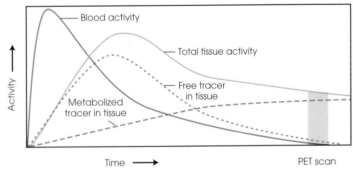

Fig. 32-30 Decay-corrected radioactivity curves for ^{18}F-FDG in tissue and blood (plasma). Injection occurs at the origin. Blood activity rapidly peaks after injection. Metabolized tracer ([^{18}F]-FDG-6-PO$_4$) slowly accumulates in tissue. Typical static PET scanning occurs after an incorporation time of 40 to 60 minutes (as shown by the *shaded box*) in which the uptake of ^{18}F-FDG is balanced with slow washout of the labeled metabolite.

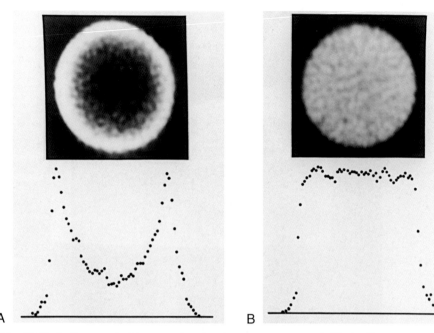

A   B

Fig. 32-31 A, Uncorrected image of a phantom homogeneously filled with water-soluble PET nuclide of ⁶⁸Ga or ¹⁸F. **B,** Attenuation-corrected image of same phantom. Cross-sectional cuts through the center of each image are shown in *lower panels.* The attenuation correction for a phantom with a diameter of 8 inches (20 cm) can be 70% in the center of the object.

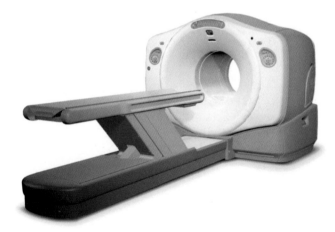

Fig. 32-32 Typical PET/CT scanner.

(Courtesy GE Medical Systems, Milwaukee, WI.)

IMAGE RECONSTRUCTION AND IMAGE PROCESSING

FOV of 6 to 8 inches (15 to 20 cm) in the axial direction is required to encompass the entire volume of the brain (from the top of the cerebral cortex to the base of the cerebellum) or the entire volume of the heart adequately. Array processors are used to perform the maximum likelihood (iterative) reconstruction that converts the raw *sinogram* data into PET images. This technique is similar to the technique employed for CT image reconstruction. Faster and less costly desktop computers are replacing array processor technology and greatly simplifying software requirements for image reconstruction.

Three important corrections need to be made during image reconstruction to ensure an accurate and interpretable scan. First, the disintegration of radionuclides follows Poisson statistics. As a result of this random process, photons from the different annihilation events may strike the tomograph detectors simultaneously. Although these are registered as true events because they occur within the coincidence time window, they degrade the overall image quality. A simple approximation allows for the subtraction of the random events after image acquisition and is based on the individual count rates for each detector and the coincidence resolving time (8 to 12 nsec) of the tomograph electronics.

Second, photons traversing biologic tissues also undergo absorption and scatter. As shown in Fig. 32-31, an attenuation correction is applied to account for photons that should have been detected but were not. In the past, the correction was typically based on a transmission scan acquired under computer control using a radioactive rod or pin source of ⁶⁸Ge (germanium; 271-day half-life) that circumscribed the portion of the patient's body within the PET scanner. At the present time, PET/CT scanners use the CT data to correct for attenuation more accurately (Fig. 32-32).

Lastly, count rates from the detectors also need to be corrected for deadtime losses. At high count rates, the detector electronics cannot handle every incoming event; some events are lost because the electronics are busy processing prior events. Measuring the tomograph response to known input count rates allows empiric formulations for the losses to be determined and applied to the image data. Valid corrections for deadtime losses can approach 100%.

Clinical Positron Emission Tomography

PET is unique in its ability to measure in vivo physiology because its results are quantitative, rapidly repeatable, and validated against the results of accurate but much more invasive techniques. It is, however, relatively costly and best used for answering complex questions that involve locating and quantitatively assessing tissue function (Figs. 32-33 and 32-34). Anatomic imaging, such as CT, is often limited in its ability to determine whether found masses are of malignant or benign etiology. Traditional anatomic imaging modalities also have difficulty determining malignancy in small masses or lymph nodes. Because PET is a functional modality, it can often be used to determine malignancy, even in very small nodes or masses.

Patient preparation for PET studies can be detailed and is imperative for optimal imaging. In most cases, the area that is to be examined must be free of metallic objects to avoid creating artifacts on the reconstructed images. This is especially important when using a PET/CT scanner because metallic objects may cause false-positive results in the final images owing to attenuation overcorrection in that area. The waiting time between dose administration and imaging varies with each study, as does the total imaging time. After completion of a routine procedure, patients may resume all normal activities. Technical summaries of commonly performed PET procedures follow.

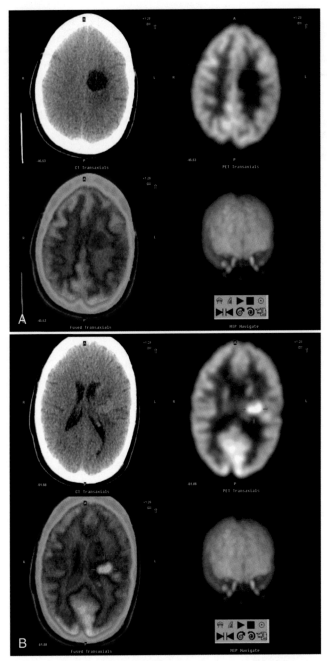

Fig. 32-33 A, PET FDG brain imaging with CT fusion shows left subcortical resection site consistent with prior tumor resection. **B,** At inferior and lateral margins of resection site, in the adjacent white matter, a hypermetabolic mass is identified. This case represents recurrent high-grade malignancy located in the left periventricular white matter at the frontoparietal junction adjacent to previous resection site.

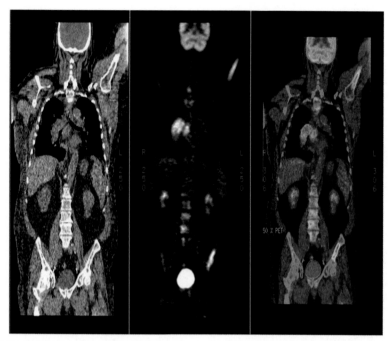

Fig. 32-34 PET FDG image with CT fusion shows large hypermetabolic right lung mass. Many PET FDG studies are done for lung cancer because of its high glucose metabolism.

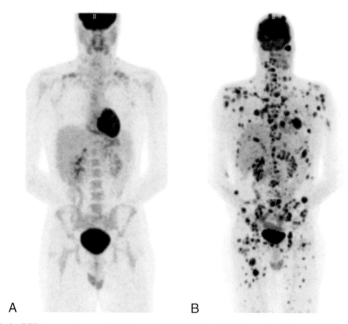

A   B

Fig. 32-35 A, PET image to evaluate a patient with a history of melanoma on the scalp. Scan shows no definite evidence for recurrence. **B,** Image 6 months later shows profound and widely disseminated hypermetabolic metastases throughout the body.

PET ONCOLOGY IMAGING

Clinically, 70% to 80% of PET scans are done to diagnose, stage, or restage cancer (Fig. 32-35), specifically cancer of the lung, breast, colon, lymph system, liver, esophagus, and thyroid. ^{18}F-FDG is the radiopharmaceutical of choice. PET plays an important role in differentiating benign from malignant processes, and it is used for image-guided biopsy. PET is an important modality for detecting cancer recurrence in patients who have undergone surgery, chemotherapy, or radiation treatments. It is also very effective in monitoring therapeutic interventions by rapidly yet noninvasively assessing the metabolic response of the tissues to drugs.

With new reimbursement policies in effect, most malignant tumors are being imaged with ^{18}F-FDG in PET. The most common cancers imaged include lung, colorectal, head and neck, lymphoma, thyroid, esophageal, breast, ovarian, melanoma, testicular, and bladder.

^{18}F-FDG ONCOLOGIC STUDY
Principle

Although ^{18}F-FDG is currently the prevailing radiopharmaceutical in tumor PET imaging, it was initially developed as a tracer to study glucose metabolism in the brain. In the late 1980s, successful reports of ^{18}F-FDG tumor imaging began to surface. It became apparent that certain tumors had a much greater uptake of ^{18}F-FDG than surrounding tissues. Tumor cells tend to have a much greater affinity for glucose than cells of surrounding tissues because of their higher glucose metabolism. This distinction is paramount in understanding how ^{18}F-FDG PET is able to detect metastatic disease.

Although there are many considerations to take into account when performing ^{18}F-FDG PET, the most important is in the regulation of the patient's blood glucose. Generally, a blood glucose level of less than 180 mg/dL is required for optimal imaging and can be achieved with a 4-hour fast. Patients with high glucose levels generally have poor ^{18}F-FDG uptake because of the already overabundant presence of glucose in their blood. In cases in which the glucose level is less than 150 mg/dL, it is still important to have the patient fasting for approximately 4 hours before the injection of ^{18}F-FDG because postprandially the insulin response is still strong enough to push the ^{18}F-FDG into more soft tissue than is normally seen in a fasting patient. The result is an image that appears to have a low target-to-background ratio. There are many other protocols that various institutions follow to increase ^{18}F-FDG uptake by the tumor, including having the patient eat low-carbohydrate meals the day before and the day of the scan.

Radiopharmaceutical

The adult dose of ^{18}F-FDG is 0.214 mCi/ kg with a minimum of 15 mCi and a maximum of 20 mCi. Pediatric doses are adjusted according to the patient's weight.

Scanning

^{18}F-FDG studies require a 60- to 90-minute uptake period after injection for incorporation of the radiopharmaceutical into the body. Some protocols suggest that imaging tumors after 90 minutes of ^{18}F-FDG incorporation may lead to significantly better signal-to-noise values in the tumor compared with surrounding tissues. During the uptake phase of the protocol, it is important that the patient be still and relaxed. Any motion, especially in the area of interest, would cause the muscles in that area to accumulate FDG and make interpretation of the images difficult. No reading, talking on the phone, or other activity is allowed. The patient must also be kept warm. If the patient develops a shiver, muscle uptake can also be increased. Depending on the dose injected and PET scanner sensitivity, approximately 3 minutes per bed position is required for the emission scan to measure the almost static distribution of ^{18}F-FDG glucose metabolism in tissue. When using a CT scan for attenuation correction, the total time for a whole-body (generally orbits through proximal femora) scan is about 20 minutes.

PET NEUROLOGIC IMAGING
Metabolic neurologic study
Principle

Because the brain uses about 25% of the body's total metabolic energy, it provides an excellent gateway for functional imaging of glucose metabolism using ^{18}F-FDG. Most clinical PET brain imaging is currently done with ^{18}F-FDG. Most PET brain scanning is done to differentiate necrotic tissue from recurrent disease, facilitate a diagnosis of cognitive status, and monitor cerebrovascular disease. Another use that is proving to be beneficial is using PET imaging in patients with temporal lobe epilepsy. The identification and location of brain tumors are difficult to assess with ^{18}F-FDG because of the high metabolic uptake of ^{18}F-FDG in the brain.

When using a PET/CT system, the anatomic information provided by the CT scan can be especially helpful in determining the effects of therapy. The guiding principle in ^{18}F-FDG PET brain imaging is that the healthy brain has high glucose metabolism and high blood flow to the cerebral cortex, which demonstrates the concentration of ^{18}F-FDG within the brain. PET is also routinely used in monitoring response to therapy and the progression of cognitive disease. With the progression of cognitive decline, glucose metabolism in the brain declines. ^{18}F-FDG assesses temporal lobe epilepsy by evaluating brain blood flow.

Radiopharmaceutical

The adult dose of ^{18}F-FDG is 0.214 mCi/ kg with a minimum of 15 mCi and a maximum of 20 mCi. Pediatric doses are adjusted according to the patient's weight.

Scanning

Before and after injection with ^{18}F-FDG, the patient should follow the same procedure as though undergoing an ^{18}F-FDG whole-body scan. The main difference is the importance of having no visual or auditory stimulation if possible. The visual cortex has a high rate of glucose metabolism during stimulation, which can make the images more difficult to interpret. Generally, the patient is injected with ^{18}F-FDG in a darkened room and is given instructions to remain still and to try to stay awake for a 30-minute uptake period. At the end of this period, the scan is performed in three-dimensional mode, meaning without collimation, with an emission time of 8 minutes. The transmission is generally done for 5 minutes, unless an elliptic or contoured attenuation correction is done. When done on a PET/ CT scanner, the CT scan is used to determine positioning of the brain and for the attenuation map. The time savings of using the CT scan for the attenuation correction can be very helpful, especially in pediatric patients or claustrophobic patients who may have difficulty staying still for any length of time.

Amyloid neurologic study
Principle

β-amyloid protein is a type of protein that forms in patients with Alzheimer's Disease (AD) and some other cognitive disorders. Thioflavin binds to beta-amyloid histologically and fluoresces. Amyloid radiotracers are thioflavin derivatives. Patients with AD have a buildup of beta-amyloid proteins between nerve cells that form plaques. Amyloid radiotracers target these plaques and identify their presence. White (neural signals) and gray matter (neuronal cell bodies) is clearly defined using ^{18}F-Florbetapir in patients with a negative AD diagnosis. Patients with AD will have increased uptake of ^{18}F-Florbetapir as it targets beta-amyloid plaque.

Radiopharmaceutical

The adult dose of ^{18}F-Florbetabir is 10 mCi (370 MB1) with a total volume of 10 mL or less.

Scanning

Because ^{18}F-Florbetabir does not rely on glucose metabolism for distribution, blood glucose does not need to be assessed. A 10-minute, dynamic acquisition should be acquired after a 30- to 50-minute uptake period with the patient laying supine and head positioned in a head holder to eliminate patient movement and thereby ensure adequate PET/CT data fusion. The FOV should include the cerebellum, and attenuation correction should be applied to the images.

Other brain studies

Other brain imaging is now being done for Parkinson disease with ^{18}F-fluorodopa, which traces dopamine synthesis in the brain. There are also a few ^{15}O radiotracers in use, such as $H_2^{15}O$, which are employed to assess cerebral blood flow quantitatively.

PET CARDIOLOGY IMAGING

PET is a highly valuable diagnostic tool in the determination of myocardial viability and coronary flow reserve. Because of its higher temporal and spatial resolution and its built-in attenuation correction,

PET is able to offer higher diagnostic accuracy than conventional nuclear medicine techniques. Because PET tracers emit higher energy gamma rays (511 keV) compared with conventional nuclear tracers (^{201}Tl at 80 keV and ^{99m}Tc sestamibi at 140 keV), PET is able to measure tracer uptake in the body more accurately. At the present time, clinical application of PET imaging in cardiology can be divided into two main categories: detection of myocardial viability and assessment of coronary flow reserve.

Cardiac viability

Principle

PET imaging for cardiac viability is an invaluable tool in the assessment of viable tissue in the left ventricle. The use of ^{18}F-FDG as an indicator of glucose metabolism allows the clinician to assess the likelihood of successful coronary revascularization. Patients with moderate to severe left ventricular dysfunction yet high myocardial viability are the most likely to benefit from revascularization. Patients who are found to have minimally viable tissue would not benefit from revascularization and may undergo the procedure needlessly if no noninvasive testing is done. Normal protocols stipulate that patients undergo a resting cardiac perfusion scan before cardiac ^{18}F-FDG PET. Traditional patterns of myocardial viability include decreased resting blood perfusion in the presence of enhanced metabolic uptake.

Radiopharmaceutical

The adult dose of ^{18}F-FDG is 0.214 mCi/kg with a minimum of 15 mCi and a maximum of 20 mCi. The ^{13}N-ammonia dose is calibrated to 20 mCi in adult patients.

Scanning

The day of the scan, all patients are to fast and refrain from caffeine and nicotine intake. Upon arrival, patients have two intravenous lines placed, one in each arm. One line is for the radiopharmaceutical injection; the other is for the insulin and dextrose infusion. A rest perfusion scan with ^{13}N-ammonia is usually performed first, and the protocol is the same as for the resting portion of the coronary flow reserve study. After completion of the scan, the patient is given intravenous insulin and dextrose to prepare the heart for maximal ^{18}F-FDG uptake. When the patient's blood glucose level reaches an optimal level, ^{18}F-FDG is injected. At 30 minutes after injection, the patient is moved onto the scanner and positioned for the transmission scan. A transmission scan of 10 to 15 minutes ensues with a 10- to 15-minute emission scan to follow. When the scan is completed, patients are fed a light lunch, and their blood glucose levels are monitored until they reach normal levels.

Coronary flow reserve

Principle

PET is now commonly used to facilitate diagnosis of coronary artery disease and to assess coronary flow reserve. It is especially helpful in differentiating between stress-induced coronary ischemia and necrosis. These studies are most often done using ^{13}N-ammonia, but the advantages of other radioisotopes such as ^{82}Ru and ^{15}O are making their use more common. The advantage of ^{82}Ru is that it is generator-produced and acts as a potassium analog, similar to ^{201}Tl. It is expensive and requires a large patient load to make it cost-effective. The benefit of ^{15}O is that it is freely diffusible in the myocardium and is independent of metabolism, making it an excellent choice for quantitative studies. It does present other problems, however, because its short half-life and short imaging time can lead to grainy images, making it a poor choice for qualitative studies. Use of ^{13}N-ammonia is most common because of its relatively short half-life (10 minutes) and because it is trapped by the myocardium in the glutamine synthesis reaction.

Radiopharmaceutical

^{13}N-ammonia is injected at a dose of approximately 10 to 20 mCi. Because of its 10-minute half-life and because it is cyclotron-produced, it can be difficult to obtain an exact dose. This is especially true during the stress portion of the test.

Scanning

Patients are asked to eat a light meal approximately 2 hours before the test and to avoid caffeine and nicotine products for 24 hours before the test. This is because caffeine may affect the adenosine, which is the pharmacologic stress agent of choice for PET coronary flow reserve studies. In patients with asthma or other contraindications to adenosine, dobutamine may be preferred. The test consists of two portions: rest imaging and stress imaging. The rest imaging is initiated by using the transmission scan to locate and position the heart in the center of the FOV. If the imaging is being done on a PET/CT system, this is done using the CT scan as a scout. When the heart is centered, a transmission scan of 10 to 15 minutes, based on patient girth, is performed for attenuation purposes. On completion of the transmission scan, ^{13}N-ammonia may be injected. The emission scan generally takes 10 to 15 minutes, and it may be done as a gated acquisition if desired. After approximately 50 minutes (five ^{13}N half-lives), the stress study may begin. The stress agent, usually adenosine, is infused for 7 minutes total with ^{13}N-ammonia injected 3 minutes into the infusion (other stress agents such as dobutamine or dipyridamole may also be used). Emission imaging should begin immediately. If the patient needed to use the restroom or had any movement between the rest and stress image, another transmission image would need to be acquired. On completion of the examination, the patient may be discharged and allowed to resume normal activity.

Future of Nuclear Medicine

RADIOIMMUNOTHERAPY

Several radioimmunotherapy protocols have come into clinical use in recent years. Monoclonal antibodies specifically designed to localize on the surface of different types of cancer cells can now be tagged with a radioisotope and then imaged. If the monoclonal antibody successfully localizes on the tumor site, the radioisotope may be replaced with a beta-emitting therapeutic radioisotope such as ^{131}I or ^{90}Y. Current studies are looking to treat osteosarcoma with ^{153}Sm-EDTMP and refractory low-grade transformed B-cell non-Hodgkin lymphoma with ^{90}Y–ibritumomab tiuxetan (Zevalin) or ^{131}I-tositumomab (Bexxar). These studies provide convincing evidence that more diseases may be treatable in the future using radioimmunotherapy.

HYBRID IMAGING

Considerable research into the fusion of functional (SPECT and PET) and anatomic (CT and MRI) imaging has led to the introduction of dual-modality, or hybrid, imaging systems. This is one of the most exciting developments in the field of nuclear medicine. The combined PET/CT camera shown in Fig. 32-32 couples the functional imaging capabilities of PET with the superb anatomic imaging of CT. Images from each modality are coregistered during the acquisition process and in near-simultaneity. Because the images can be overlaid one on another, the position of suspected tumors can be identified easily. Suspicious metabolically active areas can now be identified anatomically from the CT information. These features have improved the reliability of SPECT and PET interpretation. Metabolic and anatomic evaluation after therapy can be accomplished in one imaging session, which is likely to improve patient acceptance of the procedures significantly. For all these reasons, SPECT/CT and PET/CT are becoming among the most useful diagnostic procedures for staging disease and evaluating the treatment of cancer. All of the advantages of the integration between PET and MRI have not been identified. Continued research utilizing PET/MRI in the areas of oncology, neurology, and cardiology will lead radiologic imaging into a new era. With the hybridization of PET/CT and PET/MRI, molecular imaging has made tremendous advancements toward improving diagnostic care for all patients.

POSITRON EMISSION TOMOGRAPHY

PET technology is advancing on many fronts. ^{18}F-FDG is routinely being produced in distribution centers throughout the United States and Europe. One or more cyclotrons at each distribution site are continuously producing ^{18}F-fluoride for incorporation into ^{18}F-FDG. Unit doses are shipped via common commercial carriers, which also include chartered air and special ground couriers from a network of registered pharmacy distribution centers to individual PET centers that do not have cyclotrons. Clinical PET imaging no longer requires the high financial commitment to own and operate a nuclear accelerator to produce PET radiopharmaceuticals at a local site.

New radiopharmaceuticals are also being developed. As PET radiopharma-ceutical distribution centers expand and are able to handle the daily demands of providing ^{18}F-FDG to the existing and new PET centers, production of ^{18}F-labeled radiopharmaceuticals specifically for tumor imaging is likely to become available. FDA approval would be required before clinical imaging, but several PET manufacturers and the PET radiopharmaceutical distribution centers are sponsoring drug clinical trials to accelerate the deployment of new and viable clinical PET imaging agents. Radiolabeled choline, thymidine, fluorodopa, estrogen receptors, and numerous other biomolecules are likely candidates for new PET clinical tracers.

Mobile PET units are a reality, as shown in Figs. 32-36 and 32-37. PET scanner technology has matured to the point that the original frailty of the electronics and detector systems has been eliminated. Robust mobile units travel to community hospitals that need PET imaging but not at the level that necessitates a dedicated in-house PET scanner. By spending 1 or 2 days per week at several different hospitals in smaller communities or rural settings, the mobile PET camera best serves the needs of their oncology patients. The ^{18}F-FDG distribution centers are necessary in this scenario because the mobile PET camera unit needs a supply of radiotracer to carry out the PET imaging study. Until nationwide ^{18}F-FDG distribution centers became a reality, as they now are, the use of mobile PET was extremely limited.

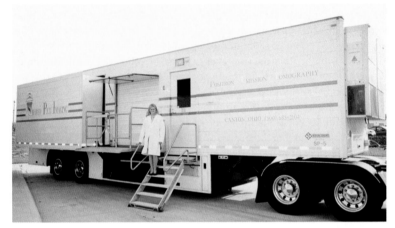

Fig. 32-36 Mobile PET coach showing operator on staff stairs and elevator platform in the elevated position. Elevator used to transport patients from ground level to floor level of the PET scanner unit.

(Courtesy Shared PET Imaging, LLC.)

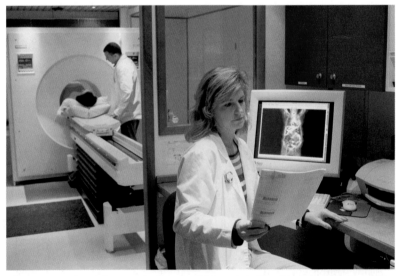

Fig. 32-37 Interior of mobile coach showing PET workstation (*foreground*) and PET scanner (*background*).

(Courtesy Shared PET Imaging, LLC.)

Conclusion

Nuclear medicine technology is a multidisciplinary field in which medicine is linked to quantitative sciences, including chemistry, radiation biology, physics, and computer technology. Since the early 20th century, nuclear medicine has expanded to include molecular nuclear medicine, in vivo and in vitro chemistry, and physiology. The spectrum of nuclear medicine technology skills and responsibilities varies. The scope of nuclear medicine technology includes patient care, quality control, diagnostic procedures, computer data acquisition and processing, radiopharmaceuticals, radionuclide therapy, and radiation safety. Many clinical procedures are performed in nuclear medicine departments across the United States and throughout the world. Nuclear medicine procedures complement other imaging methods in radiology and pathology departments.

The evolution of PET has provided the nuclear medicine department with a complex diagnostic imaging procedure. PET is a clinical tool and a research tool. PET requires the multidisciplinary support of the physician, physicist, physiologist, chemist, engineer, software programmer, and radiographer. This imaging procedure allows numerous biologic parameters in the working human body to be examined without disturbing normal-equilibrium physiology. PET measures regional function that cannot be determined by any other means, which includes CT and MRI. Current PET studies of the brain involve the imaging of patients with epilepsy, Huntington disease, stroke, schizophrenia, brain tumors, Alzheimer's disease, and other disorders of the central nervous system. PET studies of the heart are providing routine diagnostic information on patients with coronary artery disease by identifying viable myocardium for revascularization. The greatest impact PET has made is the ability to identify highly metabolic tumors. PET scanning is critically involved in the determination of the effects of therapeutic drug regimens on tumors and the differentiation of necrosis from viable tumor. Nearly 80% of all PET imaging today is directed at tumor detection and evaluation of therapeutic intervention. Overall, human physiology will become better understood as the technology advances, yielding higher resolution instruments, new radiopharmaceuticals, and improved analysis of PET data.

The future of nuclear medicine may lie in its unique ability to identify functional or physiologic abnormalities. With the continued development of new radiopharmaceuticals and imaging technology, nuclear medicine will continue to be a unique and valuable tool for diagnosing and treating disease.

Definition of Terms

alpha particle Nucleus of a helium atom, consisting of two protons and two neutrons, having a positive charge of 2.

analog PET radiopharmaceutical biochemically equivalent to a naturally occurring compound in the body.

annihilation Total transformation of matter into energy; occurs after the antimatter positron collides with an electron. Two photons are created; each equals the rest mass of the individual particles.

arterialized venous blood Arterial blood passed directly to the venous system by shunts in the capillary system after surface veins are heated to 104°F to 108°F (40°C to 42.2°C). Blood gases from the vein under these conditions reflect near-arterial levels of P_{O_2}, P_{CO_2}, and pH.

atom Smallest division of an element that exhibits all the properties and characteristics of the element; composed of neutrons, electrons, and protons.

attenuation coefficient Number that represents the statistical reduction in photons that exit a material *(N)* from the value that entered the material *(N_o)*. The reduced flux is the result of scatter and absorption, which can be expressed in the following equation: $N = N_o e - \mu\chi$, where μ is the attenuation coefficient and l is the distance traversed by the photons.

becquerel (Bq) Unit of activity in the International System of Units; equal to 1 disintegration per second (dps): 1 Bq = 1 dps.

beta particle Electron whose point of origin is the nucleus; electron originating in the nucleus by way of decay of a neutron into a proton and an electron.

BGO scintillator Bismuth germanate ($Bi_4Ge_3O_{12}$) scintillator with an efficiency twice that of sodium iodide. BGO is used in nearly all commercially produced PET scanners.

bit Term constructed from the words *binary digit* and referring to a single digit of a binary number; for example, the binary of 101 is composed of 3 bits.

blood-brain barrier Anatomic and physiologic feature of the brain thought to consist of walls of capillaries in the central nervous system and surrounding glial membranes. The barrier separates the parenchyma of the central nervous system from blood. The blood-brain barrier prevents or slows the passage of some drugs and other chemical compounds, radioactive ions, and disease-causing organisms such as viruses from the blood into the central nervous system.

byte Term used to define a group of bits, usually eight, being treated as a unit by the computer.

CM line Canthomeatal line, defined by an imaginary line drawn between the lateral canthus of the eye and meatus of the ear.

cold spot Lack of radiation being received or recorded, not producing any image and resulting in an area of no, or very light, density; may be caused by disease or artifact.

collimator Shielding device used to limit the angle of entry of radiation; usually made of lead.

curie Standard of measurement for radioactive decay; based on the disintegration of 1 g of radium at 3.731010 disintegrations per second.

cyclotron Device for accelerating charged particles to high energies using magnetic and oscillating electrostatic fields. As a result, particles move in a spiral path with increasing energy.

daughter Element that results from the radioactive decay of a parent element.

deadtime Time when the system electronics are already processing information from one photon interaction with a detector and cannot accept new events to be processed from other detectors.

decay Radioactive disintegration of the nucleus of an unstable nuclide.

detector Device that is a combination of a scintillator and photomultiplier tube used to detect x-rays and gamma rays.

deuteron Ionized nucleus of heavy hydrogen (deuterium), which contains one proton and one neutron.

dose Measure of the amount of energy deposited in a known mass of tissue from ionizing radiation. *Absorbed dose* is described in units of rads; 1 rad is equal to 10–2 joules/kg or 100 ergs/g.

ejection fraction (cardiac) Fraction of the total volume of blood of the left ventricle ejected per contraction.

electron Negatively charged elementary particle that has a specific charge, mass, and spin.

electron capture Radioactive decay process in which a nucleus with an excess of protons brings an electron into the nucleus, creating a neutron out of a proton, decreasing the atomic number by 1. The resulting atom is often unstable and gives off a gamma ray to achieve stability.

external radiation detector Instrument used to determine the presence of radioactivity from the exterior.

^{18}F-FDG Radioactive analog of naturally available glucose. It follows the same biochemical pathways as glucose; however, in contrast to glucose, it is not totally metabolized to carbon dioxide and water.

fission Splitting of a nucleus into two or more parts with the subsequent release of enormous amounts of energy.

functional image See *parametric image*.

gamma camera Device that uses the emission of light from a crystal struck by gamma rays to produce an image of the distribution of radioactive material in a body organ.

gamma ray High-energy, short-wavelength electromagnetic radiation emanating from the nucleus of some nuclides.

ground state State of lowest energy of a system.

half-life (T$\frac{1}{2}$) Term used to describe the time elapsed until some physical quantity has decreased to half of its original value.

homeostasis State of equilibrium of the body's internal environment.

image coregistration Computer technique that permits realignment of images that have been acquired from different modalities and have different orientations and magnifications. With realignment, images possess the same orientation and size. Images can then be overlaid, one on the other, to show similarities and differences between the images.

in vitro Outside a living organism.

in vivo Within a living organism.

isotope Nuclide of the same element with the same number of protons but a different number of neutrons.

isotropic Referring to uniform emission of radiation or particles in three dimensions.

kinetics Movement of materials into, out of, and through biologic spaces. A mathematic expression is often used to describe and quantify how substances traverse membranes or participate in biochemical reactions.

light pipe Tubelike structure attached to the scintillation crystal to convey the emitted light to the photomultiplier tube.

local cerebral blood flow (LCBF) Description of the parametric image of blood flow through the brain. It is expressed in units of milliliters of blood flow per minute per 100 g of brain tissue.

magnetic resonance imaging (MRI) Technique of nuclear magnetic resonance (NMR) as it is applied to medical imaging. Magnetic resonance is abbreviated *MR*.

metastable Describes the excited state of a nucleus that returns to its ground state by emission of a gamma ray; has a measurable lifetime.

neutron Electrically neutral particle found in the nucleus; has a mass of 1 mass unit.

nuclear particle accelerator Device to produce radioactive material by accelerating ions (e.g., electrons, protons, deuterons) to high energies and projecting them toward stable materials. Accelerators include linac, cyclotron, synchrotron, Van de Graaff accelerator, and betatron.

nuclear reactor Device that under controlled conditions is used for supporting a self-sustained nuclear reaction.

nuclide General term applicable to all atomic forms of an element.

parametric image Image that relates anatomic position (the *x* and *y* position on an image) to a physiologic parameter such as blood flow (image intensity or color). It may also be referred to as a *functional image*.

parent Radionuclide that decays to a specific daughter nuclide either directly or as a member of a radioactive series.

particle accelerator Device that provides the energy necessary to enable a nuclear reaction.

pharmaceutical Relating to a medicinal drug.

photomultiplier tube (PMT) Electronic tube that converts light photons to electrical pulses.

photopenia See *cold spot*.

pixel (picture element) Smallest indivisible part of an image matrix for display on a computer screen. Typical images may be 128 × 128, 256 × 256, or 512 × 512 pixels.

positron Positively charged particle emitted from neutron-deficient radioactive nuclei.

positron emission tomography (PET) Imaging technique that creates transaxial images of organ physiology from the simultaneous detection of positron annihilation photons.

proton Positively charged particle that is a fundamental component of the nucleus of all atoms. The number of protons in the nucleus of an atom equals the atomic number of the element.

pulse height analyzer Instrument that accepts input from a detector and categorizes the pulses on the basis of signal strength.

pyrogen-free Free of a fever-producing agent of bacterial origin.

quantitative Type of PET study in which the final images are not simply distributions of radioactivity but rather correspond to units of capillary blood flow, glucose metabolism, or receptor density. Studies between individuals and repeat studies in the same individual permit comparison of pixel values on an absolute scale.

radiation Emission of energy; rays of waves.

radioactive Exhibiting the property of spontaneously emitting alpha, beta, and gamma rays by disintegration of the nucleus.

radioactivity Spontaneous disintegration of an unstable atomic nucleus resulting in the emission of ionizing radiation.

radioisotope Synonym for *radioactive isotope*. Any isotope that is unstable undergoes decay with the emission of characteristic radiation.

radionuclide Unstable nucleus that transmutes via nuclear decay.

radiopharmaceutical Refers to a radioactive drug used for diagnosis or therapy.

radiotracer Synonym for *radiopharmaceutical*.

ray Imaginary line drawn between a pair of detectors in the PET scanner or between the x-ray source and detector in a CT scanner.

reconstruction Mathematic operation that transforms raw data acquired on a PET tomograph (sinogram) into an image with recognizable features.

rectilinear scanner Early imaging device that passed over the area of interest, moving in or forming a straight line.

region of interest (ROI) Area that circumscribes a desired anatomic location on a PET image. Image-processing systems permit drawing of ROI on images. The average parametric value is computed for all pixels within the ROI and returned to the radiographer.

resolution Smallest separation of two point sources of radioactivity that can be distinguished for PET or SPECT imaging.

scintillation camera See *gamma camera.*

scintillation detector Device that relies on the emission of light from a crystal subjected to ionizing radiation. The light is detected by a photomultiplier tube and converted to an electronic signal that can be processed further. An array of scintillation detectors is used in a gamma camera.

scintillator Organic or inorganic material that transforms high-energy photons such as x-rays or gamma rays into visible or nearly visible light (ultraviolet) photons for easy measurement.

septa High-density metal collimators that separate adjacent detectors on a ring tomograph to reduce scattered photons from degrading image information.

single photon emission computed tomography (SPECT) Nuclear medicine scanning procedure that measures conventional single photon gamma emissions (^{99m}Tc) with a specially designed rotating gamma camera.

sinogram Two-dimensional raw data format that depicts coincidence detectors against possible rays between detectors. For each coincidence event, a specific element of the sinogram matrix is incremented by 1. The sum of all events in the sinogram is the total number of events detected by the PET scanner minus any corrections that have been applied to the sinogram data.

target Device used to contain stable materials and subsequent radioactive materials during bombardment by high-energy nuclei from a cyclotron or other particle accelerator. The term is also applied to the material inside the device, which may be solid, liquid, or gaseous.

tracer Radioactive isotope used to allow a biologic process to be seen. The tracer is introduced into the body, binds with a specific substance, and is followed by a scanner as it passes through various organs or systems in the body.

transmission scan Type of PET scan that is equivalent to a low-resolution CT scan. Attenuation is determined by rotating a rod of radioactive 68Ge around the subject. Photons that traverse the subject either impinge on a detector and are registered as valid counts or are attenuated (absorbed or scattered). Ratio of counts with and without the attenuating tissue in place provides the factors to correct PET scans for the loss of counts from attenuation of the 0.511-MeV photons.

washout End of the radionuclide procedure, during which time the radioactivity is eliminated from the body.

Selected bibliography

Christian PE et al: *Nuclear medicine and PET technology and techniques,* ed 7, St Louis, 2012, Mosby.

Steves AM: *Review of nuclear medicine technology,* Reston, VA, 2004, Society of Nuclear Medicine.

Wieler HJ, Coleman RE: *PET in clinical oncology,* Darmstadt, 2000, Steinkopff Verlag.

Definition of Terms

33

BONE DENSITOMETRY

SHARON R. WARTENBEE

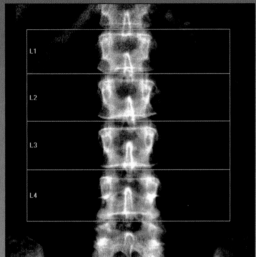

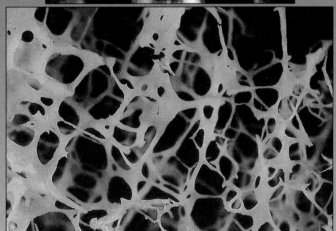

OUTLINE

Principles of Bone Densitometry, 442
History of Bone Densitometry, 443
Bone Biology and Remodeling, 445
Osteoporosis, 447
Physical and Mathematic Principles
 of Dual Energy X-Ray
 Absorptiometry, 451
Pencil-Beam and Array-Beam
 Techniques, 454
Dual Energy X-Ray Absorptiometry
 Scanning, 458
Other Bone Densitometry
 Techniques, 469
Conclusion, 476

Principles of Bone Densitometry

*Bone densitometry** is a general term that encompasses the art and science of measuring the *bone mineral content* (BMC) and *bone mineral density* (BMD) of specific skeletal sites or the whole body. The bone measurement values are used to assess bone strength, assist with diagnosis of diseases associated with low bone density (especially *osteoporosis*), monitor the effects of therapy for such diseases, and predict risk of future fractures.

---

*Almost all italicized words on the succeeding pages are defined at the end of this chapter.

Several techniques are available to perform bone densitometry using ionizing radiation or ultrasound. The most versatile and widely used is *dual energy x-ray absorptiometry* (DXA) (Fig. 33-1).[1] This procedure has the advantages of low radiation dose, wide availability, ease of use, short scan time, high-resolution images, good *precision,* and stable calibration. DXA is the focus of this chapter, but summaries of other procedures are also presented.

---

[1]Gowin W, Felsenberg D: Acronyms in osteodensitometry, *J Clin Densitometry* 1:137, 1998.

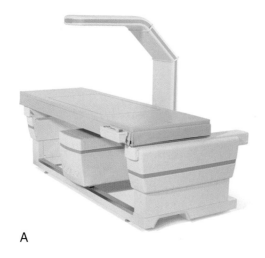

A

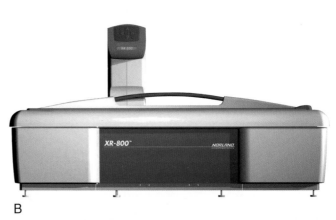

B

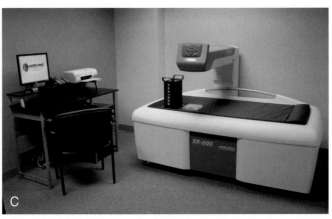

C

Fig. 33-1 A, DXA spine scan being performed on a Hologic model, Horizon. **B,** DXA spine scan being performed on a GE Lunar model, Advance. **C,** DXA whole-body scan being performed on a Norland model, XR-46.

(**A,** Courtesy Hologic, Inc, Bedford, MA. **B,** Courtesy GE Lunar Corp, Madison, WI. **C,** Courtesy Norland/Swissray Inc, Ft. Atkinson, WI.)

DUAL ENERGY X-RAY ABSORPTIOMETRY AND CONVENTIONAL RADIOGRAPHY

The differences between DXA and conventional radiography are as follows:

1. DXA can be conceptualized as a *subtraction technique*. To quantitate BMD, it is necessary to eliminate the contributions of soft tissue and measure the x-ray attenuation of bone alone. This is accomplished by scanning at two different x-ray photon energies (hence the term *dual energy x-ray*) and mathematically manipulating the recorded signal to take advantage of the differing attenuation properties of soft tissue and bone at the two energies. The density of the isolated bone is calculated on the basis of the principle that denser, more mineralized bone attenuates (absorbs) more x-ray. Adequate amounts of artifact-free soft tissue are essential to help ensure the reliability of the bone density results.

2. The bone density results are computed by proprietary software from the x-ray attenuation pattern striking the detector, not from the scan image. Scan images are only for the purpose of confirming correct positioning of the patient and correct placement of the *regions of interest* (ROI). The images may not be used for diagnosis, and any medical conditions apparent on the image must be followed up by appropriate diagnostic tests.

3. In conventional radiography, x-ray machines from different manufacturers are operated in essentially the same manner and produce identical images. This is not the case with DXA. Three DXA manufacturers are in the United States (see Fig. 39-1), and technologists must be educated about the specific scanner model in their facility. The numeric bone density results cannot be compared among manufacturers. This chapter presents general scan positioning and analysis information, but the manufacturers' specific procedures must be used when actual scans are performed and analyzed.

4. The effective radiation dose for DXA is considerably lower than the radiation dose for conventional radiography. The specific personnel requirements vary among states and countries. All bone density technologists should be instructed in core competencies, including radiation protection, patient care, history taking, basic computer operation, knowledge of scanner quality control, patient positioning, scan acquisition and analysis, and proper (record) keeping and documentation.

History of Bone Densitometry

Osteoporosis was an undetected and overlooked disease until the 1920s, when the advent of x-ray film methods allowed the detection of markedly decreased density in bones. The first publications indicating an interest in *bone mass* quantification methods appeared in the 1930s, and much of the pioneering work was performed in the field of dentistry. *Radiographic absorptiometry* involved taking a radiograph of bone with a known standard, placing it in the ROI, and optically comparing the densities.

Radiogrammetry was introduced in the 1960s, partly in response to the measurements of bone loss performed in astronauts. As bone loss progresses, the thickness of the outer shell of phalanges and metacarpals decreases and the inner cavity enlarges. Indices of bone loss are established by measuring and comparing the inner and outer diameters.

In the late 1970s, the emerging technique of computed tomography (CT) (see Chapter 29) was adapted, through the use of specialized software and reference phantoms, enabling quantitative measurement of the central area of the vertebral body, where early bone loss occurs. This technique, called *quantitative computed tomography* (QCT), is still used.

The first scanners dedicated to bone densitometry appeared in the 1970s and early 1980s. *Single photon absorptiometry* (SPA) (Fig. 33-2) and *dual photon absorptiometry* (DPA) are based on physical principles similar to those for DXA. The SPA approach was not a subtraction technique but relied on a water bath or other medium to eliminate the effects of soft tissue. SPA found application only in the peripheral skeleton. DPA used photons of two energies and was used to assess sites in the central skeleton (lumbar spine and proximal femur). The radiation source was a highly collimated beam from a radioisotope (^{125}I [iodine-125] for SPA and ^{153}Gd [gadolinium-153] for DPA). The intensity of the attenuated beam was measured by a collimated *scintillation counter,* and the bone mineral was quantified.

The first commercial DXA scanner was introduced in 1987. In this scanner, the expensive, rare, and short-lived radioisotope source was replaced with an x-ray tube. Improvements over time have included the choice of *pencil-beam* or *array-beam collimation;* a rotating C-arm to allow supine lateral spine imaging; shorter scan time; improved detection of low bone density; improved image quality; and enhanced computer power, multimedia, and networking capabilities.

Since the late 1990s, renewed attention has been given to smaller, more portable, less complex techniques for measuring the peripheral skeleton. This trend has been driven by the introduction of new therapies for osteoporosis and the resultant need for simple, inexpensive screening tests to identify persons with osteoporosis who are at increased risk for fracture. DXA of the hip and spine is still the most widely accepted method for measuring bone density, however, and it remains a superior procedure for monitoring the effects of therapy.

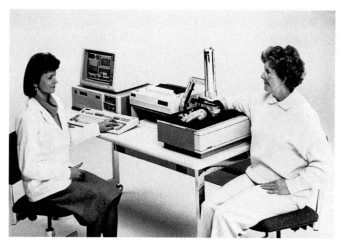

Fig. 33-2 SPA wrist scan being performed on a Lunar model, SP2. This form of bone densitometry is obsolete.

(Courtesy GE Lunar Corp, Madison, WI.)

Bone Biology and Remodeling

The skeleton serves the following purposes:

- Supports the body and protects vital organs so that movement, communication, and life processes can be carried on
- Manufactures red blood cells
- Stores the minerals that are necessary for life, including calcium and phosphate

The two basic types of bone are *cortical* (or compact) and *trabecular* (or cancellous). Cortical bone forms the dense, compact outer shell of all bones and the shafts of the long bones. It supports weight, resists bending and twisting, and accounts for about 80% of the skeletal mass. Trabecular bone is the delicate, latticework structure within bones that adds strength without excessive weight. It supports compressive loading in the spine, hip, and calcaneus, and it is also found at the ends of long bones, such as the distal radius. The relative amounts of trabecular and cortical bone differ by bone densitometry technique used and anatomic site measured (Table 33-1).

Bone is constantly going through a remodeling process in which old bone is replaced with new bone. With this *bone remodeling* process (Fig. 33-3), the equivalent of a new skeleton is formed about every 7 years. Bone-destroying cells called *osteoclasts* break down and remove old bone, leaving pits. This part of the process is called *resorption*. Bone-building cells called *osteoblasts* fill the pits with new bone. This process is called *formation*. The comparative rates of resorption and formation determine whether bone mass increases (more formation than resorption), remains stable (equal resorption and formation), or decreases (more resorption than formation).

Osteoclasts and osteoblasts operate as a bone-remodeling unit. A properly functioning bone remodeling cycle is a tightly coupled physiologic process in which resorption equals formation, and the net bone mass is maintained. The length of the resorption process is about 1 week compared with a longer formation process of about 3 months. At any point in time, millions of remodeling sites within the body are in different phases of the remodeling cycle or at rest.

TABLE 33-1

Bone densitometry regions of interest: estimated percentage of trabecular and cortical bone and preferred measurement sites

Region of interest	Trabecular bone (%)	Cortical bone (%)	Preferred measurement site
PA spine (by DXA)	66	34	Cushing disease, corticosteroid use
PA spine (by QCT)	100		
Femoral neck	25	75	Type II osteoporosis
			Second choice for hyperparathyroidism
Trochanteric region	50	50	
Calcaneus	95	5	
33% radius	1	99	First choice for hyperparathyroidism
Ultradistal radius	66	34	
Phalanges	40	60	
Whole body	20	80	Pediatrics

Data from Bonnick SL: *Bone densitometry in clinical practice: application and interpretation*, Totowa, NJ, 1998, Humana Press.

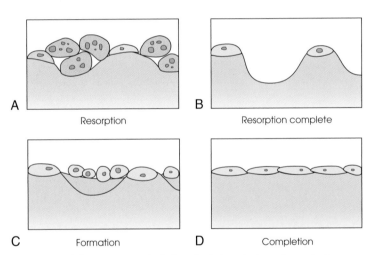

Fig. 33-3 Bone remodeling process. **A,** Osteoclasts break down bone in the process of resorption. **B,** Pits in the bone. **C,** Osteoblasts form new bone. **D,** With equal amounts of resorption and formation, the bone mass is stable.

(From National Osteoporosis Foundation: *Boning up on osteoporosis*, Washington, DC, 1997, National Osteoporosis Foundation.)

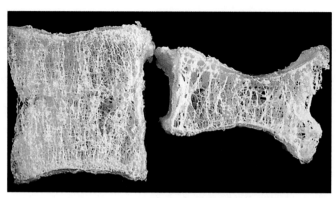

Fig. 33-4 Osteoporotic vertebral body (right) shortened by compression fractures, compared with a normal vertebral body. The osteoporotic vertebra exhibits a characteristic loss of horizontal trabeculae and thickened vertical trabeculae.

(From Kumar V, et al: *Robbins and Cotran pathologic basis of disease,* ed 8, Philadelphia, 2010, Saunders/Elsevier.)

When the cycle becomes uncoupled, the result is a net loss of bone mass. Some reasons for uncoupling are enhanced osteoclastic recruitment; impaired osteoblastic activity; and increased number of cycles, which results in shorter time for each cycle. The increased number of cycles favors the shorter resorption phase over the longer formation phase.

Bone mass increases in youth until *peak bone mass* is reached at approximately 20 to 30 years of age. This is followed by a stable period in middle age. A period of decreasing bone mass starts at approximately age 50 in women and approximately age 65 in men. The decrease in bone mass becomes pronounced in women at menopause because of the loss of bone-preserving estrogen. If the peak bone mass is low or the resorption rate is excessive, or both, at menopause, osteoporosis may result (Fig. 33-4).

Osteoporosis

Osteoporosis is a disease characterized by low bone mass and structural deterioration of bone tissue. This decrease in bone mass and degradation of bone architecture may not support the mechanical stress and loading of normal activity. As a result, the bones are at increased risk for *fragility fractures.* An estimated 10 million Americans have osteoporosis; 80% (8 million) are women. Another 48 million Americans have *low bone mass,* putting them at risk of developing osteoporosis and related fractures. By 2030, the numbers are expected to increase to 11 million adults with osteoporosis and 64.3 million with low bone mass. Persons with osteoporosis may experience decreased quality of life from the pain, deformity, and disability of fragility fractures. An increased risk of morbidity and mortality exists, especially from hip fractures. In the United States, annual medical costs for osteoporosis, including hospitalization for osteoporotic hip fractures, were $19 billion in 2005, and the cost is increasing. By 2025, it is expected to be $25.3 billion.

Many risk factors for osteoporosis have been identified and studied. The following are considered primary risk factors:

- Female gender
- Increased age
- Estrogen deficiency
- Caucasian race
- Low body weight (<127 lb [<58 kg]), low body mass index (BMI) (weight in kg divided by height in meters squared), or both
- Family history of osteoporosis or fracture
- History of prior fracture as an adult
- Smoking tobacco

Osteoporosis is often overlooked in older men because it is considered a woman's disease; however, the National Osteoporosis Foundation found that 2 million American men have osteoporosis, and another 12 million are at risk. Of Americans diagnosed with osteoporosis, 20% are men. Men older than 50 are more likely to break a hip due to osteoporosis than they are to get prostate cancer.

The exact cause of osteoporosis is unknown, but it is clearly a multifactorial disorder. Major contributors are genetics, metabolic factors regulating internal calcium equilibrium, lifestyle, aging, and menopause. Peak bone mass attained in young adulthood, coupled with the rate of bone loss in older age, determines whether an individual's bone mass becomes low enough to be diagnosed as osteoporosis. Genetic factors are estimated to account for 70% of the peak bone mass attained, which is why family history is an important risk factor for osteoporosis and fracture. Calcium equilibrium is maintained by a complex mechanism involving hormones (parathyroid, calcitonin, and vitamin D) controlling key ions (calcium, magnesium, and phosphate) within target tissues (blood, intestine, and bone). Calcium and phosphate enter the blood from the intestine and are stored in bone. The process also occurs in reverse, moving calcium out of the bones for other uses within the body. Nutritional and lifestyle factors can upset the balance and cause too much calcium to move out of bone. In the course of normal aging, the loss of estrogen at menopause tends to increase the rate of bone turnover, which increases the number of remodeling cycles and shortens the length of each cycle. Enough time is allowed for the shorter resorption process, but the longer formation process is cut short. Various combinations of these factors can result in a net loss of bone mass and increase the risk of osteoporosis and fracture.

Two points are important to note about osteoporosis. First, an older person with a normal rate of bone loss may still develop osteoporosis if his or her peak bone mass was low. Second, it is a common misconception that proper exercise and diet at menopause prevent bone loss associated with the decrease in estrogen. Persons concerned about their risk of osteoporosis should consult their physician.

Osteoporosis can be classified as primary or secondary. A DXA scan result does not automatically lead to a diagnosis of primary osteoporosis. Secondary causes of systemic or localized disturbances in bone mass must be ruled out before a final diagnosis can be made. Proper choice of treatment should be based on the type of osteoporosis and the underlying cause, if secondary osteoporosis is present (see Table 33-1).

Primary osteoporosis can be *type I* (postmenopausal), *type II* (senile or age related), or both. Type I osteoporosis is caused by bone resorption exceeding bone formation owing to estrogen deprivation in women. Type II osteoporosis occurs in aging men and women and results from a decreased ability to build bone.

Secondary osteoporosis is osteoporosis caused by a heterogeneous group of skeletal disorders resulting in imbalance of bone turnover. Disorder categories include genetic, endocrine and metabolic, hypogonadal, connective tissue, nutritional and gastrointestinal, hematologic, malignancy, and use of certain prescription drugs. Common causes of secondary osteoporosis include *hyperparathyroidism;* gonadal insufficiency (including estrogen deficiency in women and hypogonadism in men); *osteomalacia* (rickets in children); rheumatoid arthritis; anorexia nervosa; gastrectomy; celiac disease (hypersensitivity to gluten [wheat protein]); multiple myeloma; and use of corticosteroids, heparin, anticonvulsants, or excessive thyroid hormone treatment.

Several prescription medications arrest bone loss and may increase bone mass, including traditional estrogen or hormone replacement therapies, bisphosphonates, selective estrogen receptor modulators, parathyroid hormone, Receptor activator of nuclear factor kappa-B ligand (RANKL) inhibitors, and calcitonin. Other therapies are in clinical trials and may be available in the future (Table 33-2). The availability of therapies beyond the traditional estrogens has led to the widespread use of DXA to diagnose osteoporosis.

Laboratory tests for *biochemical markers* of bone turnover may be used in conjunction with DXA to determine the need for or the effectiveness of therapy. Problems of poor precision and individual variability have limited their use. Some markers of bone formation found in blood are alkaline phosphatase, osteocalcin, and C- and N-propeptides of type I collagen. Some markers of bone resorption excreted in urine are pyridinium cross-links of collagen, C- and N-telopeptides of collagen, galactosyl hydroxylysine, and hydroxyproline.

TABLE 33-2

Osteoporosis medicines—National Osteoporosis Foundation 2014

FDA approved for:	Postmenopausal women	Men	Prevents osteoporosis	Treats osteoporosis	Prevents osteoporosis caused by steroid medicines	Treats osteoporosis caused by steroid medicines
Bisphosphonates						
Alendronate (Fosamax®, Fosamax Plus D™)	■	■*	■	■		■
Ibandronate (Boniva®)	■		■	■†		
Risedronate (Actonel®, Actonel® with Calcium)	■	■*	■	■	■	■
Zoledronic Acid (Reclast®)	■	■		■	■	■
Calcitonins						
Calcitonin (Fortical®)	■			■		
Calcitonin (Miacalcin®)	■			■		
Estrogen Agonists/Antagonists						
Raloxifene (Evista®)	■		■	■		
Estrogen Therapy (ET) and Hormone Therapy (HT)						
Many brands	■		■			
Parathyroid Hormone						
Teriparatide (Forteo®)	■	■		■		
RANK Ligand (RANKL)						
Denosumab (Prolia)	■			■		

*For men, alendronate and risedronate are approved for treatment only.
†Ibandronate as an intravenous (IV) injection is approved for treatment only.

FRACTURES AND FALLS

Fractures occur when bones encounter an outside force that exceeds their strength. Fragility fractures occur with minimal trauma from a standing height or less. A small percentage of fragility fractures are spontaneous, meaning that they occur with no apparent force being applied. The most common sites for fractures associated with osteoporosis are the hip, spinal vertebrae, wrist (Colles fracture), ribs, and proximal humerus, but other bones can be affected. Current estimates of fracture in the United States are that approximately 1.5 million osteoporotic fractures occur each year; these include 700,000 vertebral (only one third are clinically diagnosed), 300,000 hip, 250,000 wrist, and 300,000 other fractures.

One in two women and one in four men older than age 50 have an osteoporotic fracture in their remaining lifetime. Risk factors for fracture include being female, low bone mass, personal history of fracture as an adult, history of fracture in a first-degree relative, current cigarette smoking, and low body weight (<127 lb [<58 kg]).

Hip fractures account for 20% of osteoporotic fractures and are the most devastating for the patient and in terms of health costs. Important points about hip fracture include the following:

- The overall 1-year mortality rate after hip fracture is one in five.[1]
- Two to three times as many women as men sustain hip fractures, but the 1-year mortality rate for men is twice as high.
- Two thirds of patients with hip fracture never regain their preoperative activity status. One fourth require long-term care.
- A woman's risk of hip fracture is equal to her combined risk of breast, uterine, and ovarian cancer.
- Protective undergarments with side padding, called *hip pads,* have proven effective in preventing hip fracture from a fall in elderly adults. Resistance to wearing the garment is the only limitation.

Vertebral fractures are the most common osteoporotic fracture, but only approximately one third are clinically diagnosed. The effects of vertebral fractures have traditionally been underestimated but are beginning to be recognized and quantified. These fractures cause pain, disfigurement, and dysfunction and decrease the quality of life. More recent studies link them to an increased risk of mortality. Vertebroplasty is a minimally invasive procedure for managing acute painful vertebral fractures. This procedure involves injecting bone cement into the fractured vertebra under fluoroscopic guidance (see Fig. 24-27). Balloon kyphoplasty is a minimally invasive procedure that can reduce back pain and restore vertebral body height and spinal alignment. This procedure involves reducing the vertebral compression and injecting the cement into this space created within the vertebral body (Fig. 33-5). Fluoroscopic guidance is also used for this procedure.

The presence of one osteoporotic vertebral fracture significantly increases the risk of future vertebral fractures and progressive curvature of the spine. Most osteoporotic fractures are caused by falls. Identifying elderly persons at increased risk for falls and instituting fall prevention strategies are important goals. Some risk factors for falling are use of some medications including sedatives, sleep aids, and antidepressants; impaired muscle strength, range of motion, balance, and gait; impaired psychological functioning, including dementia and depression; and environmental hazards, including lighting, rugs, furniture, bathroom, and stairs. Fall prevention strategies through a physical therapy program include balance, gait, and strengthening exercises. Addressing psychological issues, reviewing medication regimens, and counseling patients on correct dosing are other prevention methods. Homes and living areas should be inspected for hazards, and safety measures should be implemented.

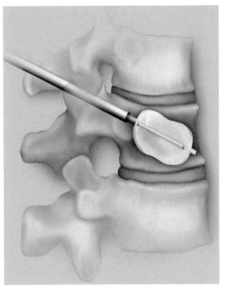

Fig. 33-5 Diagram of balloon kyphoplasty.

[1]National Institutes of Health Consensus Development Panel on Osteoporosis Prevention, Diagnosis, and Therapy: Osteoporosis prevention, diagnosis, and therapy, *JAMA* 285:785, 2001.

BONE HEALTH RECOMMENDATIONS

The National Osteoporosis Foundation's Bone Health and Prevention Recommendations are as follows:

- Obtain daily recommended amounts of calcium and vitamin D.
- Engage in regular weight-bearing and resistance exercise.
- Avoid smoking and excessive alcohol.
- Talk to a health care provider about bone health.
- Have a bone density test and take medication when appropriate.

Surgeon general's report on bone health and osteoporosis

The Surgeon General's Report on Bone Health and Osteoporosis includes an extensive review of the factors affecting bone health, including the health consequences associated with poor bone health. The report provides the following list of recommendations to promote better bone health and health status in general:

- Getting adequate levels of calcium and vitamin D
- Engaging in physical activity
- Reducing hazards in the home that can lead to fractures and falls

- Talking with a physician about preventive strategies to promote bone health
- Maintaining a healthy weight
- Not smoking
- Limiting alcohol use

Many Americans fail to meet currently recommended guidelines for optimal calcium intake. The Surgeon General's office recommends the following calcium intake: 1000 mg/daily for women 19-50 years of age and 1000 mg/daily for males 51-70 years of age. Dietary calcium is the best source including yogurt, milk, and some cheeses. Dietary shortfall should be met with calcium supplements with the USP designation that supply the appropriate amount of elemental calcium. The individual needs to check the number of pills to meet the serving size and whether or not to take with food (Table 33-3).

Adequate intake of vitamin D (the National Osteoporosis Foundation recommends at least 1000 IU/day for adults >50 years old) is essential for calcium absorption and bone health. Some calcium supplements and most multivitamins contain vitamin D. Dietary sources are vitamin D–fortified milk and cereals, egg yolks, saltwater fish, and liver.

Weight-bearing exercise occurs when bones and muscles work against gravity as the feet and legs bear the body's weight. Some examples are weight lifting to improve muscle mass and bone strength, low-impact aerobics, walking or jogging, tennis, dancing, stair climbing, gardening, and household chores.

TABLE 33-3

Daily recommended needs for calcium intake

Your body needs calcium	
If this is your age	then you need this much calcium each day (mg)
0 to 6 months	200
6 to 12 months	260
1 to 3 years	700
4 to 8 years	1,000
9 to 18 years	1,300
19 to 50 years	1,000
51- to 70-year-old males	1,000
51- to 70-year-old females	1,200
>70 years old	1,200

(A cup of milk or fortified orange juice has about 300 mg of calcium.)
From the Office of the Surgeon Generals Report

Physical and Mathematic Principles of Dual Energy X-Ray Absorptiometry

The measurement of bone density requires separation of the x-ray attenuating effects of soft tissue and bone. The mass attenuation coefficients of soft tissue and bone differ and depend on the energy of the x-ray photons. The use of two different photon energies (dual energy x-ray) optimizes the differentiation of soft tissue and bone. GE Lunar model Advance (GE Lunar Corp, Madison, WI) and Norland model XR-46 (Norland/Swissray, Inc, Ft. Atkinson, WI) use a different method of producing the two energies than Hologic model Horizon (Hologic, Inc, Bedford, MA).

GE Lunar and Norland use a rare-earth, filtered x-ray source. The primary x-ray beam is passed through selected rare-earth filters to produce a spectrum with peaks near 40 kiloelectron volts (keV) and 70 keV compared with the usual continuous spectrum with one peak near 50 keV (Fig. 33-6, *A* and *B*). Sophisticated pulse-counting detectors are used to separate and measure the low-energy and high-energy photons (Fig. 33-7). Calibration must be performed externally by scanning a calibration phantom on a regular basis.

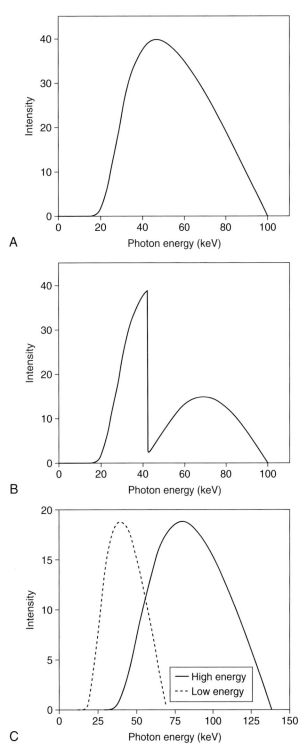

Fig. 33-6 Energy spectra (keV) for x-ray sources used in bone densitometry instruments. **A,** Continuous spectrum from x-ray tube. **B,** Continuous x-ray spectrum modified by K-edge filter. **C,** High-energy and low-energy spectra from kV-switching system.

(From Blake G et al: *The evaluation of osteoporosis: dual energy x-ray absorptiometry and ultrasound in clinical practice,* London, 1998, Martin Dunitz.)

Hologic scanners use an energy-switching system that synchronously switches the x-ray potential between 100 kVp and 140 kVp. This system produces a primary beam with two photon energies with peaks near 40 keV and 80 keV (see Fig. 33-6, *C*). The energy-switching system continuously calibrates the beam by passing it through a calibration wheel or drum (Fig. 33-8) containing three sectors for an open-air gap, a soft tissue equivalent, and a bone equivalent. Each sector is divided so that it can differentiate and measure the low-energy and high-energy photons. This permits the use of a relatively simple current-integrating detector that does not have to separate the photons.

Common physics problems of DXA are as follows:

- *Beam hardening in energy-switching systems.* With increasing body thickness, a higher proportion of low-energy photons are absorbed within the body, shifting the spectral distribution toward high-energy photons.
- *Scintillating detector pileup in K-edge filtration systems.* A detector can process only one photon at a time and assign it to the high-energy or low-energy channel. An incoming photon may be missed if the preceding photon has not yet been processed. Digital detectors do not have this problem.
- *Crossover in K-edge filtration systems.* Some high-energy photons lose energy passing through the body and are counted as low-energy photons by the detector. This problem is solved by subtracting a fraction of the high-energy counts from the low-energy channel, depending on body thickness.

The low-energy and high-energy x-rays are attenuated differently within each patient, producing a unique attenuation pattern at the detector, which is transmitted electronically to the computer. Mathematic computations are then performed to subtract the soft tissue signals, producing a profile of the bone (Fig. 33-9). Proprietary bone edge detection algorithms are next applied, and a two-dimensional area is calculated. The average BMD is calculated for all areas, and finally the *BMD* is calculated as BMD = BMC/Area. The three bone densitometry parameters reported on the DXA printouts are area in centimeters squared (cm^2), BMC in grams (g), and BMD in g/cm^2. BMD is the most widely used parameter because it reduces the effect of body size.

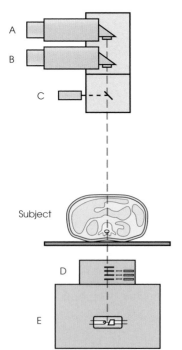

Fig. 33-7 Schematic drawing of a Norland model XR-35 illustrating the principle of operation of a rare-earth filtered system. **A,** High-energy detector. **B,** Low-energy detector. **C,** Laser indicator. **D,** Samarium filter module (one fixed, three selectable). **E,** Ultrastable 100 kV x-ray source.

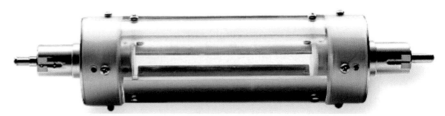

Fig. 33-8 Calibration drum used as internal reference standard in Hologic energy-switching instruments. Different segments represent bone standard, soft tissue standard, and empty segment for air value.

BMD can be calculated if BMC and area are known by the equation BMD = BMC/Area. This equation can be used to determine if a change in BMD is due to a change in BMC, area, or both. A decrease in BMC results in a decrease in BMD; conversely, a decrease in area results in an increase in BMD. If BMC and area move proportionally in the same direction, BMD remains unchanged. Generally, a change in a patient's BMD over time should be from a change in BMC, not area. A change in area could be from the technologist not reproducing the baseline positioning or from a change in the software's bone edge detection. Changes in area over time should be investigated and corrected, if possible.

BMD is based on a two-dimensional area, not a three-dimensional volume, making DXA a *projectional,* or *areal, technique.* Techniques to estimate *volumetric density* from DXA scans have been developed but have not been shown to have any improved diagnostic sensitivity over traditional areal density. Fig. 33-10 shows the lateral spine areal and estimated volumetric BMDs.

BMD values from scanners made by different manufacturers cannot be directly compared.

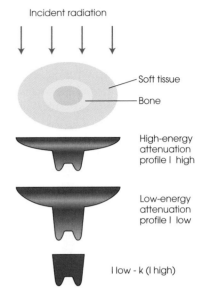

Fig. 33-9 Soft tissue compensation using DXA. By obtaining data at two energies, the soft tissue attenuation can be mathematically eliminated. The remaining attenuation is due to the amount of bone present.

(From Faulkner KG: *DXA basic science, radiation use and safety, quality assurance, unpublished certification report,* personal communication, 1996, Madison, WI.)

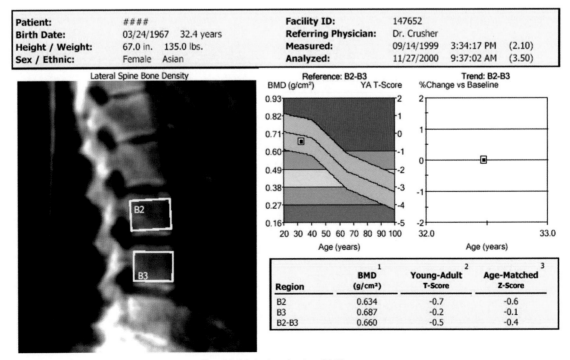

Patient:	####		Facility ID:	147652	
Birth Date:	03/24/1967	32.4 years	Referring Physician:	Dr. Crusher	
Height / Weight:	67.0 in.	135.0 lbs.	Measured:	09/14/1999	3:34:17 PM (2.10)
Sex / Ethnic:	Female	Asian	Analyzed:	11/27/2000	9:37:02 AM (3.50)

Region	BMD (g/cm²) [1]	Young-Adult T-Score [2]	Age-Matched Z-Score [3]
B2	0.634	-0.7	-0.6
B3	0.687	-0.2	-0.1
B2-B3	0.660	-0.5	-0.4

Fig. 33-10 Lateral spine BMD scan.

Pencil-Beam and Array-Beam Techniques

The original DXA scanners employed a pencil-beam system. With this system, a circular pinhole x-ray collimator produces a narrow (or pencil-beam) stream of x-ray photons that is received by a single detector. The pencil-beam of x-ray moves in a serpentine (also called *rectilinear* or *raster*) fashion across or along the length of the body (Fig. 33-11). This system has good resolution and reproducibility, but the early scanners had relatively long scan times of 5 to 7 minutes.

The array-beam (also called fan-beam) system has a wide "slit" x-ray collimator and a multielement detector (Fig. 33-12). The scanning motion is reduced to only one direction, which greatly reduces scan time and permits supine lateral lumbar spine scans to be performed. The array-beam system introduces geometric magnification and a slight geometric distortion at the outer edges. Consequently, careful centering of the object of interest is necessary to avoid parallax (Fig. 33-13). The software takes into account the known degree of magnification and produces an *estimated* BMC and estimated area.

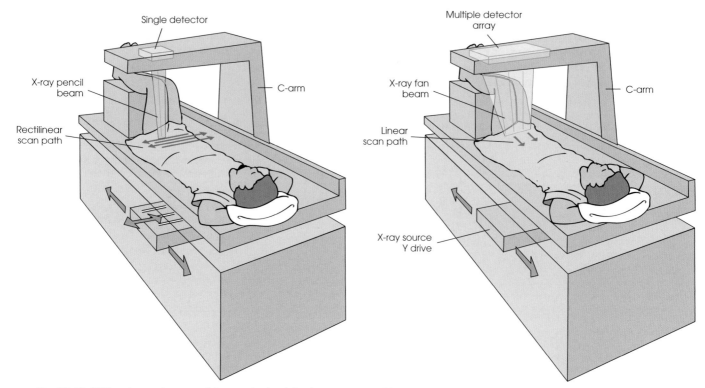

Fig. 33-11 DXA system using pencil-beam single detector.

Fig. 33-12 DXA system using an array-beam multiple detector.

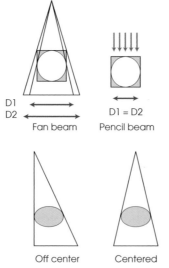

Fig. 33-13 Potential array-beam errors including magnification (*top*) and parallax (*bottom*). Area and BMC are influenced by magnification to the same degree, such that BMD is not significantly affected. Parallax errors can cause changes in BMD by altering the beam path through the object being measured.

(From Faulkner KG: *DXA basic science, radiation use and safety, quality assurance, unpublished certification report,* personal communication, 1996, Madison, WI.)

Bone Densitometry

ACCURACY AND PRECISION

Three statistics are particularly important in bone densitometry: mean, standard deviation (SD), and percent coefficient of variation (%CV).

1. The mean is commonly called the average. It is the sum of the data values divided by the number of values.

2. The SD is a measure of variability that measures the spread of the data values around their mean. It takes into account the average distance of the data values from the mean. The smaller the average distance or the spread, the smaller the SD. This is the goal in bone densitometry—a smaller SD is better. Fig. 33-14 plots two sets of phantom BMD data measured over 6 months. The means are the same (1.005 g/cm²), but the red data set has an SD that is twice as large as that of the green data set (0.008 g/cm² versus 0.004 g/cm²). It is better to have phantom BMD data that look like the green data set.

3. The %CV is a statistic that allows the comparison of variability between different data sets, whether or not they have the same mean. A smaller %CV means less variability and is preferred

in bone densitometry. The %CV is calculated using the following equation:

$$\%CV = (SD/Mean) \times 100$$

In Fig. 33-14, the green data set has a %CV of 0.35, and the red data set has a %CV of 0.81. This is the %CV that must be checked on a Hologic spine phantom plot (Fig. 33-15). The red data set would not pass the criteria that the %CV should be less than or equal to 0.6. The %CV is also used to express precision.

Bone densitometry differs from diagnostic radiology in that good image quality, which can tolerate variability in technique, is not the ultimate goal although it is very important. With bone densitometry the goal is accurate and precise quantitative measurement by the scanner software, which requires stable equipment and careful, consistent work from the technologist. Two important performance measures in bone densitometry are *accuracy* and *precision*. Accuracy relates to the ability of the system to measure the true value of an object. Precision relates to the ability of the system to reproduce the

same (but not necessarily accurate) results in repeat measurements of the same object. A target may be used to illustrate this point. In Fig. 33-16, *A*, the archer is precise but not accurate. In Fig. 33-16, *B*, the archer is accurate but not precise. Finally, in Fig. 33-16, *C*, the archer is precise and accurate.

In bone densitometry practice, accuracy is most important at baseline when the original diagnosis of osteoporosis is made. Accuracy is determined primarily by the calibration of the scanner, which is set and maintained by the manufacturer. Preventive maintenance once or twice a year is recommended. Precision is followed closely because it is easy to determine and is the most important performance measure in following a patient's BMD over time. Precision can be measured in vitro (in an inanimate object, e.g., phantom) or in vivo (in a live body). Precision is commonly expressed as %CV, and a smaller value indicates better precision.

In vitro precision is the cornerstone of the quality control systems built into the scanners to detect drifts or shifts (variations) in calibration. Each manufacturer provides a unique phantom for this purpose.

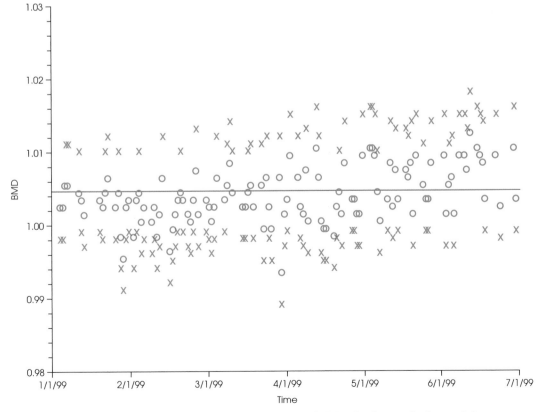

Fig. 33-14 Two datasets of longitudinal phantom BMD (*blue line* is mean). *Green data set* has mean = 1.005 g/cm², SD = 0.004 g/cm², and %CV = 0.35. *Red data set* has mean = 1.005 g/cm², SD = 0.008 g/cm², and %CV = 0.81.

In vivo precision has two main aspects in bone densitometry:

1. The variability within a patient that makes it easy or difficult to obtain similar BMD results from several scans on the same patient, on the same day, with repositioning between scans. (Patients with abnormal anatomy, very low bone mass, or thick or thin bodies are known to reflect a larger precision error.)
2. The variability related to the skill of the technologist and how attentive he or she is to obtaining the best possible baseline scan and then reproducing the positioning, scanning parameters, and placement of ROI on all *follow-up scans.*

The primary factors affecting precision are as follows:

- Reproduction of positioning, acquisition parameters (e.g., mode, speed, current), and ROI placement
- Anatomic variations and pathology and their degeneration over time
- Body habitus (e.g., excessive thickness or thinness)
- Large weight changes over time
- Geometric factors on array scanners
- Stability of scanner calibration and bone edge detection

Performing precision assessment

Each DXA laboratory should determine its precision error and calculate the *least significant change* (LSC). This precision is used to determine the magnitude of change in BMD that must occur over time to ensure the change is due to a change in the patient's BMD and not to the precision error of the technologist and scanner. The precision error supplied by the manufacturer should not be used because it is the error rate for the machine and not the technologist. If a DXA laboratory has more than one technologist, an average precision error that combines the data from all technologists should be used to establish the precision error and LSC for the facility. Every technologist should perform an in vivo precision assessment using patients who are representative of the patient population of the facility. Each technologist should do one complete precision assessment after basic scanning skills have been learned and after having performed at least 100 patient scans. If a new DXA system is installed, a repeat precision assessment should be done. A repeat assessment should also be done if a technologist's skill level has changed (International Society for Clinical Densitometry [ISCD] 2013 Position Statements).

Procedure to determine precision error for each technologist

Measure 15 patients three times or 30 patients two times, repositioning the patient after each scan. Use the ISCD Precision Assessment tool (www.iscd.org) to calculate precision. Calculate LSC for the group at 95% confidence interval. The clinician uses this information to interpret all serial scans. The minimum acceptable

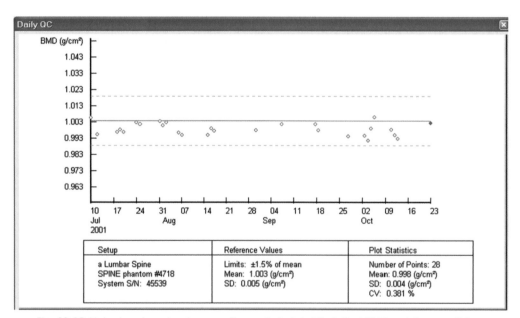

Fig. 33-15 Hologic spine phantom quality control plot. All plotted BMD points are within the control limits (*dotted lines*), which indicate 1.5% of the mean. The coefficient of variation (CV) (under *Plot Statistics*) is within acceptable limits at 0.43%.

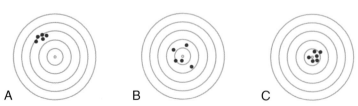

Fig. 33-16 Illustration of accuracy versus precision, assuming an archer is shooting for the center of the target. **A,** Precise but not accurate. **B,** Accurate but not precise. **C,** Accurate and precise.

precision values for an individual technologist are as follows:

- Lumbar spine: 1.9% (LSC = 5.3%)
- Total hip: 1.8% (LSC = 5.0%)
- Femoral neck: 2.5% (LSC = 6.9%)

Retraining is required if a technologist's precision is worse than these values.

Precision assessment should be standard clinical practice. It is not research and may potentially benefit patients. It should not require approval from an institutional review board. Adherence to local or state radiologic safety regulations is necessary. A precision assessment requires the consent of participating patients (ISCD 2013 Position Statements).

CROSS-CALIBRATION OF DUAL ENERGY X-RAY ABSORPTIOMETRY MACHINES

- It is impossible to compare BMD quantitatively or to calculate LSC between facilities without cross-calibration of the machines.
- DXA facilities should always cross-calibrate machines when changing hardware, replacing a system with the same technology, changing the entire system, or changing to a system by a different manufacturer.
- Scan patients as suggested in ISCD position statements. Calculate the average BMD relationship and LSC between the initial machine and new machine using the ISCD Machine Cross-Calibration tool (www.iscd.org).
- If a cross-calibration assessment is not performed, no quantitative comparison to the prior machine can be made. Consequently, a new baseline BMD and intrasystem LSC should be established (ISCD 2013 Position Statements).

Z-SCORES AND T-SCORES

A BMD measurement from a patient is most useful when it is compared statistically with an appropriate sex-matched *reference population*. The three DXA manufacturers have separately collected reference population databases, which vary because different populations, entrance criteria, and statistical methods were used. To correct this problem, the Third National Health and Nutrition Examination Survey (NHANES III) DXA total hip database was adapted to provide a *standardized hip* reference database for all manufacturers. This database is widely used today. All reference databases are separated by gender and provide the BMD mean and SD at each age; however, the lumbar spine database is manufacturer specific.

To compare a patient's BMD with the reference population BMD, two standardized scores have been developed called the *Z-score* and *T-score* (see Fig. 33-10). In older adults, the Z-score is greater than the T-score.

The Z-score indicates the number of SDs the patient's BMD is from the average BMD for the patient's respective age and sex group. The Z-score is used to determine if the measured BMD is reasonable and if evaluation for secondary osteoporosis is warranted. It is calculated using the following equation:

$$\text{Z-score} = (\text{measured BMD} - \text{age-matched mean BMD})/\text{age-matched SD}$$

The T-score indicates the number of SDs the patient's BMD is from the average BMD of young, normal, sex-matched individuals with peak bone mass. The T-score is used to assess fracture risk, diagnose osteoporosis and low bone mass *(osteopenia)*, and determine if therapy is recommended. The T-score is calculated using the following equation:

$$\text{T-score} = (\text{measured BMD} - \text{young adult mean BMD})/\text{young adult SD}$$

The Z-score, T-score, or both may also be adjusted for ethnicity, weight, or both. It is incorrect to assume that because ethnicity and weight have been entered into the scan biographic information that the standardized scores have been adjusted. Some manufacturers allow an ethnicity to be entered for which there is no reference database; these patients are compared with whites. Some manufacturers adjust for weight and ethnicity on the Z-score but not the T-score. To determine what adjustments have been made, first carefully check the information on the scan printout including footnotes. If a question remains, call the manufacturer's customer service line and ask.

As of November 1, 2003, the International Society of Clinical Densitometry (ISCD) recommends use of a uniform white (non–race adjusted) female and male normative database for women and men of all ethnic groups. All manufacturers' defaults may not be adjusted to this recommendation. The technologist needs to be familiar with the defaults of the specific equipment and know how to make adjustments.

Bone mass is normally distributed (i.e., has a bell-shaped curve) in the population, and no one exact cut point exists below which a person has osteoporosis. However, with the widespread availability of DXA and T-scores, there was pressure to declare such a cut point. In 1994, the World Health Organization (WHO) recommended that the classifications presented in Table 33-4 be used in DXA studies of postmenopausal Caucasian women.

Discordance refers to the issue of different T-scores occurring at anatomic sites within a patient, within populations, and between modalities. It makes the diagnosis of osteoporosis more complicated than simply applying T-score criteria, and the problems are being researched to find more standardized diagnostic criteria. A patient may be found to have a low T-score at the hip but not at the spine, and a QCT scan of the spine is likely to produce a lower T score than a DXA scan of the spine in the same patient.

The WHO classifications have become widely used in clinical practice. Applying the T-score criteria designed for DXA to other modalities (e.g., quantitative ultrasound [QUS], QCT) has proved to be problematic, however. The best practice is to apply the T-score criteria only to DXA until ongoing research provides acceptable criteria for other modalities. The T-score is one important risk factor for osteoporosis, but the patient's medical history, lifestyle, medications, and other risk factors must also be considered in a complete clinical evaluation. Physicians who interpret bone density scans need to be educated in the complexities of the task.

Large epidemiologic studies have investigated the clinical value of BMD in elderly women and have yielded information on the relationship of BMD and T-scores to fracture risk. A gradient of risk has been observed between BMD and fracture incidence, with lower BMD or T-score conferring increased risk of fracture. For each 1 SD decrease in T-score, the risk for fracture increases 1.5-fold to 2.5-fold. A woman with a T-score of −2 has roughly twice the risk of fracture compared with a woman with a T-score of −1, all other factors being equal. This information helps clinicians explain the meaning of a bone density test to patients. Patients can then make informed decisions about the level of fracture risk they are willing to accept and whether to begin or continue therapy.

Dual Energy X-Ray Absorptiometry Scanning

RADIATION PROTECTION

Radiologic technologists receive extensive instruction in radiation physics, biology, and protection during their professional education. Practicing proper radiation protection and achieving the goal of *ALARA* (as low as reasonably achievable) is relatively simple for DXA. The effective radiation dose in *sieverts* (Sv) for DXA scans is low compared with conventional radiography doses and similar to natural background radiation (Table 33-5). If the positioning or acquisition parameters of a scan are questionable, the scan should be repeated because the risk from the additional radiation dose is negligible compared with the risk of an incorrect medical diagnosis.

Time, distance, and shielding relate to DXA in the following ways:

1. The manufacturer sets the time for the scan based on the array or scan mode appropriate for the thickness of the body part being scanned.
2. The manufacturer sets the distance from the x-ray tube to the patient. This is a fixed distance.
3. Distance is the best form of protection for the technologist. The technologist's console should be at least 3 ft (1 m) from the x-ray source (x-ray tube) scanner for pencil-beam scanners and up to 9 ft (3 m) from heavily used array-beam scanners (array-beam produces higher dose than pencil-beam). If these distances cannot be accommodated, a mobile radiation shield can be used.

Shielding is built into the scanner via collimation. Additional lead shielding should not be used on DXA patients.

Other important radiation safety points include the following:

- The technologist should wear an individual dosimetry device (film badge, thermoluminescent dosimeter, or optically stimulated luminescence device) at the collar on the side adjacent to the scanner. Another monitor can be placed outside the scan room. A staff member should be charged with understanding and monitoring the dosimetry records and performing any necessary follow-up. A radiation warning sign should be posted and highly visible.
- The technologist should remain in the room during the scan and monitor the acquisition image, allowing the scan to be aborted as soon as the need for repositioning and rescanning is obvious.
- The technologist should have adequate instruction and experience to minimize repositioning and repeated scans. It is important to know how to prepare the patient to eliminate artifacts. Any questionable scan should be repeated.
- The technologist should follow proper procedures to avoid scanning a pregnant patient and place documentation in the permanent record. If a woman of childbearing age will not sign that she is not pregnant, the "10-day rule" allows scanning during the first 10 days after the first day of her last menstrual period.
- Patients should be screened at scheduling for problems that require postponement of scanning, such as pregnancy and recent barium, contrast, or nuclear medicine examinations.

The most effective radiation safety practice is a knowledgeable, well-educated, and conscientious DXA technologist. It is essential for DXA technologists to receive instructions from the manufacturer of a specific model of scanner. This might consist of review of DVDs and a 1- or 2-day session with a field applications specialist and review of performed scans. When experience is obtained, a technologist can be certified by the International Society for Clinical Densitometry (ISCD). Another certification is available through the American Registry of Radiologic Technologists (ARRT). Both of these credentials can be obtained by technologists who are educationally prepared and clinically competent. Technologists must obtain continuing education in bone densitometry to meet the qualifications of a current status in this ever-changing field.

TABLE 33-4

World Health Organization classifications of bone density by T score

Classification	Criteria
Normal	BMD or BMC T score of ≥–1
Low bone mass (osteopenia)	BMD or BMC T score between –1 and –2.5
Osteoporosis	BMD or BMC T score of ≤2.5
Severe osteoporosis	BMD or BMC T score of ≤2.5 and ≥1 fragility fractures

Data from Kanis JA: World Health Organization (WHO) Study Group: assessment of fracture risk and its application to screening for postmenopausal osteoporosis: a synopsis of the WHO report, *Osteoporos Int* 4:358, 1994.

TABLE 33-5

Bone densitometry radiation doses compared with other commonly acquired doses

Type of radiation exposure	Effective dose (mSv)
Daily natural background radiation	5-8
Round-trip air flight across the United States	60
Lateral lumbar spine radiograph	700
PA chest radiograph	50
QCT with localizer scan (from scanner offering low kV and mAs; may be 10 times higher for other scanners)	60
DXA scan (range allows for different anatomic sites; Lunar EXPERT-XL may be higher)	1-5
SXA scan	≤1
QUS	0

Data from Kalender WA: Effective dose values in bone mineral measurements by photon absorptiometry and computed tomography, *Osteoporos Int* 2:82, 1992.

PATIENT CARE AND EDUCATION

Typical DXA patients are ambulatory outpatients; however, many are frail and at increased risk for fragility fractures. Patient care and safety requires attention to the following points of courtesy and common sense:

- All areas of the laboratory, including the front entrance, waiting room, and scan room, should be monitored daily and modified for patient safety. The location of floor-level cables in the scan room should be checked.
- The technologist should maintain professionalism at all times by introducing himself or herself and other staff members to the patient and explaining the procedure.
- The technologist needs to remove all external artifacts. Some DXA laboratories have all patients gowned for consistency. It is possible, however, to scan a patient who is wearing loose cotton clothing with no buttons, snaps, or zippers (i.e., "sweats"). If clothing is not removed, the bra must be undone, and all hooks and underwires must be removed from the scan field. Considering that shoes must be removed for proper height measurement, a long-handled shoehorn would be a practical aid.
- The technologist should provide a simple explanation of the expected action of the scan-arm, the proximity of the scan-arm to the patient's face and head, the noise of the motor, and the length of time for the scan. This information may reduce the patient's anxiety.
- The technologist must listen to any concerns the patient may have about the procedure and be ready to answer questions about radiation exposure, the length of the examination, and the reporting protocol used by the laboratory.
- Although the scan tables are not more than 3 ft (about 1 m) in height, a steady footstool with a long handle is recommended. All patients should be assisted on and off the table.
- On completion of the examination, the technologist should ensure the scan arm has returned to the home position, clearing the patient's head. The patient should sit upright for several seconds to regain stability before descending from the scanner.

In some institutions, it is the responsibility of the DXA technologist to provide education to the patient and the family. Topics may include osteoporosis prevention, proper nutrition, calcium supplementation, weight-bearing exercise, and creating a hazard-free living environment. Many technologists give community educational programs, staff in-service seminars, and participate in health fairs.

PATIENT HISTORY

Each bone density laboratory should develop a patient questionnaire customized for the types of patients referred and the needs of the referring and reporting physicians. Before scanning is performed, any information that could postpone or cancel the scan should be identified. The questionnaire should be directed at obtaining information in four basic categories. Sample questions include the following:

1. *Scanning criteria:*
   - Is there a possibility of pregnancy?
   - Is it impossible for you to lie flat on your back for several minutes?
   - Have you had a nuclear medicine, barium, or contrast x-ray examination performed in the last week?
   - Have you had any previous fractures or surgeries in the hip, spine, abdomen, or forearm areas?
   - Do you have any other medical conditions affecting the bones, such as osteoporosis, curvature of the spine, or arthritis?

2. *Patient information:* This includes identifying information, referring physician, current standing height and weight, and medical history including medications.

3. *Insurance information:* Because DXA scans are not universally covered by insurance, it is important to obtain information on the insurance carrier, the need for prior approval, and the information necessary for insurance coding. In 1998, the U.S. Congress passed the Bone Mass Measurement Act (BMMA) dealing with reimbursement for Medicare patients. Central and peripheral technologies are covered. Medicare does not cover screening, so a qualified individual must meet at least one of the following requirements:
   - Estrogen-deficient woman at clinical risk of osteoporosis
   - Individual with hyperparathyroidism
   - Individual receiving long-term glucocorticoid (steroid) therapy
   - Individual with vertebral abnormalities by radiograph
   - Individual being monitored on osteoporosis therapy that has been approved by the U.S. Food and Drug Administration (FDA)

4. *Reporting information:* The type and scope of the report that is provided determines how much information is necessary about the patient's risk factors for, and history of, low bone mass, fragility fractures, and bone diseases.

REPORTING, CONFIDENTIALITY, RECORD KEEPING, AND SCAN STORAGE

When the scan has been completed, the following guidelines should be observed:

- The technologist should end the examination by telling the patient when the scan results will be available to the referring physician. If a patient asks for immediate results, the technologist should explain that it is the ordering physician's responsibility to give the results to the patient after the scan has been interpreted by an educationally prepared and clinically competent DXA clinician.
- DXA scan results are confidential medical records and should be handled according to the institution's rules for such records. Results should not be discussed with other staff members or patients, and printed results, whether on hard copy or a computer screen, should be shielded from inappropriate viewing. As of April 2005, the guidelines of the American Health Insurance Portability and Accountability Act of 1996 (HIPAA) must be integrated in the DXA laboratory. Manufacturers have HIPAA-compliant software upgrades available. Manufacturers use privacy tools or HIPAA-secure tools to ensure patient confidentiality.
- Complete records must be kept for each patient. If a patient returns for *follow-up* scans, the positioning, acquisition parameters, and placement of the ROI must be reproduced as closely as possible to the original scans. The tech-

nologist should keep electronic records with the patient's identifying information and date, the file name, and the archive location of each scan. The electronic record should also identify any special information about why particular scans were or were not performed (e.g., the right hip was scanned because the left hip was fractured, or the forearm was not scanned because of the patient's severe arthritis) and any special procedures done for positioning (e.g., the femur was not fully rotated because of pain) or scan analysis (e.g., the bone edge was manually placed for the radial ultradistal region). The patient questionnaire, log sheet, and complete scan printouts should be kept electronically. All scan archive media must be clearly labeled and accessible.

- The general consensus is that DXA scan results should be kept electronically indefinitely because all serial studies are compared with the baseline.

COMPUTER COMPETENCY

DXA scan acquisition, analysis, and archiving is controlled with a personal computer (PC). DXA technologists must be familiar with the basic PC components and how they work, such as the disk drives and storage media, keyboard, monitor, printer, and mouse. Digital networking allows a scan to be performed at one location and be sent electronically to a remote location for reading or review by an interpreting or referring physician. A technologist must be able to back up, archive, locate, and restore patient scan files. Daily

backup and archival is recommended to preserve patient scan files and data. A third copy of data should be stored offsite to ensure retrieval of patient data and to be able to rebuild databases if there is a computer failure, fire, flood, or theft. Most facilities have access to *picture archiving communications systems (PACs)* where all scans are stored electronically and can be retrieved when needed.

Manufacturers frequently upgrade software versions, and the technologist is responsible for performing this task. Records of upgrades and software installation should be maintained. Current software media should be accessible to service engineers at the time of preventive maintenance and repairs.

Computers consist of software and hardware.* Software consists of programs written in code that instruct the computer how to perform tasks. The DXA manufacturer's software controls many aspects of DXA scanning from starting the scan to calculating and reporting the results. Hardware comprises the physical components for central processing, input, output, and storage.

---

*After the introduction of the computer in medicine, the practice and development of radiologic procedures expanded rapidly. In bone densitometry, the computer assisted in major advancements. Because of space considerations in this edition of *Merrill's Atlas*, the "Computer Fundamentals and Applications in Radiology" chapter has been deleted. For individuals interested in learning more about computer fundamentals, see Volume 3, Chapter 32, of the eighth or ninth edition of this atlas.

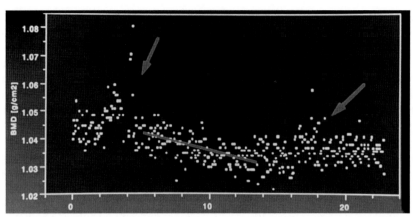

Fig. 33-17 Plot of spine phantom BMD and time (in months). Two *arrows* show abrupt shifts in BMD. *Straight line* shows a slow drift downward in BMD. These indicate changes in scanner calibration.

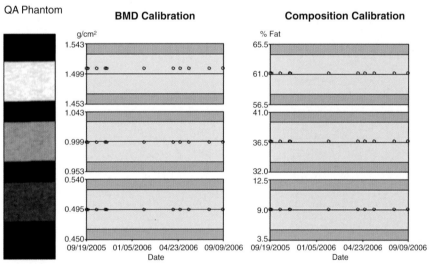

GE Healthcare
Lunar DXA
Madison, WI 53717

QA Phantom Report

08/07/2006
8:56:22 AM

Lunar iDXA
ME+00001
(10.50)

QA Phantom

QA Phantom			QC Tests	
BMD	0.994 g/cm²	Pass	X-ray and Detector Status	Pass
BMC	24.93 g	Pass	Mechanical Tests	Pass
Area	25.09 cm²	Pass	Calibration Status	Pass

Precision

BMD CV	0.00%

System Status: Pass

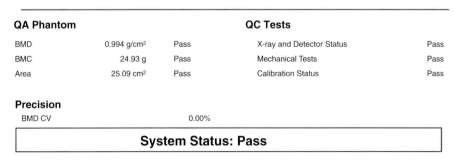

GE Healthcare

Lunar iDXA
ME+00001
(10.50)

Fig. 33-18 GE Lunar quality assurance results printout. The technologist must perform and review the data before performing clinical patient scans.

(Courtesy GE Lunar, Madison, WI.)

DUAL ENERGY X-RAY ABSORPTIOMETRY SCANNER LONGITUDINAL QUALITY CONTROL

Longitudinal quality control procedures are performed in accordance with the manufacturer's recommendation. Manufacturers' instructions in operator manuals must be followed exactly. These procedures have the common goal of ensuring that patients are scanned on properly functioning equipment with stable calibration. Unstable calibration can take the form of abrupt shifts or slow drifts in BMD, as seen on plots of phantom scan results (Fig. 33-17). These problems make the patient's BMD values too high or too low and prohibit a valid comparison between baseline and follow-up scans.

The procedures use either external or internal instruments to track the calibration of the DXA scanner over time. Lunar and Norland systems necessitate scanning an external calibration block to perform a calibration check. The technologist must observe the procedure; he or she should review the report and note whether the system passed all tests of internal parameters (Fig. 33-18). Hologic systems perform an automatic internal calibration check when the system is turned on.

Manufacturers also provide semi-anthropomorphic and aluminum phantoms for tracking calibration over time. Hologic systems require that daily QC be performed before patient scanning (Fig. 33-19).

When not recommended by the manufacturer, the International Society for Clinical Densitometry (ISCD) advises the following procedures. Periodic (at least once per week) phantom scans should be performed for any DXA system as an independent assessment of system calibration. The BMD is plotted, monitored, and checked with statistical and quality control rules. The quality control rule used to check DXA scanners is modified from Shewhart Control Chart rules. Shewhart rules are a classic method of checking that a quality parameter is stable and within acceptable limits of 3 SDs. For DXA, the value of the control limits is modified to *1.5%* of the mean, to provide more uniformity across scanners.

The mean and SD are calculated from the first 25 measurements of the parameter. A graph is created displaying the mean and the control limits 1.5 SDs above and below the mean. The parameter measurements are plotted over time and checked for violation of rules, such as one measurement more than 1.5 SDs from the mean. DXA control charts display the mean as the center line with control limits (1.5% of the mean) above and below. The Hologic software produces this graph automatically (see Fig. 33-15). For other manufacturers, the graph and plotting must be done by hand. The technologist must verify the phantom BMD after any service is performed on the scanner. When the phantom BMD value falls outside the control limits, the scan should be repeated once; if it fails, service should be called and patient scans should be cancelled. If the BMD remains outside the control limits, the manufacturer must be contacted. No patients should be scanned until the equipment has been repaired and is operating within the known values.

Ten phantom scans should be performed and plotted before and after scanner preventive maintenance, repair, relocation, and software or hardware upgrades. This practice is to ensure that the calibration has not been altered and proper adjustments can be made. These phantoms and values should be reviewed before the service engineer leaves the DXA laboratory. Recalibration adjustments should be made before scanning any patients. The technologist is required to oversee this operation.

Inconsistent phantom scanning, analysis, or interpretation of the results may lead to false precision and patient outcomes. The DXA technologist must understand the quality control procedures and follow them consistently. DXA laboratories should have written procedures and documented instructions to ensure consistency among technologists. The technologist is required to maintain service logs and compliance with government inspections, radiation surveys, and regulatory requirements.

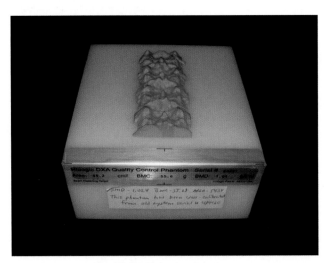

Fig. 33-19 Hologic phantom.

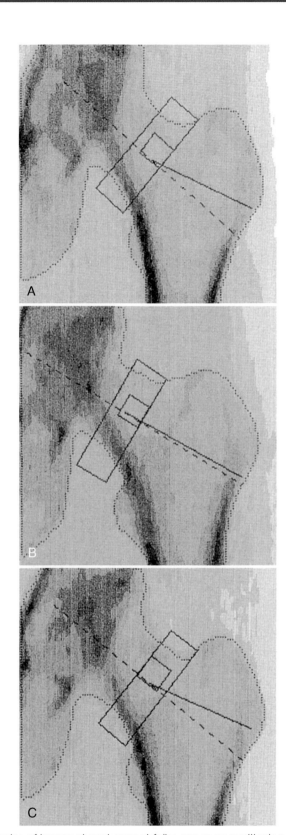

Fig. 33-20 Examples of incorrect and correct follow-up scan positioning. Note difference in BMD between the scans. **A,** Baseline hip scan. **B,** Incorrectly positioned follow-up scan. Size and shape of lesser trochanter and angle of femoral body do not match baseline. **C,** Correctly positioned follow-up scan.

ANATOMY, POSITIONING, AND ANALYSIS

Radiologic technologists receive extensive instruction in anatomy during their radiology training. DXA scanning requires knowledge of DXA specific anatomy. This anatomy relates to positioning the patient properly for scan acquisition. The points presented in this section generally apply to all DXA scanners; however, instruction from the specific manufacturer is required before operating the scanner. The operator's manual that accompanies the equipment is the referred guideline.

Similar to all technologies, DXA has operating limits. Accuracy and precision may be impaired if the bone mass is low, the patient is too thick or thin, the anatomy is abnormal, or there have been significant changes in soft tissue between serial scans. The added value of an experienced DXA technologist is recognition and adaptation to abnormal situations. Any anomaly or protocol variation that may compromise the scan results must be noted by the technologist and taken into consideration by the interpreting physician.

DXA calculations are based on soft tissue and bone. Adequate amounts of soft tissue are essential for valid results.

Serial scans

DXA is a qualitative instrument used to monitor BMD change over time. True comparison of BMD results requires that serial scans be performed on the same scanner that was used for the baseline scans.

Scan results are more precise with less intervention from the technologist and the DXA equipment, reflecting a true biologic change. It is imperative that the patient positioning be exactly the same for baseline and serial scans. The same scan settings (e.g., field size, mode, or speed and current) and ROI should be placed identically on the images. These steps ensure that scan results are comparable over time. When recommended, the software's *compare feature or copy* should be used. The baseline printouts should be available at the time of the patient's appointment. Documentation of any procedures out of the range of the laboratory's standard operating procedure needs to be available when performing serial scans.

Fig. 33-20 shows the comparison of a patient's hip scans from 1995 (see

Fig. 33-20, *A*) and 2001 and is an example of why follow-up positioning must match baseline if the BMD measurements are to be compared. The first follow-up scan (see Fig. 33-20, *B*) did not reproduce the baseline positioning. The rotation of the femoral neck was different, as indicated by the larger lesser trochanter and the femoral shaft being more abducted, and resulted in the midline being placed differently by the software and a different angle for the neck ROI. The scan was repeated (see Fig. 33-20, *C*) to reproduce the baseline positioning correctly. The difference in total hip BMD between scans *A* and *B* is −13% compared with a difference of −10% between scans *A* and *C*.

PA lumbar spine

Spine scans are most appropriate for predicting vertebral fracture risk. Underestimation of fracture risk occurs in patients older than 65 years who present with degenerative changes that can artificially elevate spinal BMD. The following points can help with positioning patients for posteroanterior (PA) lumbar spine DXA scans, analyzing the scan results, and evaluating the validity of the scans:

1. Degenerative changes in the spine, such as *osteophytosis,* overlying calcification, compression fractures (Fig. 33-21), or scoliosis greater than 15 degrees (Fig. 33-22), can falsely elevate the BMD. Artifacts in the vertebral bodies or very dense artifacts in the soft tissue may also affect the BMD, depending on the model of the scanner and version of the software. The interpreting physician should develop policies and protocols for the technologist in these circumstances (e.g., do not include the spine but include another site, such as forearm).

2. The lumbar spine is centered in the scan field. In a patient with scoliosis, L5 may need to be off center so that adequate and relatively equal amounts of soft tissue are on either side of the spine throughout the scan.

3. Some visualization of iliac crests should be acquired in the scan region. This ensures the inclusion of all of L4. The iliac crest is an excellent landmark for consistent placement of the intervertebral markers at baseline and follow-up scanning.

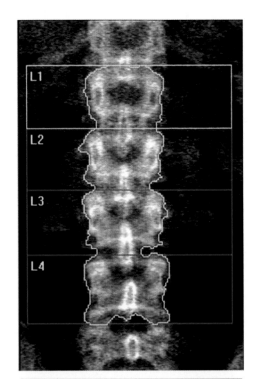

Region	Area(cm²)	BMC(g)	BMD(g/cm²)
L1	13.56	10.07	0.743
L2	13.75	11.63	0.846
L3	14.56	11.83	0.812
L4	16.44	14.34	0.872
TOTAL	58.31	47.87	0.821

A

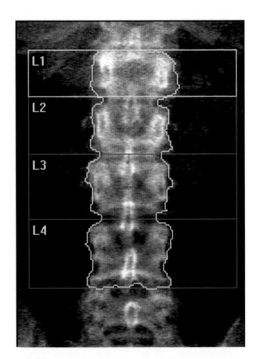

Region	Area(cm²)	BMC(g)	BMD(g/cm²)
L1	11.45	10.88	0.951
L2	12.97	11.72	0.903
L3	14.95	11.80	0.789
L4	16.50	14.35	0.870
TOTAL	55.87	48.75	0.873

B

Fig. 33-21 Use of Hologic compare feature indicates that L1 bone map and ROI from baseline scan (**A**) no longer fit the follow-up scan (**B**) because of a compression fracture of L1. Both scans should be analyzed to exclude L1 before comparing total BMD. Note differences in BMD and area measurements.

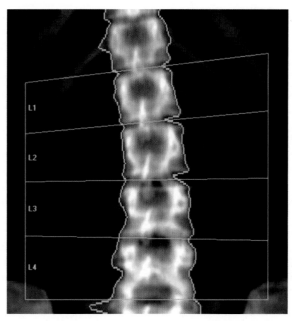

Fig. 33-22 DXA PA spine scan with scoliosis and scoliosis analysis technique.

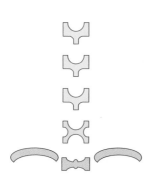

Fig. 33-23 Characteristic shapes of L1-5 and their relationship to the iliac crests as seen on DXA PA spine scan.

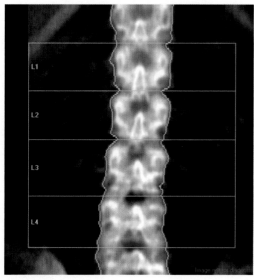

Fig. 33-24 Six lumbar vertebrae. Vertebral labeling is done from the bottom to the top according to the shape of the vertebrae.

4. The PA spine scan image displays the posterior vertebral elements, which have unique characteristic shapes, contrast to a general lumbar radiograph. These shapes can be used to differentiate placement of the intervertebral markers. When degenerative disease has obscured the intervertebral spaces, these shapes can aid in determining proper labeling of the vertebral levels. L1, L2, and L3 have a U shape; L4 has an H or X shape and appears to have "feet"; and L5 looks like a sideways I or "dog bone" (Fig. 33-23). Another aid is that L3 typically has the widest transverse processes. L1, L2, and L3 are approximately the same height. L4 is a bit taller than the others, whereas L5 is the shortest in height. The iliac crest usually lies at the level of L4-5 intervertebral space.

5. A small percentage of patients appear to have four or six lumbar vertebrae rather than five, which is most commonly seen. The vertebrae can be labeled by locating L5 and L4 on the basis of their characteristic shapes and then counting upward (Fig. 33-24). The procedure of counting from the bottom superiorly biases toward a higher BMD and avoids including T12 without a rib, which significantly lowers the BMD. This procedure ensures a conservative diagnosis of low BMD.

6. Do not adjust the bone edges or angle or move the intervertebral markers unless absolutely necessary. These techniques should be performed in a fashion that is easy to reproduce for serial scans. Variations to protocol should be documented.

7. Check that the patient is lying straight by observing from the head or foot end of the table. If a patient is lying straight on the table but the spine is not straight on the scan, do not attempt to twist the patient to get the image straight. This unusual positioning would not be reproducible at follow-up. Make a note in the record that the patient was positioned straight on the table.

8. The purpose of the leg-positioning block is to reduce the lordotic curve, open up the intervertebral spaces, and reduce the part-image distance. Consistency in using the same height of the leg-positioning block when a patient returns for serial scans is important. Document the block height.

9. A checklist for a good PA spine scan (see Fig. 33-21, *A*) includes the following:
   - The spine is straight and centered in the scan field. Patients with scoliosis should have equal amounts of soft tissue on either side of the spine if possible.
   - The scan contains a portion of the iliac crest and half of T12; the last set of ribs is shown, when applicable.
   - The entire scan field is free of external artifacts.
   - The intervertebral markers are properly placed.
   - The vertebral levels are properly labeled.
   - The bone edges are correct.

Proximal femur

The hip scan is perhaps the most important because it is the best predictor of future hip fracture, which is the most devastating of the fragility fractures. Compared with the spine scan, the hip scan is more difficult to perform properly and precisely because of variations in anatomy and the small ROI. The following points can help in positioning patients for hip DXA scans, analyzing the results, and evaluating the validity of the scans:

1. With the patient in a supine position, rotate the entire leg 15 to 25 degrees internally to place the femoral neck parallel with the tabletop and perpendicular to the x-ray beam. Successful rotation is achieved when the lesser trochanter is diminished in size and only slightly visible (or not visible). A large, pointed lesser trochanter may indicate too little rotation (see Fig. 33-20, *B,* and *C*). Patient anatomy is not always as shown in textbooks, however. Patients can have a prominent lesser trochanter, and proper rotation is achieved when the femoral neck region is free of overlapping ischium, and appropriate pelvis separation is visualized. This positioning allows proper placement of the femoral neck ROI. All scanners come with positioning aids that should be used according to the manufacturer's instructions.

2. The shaft of the femur must be straight and parallel to the long axis of the table.

3. A few patients have little or no space between the ischium and femoral neck. In some cases, part of the ischium lies under the femoral neck, elevating the BMC and falsely elevating the femoral neck BMD (Fig. 33-25). This could be caused by the ischium (pelvis) being rotated. The patient should be removed from the table and repositioned. If the problem persists, slightly adjust the leg until the ischium and neck are separated. Variations in positioning should be noted and reproduced at the time of the serial scan.

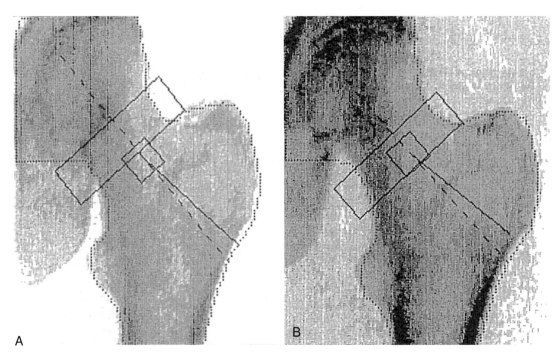

A   B

Fig. 33-25 A, Despite use of the software tool to "cut out the ischium," bone from the ischium underlies the femoral neck ROI. The BMC is increased, increasing the BMD. **B,** The same patient was positioned for a follow-up scan 1 year later. The pelvis is no longer rotated, as indicated by the narrower width of the ischium. Adequate space exists between the neck and ischium, and there is no ischium beneath the neck ROI. This is an example of poor pelvis positioning in **A;** the patient must be lying flat on the pelvis as in **B.** These two scans *cannot* be compared for rate of bone loss. The scan in **B** should be considered a new baseline and compared with a properly performed follow-up scan in the future.

4. To compare proximal femur BMD over time, the positioning must be exactly reproduced, and the angle of the neck box ROI must be the same (see Fig. 33-20). Check these points on the baseline and serial scan images:
   - The lesser trochanter must be the same size and shape. If not, change the hip rotation. More rotation would make the lesser trochanter appear smaller.
   - The femoral shaft must be abducted the same amount. Adjust the abduction or adduction accordingly.
   - The neck box ROI is automatically placed perpendicular to the midline, so the midline must be at the same angle in each scan. If it is not, reposition as required. If positioning is not the problem, proper software adjustments must be made according to the manufacturer's guidelines.
5. Manufacturers provide dual-hip software that scans both hips without repositioning. Scoliosis, diseases that cause unilateral weakness (e.g., polio, stroke), or unilateral osteoarthritis of the hip may cause left-right differences, however. If arthritis is present, the less affected hip should be scanned because arthritis can cause increased density in the medial hip and shortening of the femoral neck (Fig. 33-26). In cases of unilateral disease, scan the less affected hip. A fractured hip with orthopedic hardware should not be scanned. The DXA diagnosis should always be based on the lowest BMD value.
6. The limits of the technology are taxed by patients who are very thin or thick or have very low bone mass. These problems are revealed by poor bone edge detection, a mottled appearance of the image, or both. Some images show the bone edges, and it is obvious when the proper edge cannot be detected. For images that do not show the bone edges, the area values must be checked and compared. The operator's manual may not adequately cover these problems. The technologist is responsible for recognizing problems and querying the manufacturer's applica-

tions department about the best ways to handle such difficulties. If a patient is deemed unsuitable for a DXA hip scan, a physician can suggest alternative scans using DXA or other technologies. Newer software and improved technologies are minimizing the incidence of these situations.
7. A basic checklist for a good DXA hip scan (see Fig. 33-20, *A*) includes the following:
   - The lesser trochanter is small or barely visible.
   - The midline of the femoral shaft is parallel to the lateral edge of the scan.
   - Adequate space is present between the ischium and femoral neck.
   - The midline through the femoral neck is reasonably placed, resulting in a reasonable angle for the femoral neck box.
   - The proximal, distal, and lateral edges of the scan field are properly located.
   - No air is present in the scan field on GE Lunar scans.

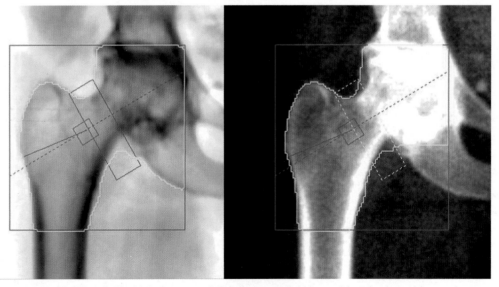

Fig. 33-26 Hip arthritis. Note increased density in medial hip and foreshortened femoral neck. The technologist may be required to intervene in this situation. Notation of difficulty with positioning and known arthritis should be mentioned on the patient's history form.

Forearm

Two important ROIs are present on the DXA forearm scan: the ultradistal region, which is the site of the common Colles fracture, and the one-third (33%) region, which measures an area that is primarily cortical bone near the mid-forearm (see Table 33-1). Although the ulna is used for forearm length measurement and available for analysis, only the one-third (33%) region of the radius is reported. The following guidelines can aid in positioning, acquisition, and analysis of forearm DXA scans and evaluating the validity of the scans:

1. The nondominant forearm is scanned because it is expected to have slightly lower BMD than the dominant arm. A forearm should not be scanned in patients with a history of wrist fracture, internal hardware, or severe deformity resulting from arthritis. If both forearms are unsuitable for scanning, other anatomic sites should be considered.

2. The same chair should be used for all patients to ensure consistency over time. The chair should have a back but no wheels or arms. Selection of the chairs varies from manufacturer to manufacturer.

3. At the time of the baseline scan, the forearm should be measured according to the manufacturer's instructions. The ulna is measured from the ulnar styloid to the olecranon process. The distal one third of this measurement is used to place the one-third, or 33%, ROI. One manufacturer estimates the forearm length based on the height. The directions for determining the starting and ending locations of the scan must be followed exactly (Fig. 33-27, A).

4. The forearm must be straight and centered in the scan field (see Fig. 33-27, A). Correct use of the appropriate positioning aids must be applied. For Hologic models, the forearm scan requires adequate amounts of air in the scan field. Soft tissue must surround the ulna and radius, and several lines of air must be present on the ulnar side. If the forearm is wide, the scan must be manually set for a wider scan region so that adequate air is included.

5. Motion is a common problem in forearm scan acquisition (see Fig. 33-27, A). The patient should be in a comfortable position so that the arm does not move during the scan. The hand and proximal forearm can be secured with straps or tape placed outside the scan field. Avoid unnecessary conversation during the scan to minimize movement.

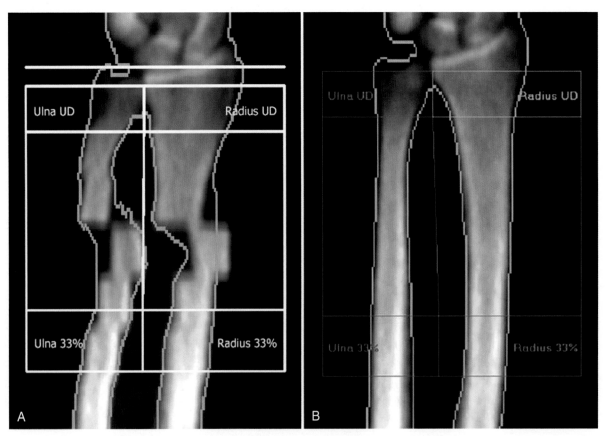

Fig. 33-27 DXA forearm scans. **A,** DXA forearm scan shows several positioning and acquisition mistakes: The forearm is not straight or centered in the scan field, and motion has occurred in the radius and ulna. **B,** Scan shows good patient positioning, scan acquisition, and scan analysis.

6. The placement of the ultradistal ROI should be just below the radial end plate. This placement is easy to reproduce on serial scans. The ultradistal ROI is subject to low BMD, which could create bone edge detection problems. The bone edge should be adjusted if necessary. Baseline and serial scan bone edges must match for proper analysis, comparison, and report of percent change over time.

7. A basic checklist for a good DXA forearm scan (Fig. 33-27, *B*) includes the following:
   - The forearm is straight and centered in the scan field.
   - Adequate amounts of soft tissue and air are included.
   - No motion is present.
   - The proximal and distal ends of the scan field are properly placed.
   - Bone edges are properly and consistently placed.
   - No artifacts are present in the scan field.

Other Bone Densitometry Techniques

CENTRAL (OR AXIAL) SKELETAL MEASUREMENTS

QCT is an established method using cross-sectional CT images from commercial scanners equipped with QCT software and a bone mineral reference standard. QCT has the unique ability to provide separate BMD measurements of trabecular and cortical bone and true volumetric density measurements in grams per cubic centimeter (g/cm^3). QCT of the spine is used to measure the trabecular bone within the vertebral bodies to estimate vertebral fracture risk and age-related bone loss; it is also used for follow-up of osteoporosis and other metabolic bone diseases and their therapies (Fig. 33-28). Other current uses of QCT involve measuring BMD at the hip and producing high-resolution three-dimensional images to analyze trabecular bone architecture.

Lateral lumbar spine DXA scans can be performed with the patient in the decubitus lateral position using fan beam technology. Decubitus lateral scans are obtained with fixed-arm scanners. Lateral spine DXA allows partial removal of the outer cortical bone and gives a truer measurement of the inner trabecular bone, which experiences earlier bone loss and is more responsive to therapy (see Fig. 33-10). Lateral spine DXA is often confounded, however, by superimposition of the ribs and iliac crest with the vertebral bodies and has poorer precision than PA spine DXA. Lateral DXA is being more widely used in clinical practice for early detection of vertebral fractures and abdominal aortic calcifications.

The term *vertebral fracture assessment (VFA)* encompasses looking at the spine "morphometrically" in the lateral projection, which means visualizing the shapes of the vertebral bodies of the lumbar and thoracic spine to determine if there has been some deformity with resultant

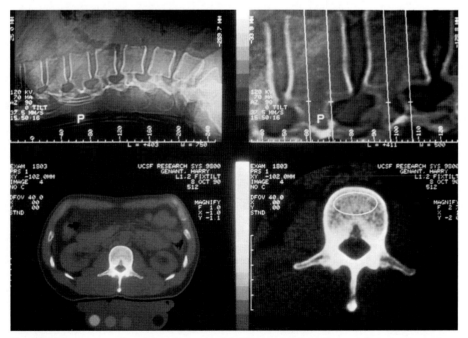

Fig. 33-28 Examples of various elements of QCT examination. *Upper left,* Lateral scout image of lumbar spine. *Upper right,* Localizer lines for midvertebral slices through L1 and L2. *Lower left,* CT slice showing calibration phantom below the patient. *Lower right,* Elliptic ROI positioned in the trabecular bone of the vertebral body.

compression of the vertebral bodies. Dual energy vertebral assessment (DVA), lateral vertebral assessment (LVA), instant vertebral analysis (IVA), and radiologic vertebral assessment (RVA) are synonymous for this process. The manufacturers of bone densitometers have devised their own way of either enhancing the image or improving the scan acquisition and analysis. Images are obtained in dual energy acquisition and the single energy method. Both methods are comparable.

In contrast to traditional lateral spine x-rays, VFA has the capability of visualizing the lumbar and the thoracic spine as one continuous image. This capability aids the interpreting physician in identifying the vertebral level where abnormalities are present. PA views can also be incorporated into a VFA study. For an accurate representation of the vertebral bodies, the patient's spine must be as straight as possible.

The PA view can help identify artifacts and deformities, such as scoliosis. Scoliosis is the one condition that can cause the greatest challenge in VFA and possibly make a study "unreadable." VFA also exposes the patient to about $\frac{1}{100}$ the radiation dose of just a single lateral x-ray image. VFA is an adjunct to DXA scanning in cases when a patient might not have been x-rayed for vertebral fracture beforehand. General spine x-ray is still the gold standard for visualizing abnormalities in the spine.

VFA uses single energy x-ray absorptiometry (for image only) or DXA (for image and BMD) lateral scans of the thoracic and lumbar spines from the level of about T4 to L5 (Fig. 33-29). The images are used to determine abnormalities in vertebral shape that may indicate vertebral fragility fractures, which are a strong risk factor for future vertebral fractures. The upper right corner of Fig. 33-29 shows the Genant grading system. The three columns on the right show the types of fracture, and the rows show the grades of severity. Seeing a severe fracture is easy, and seeing a moderate fracture is relatively easy, but it is difficult to determine if a mild deformity is normal for the patient or the beginning of a problem. VFA should be interpreted by a trained physician who is viewing the images on the scan monitor (Fig. 33-30).

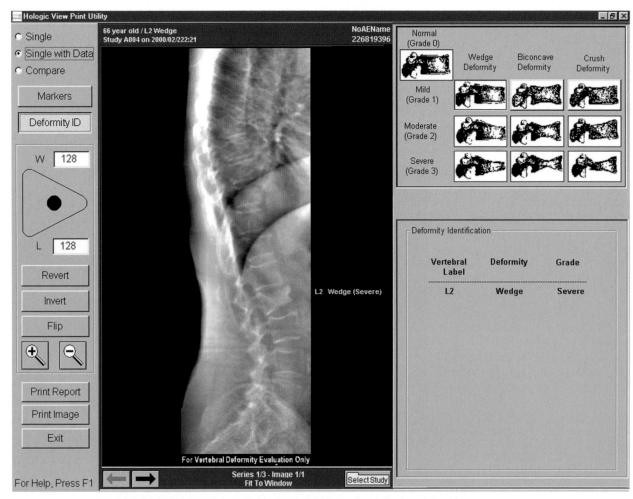

Fig. 33-29 Morphometric x-ray absorptiometry scan to detect vertebral shape abnormalities. Genant grading system is in the *upper right corner.*

(Courtesy Hologic, Inc, Bedford, MA.)

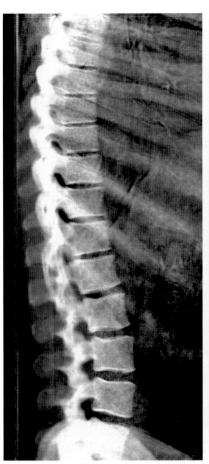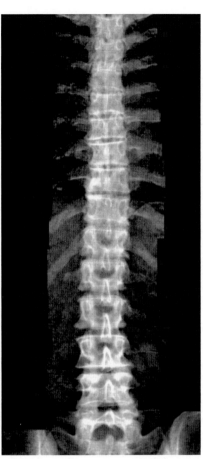

Fig. 33-30 Dual VFA.

Total body and body composition

Whole-body DXA measures bone mass (i.e., area, BMC, BMD) and *body composition* for the total body and subregions of the body (e.g., arms, legs, trunk). Body composition can be measured as fat and fat-free mass (with or without BMC) in grams or percent body fat (Fig. 33-31). Careful positioning is required to separate the bones of the forearm and lower leg. Obese patients present a problem when not all of the body fits in the scan field. The ROI must be carefully placed according to the manufacturer's instructions. Having internal or external artifacts that cannot be removed is not unusual; the effect of such artifacts depends on size, density, and location. Hip joint replacement hardware would have more effect than a woman's thin wedding band. Each DXA laboratory should have written procedures so that all patients are scanned and analyzed consistently. All deviations from normal and artifacts should be noted for the interpreting physician. Whole-body DXA data are useful for studying energy expenditure, energy stores, protein mass, skeletal mineral status, and relative hydration. These measurements have been used in research studies and clinical trials of osteoporosis therapies, obesity and weight change, fat and lean distribution, and diabetes. Clinically, whole-body scans are used routinely in pediatrics and for body fat analysis in athletes and patients with underweight disorders (e.g., anorexia nervosa).

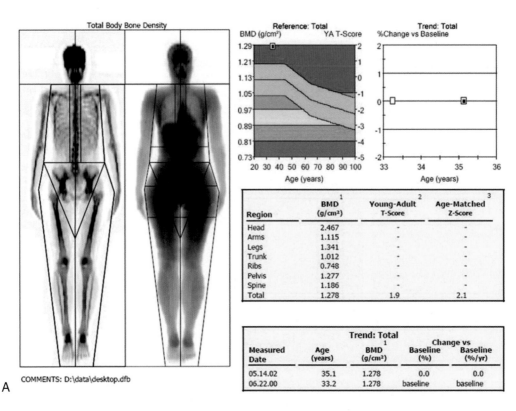

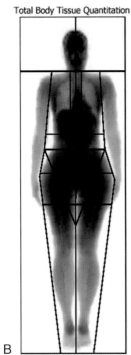

Total Body Bone Density

COMMENTS: D:\data\desktop.dfb

A

Region	BMD[1] (g/cm²)	Young-Adult[2] T-Score	Age-Matched[3] Z-Score
Head	2.467	-	
Arms	1.115	-	-
Legs	1.341	-	-
Trunk	1.012	-	-
Ribs	0.748	-	-
Pelvis	1.277	-	-
Spine	1.186	-	-
Total	1.278	1.9	2.1

Trend: Total

Measured Date	Age (years)	BMD[1] (g/cm²)	Change vs Baseline (%)	Change vs Baseline (%/yr)
05.14.02	35.1	1.278	0.0	0.0
06.22.00	33.2	1.278	baseline	baseline

Total Body Tissue Quantitation

Trend: Total

Measured Date	Age (years)	Tissue (%Fat)	Centile[2,3]	T.Mass (kg)	Region (%Fat)	Tissue (g)	Fat (g)	Lean (g)	BMC (g)	Fat Free (g)
05.14.02	35.1	32.3	58	62.9	30.8	59,950	19,346	40,603	2,956	43,559
06.22.00	33.2	32.5	61	63.2	31.0	60,256	19,560	40,697	2,922	43,618

Trend: Fat Distribution

Measured Date	Age (years)	Android (%Fat)	Gynoid (%Fat)	A/G Ratio	Total Body (%Fat)
05.14.02	35.1	24.7	44.5	0.55	32.3
06.22.00	33.2	26.3	45.0	0.58	32.5

B

Fig. 33-31 A, Hologic DXA whole-body scan with printout of total body composition results. **B,** Percent body fat (% Fat) is reported.

SKELETAL HEALTH ASSESSMENT IN CHILDREN FROM INFANCY TO ADOLESCENCE

Fracture prediction and definition of osteoporosis

- Evaluation of bone health should identify children and adolescents who may benefit from interventions to decrease their elevated risk of a clinically significant fracture.
- The finding of one or more vertebral compression (crush) fractures is indicative of osteoporosis, in the absence of local disease or high-energy trauma. In such children and adolescents, measuring BMD adds to the overall assessment of bone health.
- The diagnosis of osteoporosis in children and adolescents should not be made on the basis of densitometric criteria alone.
- In the absence of vertebral compression (crush) fractures, the diagnosis of osteoporosis is indicated by the presence of both a clinically significant fracture history and BMD Z-score ≤−2.0. A clinically significant fracture history is one or more of the following: (1) two or more long bone fractures by age 10 years; (2) three or more long bone fractures at any age up to age 19 years. A BMC/BMD Z-score >−2.0 does not preclude the possibility of skeletal fragility and increased fracture risk.

DXA assessment in children and adolescents with disease that may affect the skeleton

- DXA measurement is part of a comprehensive skeletal health assessment in patients with increased risk of fracture.
- In patients with primary bone disease, or at risk for a secondary bone disease, a DXA should be performed when the patient may benefit from interventions to decrease their elevated risk of a clinically significant fracture, and the DXA results will influence that management.
- DXA should not be performed if safe and appropriate positioning of the child cannot be ensured.

QCT in children and adolescents

There is no preferred method for QCT for clinical application in children and adolescents. QCT, pQCT, and HR-pQCT are primarily research techniques used to characterize bone deficits in children. They can be used clinically in children when appropriate reference data and expertise are available. It is imperative that QCT protocols in children using general CT scanners use appropriate exposure factors, calibration phantoms, and software to optimize results and minimize radiation exposure.

Densitometry in infants and young children

DXA is an appropriate method for clinical densitometry of infants and young children. DXA lumbar spine measurements are feasible and can provide reproducible measures of BMC and aBMD for infants and young children 0-5 years of age. DXA whole body measurements are feasible and can provide reproducible measures of BMC and aBMD for children 3 years or older. DXA whole body BMC measurements for children under 3 years of age are of limited clinical utility due to feasibility and lack of normative data. Areal BMD should not be utilized routinely due to difficulty in appropriate positioning. Forearm and femur measurements are technically feasible in infants and young children, but there is insufficient information regarding methodology, reproducibility, and reference data for these measurements sites to be clinically useful at this time. In infants and children below 5 years of age, the impact of growth delay on the interpretation of the DXA results should be considered, but it is not currently quantifiable (Fig. 33-32) (ISCD 2013 Position Statements).

DXA interpretation and reporting in children and adolescents

- DXA is the preferred method for assessing BMC and areal BMD.

- The posterior-anterior (PA) spine and total body less head (TBLH) are the preferred skeletal sites for performing BMC and areal BMD measurements in most pediatric subjects. Other sites may be useful depending on the clinical need.
- Soft tissue measures in conjunction with whole body scans may be helpful in evaluating patients with chronic conditions associated with malnutrition or with muscular and skeletal deficits.
- The hip is not a preferred measurement site in growing children due to variability in skeletal development.
- If a follow-up DXA scan is indicated, the minimum interval between scans is 6 to 12 months.
- In children with short stature or growth delay, spine and TBLH BMC and areal BMD results should be adjusted. For the spine, adjust using either BMAD or the height Z-score. For TBLH, adjust using the height Z-score.
- An appropriate reference data set must include a sample of healthy representatives of the general population sufficiently large to capture variability in bone measures that takes into consideration gender, age, and race/ethnicity.
- When upgrading densitometer instrumentation or software, it is essential to use reference data valid for the hardware and software technological updates.
- Baseline DXA reports should contain the following information:
  - DXA manufacturer, model, and software version
  - Referring physician
  - Patient age, gender, race-ethnicity, weight, and height

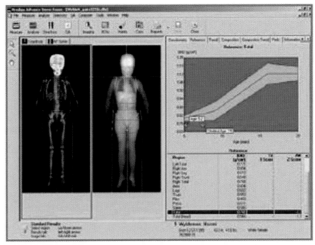

Fig. 33-32 Pediatric BMD and soft tissue assessment.

- Relevant medical history including previous fractures
- Indication for study
- Tanner Stage or Bone age results, if available
- Technical quality
- BMC and areal BMD
- BMC and/or areal BMD Z-score
- Source of reference data for Z-score calculation
- Adjustments made for growth and interpretation
- Recommendations for the necessity and timing of the next DXA study are optional
- Serial DXA reports should include the same information as for baseline testing. Additionally, indications for follow-up scan, technical comparability of studies, changes in height and weight, and changes in BMC and areal BMD Z-scores should be reported.
- Terminology
  - T-scores should not appear in pediatric DXA reports.
  - The term "osteopenia" should not appear in pediatric DXA reports.
  - The term "osteoporosis" should not appear in pediatric DXA reports without a clinically significant fracture history.
  - "Low bone mineral mass or bone mineral density" is the preferred term for pediatric DXA reports when BMC or areal BMD Z-scores are less than or equal to −2.0 SD.

(ISCD 2013 Position Statements)

PERIPHERAL SKELETAL MEASUREMENTS

Peripheral bone density measurements include scans at the hand, forearm, heel, and tibia. Other skeletal sites are being investigated. The scanners are smaller (some are portable), making the scans more available to the public and less expensive than conventional DXA. Peripheral measurements can predict *overall risk of fragility fracture* to the same degree as measurements at central skeletal sites but are not generally accepted for following skeletal response to therapy.

Radiographic absorptiometry is a modern adaptation of the early bone density technique. Digital radiographic absorptiometry uses a hand radiograph that is scanned (digitized) into a computer (Fig. 33-33, *A*). ROI are placed on the digital image of the metacarpals, and estimated BMD is reported (Fig. 33-33, *B*).

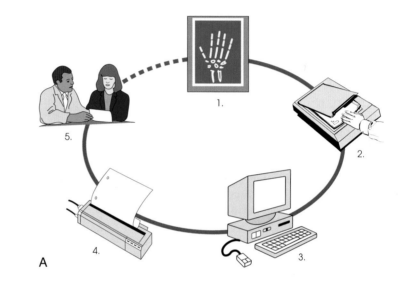

A

Selected Measurement

Date of recording	1/28/01
Est. BMD	0.480 g/cm²
T-Score	-2.18
Z-Score	-2.51
T-Score (% of H.Y.A)	82
Z-Score (%)	81
Porosity (1-19)	8.2

B

Fig. 33-33 Pronosco X-posure System for digital BMD estimates. **A,** Five steps of acquiring and digitizing a standard hand x-ray, keying in patient data, receiving a printout, and discussing results with the patient. **B,** Partial report showing automatically placed ROI on the metacarpals, estimated BMD, T score and Z score, and a unique porosity measurement.

(Courtesy Pronosco A/S, Vedbaek, Denmark.)

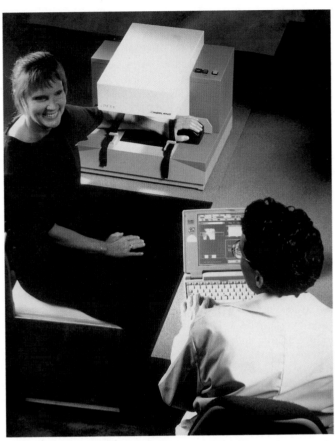

Fig. 33-34 Norland model peripheral DXA performs peripheral DXA bone mineral analysis of the wrist.

(Courtesy Norland/Swissray, Ft. Atkinson, WI.)

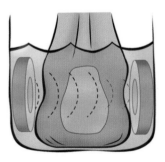

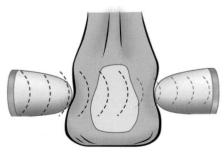

Fig. 33-35 QUS of the heel uses either water as a coupling mechanism (*top*) or a dry system using a gel on the transducers (*bottom*).

(Courtesy GE Lunar, Madison, WI.)

Single energy x-ray absorptiometry, peripheral DXA, and peripheral QCT are adaptations of DXA or QCT for measuring the thinner, easier to penetrate, peripheral skeletal sites. Most scanners measure the wrist (Fig. 33-34) or the heel.

With *QUS* of the heel, ultrasound waves are transmitted laterally through the calcaneus using water, gel, or alcohol (dry system) as a coupling medium (Fig. 33-35). Attenuation increases as the velocity of the ultrasound waves increases, and normal bone attenuates more than osteoporotic bone. These properties of bone and ultrasound signals permit the assessment of the QUS parameters of broadband ultrasound attenuation (BUA) and speed of sound (SOS). BUA, SOS, and proprietary combinations of the two (e.g., stiffness) characterize the mechanical properties of bone relating to elasticity, strength, and consequently fracture risk. QUS measurements at the heel have been found to be good predictors of spine fractures in elderly adults when degenerative disease compromises the DXA spine scan. Other measurement sites, some of which are under investigation, include the finger, tibia, iliac crest, vertebral arch and spinous processes, and femoral neck and greater trochanter.

FRACTURE RISK MODELS

The WHO has developed the *FRAX* tool to evaluate the fracture risk of patients. It is based on individual patient models that integrate the risks associated with clinical risk factors and BMD at the femoral neck. The FRAX algorithm gives the 10-year probability of fracture. The FRAX tool and other fracture risk models may assist physicians in making decisions about who to treat, especially patients with low bone mass. Fracture prediction models should be used judiciously in managing individual patients (www.shef.ac.uf/FRAX).

Conclusion

The main purpose of bone densitometry is to assist the diagnosis of osteoporosis by detecting low bone mass before fractures occur. Osteoporosis is a preventable and treatable disease. Patients concerned about their risk of this disease should consult their physicians for a complete evaluation.

DXA scans of the hip and spine are the most widely performed techniques, but simpler, less expensive peripheral scans of the extremities are also available. Radiographers using bone densitometry equipment must be properly trained in scanner quality control, patient scan positioning, acquisition, and analysis. This training ensures accurate and precise bone density results.

Knowledge of current treatments and expected changes is important for complete technical evaluation of the scan results. History taking and data input are valuable tools for completion of this examination. Technologists are frontline educators to patients, and knowledge in the field is ever changing. The technologist must keep informed about the treatment options and their effects on bone density.

Quality assurance is a key factor in accurate and precise DXA acquisition and analysis. Technology changes frequently, so it is important for the technologist to understand the changes within the industry. The technologist must be able to oversee these applications to maintain and update equipment properly.

Definition of Terms

anthropomorphic Simulating human form.

ALARA (as low as reasonably achievable) achievable Principle of reducing patient radiation exposure and dose to lowest reasonable amounts.

areal technique See *projectional technique.*

array-beam collimation Dual energy x-ray absorptiometry system that uses a narrow "slit" x-ray collimator and a multi-element detector. The motion is in one direction only, which greatly reduces scan time and permits supine lateral spine scans. It introduces a slight geometric distortion at the outer edges, which necessitates careful centering of the object of interest.

biochemical markers Laboratory tests on blood and urine to detect levels of bone formation or resorption.

body composition Results from whole-body scans obtained by dual energy x-ray absorptiometry; reported as lean mass in grams, percent body fat, and bone mineral density of the total body and selected regions of interest.

bone densitometry Art and science of measuring bone mineral content and density of specific anatomic sites or the whole body.

bone mass General term for amount of mineral in a bone.

bone mineral content (BMC) Measure of bone mineral in the total area of a region of interest.

bone mineral density (BMD) Measure of bone mineral per unit area of a region of interest.

bone remodeling Process of bone resorption by osteoclasts, followed by bone formation by osteoblasts. The relative rates of resorption and formation determine whether bone mass increases, remains stable, or decreases.

celiac disease Disease characterized by hypersensitivity to gluten (wheat protein).

compare feature Software feature of dual energy x-ray absorptiometry that replicates the size and placement of regions of interest from the reference scan to the follow-up scan.

cortical bone Dense, compact outer shell of all bones and the shafts of the long bones; supports weight, resists bending and twisting, and accounts for about 80% of the skeletal mass.

cross-calibration Cross-calibration of numbers is needed to calculate the average BMD relationship and least significant change between the initial machine and new machine of a DXA facility. It is not possible to quantitatively compare BMD or to calculate LSC between facilities without cross-calibration.

discordance Patient may have T score indicating osteoporosis at one anatomic site but not at another site or by one modality but not by another.

dual energy x-ray absorptiometry (DXA) Bone density measurement technique using an x-ray source separated into two energies. It has good accuracy and precision and can scan essentially any anatomic site, making it the most versatile of the bone density techniques.

dual photon absorptiometry (DPA) Obsolete method of measuring bone density at the hip or spine using a radioisotope source that produces two sources of photons; replaced by dual energy x-ray absorptiometry.

fragility fractures Nontraumatic fractures resulting from low bone mass, usually at the hip, spinal vertebrae, wrist, proximal humerus, or ribs.

FRAX Fracture risk assessment tool developed by the World Health Organization.

HIPAA The American Health Insurance Portability and Accountability Act of 1996 (HIPAA) is a set of rules to be followed by health plans, physicians, hospitals, and other health care providers. HIPAA took effect on April 14, 2003. In the health care and medical profession, the great challenge that HIPAA has created is the assurance that all patient account handling, billing, and medical records are HIPAA compliant.

hyperparathyroidism Disease caused by excessive secretion of parathyroid hormone (PTH) from one or more parathyroid glands, resulting in excessive calcium in the blood; affects cortical bone more than trabecular bone.

kyphosis Exaggerated outward curvature of the thoracic spine, also called *dowager's hump.*

least significant change (LSC) Amount of change in bone density needed to be statistically confident that a real change has occurred.

longitudinal quality control Manufacturer-defined procedures performed on a regular basis to ensure that patients are scanned on properly functioning equipment with stable calibration. Scanning must be postponed until identified problems are corrected.

mean Statistic commonly called the *average;* sum of the data values divided by the number of data values.

morphometric x-ray absorptiometry (MXA) Lateral scans of the thoracic and lumbar spine using single energy or dual energy x-ray absorptiometry to determine vertebral abnormalities or fractures from the shapes of the vertebrae.

osteoblasts Bone-building cells that fill the pits left by resorption with new bone.

osteoclasts Bone-destroying cells that break down and remove old bone, leaving pits.

osteomalacia Bone disorder characterized by variable amounts of uncalcified osteoid matrix.

osteopenia/low bone mass Reduction in bone mass, putting a person at increased risk of developing osteoporosis. By World Health Organization criteria, it is a bone mineral density or bone mineral content T score between −1 and −2.5. *Low bone mass* or *low bone density* is the preferred term.

osteophytosis Form of degenerative joint disease resulting from mechanical stress that increases measured spinal bone mineral density.

osteoporosis Systemic skeletal disease characterized by low bone mass and deterioration of bone structure, resulting in decreased mechanical competence of bone and an increase in susceptibility to fracture. By World Health Organization criteria, it is a bone mineral density or bone mineral content T score of less than −2.5.

overall risk of fragility fracture Risk of sustaining an unspecified fragility fracture. The risk for hip fracture specifically is best measured at the hip.

peak bone mass Maximum bone mass, usually achieved between 20 and 30 years of age. Population mean peak bone mass is used as a reference point for the T score.

pencil-beam collimation Dual energy x-ray absorptiometry system using a circular pinhole x-ray collimator that produces a narrow x-ray stream, which is received by a single detector. Its motion is serpentine (or raster) across or along the length of the body. Modern systems have improved scan time and image quality. Off-centering of the object does not cause geometric distortion.

percent coefficient of variation (%CV) Statistic used to compare standard deviations from different data sets, which may have different means; also a measure of precision; calculated as SD ÷ mean × 100. A smaller %CV indicates better precision.

peripheral dual energy x-ray absorptiometry (pDXA) Dual energy x-ray absorptiometry system designed to scan only the peripheral skeleton; smaller and simpler to operate than DXA scanners.

peripheral quantitative computed tomography (pQCT) Dedicated QCT system designed to measure bone density on the peripheral skeleton, usually the forearm.

picture archiving communication system (PACS) Medical imaging technology that provides economical storage and convenient access to images from multiple modalities.

primary osteoporosis Osteoporosis not caused by an underlying disease, classified as type I or type II.

projectional (or areal) technique Two-dimensional representation of a three-dimensional object.

quantitative computed tomography (QCT) System for quantitative CT measurements of bone density, allowing true measurement of volume and separation of trabecular and cortical bone; usually measured at the spine or forearm, sometimes at the hip.

quantitative ultrasound (QUS) Quantitative measurement of bone properties related to mechanical competence using ultrasound. The results are reported in terms of broadband ultrasound attenuation (BUA); speed of sound (SOS); and a nonstandardized proprietary mathematic combination of the two, called the *stiffness* or *quantitative ultrasound index* (QUI). It predicts overall or spine fracture risk without using ionizing radiation and is usually measured at the calcaneus.

radiogrammetry Older method of measuring bone loss by comparing the outer diameter and inner medullary diameter of small tubular bones, usually the finger phalanges, or metacarpals.

radiographic absorptiometry (RA) Visual comparison of hand x-ray density with a known standard in the exposure field.

reference population Large, sex-matched, community-based population used to determine the average bone mineral density and standard deviation at each age; used as reference base for T scores and Z scores; may also be matched on ethnicity and weight.

regions of interest (ROI) Defined portion of bone density scans where the bone mineral density is calculated; may be placed manually or automatically by computer software.

scintillation counter Counter employing a photomultiplier tube for detection of radiation.

secondary osteoporosis Osteoporosis caused by an underlying disease.

serial scans Sequential scans, usually performed 12, 18, or 24 months apart, to measure changes in bone density. Scans are best done on the same scanner or on a new scanner cross-calibrated to the original scanner.

Shewhart Control Chart rules Classic quality control rules based on comparing a data value with the mean and standard deviation of a set of similar values.

sieverts (Sv) Measurement of effective radiation dose to a patient. Bone density doses are measured in microsieverts (μSv), which are one millionth of 1 sievert.

single energy x-ray absorptiometry (SXA) Bone density technique for the peripheral skeleton using a single energy x-ray source and an external medium, such as water, to correct for the effects of soft tissue attenuation. Scanners are smaller and simpler to operate than dual energy x-ray absorptiometry scanners.

single photon absorptiometry (SPA) Obsolete method of measuring bone density at the forearm using a single radioisotope source; replaced by single energy x-ray absorptiometry.

standard deviation (SD) Measure of the variability of data values around the mean value.

subtraction technique Removal of the density attributable to soft tissue so that the remaining density belongs only to bone.

T-score Number of standard deviations an individual's bone mineral density (BMD) is from the average BMD for sex-matched, young normal peak bone masses.

total body less head (TBLH) Total body scanning less head analysis.

trabecular bone Delicate, lattice-work structure within bones that adds strength without excessive weight; supports compressive loading at the spine, hip, and calcaneus and is found in the ends of long bones, such as the distal radius.

type I osteoporosis Primary osteoporosis related to postmenopausal status.

type II osteoporosis Primary osteoporosis related to aging.

vertebral fracture assessment (VFA) Encompasses looking at the spine "morphometrically" in the lateral projection. Common synonymous terms are *dual-energy vertebral assessment (DVA), lateral vertebral assessment (LVA), instant vertebral assessment (IVA),* and *radiologic vertebral assessment (RVA).*

volumetric density Bone mineral density calculated by dividing by the true three-dimensional volume.

Ward's triangle Region on proximal femur lying on the border of the femoral neck and greater trochanter; has low bone mineral density. Cannot be used in diagnosis.

Z-score Number of standard deviations the individual's bone mineral density (BMD) is from the average BMD for a sex-matched and age-matched reference group.

Resources for information and instruction

American College of Radiology: *ACR standard for the performance of adult dual or single x-ray absorptiometry (DXA/pDXA/ SXA)*. Contact the Standards & Accreditation Department, American College of Radiology, 1891 Preston White Drive, Reston, VA 22091.

American Registry of Radiologic Technologists: Provides a postprimary examination leading to a certificate of added qualifications in bone densitometry. For details, see the *Examinee handbook for bone densitometry*. Contact the American Registry of Radiologic Technologists, 1255 Northland Drive, St Paul, MN 55120-1155. Web site: www.arrt.org.

American Society of Radiologic Technologists: Approved elective curriculum in bone densitometry for radiography programs. Contact the American Society of Radiologic Technologists, 15000 Central Avenue SE, Albuquerque, NM 87123. Web site: www.asrt.org.

International Society for Clinical Densitometry: Certification courses, annual and regional meetings, continuing education, newsletter, *Journal of Clinical Densitometry,* and web site with links to Official Positions and Pediatric Official Positions. Contact International Society for Clinical Densitometry 955 South Main St. Building C Middletown, CT 06457. Web site: www.iscd.org.

Mindways.com.

National Osteoporosis Foundation: Excellent source of osteoporosis information and educational materials for technologists, physicians, and patients. Contact the National Osteoporosis Foundation, 1232 22nd Street NW, Washington, DC 20037-1292. Web site: www.nof.org.

Scanner manufacturers: source for technologist instruction and answers to scanner-specific application questions. Refer to the operator's manual for contact information.

StrongerBones.org.

Surgeon General's Report. Web site: www.surgeongeneral.gov.

Selected bibliography

Blunt BA et al: Good clinical practice and audits for dual x-ray absorptiometry and x-ray imaging laboratories and quality assurance centers involved in clinical drug trials, private practice, and research, *J Clin Densitometry* 1:323, 1998.

FRAX: *WHO Fracture Risk Assessment tool,* Available at: http://www.shef.ac.uk/FRAX. Accessed August 27, 2009.

Genant HK: Development of formulas for standardized DXA measurements, *J Bone Miner Res* 9:997, 1995.

Genant HK et al: Universal standardization for dual x-ray absorptiometry: patient and phantom cross-calibration results, *J Bone Miner Res* 9:1503, 1994.

International Society for Clinical Densitometry: *Official positions,* Available at: www.iscd.org/Visitors/positions/ OfficialPositionsPowerPoint.cfm. Accessed November 24, 2014.

National Institutes of Health Consensus Development Panel on Osteoporosis Prevention, Diagnosis, and Therapy: Osteoporosis prevention, diagnosis, and therapy, *JAMA* 285:785, 2001.

National Osteoporosis Foundation, Available at: www.nof.org. Accessed November 2014.

National Osteoporosis Foundation physician's guide, Washington, DC, 1998, National Osteoporosis Foundation.

34

RADIATION ONCOLOGY

LEILA A. BUSSMAN-YEAKEL

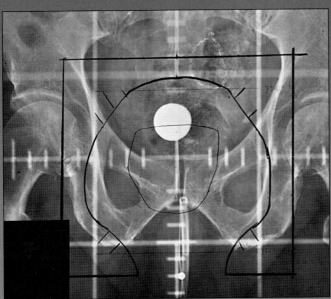

OUTLINE

Principles of Radiation
    Oncology, 480
Historical Development, 481
Cancer, 481
Theory, 484
Technical Aspects, 485
Steps in Radiation Oncology, 489
Clinical Applications, 502
Future Trends, 505
Conclusion, 505

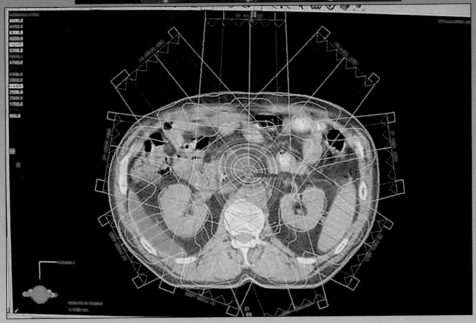

Principles of Radiation Oncology

Radiation oncology, * or *radiation therapy,* is one of three principal modalities used in the treatment of cancer. The others are surgery and chemotherapy. In radiation therapy for malignancies, *tumors* or *lesions* are treated with *cancericidal doses* of ionizing radiation as prescribed by a *radiation oncologist,* a physician who specializes in the treatment of malignant disease with radiation. The goals of the treatment are to deliver a cancericidal dose of radiation precisely to the tumor, limiting as much as possible the dose of radiation received by normal, noncancerous tissues. These dual tasks make this form of treatment complex and often challenging. Input from all members of the radiation oncology team is crucial in developing the optimal treatment plan or approach for a patient.

Cancer treatment requires a multidisciplinary approach. First, diagnostic radiologic studies such as radiographs, computed tomography (CT) scans, magnetic resonance imaging (MRI), positron emission tomography (PET) scans, and sonograms are obtained to acquire information about the location and anatomic extent of the tumor. Second, a tissue specimen *(biopsy)* is removed surgically. A *pathologist* examines the tissue to determine whether the lesion is cancerous. When cancer is diagnosed, the plan for the best treatment is determined through consultation with various *oncology* specialists (e.g., surgical *oncologist,* radiation oncologist, medical oncologist).

---

*Almost all italicized words on the succeeding pages are defined at the end of the chapter.

Although radiation oncology may be used as the only method of treatment for malignant disease, a more common approach is to use radiation in conjunction with surgery, chemotherapy, or both. Some patients with cancer may be treated only with surgery or chemotherapy; however, approximately 75% of all diagnosed cancer patients are treated with radiation. The choice of treatment can depend on many patient variables, such as the patient's overall physical and emotional condition, the histologic type of the disease, and the extent and anatomic position of the tumor. If a tumor is small and its margins are well defined, a surgical approach alone may be prescribed. If the disease is *systemic,* a chemotherapeutic approach may be chosen. Most tumors exhibit degrees of size, invasion, and spread, however, and require variations in the treatment approach that are likely to include radiation treatments administered as an adjunct to or in conjunction with surgery or chemotherapy.

Radiation is generally used after surgery when a patient is deemed to be at high risk for tumor recurrence in the *surgical bed.* The risk of recurrence is considered to be increased in the following situations:
- When the surgical margin between normal tissue and cancerous tissue is minimal (<2 cm)
- When the margin is positive for cancer (i.e., when cancerous tissue is not completely removed)
- When the tumor is incompletely resected because of its large size, its relationship with normal vital structures, or both
- When the cancer has spread to adjacent lymph nodes

Radiation can be used as the definitive (primary) cancer treatment or as an adjuvant treatment (i.e., in combination with another form of therapy). It can also be used for *palliation.*

Radiation treatments most often are delivered on a daily basis, Monday through Friday, for 2 to 8 weeks. The length of time and the total dose of radiation delivered depend on the type of cancer being treated and the purpose of treatment (*cure* or palliation). Prescribed dosages of radiation can range from 2000 centigray (cGy) for palliation to 8000 cGy

for curative intent (total doses). The delivery of a small amount of radiation per day (180 to 200 cGy) for a certain number of treatments, instead of one large dose, is termed *fractionation.* Because these smaller doses of radiation are more easily tolerated by normal tissue, fractionation can help minimize the acute toxic effect a patient experiences during treatment and the possible long-term side effects of treatment.

The precision and accuracy necessary to administer high doses of radiation to tumors while not harming normal tissue require the combined effort of all members of the radiation oncology team. Members of this team include the radiation oncologist, a physicist, dosimetrists, radiation therapists, and oncology nurses.

The radiation oncologist prescribes the quantity of radiation and determines the anatomic region or regions to be treated. The *medical physicist* is responsible for calibration and maintenance of the radiation-producing equipment. The physicist also advises the physician about dosage calculations and complex treatment techniques. The *medical dosimetrist* devises a plan for delivering the treatments in a manner to meet best the physician's goals of irradiating the tumor while protecting vital normal structures. The *radiation therapist* is responsible for obtaining radiographs or CT scans that localize the area to be treated, administering the treatments, keeping accurate records of the dose delivered each day, and monitoring the patient's physical and emotional well-being. Educating patients about potential radiation side effects and assisting patients with the management of these side effects are often the responsibilities of the oncology nurse.

The duties and responsibilities of the radiation therapist are more thoroughly described elsewhere in this chapter. In addition, more information is provided about the circumstances in which radiation is used to treat cancer. The steps necessary to prepare a patient for treatment are also described. These steps include (1) simulation, (2) development of the optimal treatment plan in dosimetry, and (3) treatment delivery. Current techniques and future trends are also discussed.

Historical Development

Ionizing radiation was originally used to obtain a radiographic image of internal anatomy for diagnostic purposes. The resultant image depended on many variables, including the energy of the beam, the processing techniques, the material on which the image was recorded, and, most important, the amount of energy absorbed by the various organs of the body. The transfer of energy from the beam of radiation to the biologic system and the observation of the effects of this interaction became the foundation of radiation oncology.

Two of the most obvious and sometimes immediate biologic effects observed during the early diagnostic procedures were epilation (loss of hair) and erythema (reddening of the skin). Epilation and erythema resulted primarily from the great amount of energy absorbed by the skin during radiographic procedures. These short-term, radiation-induced effects afforded radiographic practitioners an opportunity to expand the use of radiation to treat conditions ranging from relatively benign maladies such as hypertrichosis (excessive hair), acne, and boils to grotesque and malignant diseases such as lupus vulgaris and skin cancer.

Ionizing radiation was first applied for the treatment of a more in-depth lesion on January 29, 1896, when Grubbé is reported to have irradiated a woman with carcinoma of the left breast. This event occurred only 3 months after the discovery of x-rays by Röntgen (Table 34-1). Although Grubbé neither expected nor observed any dramatic results from the irradiation, the event is significant simply because it occurred.

In January 1902, Skinner, in New Haven, Connecticut, performed the first reported curative treatment using ionizing radiation. Skinner treated a woman who had a diagnosed malignant fibrosarcoma. Over the next 2 years and 3 months, the woman received 136 applications of the x-rays. In April 1909, 7 years after initial application of the radiation, the woman was free of disease and considered "cured."

As data were collected, the interest in radiation therapy increased. More sophisticated equipment, a greater understanding of the effects of ionizing radiation, an appreciation for time-dose relationships, and numerous other related medical breakthroughs gave impetus to the interest in radiation therapy that led to the evolution of a distinct medical specialty—radiation oncology.

Cancer

Cancer is a disease process that involves an unregulated, uncontrolled replication of cells; put more simply, the cells do not know when to stop dividing. These abnormal cells grow without regard to normal tissue. They invade adjacent tissues, destroy normal tissue, and create a mass of tumor cells. Cancerous cells can spread further by invading the lymph or blood vessels that drain the area. When tumor cells invade the lymphatic or vascular system, they are transported by that system until they become caught or lodged within a lymph node or an organ such as the liver or lungs, where secondary tumors form. The spread of cancer from the original site to different, remote parts of the body is termed *metastasis*. When cancer has spread to a distant site via blood-borne metastasis, the patient is considered incurable. Early detection and diagnosis are the keys to curing cancer.

Cancer was diagnosed in an estimated 1,660,290 individuals in the United States in 2013. This number does not include basal and squamous cell skin cancers, which have high cure rates. These types of cancer are the most common malignant diseases, with more than 3.5 million cases diagnosed in 2006. *One in two men will develop or die of cancer in their lifetime. Slightly more than one in three women will develop or die of cancer in their lifetime. Although cancer can occur in persons of any age, it is diagnosed in most patients after age 55 years.*

TABLE 34-1

Significant developments in radiation therapy

Date	Person	Event
1895	Röntgen	Discovery of x-rays
1896	Grubbé	First use of ionizing radiation in treatment of cancer
	Becquerel	Discovery of radioactive emissions by uranium compounds
1898	M. and P. Curie	Discovery of radium
1902	Skinner	First documented case of cancer "cure" using ionizing radiation
1906	Bergonié and Tribondeau	Postulation of first law of radiosensitivity
1932	Lawrence	Invention of cyclotron
1934	Joliot and Joliot-Curie	Production of artificial radioactivity
1939	Lawrence and Stone	Treatment of cancer patient with neutron beam from cyclotron
1940	Kerst	Construction of betatron
1951		Installation of first cobalt-60 teletherapy units
1952		Installation of first linear accelerator (Hammersmith Hospital, London)

The most common cancers that occur in the United States are lung, prostate, breast, and colorectal cancer. Prostate cancer is the most common malignancy in men, and breast cancer is the most common malignancy in women. The second and third most common cancers in men and women are lung and colorectal cancer (Table 34-2).

Cancer is second only to heart disease as the leading cause of death in the United States. Lung cancer is the leading cause of cancer deaths for men and women. In 2013, an estimated 28% of cancer deaths in men and 26% in women were due to lung cancer. The next most common causes of cancer death are prostate cancer and breast cancer, which account for 10% and 14% of cancer deaths in the United States.

RISK FACTORS
External Factors

Many factors can contribute to a person's potential for the development of a *malignancy*. These factors can be external exposure to chemicals, viruses, or radiation within the environment or internal factors such as hormones, genetic mutations, and disorders of the immune system. Cancer commonly is the result of exposure to a *carcinogen*, which is a substance or material that causes cells to undergo malignant transformation and become cancerous. Some known carcinogenic agents are listed in Table 34-3. Cigarettes and other tobacco products are the principal cause of cancers of the lung, esophagus, oral cavity and pharynx, and bladder. Cigarette smokers are 23 times more likely to develop lung cancer than nonsmokers. Occupational exposure to chemicals such as chromium, nickel, or arsenic can also cause lung cancer. A person who smokes and works with chemical carcinogens is at even greater risk for developing lung cancer than a nonsmoker. In other words, risk factors can have an additive effect, acting together to initiate or promote the development of cancer. Other risk factors that have been identified are obesity, physical inactivity, and poor nutrition.

The human papilloma virus (HPV) is associated with the development of cancer of the uterine cervix, oropharynx, and anus. Infection with the hepatitis B virus (HBV) and hepatitis C virus increase one's risk for the development of hepatocellular carcinoma of the liver. Vaccines do exist to prevent infection with HPV or HBV.

Another carcinogen is *ionizing radiation.* It was responsible for the development of osteogenic sarcoma in radium-dial painters in the 1920s and 1930s, and it caused the development of skin cancers in pioneer radiologists. Early radiation therapy equipment used in the treatment of cancer often induced a second malignancy in the bone. The low-energy x-rays produced by this equipment were within the photoelectric range of interactions with matter, resulting in a 3:1 preferential absorption in bone compared with soft tissue. Some patients with breast cancer who were irradiated developed an osteosarcoma of their ribs after a 15- to 20-year latency period. With advances in diagnostic and therapeutic equipment and improved knowledge of radiation physics, radiobiology, and radiation safety practices, radiation-induced malignancies have become relatively uncommon, although the potential for their development still exists. In keeping with standard radiation safety guidelines, any dose of radiation, no matter how small, significantly increases the chance of a genetic mutation.

Internal factors

Internal factors are causative factors over which persons have no control. Genetic mutations on individual genes and *chromosomes* have been identified as predisposing factors for the development of cancer. Mutations can be sporadic or hereditary, as in colon cancer. Chromosomal defects have also been identified in other cancers, such as leukemia, Wilms tumor, retinoblastoma, and breast cancer. Because of their familial pattern of occurrence, breast, ovarian, and colorectal cancer are three major areas currently under study to obtain earlier diagnosis, which increases the cure rate. Patients with a family history of breast or ovarian cancer can be tested to see whether they have inherited the altered *BRCA-1* and *BRCA-2* genes. Patients with these altered genes are at a significantly higher risk for developing breast and ovarian cancer. Women identified as carriers of the altered genes can benefit from more intensive and early screening programs in which breast cancer may be diagnosed at a much earlier and more curable stage. These patients also have the option of *prophylactic surgery* to remove the breasts or ovaries. Some women still develop cancer, however, in the remaining tissue after surgery.

TABLE 34-2
Top five most common cancers in men and women

Men	Women
1. Prostate	1. Breast
2. Lung and bronchus	2. Lung and bronchus
3. Colon and rectum	3. Colon and rectum
4. Bladder	4. Uterus (endometrium)
5. Melanoma	5. Thyroid

TABLE 34-3
Carcinogenic agents and the cancers they cause

Carcinogen	Resultant cancer
Cigarette smoking	Cancers of lung, esophagus, bladder, and oral cavity/pharynx
Arsenic, chromium, nickel, hydrocarbons	Lung cancer
Ultraviolet light	Melanoma and nonmelanomatous skin cancers
Benzene	Leukemia
Ionizing radiation	Sarcomas of bone and soft tissue, skin cancer, and leukemia

Familial adenomatous polyposis

Familial adenomatous polyposis is a hereditary condition in which the lining of the colon becomes studded with hundreds to thousands of polyps by late adolescence. A mutation in a gene identified as the adenomatous polyposis coli *(APC)* gene is considered the cause of this abnormal growth of polyps. Virtually all people with this condition eventually develop colon cancer. These individuals develop cancer at a much earlier age than the normal population. Treatment involves removal of the entire colon and rectum.

Hereditary nonpolyposis colorectal cancer syndrome

Hereditary nonpolyposis colorectal cancer syndrome is a cancer that develops in the proximal colon in the absence of polyps or with fewer than five polyps. It has a familial distribution, occurring in three first-degree relatives in two generations, with at least one person being diagnosed before age 50 years. Hereditary nonpolyposis colorectal cancer syndrome, also known as Lynch syndrome, has also been associated with the development of cancers of the breast, endometrium, pancreas, and biliary tract.

Familial cancer research

Current research to identify the genes responsible for cancer can assist in detecting cancers at a much earlier stage in high-risk patients. Many institutions have familial cancer programs to provide genetic testing and counseling for persons with strong family histories of cancer. Experts assist in educating individuals about their potential risk for developing cancer and the importance of screening and early detection. Genetic testing remains the patient's option, and many patients prefer not to be tested.

TISSUE ORIGINS OF CANCER

Cancers may arise in any human tissue. Tumors are usually categorized under six general headings according to their tissue of origin (Table 34-4). Of cancers, 90% arise from *epithelial tissue* and are classified as *carcinomas*. Epithelial tissue lines the free internal and external surfaces of the body. Carcinomas are subdivided further into squamous cell carcinomas and adenocarcinomas based on the type of epithelium from which they arise. A squamous cell carcinoma arises from the surface (squamous) epithelium of a structure. Examples of surface epithelium include the oral cavity, pharynx, bronchus, skin, and cervix. An adenocarcinoma is a cancer that develops in glandular epithelium such as in the prostate, colon and rectum, lung, breast, or endometrium.

To facilitate the exchange of patient information from one physician to another, the International Union Against Cancer and the American Joint Committee for Cancer (AJCC) Staging and End Results Reporting designed a system for classifying tumors based on anatomic and histologic considerations. The AJCC TNM classification (Table 34-5) describes a tumor according to the size of the primary lesion *(T)*, the involvement of the regional lymph nodes *(N)*, and the occurrence of metastasis *(M)*.

TABLE 34-4

Categorization of cancers by tissue of origin

Tissue of origin	Type of tumor
Epithelium	
Surface epithelium	Squamous cell carcinoma
Glandular epithelium	Adenocarcinoma
Connective tissue	
Bone	Osteosarcoma
Fat	Liposarcoma
Lymphoreticular-hematopoietic tissue	
Lymph nodes	Lymphoma
Plasma cells	Multiple myeloma
Blood cells/ bone marrow	Leukemia
Nerve tissue	
Glial tissue	Glioma
Neuroectoderm	Neuroblastoma
Tumors of more than one tissue	
Embryonic	Nephroblastoma kidney
Tumors that do not fit into above categories	
Testis	Seminoma
Thymus	Thymoma

TABLE 34-5

Application of TNM classification system

Classification	Description of tumor
Stage 0—$T_0N_0M_0$	Occult lesion; no evidence clinically
Stage I—$T_1N_0M_0$	Small lesion confined to organ of origin with no evidence of vascular and lymphatic spread or metastasis
Stage II—$T_2N_1M_0$	Tumor of <5 cm invading surrounding tissue and first-station lymph nodes but no evidence of metastasis
Stage III—$T_3N_2M_0$	Extensive lesion >5 cm with fixation to deeper structure and lymph invasion but no evidence of metastasis
Stage IV—$T_4N_3M_1$	More extensive lesion than above with invasion of bone or other adjacent structures or with distant metastasis (M_1)

Note: This is a generalization. Variations of the staging system exist for each tumor site.

Theory

The biologic effectiveness of ionizing radiation in living tissue depends partially on the amount of energy that is deposited within the tissue and partially on the condition of the biologic system. The terms used to describe this relationship are *linear energy transfer* (LET) and *relative biologic effectiveness* (RBE).

LET values are expressed in thousands of electron volts deposited per micron of tissue (keV/μm) and vary depending on the type of radiation being considered. Because of their mass and possible charge, particles tend to interact more readily with the material through which they are passing and have a greater LET value. A 5-MeV alpha particle has an LET value of 100 keV/mm in tissue; nonparticulate radiations such as 250-kilovolt (peak) (kVp) x-rays and 1.2-MeV gamma rays have much lower LET values: 2.0 keV/mm and 0.2 keV/mm.

RBE values are determined by calculating the ratio of the dose from a standard beam of radiation to the dose required of the radiation beam in question to produce a similar biologic effect. The standard beam of radiation is 250-kVp x-rays, and the ratio is set up as follows:

$$RBE = \frac{\text{Standard beam dose to obtain effect}}{\text{Similar effect using beam in question}}$$

As the LET increases, so does the RBE. RBE and LET values are listed in Table 34-6.

The effectiveness of ionizing radiation on a biologic system depends not only on the amount of radiation deposited but also on the state of the biologic system. One of the first laws of radiation biology, postulated by Bergonié and Tribondeau, stated in essence that the *radiosensitivity* of a tissue depends on the number of *undifferentiated* cells in the tissue, the degree of mitotic activity of the tissue, and the length of time that cells of the tissue remain in active proliferation. Although exceptions exist, the preceding is true in most tissues. The primary target of ionizing radiation is the DNA molecule, and the human cell is most radiosensitive during mitosis. Current research tends to indicate that all cells are equally radiosensitive; however, the manifestation of the radiation injury occurs at different time frames (i.e., acute versus late effects).

Because tissue cells are composed primarily of water, most of the *ionization* occurs with water molecules. These events are called *indirect effects* and result in the formation of free radicals such as OH, H, and HO$_2$. These highly reactive free radicals may recombine with no resultant biologic effect, or they may combine with other atoms and molecules to produce biochemical changes that may be deleterious to the cell. The possibility also exists that the radiation may interact with an organic molecule or atom, which may result in the inactivation of the cell; this reaction is called the *direct effect*. Because ionizing radiation is nonspecific (i.e., it interacts with normal cells as readily as with tumor cells), cellular damage occurs in normal and abnormal tissue. The deleterious effects are greater in the tumor cells, however, because a greater percentage of these cells are undergoing mitosis; tumor cells also tend to be more poorly *differentiated*. In addition, normal cells have a greater capability for repairing sublethal damage than tumor cells. Greater cell damage occurs to tumor cells than to normal cells for any given increment of dose. The effects of the interactions in either normal or tumor cells may be expressed by the following descriptions:

- Loss of reproductive ability
- Metabolic changes
- Cell transformation
- Acceleration of the aging process
- Cell mutation

The greater the number of interactions that occur, the greater the possibility of cell death.

The preceding information leads to a categorization of tumors according to their radiosensitivity:

1. *Very radiosensitive*
   - Gonadal germ cell tumors (seminoma of testis, dysgerminoma of ovary)
   - Lymphoproliferative tumors (Hodgkin and non-Hodgkin lymphomas)
   - Embryonal tumors (Wilms tumor of the kidney)
2. *Moderately radiosensitive*
   - Epithelial tumors (squamous and basal cell carcinomas of skin)
   - Glandular tumors (adenocarcinoma of prostate)
3. *Relatively radioresistant*
   - Mesenchymal tumors (sarcomas of bone and connective tissue)
   - Nerve tumors (glioma)

Many concepts that originate in the laboratory have little practical application, but some are beginning to influence the selection of treatment modalities and the techniques of radiation oncology. As cellular function and the effects of radiation on the cell are increasingly understood, attention is being focused on the use of drugs, or simply oxygen, to enhance the effectiveness of radiation treatments.

TABLE 34-6

Relative biologic effectiveness and linear energy transfer values for certain forms of radiation

Radiation	RBE	LET
250-kV x-rays	1	2.0
^{60}Co gamma rays	0.85	0.2
14-MeV neutrons	12	75
5-MeV alpha particles	20	100

Technical Aspects

EXTERNAL-BEAM THERAPY AND BRACHYTHERAPY

Two major categories for the application of radiation for cancer treatment are external-beam therapy and brachytherapy. For *external-beam treatment,* the patient lies underneath a machine that emits radiation or generates a beam of x-rays. Most cancer patients are treated in this fashion. Some patients may also be treated with *brachytherapy,* a technique in which the radioactive material is placed within the patient.

The theory behind brachytherapy is to deliver low-intensity radiation over an extended period to a relatively small volume of tissue. The low-intensity isotopes are placed directly into a tissue or cavity depositing radiation only a short distance, covering the tumor area but sparing surrounding normal tissue. This technique allows a higher total dose of radiation to be delivered to the tumor than is achievable with external-beam radiation alone. Brachytherapy may be accomplished in any of the following ways:

1. Mold technique—placement of a *radioactive* source or sources on or in close proximity to the lesion
2. Intracavitary implant technique—placement of a radioactive source or sources in a body cavity (i.e., uterine canal and vagina)
3. Interstitial implant technique—placement of a radioactive source or sources directly into the tumor site and adjacent tissue (i.e., sarcoma in a muscle)

Most brachytherapy applications tend to be temporary in that the sources are left in the patient until a designated tumor dose has been attained. Two different brachytherapy systems exist. They are *low-dose-rate* (LDR) and *high-dose-rate* (HDR). LDR brachytherapy has been the standard system for many years. A low-activity isotope is used to deliver a dose of radiation at a slow rate of 40 to 500 cGy per hour. This therapy requires that a patient be hospitalized for 3 to 4 days until the desired dose is delivered.

HDR systems are the more standard method of brachytherapy. This system uses a high-activity isotope capable of delivering greater than 1200 cGy per hour. The HDR system allows the prescribed dose to be delivered over minutes, which means this treatment can occur on an outpatient basis. Gynecologic tumors are one of the most common sites to be treated with HDR brachytherapy. HDR systems use a high-activity iridium-192 source.

Permanent implant therapy may also be accomplished. This is the most common type of LDR brachytherapy in practice today. An example of a permanent implant nuclide is iodine-125 and palladium-103 seeds. Permanent implant nuclides have relatively short *half-lives* of days and are left in the patient essentially forever. The amount and distribution of the radionuclide implanted in this manner depends on the total dose that the radiation oncologist is trying to deliver. Early-stage prostate cancer is commonly treated with this technique alone. In some cases of brachytherapy implantation, the implant is applied as part of the patient's overall treatment plan and may be preceded by or followed by additional external-beam radiation therapy.

EQUIPMENT

Most radiation oncology departments use linear accelerators (linacs) as their main treatment unit. Following are treatment units that may be found in a radiation oncology department:

- 120-kVp superficial x-ray unit for treating lesions on or near the surface of the patient
- 250-kVp orthovoltage x-ray unit for moderately superficial tissues
- ^{60}Co (cobalt-60) *gamma ray* source with an average energy of 1.25-MeV; Gamma Knife Unit
- 6-MV to 35-MV *linear accelerator* to serve as a source of high-energy (megavoltage) electrons and x-rays
- TomoTherapy
- CyberKnife

The dose depositions of these units are compared in Fig. 34-1.

The penetrability, or energy, of an x-ray or gamma ray totally depends on its wavelength: The shorter the wavelength, the more penetrating the photon; conversely, the longer the wavelength, the less penetrating the photon. A low-energy beam ($\leq$120 kVp) of radiation tends to deposit all or most of its energy on or near the surface of the patient and is suitable for treating lesions on or near the skin surface. In addition, with the low-energy beam, a greater amount of absorption or dose deposition occurs in bone than in soft tissue.

A high-energy beam of radiation ($\geq$1 MeV) tends to deposit its energy throughout the entire volume of tissue irradiated, with a greater amount of dose deposition occurring at or near the entry port than at the exit port. In this energy range, the dose is deposited about equally in soft tissue and bone. The high-energy (megavoltage) beam is most suitable for tumors deep beneath the body surface.

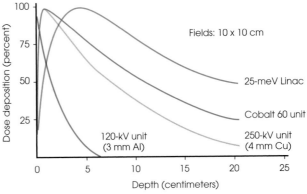

Fig. 34-1 Plot of percent of dose deposition in relation to depth in centimeters of tissue for various energies of photon beams.

The *skin-sparing* effect, a phenomenon that occurs as the energy of a beam of radiation is increased, is valuable from a therapeutic standpoint. In the superficial and orthovoltage energy range, the maximum dose occurs on the surface of the patient, and deposition of the dose decreases as the beam traverses the patient. As the energy of the beam increases into the megavoltage range, the maximum dose absorbed by the patient occurs at some point below the skin surface. The skin-sparing effect is important clinically because the skin is a radiosensitive organ. Excessive dose deposition to the skin can damage the skin, requiring treatments to be stopped and compromising treatment to the underlying tumor. The greater the energy of the beam, the more deeply the maximum dose is deposited (Fig. 34-2).

Cobalt-60 units

The ^{60}Co unit was the first skin-sparing machine. It replaced the orthovoltage unit in the early 1950s because of its greater ability to treat tumors located deeper within tissues. ^{60}Co is an artificially produced *isotope* formed in a nuclear *reactor* by the bombardment of stable cobalt-59 with neutrons. ^{60}Co emits two gamma-ray beams with an energy of 1.17 MeV and 1.33 MeV. The unit was known as a "workhorse" because it was extremely reliable, was mechanically simple, and had little downtime. It was the first radiation therapy unit to rotate 360 degrees around a patient. A machine that rotates around a fixed point, or axis, and maintains the same distance from the source of radiation is called an *isocentric machine*. All modern therapeutic units are isocentric machines. This type of machine allows the patient to remain in one position, lessening the chance for patient movement during treatment. Isocentric capabilities also assist in directing the beam precisely at the tumor while sparing normal structures.

Because ^{60}Co is a radioisotope, it constantly emits radiation as it *decays* in an effort to return to a stable state. It has a half-life of 5.26 years (i.e., its activity is reduced by 50% at the end of 5.26 years). Because the source decays at a rate of 1% per month, the radiation treatment time must be adjusted, resulting in longer treatment times as the source decays.

The use of ^{60}Co units has declined significantly since the 1980s, and ^{60}Co is rarely used for conventional external-beam radiation therapy today. This decline has been basically attributed to the introduction of the more sophisticated linac, which has greater skin-sparing capabilities and more sharply defined radiation *fields*. The radiation beam, or field, from a ^{60}Co unit also has large penumbra, which results in fuzzy field edges, another undesirable feature. ^{60}Co is still used in radiation oncology as part of a special procedure called stereotactic radiosurgery. The treatment unit is called the Gamma Knife. The Gamma Knife consists of 192 to 201 ^{60}Co sources arranged in a hemispherical array

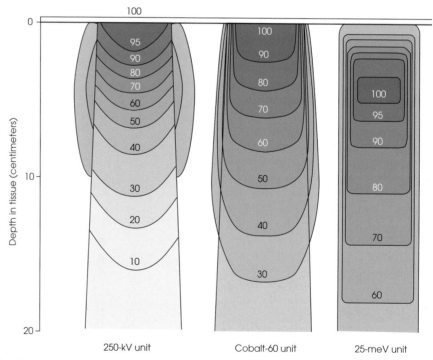

Fig. 34-2 Three isodose curves showing comparison of percent of dose deposition from three x-ray units of different energies. As the energy of the beam increases, the percentage of dose deposited on the surface of the patient decreases.

with all sources converging at a single point (Fig. 34-3). The point where the beams converge forms a treatment area of 4 to 18 mm in diameter.

The Gamma Knife is primarily used to treat small benign or malignant lesions located deep within the brain employing an external rigidly fixed stereotactic head frame. The Gamma Knife does not involve surgery. It is called radiosurgery because the radiation is delivered in such a precise, focused manner that the lesion is ablated as if removed surgically. Adjacent normal tissues receive minimal radiation and are unharmed. The stereotactic head frame provides a coordinate system that allows the lesion to be three-dimensionally localized on MRI, CT scan, or angiography so that the radiation can be planned and targeted directly to the involved area. The Gamma Knife delivers a large dose of radiation in a single treatment to one or more areas in the brain. The types of conditions treated with the Gamma Knife include benign conditions such as acoustic neuromas, pituitary adenomas, arteriovenous malformations, and trigeminal neuralgia. Malignant lesions treated with the Gamma Knife include gliomas, meningiomas, chordoma, and solitary brain metastasis.

There are many advantages of Gamma Knife radiosurgery over conventional neurosurgery. First, the patient does not have to undergo an invasive surgical procedure. The procedure can be done as an outpatient or may require an overnight stay in the hospital. There is no major recuperation period after a Gamma Knife procedure. The cost of Gamma Knife radiosurgery is much less than the cost of neurosurgery. The Gamma Knife is considered a very effective treatment for small intracranial lesions. One disadvantage of the Gamma Knife is that it can be used only for intracranial lesions. Another disadvantage is that the effects of radiation on the lesion are not immediate but occur over a period of weeks.

Linear accelerators

Linacs are the most commonly used machines for cancer treatment. The first linac was developed in 1952 and first used clinically in the United States in 1956. A linac is capable of producing high-energy beams of photons (x-rays) or electrons in the range of 4 million to 35 million volts. These megavoltage photon beams allow a better distribution of dose to deep-seated tumors with better sparing of normal tissues than their earlier counterparts—the orthovoltage or ^{60}Co units.

The photon beam is produced by accelerating a stream of electrons toward a target. When the electrons hit the target, a beam of x-rays is produced. By removing the target, the linac can also produce a beam of electrons of varying energies.

Linacs can now be purchased with a single photon energy or a dual photon machine with two x-ray beams. Typically, a dual photon energy machine consists of one low-energy (6-MeV) and one high-energy (18-MV) photon beam plus a range of electron energies (Fig. 34-4). The dual photon energy machine gives the radiation oncologist more options in prescribing radiation treatments. As the energy of the beam increases, so does its penetrating power. A lower energy beam is used to treat tumors in thinner parts of the body, whereas high-energy beams are prescribed for tumors in thicker parts of the body. A brain tumor or a tumor in a limb would most likely be treated with a 6-MeV beam; conversely, a pelvic malignancy would be better treated with an 18-MeV beam. A small oncology center can serve its patients well by purchasing one dual photon linac for a cost of approximately $1.7 million instead of having to purchase two single energy 6-MeV and 18-MeV machines for almost $2 million.

Electrons are advantageous over photons in that they are a more superficial form of treatment. Electrons are energy dependent, which means that they deposit their energy within a given depth of tissue and go no deeper, depending on the energy selected. An 18-MeV beam has a total penetration depth of 3.5 inches (9 cm). Any structure located deeper than 3.5 inches (9 cm) would not be appreciably affected. This is important when the radiation oncologist is trying to treat a tumor that overlies a critical structure.

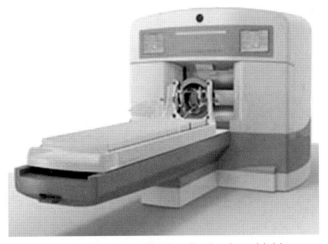

Fig. 34-3 Gamma Knife unit without a patient on the treatment table.

(From Washington CM, Leaver DT, editors: *Principles and practice of radiation therapy*, ed 3, St Louis, 2010, Mosby.)

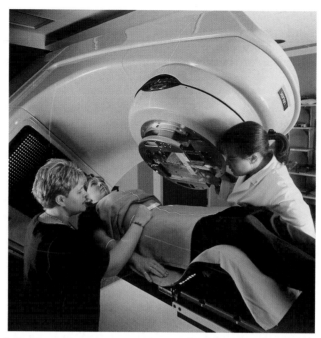

Fig. 34-4 Radiation therapists shown aligning the patient and shielding block in preparation for treatment using a modern linac. X-ray beams of 6 to 25 million V may be produced to treat tumors in the body.

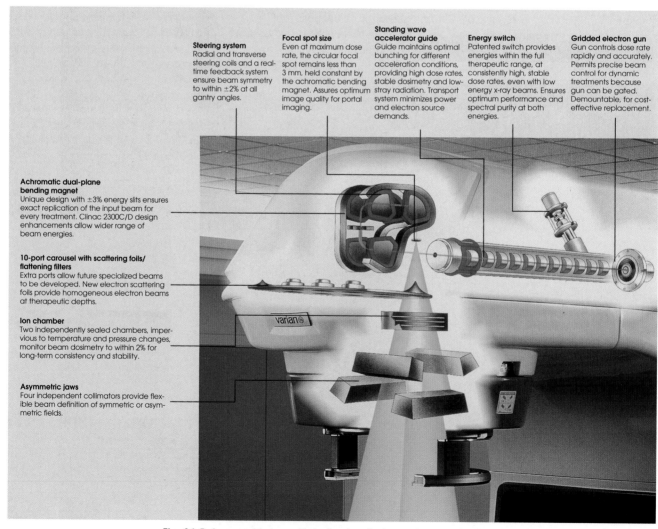

Steering system
Radial and transverse steering coils and a real-time feedback system ensure beam symmetry to within ±2% at all gantry angles.

Focal spot size
Even at maximum dose rate, the circular focal spot remains less than 3 mm, held constant by the achromatic bending magnet. Assures optimum image quality for portal imaging.

Standing wave accelerator guide
Guide maintains optimal bunching for different acceleration conditions, providing high dose rates, stable dosimetry and low-stray radiation. Transport system minimizes power and electron source demands.

Energy switch
Patented switch provides energies within the full therapeutic range, at consistently high, stable dose rates, even with low energy x-ray beams. Ensures optimum performance and spectral purity at both energies.

Gridded electron gun
Gun controls dose rate rapidly and accurately. Permits precise beam control for dynamic treatments because gun can be gated. Demountable, for cost-effective replacement.

Achromatic dual-plane bending magnet
Unique design with ±3% energy slits ensures exact replication of the input beam for every treatment. Clinac 2300C/D design enhancements allow wider range of beam energies.

10-port carousel with scattering foils/flattening filters
Extra ports allow future specialized beams to be developed. New electron scattering foils provide homogeneous electron beams at therapeutic depths.

Ion chamber
Two independently sealed chambers, impervious to temperature and pressure changes, monitor beam dosimetry to within 2% for long-term consistency and stability.

Asymmetric jaws
Four independent collimators provide flexible beam definition of symmetric or asymmetric fields.

Fig. 34-5 Asymmetric jaws. Note the four independent collimators.

(Courtesy Varian Associates, Palo Alto, CA.)

As with a diagnostic x-ray machine, the irradiated field of a linac is defined by a light field projected onto the patient's skin. This corresponding square or rectangle equals the length and width setting of the x-ray *collimators.* A modern linac is equipped with *asymmetric (independent) jaws;* this allows each of the four collimator blades that define length or width to move independently (Fig. 34-5). The jaw that defines the superior extent of the field may be 2.75 inches (7 cm) from the central axis, whereas the inferior region may be at 4 inches (10 cm). The total length would equal 6.75 inches (17 cm), but it is not divided equally because it is in a diagnostic x-ray collimator. The radiation oncologist is able to design a field that optimally covers the area of interest while sparing normal tissue. Independent collimation can also assist in reducing the total weight of lead shielding blocks generally constructed to protect normal tissues.

Multileaf collimation

Multileaf collimation (MLC) is the newest and most complex beam-defining system. Within the head of the linac, 45 to 80 individual collimator blades, about $\frac{3}{8}$ to $\frac{3}{4}$ inch (1 to 2 cm) wide, are located and can be adjusted to shape the radiation field to conform to the target volume (Fig. 34-6). The design of the field is digitized from a radiograph into a computer software program, which is transferred to the treatment room. The MLC machine receives a code that tells it how to position the individual leaves for the treatment field. Before MLC, custom-made lead blocks, or *cerrobend* blocks, were constructed to shape radiation fields and shield normal tissues from the beam of radiation. Heavy cerrobend blocks were placed within the head of the linac for each treatment field. Linacs equipped with the MLC package now receive a custom-designed field at the stroke of a computer keyboard. Today, multileaf collimators can be programmed to move across the radiation field during a treatment to alter the intensity of the radiation beam. Altering the beam intensity across the radiation field allows a lower dose to be delivered to normal structures and tissues and ensures the tumor or target receives the prescribed dose. This technique is called *intensity modulated radiation therapy* (IMRT). IMRT allows the dose of radiation to be more tightly conformed to the target areas and has greatly reduced the dose to normal tissues and structures. IMRT is widely used and has replaced the conventional treatment field approach for many cancers, such as prostate and gynecologic cancers in the pelvis and cancers of the head and neck. IMRT can be used for almost any anatomic site.

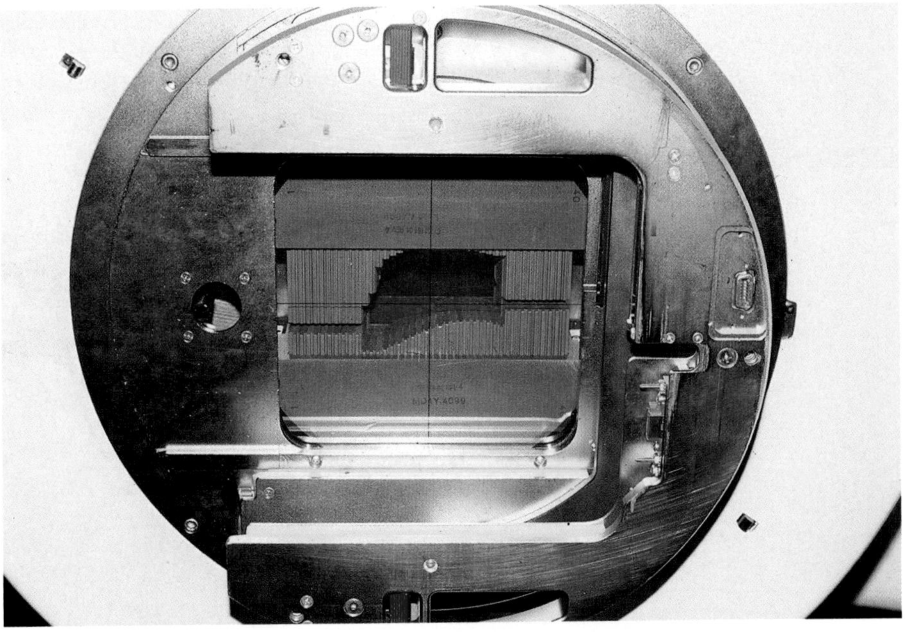

Steps in Radiation Oncology
SIMULATION

The first step of radiation therapy involves determining the volume of tissue that needs to be encompassed within the radiation field. This is done with a *CT simulator.* During simulation, the radiation oncologist uses the patient's CT images or MRI to determine the tumor's precise location and to design a treatment volume, or area. The treatment volume often includes the tumor plus a small margin, the draining lymphatics that are at risk for involvement, and a rim of normal tissue to account for patient movement.

Most centers perform virtual simulations using a CT scanner equipped with radiation oncology software tools (Fig. 34-7). Before CT simulators, the films taken with the conventional fluoroscopic simulator were done first to outline and localize areas to be treated. After the simulation, a CT scan was done with the patient in treatment position. The CT information was interfaced into the radiation oncology treatment planning computer for development of the treatment plan. CT simulation combines the two aforementioned steps into one. First, CT images necessary to plan the treatment are obtained; second, a treatment isocenter is selected. The traditional marks to be placed on the patient are made with the unit's sophisticated patient marking system, and digitally reconstructed images similar to standard simulation radiographs that depict the anatomy are processed. This system enables a more accurate design of treatment fields and facilitates the implementation of three-dimensional treatment planning.

Fig. 34-6 Multileaf collimation system on the treatment head.

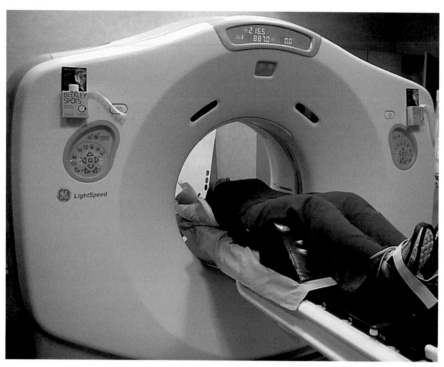

Fig. 34-7 CT simulator.

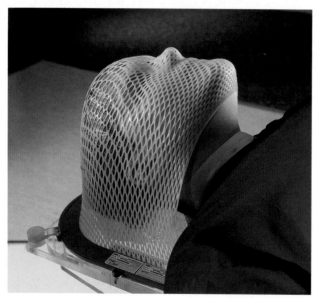

Fig. 34-8 Aquaplast mask.

CT simulation is to position the patient in a manner that is stable and reproducible for each of the 28 to 40 radiation treatments. Therapists are responsible for constructing immobilization devices to help patients hold their position. It is crucial for a patient to hold still and maintain the same position. If the patient does not maintain the planned position, critical normal tissues may be irradiated, or the tumor may not be irradiated. Immobilization devices greatly assist the radiation therapist in correctly aligning the patient for each treatment, and many patients feel more secure when supported by these devices. Immobilization devices can be constructed for any part of the body but are most important for more mobile parts, such as the head and neck region or the limbs. Many different types of immobilization systems exist. Fig. 34-8 shows a thermoplastic device that secures the head and neck against rotation or flexion-extension. Fig. 34-9 shows a vacuum bag device that may be used to secure upper body or lower extremities.

Contrast material is often administered before or during a simulation to localize the area that needs to be treated or to identify vital normal structures that are to be shielded. A small amount of meglumine diatrizoate (Gastrografin or Gastroview) for CT simulation is injected into the rectum of a patient with rectal cancer to assist in localizing the rectum on the simulation images. In Fig. 34-10, contrast material in the bladder is used to assist in localizing the prostate gland, which lies directly inferior to the bladder. Rectal contrast material is used to show the relationship of the rectum to the prostate to monitor and minimize the dose the rectum receives (Fig. 34-11).

When a CT simulation is performed, a reference isocenter is marked on the patient, and a pilot or scout scan is obtained. The radiation oncologist uses the scout or pilot image to determine the superior and inferior extent of the area to be scanned. The CT data are transferred to the virtual simulation computer workstation. From this limited scan, the physician reviews the CT images and uses imaging tools to outline the target volume and critical normal structures. The physician establishes the actual treatment isocenter. The computer software determines the change in location from the coordinates associated with the reference marks to the newly established treatment isocenter. The radiation therapist adjusts the couch and uses the laser marking system to apply these shifts to mark the treatment isocenter on the patient. The radiation therapist records all details regarding the patient's position in the treatment chart, and the patient is dismissed.

The physician creates treatment fields (length and width) electronically with the CT virtual simulation software (Fig. 34-12). The CT simulation data are transferred to the treatment planning system. In complex cases, the physician communicates preferences for treatment goals to the dosimetrist, who then designs the beam's eye view treatment fields and beam arrangement as part of the three-dimensional planning. A digitally reconstructed radiograph (DRR) for each treatment field is produced. The DRR is analogous to the radiograph taken in the conventional simulator (Fig. 34-13).

Precise measurements and details about the field dimensions, machine position, and patient positioning are recorded in the treatment chart. In some centers, the treatment parameters, such as field length, width, couch, and gantry positions, are electronically captured and transferred to the treatment unit. Recording of this information is crucial so that the radiation therapist performing the treatment can precisely reproduce the exact information.

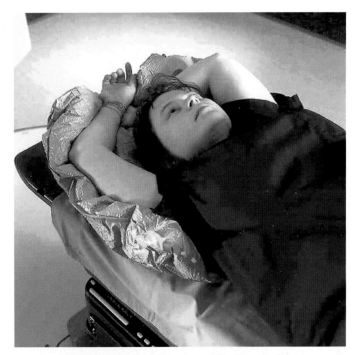

Fig. 34-9 Vacuum bag immobilization device.

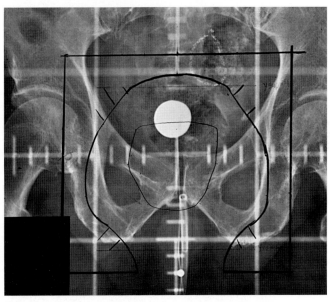

Fig. 34-10 AP pelvic radiograph from fluoro simulator showing contrast material in the bladder and relationship of bladder to the prostate gland.

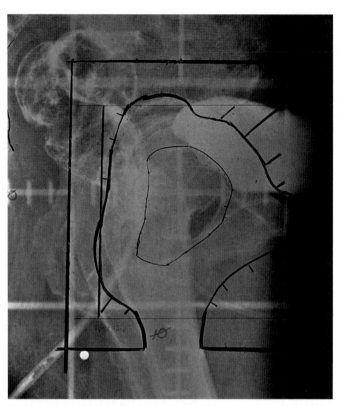

Fig. 34-11 Lateral radiograph from fluoro simulator showing contrast material in the rectum and bladder and relationship of rectum and bladder to the prostate gland.

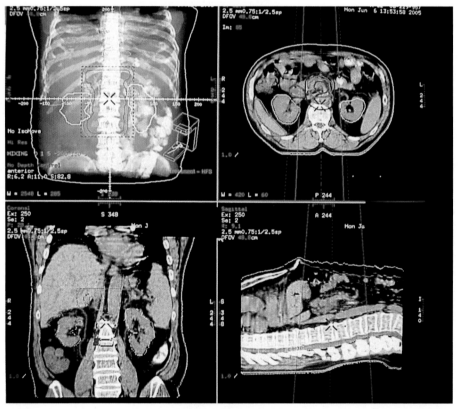

Fig. 34-12 Virtual CT simulation. Note divergent radiation beam lines indicating the path of the beam. Target volume, kidneys, and spinal cord have been outlined on CT axial image and reconstructed sagittal and coronal images. Treatment field outline is seen on DRR and coronal image.

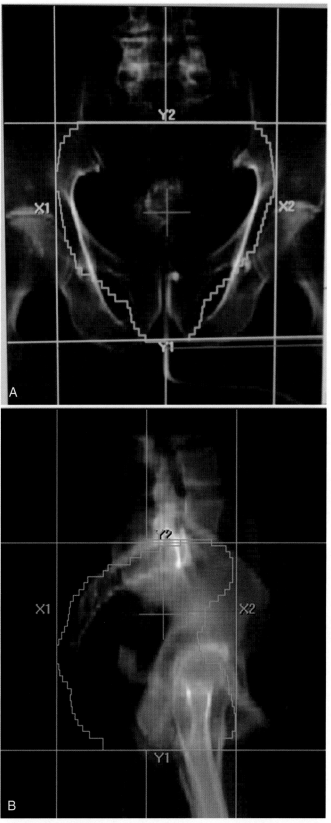

Fig. 34-13 DRR of AP and lateral pelvis. Note outlining of treatment field.

DOSIMETRY

Dosimetry refers to the measurement of radiation dose, and it shows how the radiation is distributed or *attenuated* throughout the patient's body (absorbing medium). The dosimetrist devises a treatment plan that best fulfills the physician's prescription for the desired dose to the *tumor/ target volume,* while minimizing the amount of radiation to critical normal structures or tissues.

Each organ of the body has a tolerance dose to radiation that limits the amount it can receive and still function normally. If an organ receives an excess of the tolerance dose, the organ can fail, resulting in a fatal complication. The kidneys are among the more radiosensitive structures of the body (Table 34-7). A dose greater than 2500 cGy can result in fatal radiation nephritis. The spinal cord has a higher tolerance dose, but many tumors require even higher doses for treatment to be effective.

Precise localization of dose-limiting structures and their relationship with the target volume is crucial for adequate planning. The dosimetrist must devise a plan that delivers a homogeneous dose to the tumor, while not exceeding the tolerance dose of a specific organ. This task can be quite challenging. The radiation oncologist might prescribe 6000 cGy to treat lung cancer located in the mediastinum directly over the spine but must limit the spinal cord dose to 4500 cGy to prevent

irreparable damage, which could result in paralysis. The dosimetrist must devise a plan that enables combined treatment and protection to be accomplished.

The first step in dosimetry is to obtain a contour or CT scan of the patient in treatment position. A *contour* is an outline of the external surface of the patient's body at the level of the central axis (center of treatment field). This contour is typically performed in the transverse plane, but other planes may be used. Then the tumor volume and critical dose-limiting internal structures are transferred from the simulation radiographs and drawn onto the contour. CT scans from a CT simulator are more commonly used than contours. With CT scanning, the tumor and internal structures and their relationships are directly visible. These images are interfaced with the treatment planning computer system for development of the plan.

PET and MRI with the patient in treatment position are also obtained sometimes to facilitate the planning process. Fusion of MRI or PET images onto the CT simulation data set allows a more precise delineation of the tumor volume than what would be seen on CT alone. To obtain an even distribution of radiation to the target volume, radiation is delivered from various angles, all focused on the area of interest. Three-dimensional treatment planning allows for the design of a beam that exactly conforms to the shape of the

tumor at any plane within the body. The treatment planning computer can digitally reconstruct the anatomy, which allows the dosimetrist to manipulate the image to view the tumor from any angle or plane. Important critical anatomic structures such as the kidneys and spinal cord are also more readily identified. Such a system allows the dosimetrist to plan and design beams that are coplanar and noncoplanar, tightly conforming to the target or tumor volume. This is known as *three-dimensional conformal radiotherapy* (CRT). The beam's eye view obtained by three-dimensional beams allows higher doses of radiation to be administered more safely by treating the cancer through multiple fields (more than four) on different planes, which reduces the amount of dose that normal tissues receive (Fig. 34-14).

The standard approach for a tumor located in the pelvis, such as rectal cancer, is the use of three fields— posteroanterior, right lateral, and left lateral. Using the treatment parameters established in the simulator, the dosimetrist enters this information into the treatment planning computer, designs beam's eye view conformal fields, and obtains an isodose distribution, which shows how the radiation is being deposited. An *isodose line/curve* is a summation of areas of equal radiation dosage and may be stated as percentages of the total prescribed dose or as actual radiation dosages in *gray* (Gy) units.

TABLE 34-7

Tolerance doses to radiation

Structure	Tolerance dose (cGy)
Testes	500
Ovary	500
Lung (whole lung)	1800
Kidney (whole organ)	2300
Liver (whole organ)	3000
Spinal cord (5 cm³)	4500

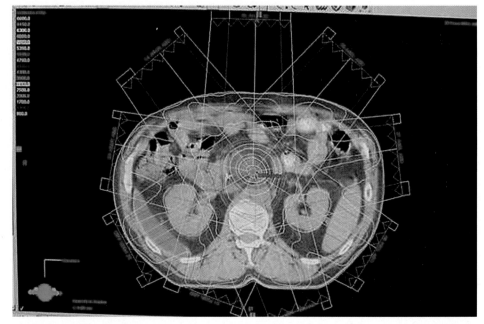

Fig. 34-14 Dosimetry plan showing nine different radiation fields used to treat pancreatic tumor.

The dosimetrist optimizes the plan by eliminating any areas of dose inhomogeneity (e.g., hot spots). A *hot spot* is an area of excessive radiation dose. One method to adjust for hot spots is to add a *wedge filter*. This wedge-shaped device is made of lead and is placed within the radiation beam to absorb the radiation preferentially, altering the shape of the isodose curve (Fig. 34-15). Another method of reducing hot spots is to change the weighting of the radiation beams by delivering a greater dose of radiation from the anterior field than from the posterior field.

Another major task of the dosimetrist is to monitor the dose that critical structures are receiving and to keep the dose within the established guidelines dictated by the physician. To avoid treating the spinal cord in the aforementioned example, the dosimetrist may angle the entry points of the radiation beams to include the target volume, while not irradiating the spinal cord. The resultant fields might be right anterior oblique and left posterior oblique (RAO/LPO) fields. The dosimetrist evaluates the dose distribution after each modifier is added and looks at different combinations of wedges, beam weighting, and beam entry points until an acceptable plan is produced. This technique is called *forward planning*. The final plan directs the radiation therapist, who treats the patient, how to proceed. For the example presented previously (i.e., lung cancer in the mediastinum directly over the spine), the plan might consist of the following:

1. Do 25 treatments anteroposterior (AP) and posteroanterior (PA) fields, RAO and LPO, 30 degrees off vertical.
2. Reduce field size to 12 cm long; do five more treatments AP, PA, RAO, and LPO, 30 degrees off vertical.

When the plan is complete, treatment of the patient can begin.

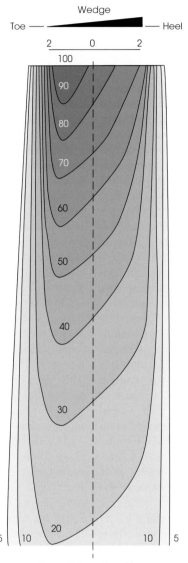

Fig. 34-15 Isodose curve obtained from ^{60}Co unit, with wedge placed between the source and absorbing material.

Another type of three-dimensional treatment planning is IMRT. The planning process begins as previously described—the physician identifies target volume and critical structures. Treatment fields are designed and arranged so that the target receives the prescribed dose, and the dose to critical structures is limited. The optimization of the dose distribution is not done, however, by trying different combinations of wedges or dose weighting as in conventional forward planning. IMRT uses a method called inverse planning. The prescribed dose to the target and the dose limit assigned to each critical structure are entered into the inverse planning system. A sophisticated mathematic algorithm creates a dose distribution that conforms to the target area, while sparing critical normal structures. This is achieved by modifying the intensity of radiation within the treatment field. This is accomplished by moving the multileaf collimator across the radiation field during a treatment from open to closed position, modulating the intensity of a beam to obtain the desired dose. The plan is computed by dividing the treatment field beam into hundreds of beamlets. Each beamlet can have an intensity level that measures from 0% to 100%. The intensity of a beamlet is changed by maintaining the multileaf collimator open for a specific amount of time and then closing it.

The IMRT planning process is time intensive and requires a comprehensive physics quality assurance check of multileaf collimator movement and dose verification before treatment is administered for the first time. IMRT has proven to be better at minimizing the dose to normal structures than conventional three-dimensional CRT and has allowed higher doses to be delivered to the target or tumor volume. IMRT was initially used for prostate cancer and cancers of the head and neck region. In prostate cancer treatment, IMRT optimized the dose to the prostate, while substantially minimizing the dose to the rectum. When treating a cancer in the head and neck region (e.g., nasopharynx), IMRT significantly reduced the dose to the parotid gland and spinal cord. IMRT is also used in the treatment of brain tumors, gastrointestinal, gynecologic, lung, breast, and soft tissue sarcomas.

The advantages of IMRT are well known—a method to deliver a highly conformal dose of radiation to the tumor while reducing the dose received by normal tissues. One disadvantage of IMRT is the total time it takes to deliver the daily session of radiation therapy. A patient with head and neck cancer might be on the table for 30 minutes each day to deliver radiation from 10 to 18 different radiation fields. The patient might move between or during the time the radiation beam is on. A new method of delivering IMRT treatment called volumetric modulated arc therapy (VMAT) has been developed. This method involves the linac rotating around the patient while the radiation beam is on and while the MLC leaves are moving for the IMRT delivery. With VMAT, the dose to the target and normal tissues is customized by altering the speed of the rotation, altering the dose rate of the linac, and simultaneously moving the MLC leaves. VMAT results in the delivery of the same highly conformal dose to the target while sparing normal tissues but in about half the time of a traditional IMRT stationary field technique. VMAT is also being used for prostate, lung, gynecologic, and gastrointestinal cancers. It is being explored for other tumor sites.

TREATMENT

On completion of the planning stage, including simulation and dosimetry, patient treatment can begin. The radiation therapist positions the patient and aligns the skin marks according to what was recorded in the treatment chart at the time of simulation. Accuracy and attention to detail are crucial for precise administration of the radiation to the patient. The radiation therapist is responsible for interpreting the radiation oncologist's prescription and calculating the correct monitor units, to achieve a desired dose of radiation for each treatment field. This responsibility also involves recording the daily administration of the radiation and the cumulative dose to date.

Precision in positioning the machine, proper selection of treatment field and MLC, accurate placement of cerrobend blocks or wedges, and implementation of any change in a patient's treatment plan are crucial for ensuring optimal treatment. Failure to do any of these may result in an overdose to normal tissue, causing long-term side effects, or underexposure of the tumor, reducing the patient's chance for cure. Most radiation oncology departments use an electronic radiation oncology medical record and computer verification system that ensures a patient's treatment parameters are correct before treatment may begin. The complexity of three-dimensional CRT and IMRT treatments with the numerous positions of the treatment couch, gantry, or collimator necessitates the use of a verification system. The computer verification system compares the machine settings with the information in the patient's electronic radiation chart. If there is a mismatch between any of the parameters in the electronic chart and what is being set up for treatment, the radiation therapist would be unable to initiate treatment. When a mismatch occurs, a computer prompt appears, highlighting the areas of disagreement. The radiation therapist must double-check parameters and patient setup, making corrections before treatment may occur. The verification and record system also records and adds the cumulative radiation doses.

Most linacs are now equipped with electronic portal imaging devices (EPIDs) and a kilovolt (kV) imager. These retractable imaging devices produce a digital image that is displayed immediately on a computer screen adjacent to the linac computer console. The EPID imager uses the 6-MV beam of the linac to obtain an image. Most radiation oncology departments have linacs equipped with a kV x-ray tube and flat panel image detector in addition to EPID. The kV imager, called an on board imager (OBI), provides a better diagnostic quality image with improved skeletal to soft tissue contrast compared with the megavoltage EPID imagers. These images can be viewed before treatment, and adjustments can be made before treating the patient, ensuring accurate and precise treatment. Some systems have computer software that compares the CT simulation image with the EPID or kV image using a registration algorithm. The computer automatically calculates the necessary adjustments (e.g., shift in couch position) to be made. The radiation therapist makes the adjustments and begins treatment.

When this treatment is used in cases of prostate cancer, gold seed markers are injected into the prostate gland before simulation. After the CT simulation is performed, the patient's treatment plan is completed, and treatment begins. The radiation therapist positions the patient, aligns the treatment machine, and takes an anterior and lateral or oblique kV image. The images are analyzed, and the computer generates any necessary shifts. These adjustments in couch or collimator position are made before initiating treatment. This process is done daily. Many treatment systems or situations also require the radiation therapist to analyze the kV images, compare skeletal anatomy to CT simulation DRR, and make adjustments to the couch position before treating the patient (Fig. 34-16).

If the patient has been positioned correctly, why do these changes or errors in treatment field position occur? Patient movement during treatment has always been a major constraint in providing accurate and precise delivery of radiation treatments. Improvements in immobilization devices have been made; however, they do not prevent internal organ movement. The prostate may move and be in a different position within the treatment field from day to day or even during treatment because of the filling of the rectum or bladder. Tumor or organ movement can also occur because of normal respiration. This movement can result in a geographic miss of the tumor or irradiation of critical normal structures.

Because movement of internal structures does occur, many technologic innovations are being developed to address this issue. Obtaining daily kV or EPID images before treatment is one method. Another means of ensuring the prostate is in the correct position is with B-mode acquisition technology (BAT). A transabdominal ultrasound scan is performed before treatment. The ultrasound wand or arm location coordinates are registered to the table and treatment isocenter. Computer algorithms similar to the kV or EPID gold seed compare images and determine whether any shifts are needed. Adjustments in couch position are made, and the treatment is delivered.

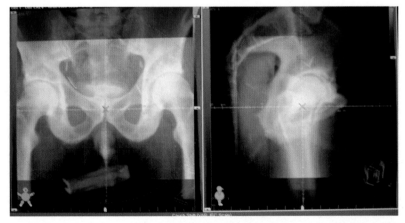

Fig. 34-16 OBI kV image overlaid on CT DRR; therapists shift couch to match skeletal anatomy.

The process of using images such as EPID, kV, or BAT to verify the treatment field position daily before treatment is known as *image-guided radiation therapy* (IGRT). Other methods of IGRT involve the use of a CT scan, an infrared camera system, or a sophisticated tracking system that uses two x-ray tubes mounted 90 degrees apart. In addition, there are two newly developed treatment units, Tomo-Therapy and the CyberKnife, which combine IGRT and innovative treatment delivery. These various IGRT methods are discussed subsequently.

The use of a CT scan before treatment as a means of IGRT is becoming quite common. A CT scan is obtained with the patient in treatment position, immediately before treatment, to verify target, isocenter, and patient position. This method is accomplished in one of two ways. One approach is to equip the linac with a kV x-ray tube and panel detector that obtains a cone-beam CT image when the accelerator gantry rotates a complete 360 degrees. The kV x-ray tube also provides a means of obtaining diagnostic quality images for treatment and patient position verification as previously discussed (Fig. 34-17). Another technique is using the linac's megavoltage beam and EPID imager to acquire a cone-beam CT image. The cone-beam CT image is obtained in the same fashion, by rotating the linac 360 degrees. The kV cone-beam CT image provides better contrast and soft tissue delineation

than megavoltage CT. The megavoltage CT images are of a high enough quality to compare target position and related bony anatomy to determine if any adjustments in patient or couch position are necessary before treatment. Another method of CT image guidance is having a CT scanner located in the actual treatment room opposite the linac, near the foot end of the treatment couch. The scanner can be moved into position to obtain a CT scan with the patient positioned for treatment. The most common method is the use of the linac to obtain a cone-beam CT image.

The infrared camera is a complex system that detects respiratory motion during simulation and treatment. This is a technique called *respiratory gating*. A reflective marker box is placed on the external surface of the patient's abdomen during simulation. The infrared camera detects the marker box, and a special computer software program connected to the infrared camera monitors the marker box movement (Fig. 34-18). The movement of the reflective marker is correlated with the patient's diaphragm position during the CT simulation. The respiratory cycle is evaluated relative to the treatment target volume and diaphragm movement. A specific portion of the respiratory cycle that has the least amount of motion is selected as the gated interval. This information is saved as a tolerance or standard to use during treatment. When the patient is treated, the reflective marker box is placed

on the same place on the abdomen, and an infrared camera is used to monitor the movement of the box. Pretreatment portal images (AP and lateral) to verify patient position, isocenter location, and gating interval are obtained with the EPID or kV imager. When approved, the radiation therapist initiates treatment. The respiratory gating computer monitors the marker box movement and automatically turns off the radiation beam if the marker moves out of the acceptable gated interval. Treatment automatically begins again when the marker box returns to the acceptable position. Respiratory gating has been done in various ways. One method is to have patients breathe freely, whereas another method is to have patients exhale and hold their breath.

The ExacTrac/Novalis Body system by BrainLab AG (Heimstetten, Germany) is a system that uses two kV x-ray tubes mounted in the floor 90 degrees apart that project a beam at 45-degree angles to the patient through the linac isocenter. The flat panel detectors are located in the ceiling. This sophisticated system is able to analyze the stereoscopic images and compare bony anatomy or implanted fiducial markers with the digital radiographs from simulation. The computer system calculates shifts in six dimensions rather than using the typical three-dimensional imaging. When the radiation therapist has acknowledged the recommended shifts, the information is sent to the robotic

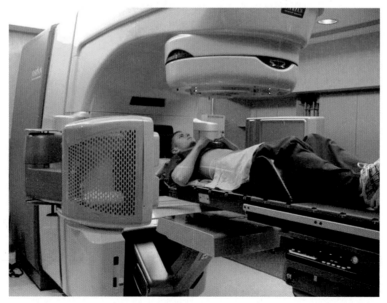

Fig. 34-17 Linac equipped with kV x-ray tube and flat panel detector. EPID is extended underneath the patient.

couch, and the adjustments are made automatically from outside the treatment room. The ExacTrac system may be used to take images anytime during treatment for real-time tracking of target motion during treatment as in respiratory gating. ExacTrac is commonly used for the treatment of head and neck cancers, prostate cancer, lung cancer, and small centrally located brain tumors and for stereotactic radiation therapy (SRT).

SRT is similar to stereotactic radiosurgery (SRS) in that the area being treated is small and surrounded by critical structures. The difference is that SRS is a large dose delivered in one treatment and is typically used for intracranial lesions. SRT is a conventional dose delivered in a fractionated manner using very focused small beams while the patient is rigidly immobilized. This technique is typically for intracranial lesions. SRT has been expanded to include tumors within the body. The treatment involves delivering larger doses of radiation per treatment than conventional treatment with a smaller number of total treatments. A patient may receive only three to five total treatments but the dose may be similar to that of conventional treatment. This new technique is called stereotactic body radiation therapy. Stereotactic body radiation therapy (SBRT) is being used for small lesions in the lung, liver, pancreas, other

bone metastasis, and spine of patients who cannot undergo surgery.

TomoTherapy

TomoTherapy is a new treatment unit that was developed at the University of Wisconsin in 2001 and was first used clinically in patients in 2004. TomoTherapy combines the principles of helical CT scanning with a 6-MV linac. The TomoTherapy unit resembles a CT scanner and operates in a similar fashion. The 6-MV gantry rotates in a continuous full circle while the couch and patient simultaneously move slowly through the aperture of the machine (Fig. 34-19). The TomoTherapy unit is equipped with computer-controlled multileaf collimators that move to modulate the radiation beam intensity. TomoTherapy provides IMRT in a helical pattern delivering highly conformal radiation to the specific prescribed anatomic regions, while sparing normal structures. The TomoTherapy unit also uses daily IGRT. Before initiating treatment, megavoltage CT of the patient is obtained. This newly acquired CT image is compared with the initial CT image used in planning the treatment to verify patient position. Any necessary shifts in isocenter location are made before treatment. TomoTherapy is another option of providing precise and conformal radiation therapy.

CyberKnife

The CyberKnife (Accuray Inc, Sunnyvale, CA) is a stereotactic radiosurgery system that uses a precise image guidance system for delivering a single treatment or two to five high-dose treatments called hypofractionated radiotherapy. The CyberKnife is a 6-MV linac housed within a robotic arm. The robotic arm has six different joints or axes that allow the delivery of radiation beams from thousands of angles from any direction around the patient (Fig. 34-20). The CyberKnife provides many more beam options to conform to the target or tumor than a traditional linac. The radiation beams are collimated to range in diameter from 5 to 60 mm. The small beams enter from various angles to conform tightly to the target, while sparing normal tissue, thereby allowing higher doses to be delivered.

The image guidance system consists of two diagnostic x-ray tubes mounted in the ceiling at 45-degree angles, offset 90 degrees from one another with two opposing amorphous silicon detectors located in the floor. The imaging system continually takes a set of images at each treatment angle and analyzes the images during treatment to track target and patient motion. The robotic arm is automatically adjusted to correct for any target or patient motion. The CyberKnife was the first system to use real-time tracking of target motion during treatment. The treatment

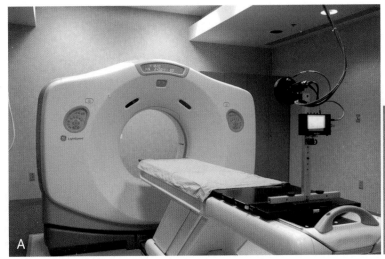
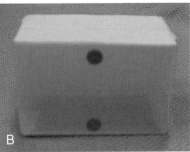

Fig. 34-18 A, Infrared camera system attached to CT simulator. **B,** Reflective marker box.

times for CyberKnife are 30 to 90 minutes. The CyberKnife is used to treat cancers of the lung, pancreas, brain, head and neck, spine, and prostate.

Even with all of these technologic advancements, the radiation therapist cannot become totally dependent or reliant on the sophisticated equipment. The radia-tion therapist must still use critical think-ing skills to analyze and assess why the couch parameters may need to be adjusted. Does the computer-generated shift make sense? Is the shift or collimator adjust-ment excessive? The radiation therapist must evaluate all aspects of the patient's setup and the computer information before automatically implementing such shifts.

The radiation therapist is also respon-sible for monitoring the patient's physical and emotional well-being. The radiation therapist is generally the only member of the radiation oncology team who sees the patient on a daily basis. The radiation

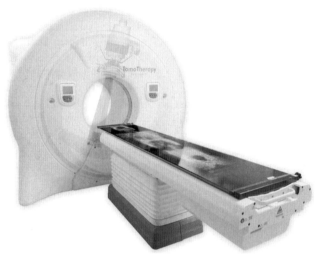

Fig. 34-19 TomoTherapy Hi-Art imaging and treatment system, which uses a megavoltage source for CT and for treatment.

(Courtesy TomoTherapy Incorporated. From Washington CM, Leaver DT, editors: *Principles and practice of radiation therapy,* ed 3, St Louis, 2010, Mosby.)

therapist monitors the patient's progress and assists in the management of any side effects. Acting as a liaison between the patient and the physician, the radiation therapist must know when to withhold treatment and when to refer the patient to be seen by the physician or oncology nurse for further evaluation. The daily interaction with the patient is the most rewarding aspect of the radiation therapist's job. Putting the patient at ease and making a cancer diagnosis and subsequent treatment a less traumatic experience is a satisfying aspect of this career. Patients often express their gratitude to radiation therapists for their care and support.

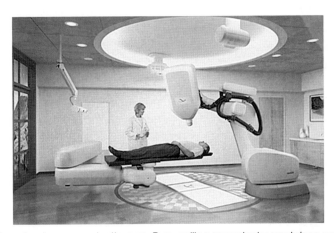

Fig. 34-20 Accelerator on a robotic arm. Two ceiling-mounted x-ray tubes are clearly shown.

(From Washington CM, Leaver DT, editors: *Principles and practice of radiation therapy,* ed 3, St Louis, 2010, Mosby.)

Clinical Applications

The amount of radiation prescribed depends on the type of tumor and the extent of the disease. Following are brief summaries of radiation therapy techniques used in the management of common forms of cancer.

LUNG CANCER

Treatment of lung cancer varies by type and stage. Radiation therapy is often used in conjunction with surgery and chemotherapy. A dose of 5000 to 6000 cGy of 10-MeV photons is often applied via a combination of AP, PA, and off-cord oblique fields. The primary tumor plus draining lymphatics are generally included in the treatment volumes (Fig. 34-21). More recently, the use of multiple oblique IMRT fields, VMAT, or a hybrid technique that incorporates both static fields and VMAT is used to treat lung cancer. These techniques provide a more conformal dose to the target volume while delivering less dose to normal lung and spinal cord than the traditional static AP-PA and oblique fields. SBRT is used for the treatment of medically inoperable patients with stage I non-small-cell lung cancers. One to five treatments with doses in the range of 1000 to 2000 cGy per treatment may be given for a total dose of 5000 to 6000 cGy.

PROSTATE CANCER

Definitive radiation therapy is a standard treatment for prostate cancer. Surgical removal of the prostate gland is another common approach to the management of this disease. Traditionally, a four-field technique of AP, PA, and right and left

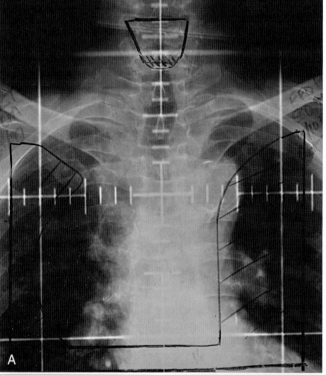

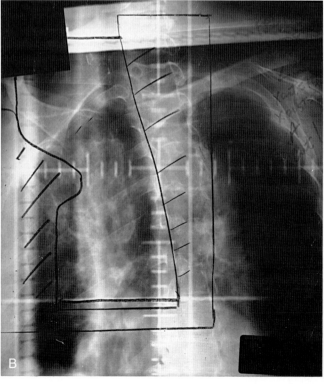

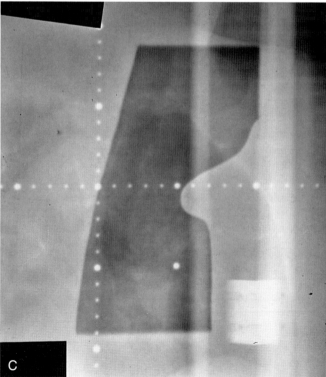

Fig. 34-21 A, AP lung field simulation radiograph. **B,** Off-cord oblique simulation radiograph. *Striped lines* in **A** and **B** indicate areas to be shielded. **C,** Off-cord oblique port radiograph.

lateral ports using a megavoltage beam of 10 MV or more is often used to deliver a dose of 7000 to 7600 cGy to the prostate gland. A series of six to eight oblique fields delivered with IMRT or VMAT to a dose of 7600 cGy is a common method of treatment for prostate cancer. Another method of treating limited, early-stage prostate cancer is a brachytherapy procedure known as prostate seed implant. This procedure involves the permanent implantation of 100 or more seeds of the radioisotope iodine-125 or palladium-103 into the prostate gland. A dose of 145 Gy is delivered with iodine-125 and a dose of 125 Gy is delivered with palladium-103.

HDR brachytherapy is another method for treating early-stage prostate cancer. This procedure is done on an outpatient basis and is a temporary implant. The patient has four HDR brachytherapy treatments. The interstitial needles are inserted early in the morning, then the patient has a morning and afternoon treatment. The patient comes back 2 to 3 weeks later for another two HDR treatments. Prostate cancer is one anatomic site that may be treated with protons.

HEAD AND NECK CANCERS

Numerous approaches may be used to treat head and neck cancers, depending on the location, size, and extent of the tumor. The most common method of treating head and neck cancer is with VMAT. VMAT allows a significant reduction in the dose to the parotid gland and spinal cord, while allowing a greater dose to be delivered to the target area. VMAT treatments are shorter in duration than the traditional IMRT technique for head and neck cancer. This makes the treatment more tolerable for the patient who is held in place on the table by a thermoplastic mask. VMAT is the newest IMRT method for delivering radiation to head and neck cancers.

CERVICAL CANCER

Early diagnosed cervical cancers can be treated with either surgery or radiation therapy. A four-field technique of AP, PA, and right and left lateral ports using a megavoltage unit, preferably 10 MV or greater, delivers 4500 to 5000 cGy in 5 weeks to an area of the primary and regional lymph nodes (Fig. 34-22). IMRT or VMAT are becoming common methods of treating cervical cancer. An intracavitary HDR implant is also included in the standard treatment of cervical cancer.

HODGKIN LYMPHOMA

The age of the patient and extent of the disease may determine treatment and prognosis for Hodgkin lymphoma. Involved field lymph node irradiation after chemotherapy is more commonly used than extended field therapy that included the lymphatic chain above or below the diaphragm. Treatment consists of chemotherapy followed by 2000 to 3000 cGy delivered through AP-PA fields or IMRT fields using a megavoltage unit. Chemotherapy may also be indicated for more advanced cases.

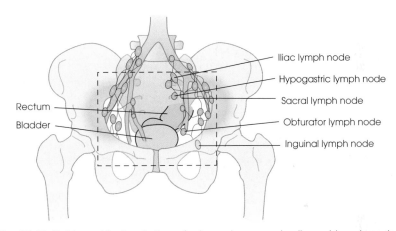

Fig. 34-22 Field used for irradiation of primary tumor and adjacent lymph nodes.

BREAST CANCER

Using two tangential fields to the chest wall or intact breast, megavoltage radiation delivers 5000 cGy in 5 weeks (Fig. 34-23). An electron boost to the site of initial lumpectomy adds an additional 1000 cGy. Irradiation of the axillary, supraclavicular, and internal mammary nodes to a dose of 5000 cGy is indicated for patients with a large primary tumor or node-positive disease. IMRT may also be used for the treatment of breast cancer. The breast is one location that respiratory gating may be utilized. A patient's breathing is monitored, and patients are instructed to hold their breath to limit internal organ motion while treatment commences. Respiratory gating limits the dose to the heart in patients with left-sided breast cancer.

Accelerated partial-breast irradiation (APBI) is a breast conservation method being studied as an alternative to whole breast irradiation. This treatment option may be offered to a subset of women who are older than 50 years of age with tumors of <3 cm located in the outer quadrant of the breast. The patient must have negative surgical margins and no lymph nodes involved. *Accelerated* is the term used because the treatment is delivered in 1 week with twice-a-day treatments using external beam or brachytherapy. The two commonly used brachytherapy applicators are MammoSite and SAVI. Both applicators are placed in the lumpectomy site. The MammoSite applicator is a balloon catheter that is placed in the lumpectomy cavity. The strut adjusted volume implant applica-tor (SAVI) has individual catheters in the shape of an eggbeater and is placed in the cavity created by the lumpectomy. The applicator used is hooked up to the HDR unit for treatment delivery. A total dose of 3400 cGy is delivered in the 1-week period. Chemotherapy, hormonal therapy, or both are also commonly used to treat breast cancer.

LARYNGEAL CANCER

Cancer of the larynx is best treated with megavoltage radiation. Tumors that are confined to the true vocal cord, with normal cord mobility, have a 90% 5-year cure rate; in addition, the voice remains useful. The method of treatment is usually accomplished by using small 2- × 2-inch (5- × 5-cm) opposing lateral wedged fields and delivering a dose of 6300 to 6500 cGy over a 6-week period.

SKIN CANCER

Carcinomas of the skin are usually squamous cell or basal cell lesions that may be treated with superficial radiation or surgery. Cure rates tend to be 80% to 90%, and basal cell lesions less than $\frac{3}{8}$ inch (1 cm) in diameter have a cure rate of almost 100%. The method of treatment is usually a single-field approach with attention given to shielding the uninvolved skin and delivering 4000 to 5000 cGy in a 3- to 4-week period.

MEDULLOBLASTOMA

Children with medulloblastoma are usually referred to the radiation oncology department after a biopsy and shunt procedure. The tumor is radiosensitive, and patients who have had treatment of the entire cerebrospinal axis have a 5-year cure rate of greater than 60%. The therapeutic approach tends to be complicated because the entire brain is irradiated with 3600 cGy, the spinal cord receives a dose of 2340 to 3600 cGy, and the cerebellum receives an additional dose of radiation to bring the total up to 5500 cGy (Fig. 34-24). This irradiation is usually accomplished with parallel opposed fields to the cranial vault and an extended single field to the spinal cord. The boost dose of 2000 cGy to the posterior fossa may be given with IMRT to provide better dose optimization to the target and less dose to critical structures. A megavoltage unit is used, with extreme care given to the areas of abutting fields. Medulloblastoma is one area that has been treated with proton therapy.

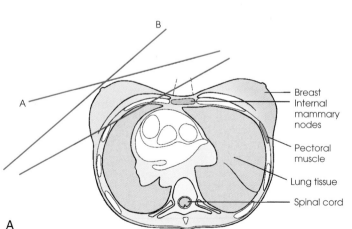

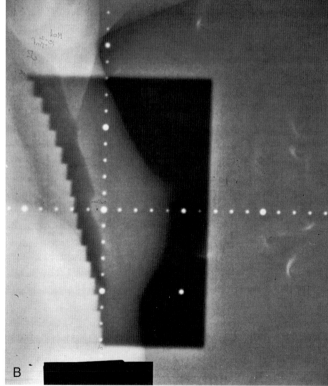

Fig. 34-23 A, Cross section of thorax showing field arrangements to irradiate the intact breast tangentially while sparing the lung (*lines A* and *B*). **B,** Port image of tangential breast field. Note sparing of lung tissue.

Future Trends

Radiation therapy has entered the electronic age with increased technologic advancement in the areas of dosimetry, simulation, and treatment. Most institutions use computer-interfaced accelerators with treatment verification software packages to ensure accurate treatment. Paperless treatment charting and filmless departments are the standard design of a facility. VMAT and IMRT are standard treatment techniques used in most facilities to treat various tumor types. Developments will continue to occur in the use of IGRT. Refinements in the application of linac cone-beam CT and other modalities, such as PET, to verify target, isocenter, and patient position before treatment will occur more routinely. Advancements and implementation of respiratory gating will permit better delineation of three-dimensional conformal target volumes, lessen the chance of a geographic miss of the target volume, and further minimize the dose to normal structures. The use of gating may permit higher doses to be prescribed and result in greater control and cure rates. The use of stereotactic body radiation therapy (SBRT) may expand for use in the treatment of other cancer sites within the body.

Linacs are the most commonly used equipment for treating malignant disease. There has been an increase more recently in the installation of proton facilities worldwide. Proton beams are not a new form of cancer treatment. The first use of a proton beam was in 1954 at the University of California in Berkeley; however, owing to the complexity, cost, and size of a cyclotron facility, protons were not widely implemented. Proton beams used therapeutically produce beams between 100 MeV and 250 MeV. The use of protons in the treatment of cancer is gaining in popularity again because of the characteristic properties of the proton beam. Proton beams have minimal scatter and deposit little energy as the beam first traverses tissue. As the protons slow down when they reach a certain depth, most (80%) of the energy or dose is deposited in tissue and then quickly falls to zero dose within millimeters.

This burst of energy deposited at a specific depth is termed the *Bragg peak*. The depth at which this peak deposition of dose occurs can be adjusted by changing the energy of the proton beam and adding beam modifiers. The principal advantage of the proton beam is the sparing of surrounding normal tissues. The proton beam can be precisely controlled to deliver the Bragg peak dose at a prescribed depth. The rapid fall-off of the beam allows treatment of the target while sparing critical structures located within millimeters of the target. Research regarding the effectiveness of protons and dosimetric planning initiatives including intensity-modulated proton therapy are currently being explored. Cost and space constraints are still a major barrier preventing many hospital-based facilities from implementing a proton therapy program. There has been an increase in the number of proton facilities in the United States with more centers under construction or in the planning stages.

Conclusion

From a questionable beginning, radiation therapy has emerged as one of the primary modalities used in the treatment of malignant disease. Radiation therapy departments are currently examining and treating approximately 75% of all patients with a new diagnosis of cancer. Radiation oncologists and radiation therapists are integral members of the health care team that discusses and selects the appropriate treatment regimens for all cancer patients.

As the factors that initiate cellular change, growth, and spread become better understood, the radiation treatments for cancer are expected to become even more effective. The irradiation techniques presently used may change dramatically based on this new information. In addition, new, more sophisticated radiation-producing equipment is currently under design and may lead to the reevaluation of presently accepted therapeutic techniques and dose levels. Finally, new chemotherapeutic agents are being produced that, when used by themselves or with other drugs, may enhance tumor sensitivity when used in conjunction with irradiation.

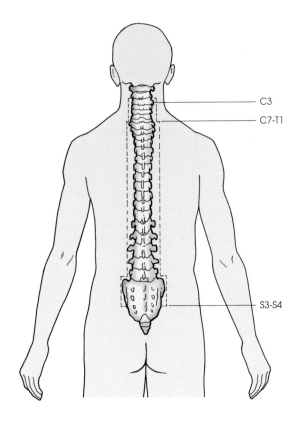

Fig. 34-24 Spinal treatment portal for medulloblastoma.

Conclusion

Definition of Terms

absorbed dose Amount of ionizing radiation absorbed per unit of mass of irradiated material.

accelerator (particle) Device that accelerates charged subatomic particles to great energies. These particles or rays may be used for direct medical irradiation and basic physical research. Medical units include linear accelerators, betatrons, and cyclotrons.

asymmetric jaws Four independent x-ray collimators that are used to define the radiation treatment field.

attenuation Removal of energy from a beam of ionizing radiation when it traverses matter, accomplished by disposition of energy in matter and by deflection of energy out of the beam.

betatron Electron accelerator that uses magnetic induction to accelerate electrons in circular path; also capable of producing photons.

biopsy Removal of a small piece of tissue for examination under the microscope.

brachytherapy Placement of radioactive nuclide or nuclides in or on a neoplasm to deliver a cancericidal dose.

cancer Term commonly applied to malignant disease; abnormal growth of cells; *neoplasm* (new growth) or *-oma* (tumor).

cancericidal dose Dose of radiation that results in the death of cancer cells.

carcinogen Any cancer-producing substance or material, such as nicotine, radiation, or ingested uranium.

carcinoma Cancer that arises from epithelial tissue—either glandular or squamous epithelium.

cerrobend block Beam-shaping device made of a lead alloy that attenuates the x-ray beam, preventing exposure of normal tissue.

chromosome Unit of genetic information that guides cytoplasmic activities of the cell and transmits hereditary information.

cobalt-60 Radioisotope with half-life of 5.26 years, average gamma ray energy of 1.25 MeV (range 1.17 to 1.33 MeV), and ability to spare skin with buildup depth in tissue of 0.5 cm.

collimator Diaphragm or system of diaphragms made of radiation-absorbing material that defines dimension and direction of beam.

conformal radiation Treatment designed to deliver radiation to the exact target volume as seen on any plane (e.g., transverse, sagittal, vertex views); requires a three-dimensional treatment planning system.

contour Reproduction of an external body shape, typically in the transverse plane at the level of the central axis of the beam; facilitates planning of radiation treatment. Other planes of interest may also be obtained.

cure Usually a 5-year period after completion of treatment during which time the patient exhibits no evidence of disease.

decay or disintegration Transformation of radioactive nucleus, resulting in emission of radiation.

differentiation Acquisition of cellular function and structure that differ from that of the original cell type.

direct effect Radiation that interacts with an organic molecule such as DNA, RNA, or a protein molecule. This interaction may inactivate the cell.

dosimetry Measurement of radiation dose in an absorbing medium.

epithelial tissue Cells that line the surfaces of serous and mucous membranes, including the skin.

etiology Study of causes of diseases.

external-beam treatment Delivery of radiation to a patient from a unit such as a linear accelerator in which the radiation enters the patient from the external surface of the body.

field Geometric area defined by collimator or radiotherapy unit at skin surface.

fractionation Division of total planned dose into numerous smaller doses to be given over a longer period. Consideration must be given to biologic effectiveness of smaller doses.

gamma ray Electromagnetic radiation that originates from radioactive nucleus and causes ionization in matter; identical in properties to x-ray.

gray (Gy) International unit for the quantity of radiation received by the patient; previously rad; 1 cGy = 1 rad.

grenz rays X-rays generated at 20 kVp or less.

half-life Time (specific for each radioactive substance) required for radioactive material to decay to half its initial activity; types are biologic and physical.

half-value layer Thickness of attenuating material inserted in beam to reduce beam intensity to half of the original intensity.

high-dose-rate brachytherapy Use of a high-activity radionuclide placed within the body for the treatment of cancer. Delivers more than 1200 cGy per hour.

image-guided radiation therapy (IGRT) Use of images to verify treatment isocenter, target, and patient positioning before initiating radiation treatment.

independent jaws X-ray collimator with four individual blades that can be moved independently of one another (see *asymmetric jaws*).

indirect effect Interaction of radiation with water molecules within the cell; results in the formation of free radicals OH, H, and HO_2, which can damage the cell.

intensity-modulated radiation therapy (IMRT) Modification of beam intensity to deliver nonuniform exposure across radiation field.

ionization Process in which one or more electrons are added to or removed from atoms, creating ions; can be caused by high temperatures, electrical discharges, or nuclear radiations.

ionizing radiation Energy emitted and transferred through matter that results in the removal of orbital electrons (e.g., x-rays or gamma rays).

isocentric Refers to rotation around a fixed point.

isodose line curve Curve or line drawn to connect points of identical amounts of radiation in a given field.

isotope Atoms that have the same atomic number but different mass numbers.

lesion Morbid change in tissue; mass of abnormal cells.

linear accelerator (linac) Device for accelerating charged particles, such as electrons, to produce high-energy electron or photon beams.

linear energy transfer (LET) Rate at which energy is deposited as it travels through matter.

low-dose-rate brachytherapy Use of a low-activity radionuclide placed within the body for treatment of cancer. Dose is slowly delivered, 40 to 500 cGy per hour, to a small volume of tissue over a period of days.

malignancy Cancerous tumor or lesion.

medical dosimetrist Person responsible for calculation of proper radiation treatment dose who assists the radiation oncologist in designing individual treatment plans.

medical physicist Specialist in the study of the laws of ionizing radiation and their interactions with matter.

metastasis Transmission of cells or groups of cells from primary tumor to sites elsewhere in body.

multileaf collimator (MLC) Individual collimator rods within the treatment head of the linear accelerator that can slide inward to shape radiation field.

oncologist Physician specializing in the study of tumors.

oncology Study of tumors.

palliation To relieve symptoms; not for cure.

pathologist Specialist in the study of the microscopic nature of disease.

prophylactic surgery Preventive surgical treatment.

radiation oncologist Physician who specializes in the use of ionizing radiation in treatment of disease.

radiation oncology Medical specialty involving the treatment of cancerous lesions using ionizing radiation.

radiation therapist Person trained to assist and take directions from the radiation oncologist in the use of ionizing radiation for treatment of disease.

radiation therapy Older term used to define the medical specialty involving treatment with ionizing radiation.

radioactive Pertaining to atoms of elements that undergo spontaneous transformation, resulting in emission of radiation.

radiocurable Susceptibility of neoplastic cells to cure (destruction) by ionizing radiation.

radiosensitivity Responsiveness of cells to radiation.

radium (Ra) Radionuclide (atomic number 88, atomic weight 226, half-life 1622 years) used clinically for radiation therapy. In conjunction with its subsequent transformations, radium emits alpha and beta particles and gamma rays. In encapsulated form, it is used for various intracavitary radiation therapy applications (e.g., for cervical cancer).

reactor Cubicle in which isotopes are artificially produced.

relative biologic effectiveness (RBE) Compares radiation beams with different LETs and their ability to produce a specific biologic response. Dose in gray from 250 kVp beam of x-rays/dose from another type of radiation to produce the same effect.

simulator Diagnostic x-ray machine that has the same geometric and physical characteristics as a radiation therapy treatment unit.

skin sparing In megavoltage beam therapy, reduced skin injury per centigray (cGy) exposure because electron equilibrium occurs below skin; occurs $\frac{1}{4}$ to 2 inches (0.6 to 5 cm) deep, depending on energy.

stereotactic radiation therapy Use of small focused radiation beams to treat small extracranial or intracranial lesions; delivered with conventional fractionation or in two to five treatments instead of a single treatment as in stereotactic radiosurgery. Rigid immobilization of involving patient is required.

stereotactic radiosurgery Use of multiple, narrow, highly focused radiation beams to deliver a large dose in a single treatment to a small intracranial lesion. The patient is immobilized with a fixed stereotactic head frame.

surgical bed Area of excision and adjacent tissues manipulated during surgery.

systemic Throughout the human body.

teletherapy Radiation therapy technique for which the source of radiation is at some distance from the patient.

treatment field Anatomic area outlined for treatment (e.g., AP or RL pelvis).

tumor/target volume Portion of anatomy that includes tumor and adjacent areas of invasion.

undifferentiation Lack of resemblance of cells to cells of origin.

wedge filter Wedge-shaped beam attenuating device used to absorb beam preferentially to alter the shape of the isodose curve.

Selected bibliography

Accuray, Available at: www.accuray.com. Accessed June 6, 2009.

American Cancer Society: *Cancer facts and figures 2013*, Atlanta, 2013, American Cancer Society.

Berson AM et al: Clinical experience using respiratory gated radiation therapy: comparison of free-breathing and breath-hold techniques, *Int J Radiat Oncol Biol Phys* 60:419, 2004.

Boyer AL: The physics of intensity-modulated radiation therapy, *Phys Today* 55:38, 2002.

BrainLab, Available at: www.BrainLab.com. Accessed June 6, 2009.

Brenner DJ: Dose, volume, and tumor-control predictions in radiotherapy, *Int J Radiat Oncol Biol Phys* 26:171, 1993.

Chan OS et al: The superiority of hybrid-volumetric arc therapy (VMAT) technique over double arcs VMAT and 3D-conformal technique in the treatment of locally advanced non-small cell lung cancer—a planning study, *Radiother Oncol* 101:298, 2011.

Chang JY et al: Image-guided radiation therapy for non-small cell lung cancer, *J Thorac Oncol* 3:177, 2008.

Chang SD et al: An analysis of the accuracy of the Cyberknife: a robotic frameless stereotactic radiosurgical system, *Neurosurgery* 52:140, 2003.

Cheng J et al: Comparison of intensity modulation radiation therapy treatment techniques for nasopharyngeal carcinoma, *Int J Radiat Oncol Biol Phys* 96:126, 2001.

Chirag S et al: The American Brachytherapy Society consensus statement for accelerated partial breast irradiation, *Brachy* 12:267, 2013.

Chuong MA et al: Stereotactic body radiation therapy for locally advanced and borderline resectable pancreatic cancer is effective and well tolerated, *Int J Radiat Oncol Biol Phys* 86:516, 2013.

Coleman A: Treatment procedures. In Washington CM, Leaver DT, editors: *Principles and practices of radiation therapy,* ed 3, St Louis, 2010, Mosby.

Damien C et al: Intensity modulated proton and photon therapy for early prostate cancer with or without transperineal injection of a polyethylene glycol spacer: a treatment planning comparison study, *Int J Radiat Oncol Biol Phys* 84:e311, 2012.

Das IJ et al: Intensity-modulated radiation therapy dose prescription, recording and delivery: patterns of variability among institutions and treatment planning systems, *J Natl Cancer Inst* 100:300, 2008.

Dawson LA, Jaffray DA: Advances in image-guided radiation therapy, *J Clin Oncol* 25:938, 2007.

Dieterich SP Pawlicki TP: CyberKnife image-guided delivery and quality assurance, *Int J Radiat Oncol Biol Phys* 71:126, 2008.

Dische S: Radiotherapy in the nineties: increase in cure, decrease in morbidity, *Acta Oncol* 31:501, 1992.

Elekta, Available at: http://www.elekta.com/healthcare_international_gamma_knife_surgery.php. Accessed June 6, 2009.

Furlow B: Three-dimensional conformal radiation therapy, *Radiat Therapist* 12:131, 2003.

Gierga DP et al: The correlation between internal and external markers for abdominal tumors: implications for respiratory gating, *Int J Radiat Oncol Biol Phys* 61:1551, 2005.

Gillin MT: Special procedures. In Washington CM, Leaver DT, editors: *Principles and practices of radiation therapy,* ed 3, St Louis, 2010, Mosby.

Goetein M et al: Treating cancer with protons, *Phys Today* 55:45, 2002.

Grabowski CM et al: Factors predictive of completion of treatment and survival after palliative radiation therapy, *Radiology* 184:329, 1992.

Greenlee RT et al: Cancer statistics 2001, *CA Cancer J Clin* 51:15, 2001.

Hovington JA et al: Treatment of stage I and II non-small cell lung cancer, *Chest* 143(Suppl):e2788, 2013.

Jaffray DA et al: Flat-panel cone-beam computed tomography for image-guided radiation therapy, *Int J Radiat Oncol Biol Phys* 53:1337, 2002.

Jessup JM et al: Diagnosing colorectal carcinoma: clinical and molecular approaches, *CA Cancer J Clin* 47:70, 1997.

Landis SH et al: Cancer statistics, 1998, *CA Cancer J Clin* 48:6, 1998.

Leaver D: Intensity modulated radiation therapy: part 2, *Radiat Therapist* 12:17, 2003.

Leaver D et al: Simulation procedures. In Washington CM, Leaver DT, editors: *Principles and practices of radiation therapy,* ed 3, St Louis, 2010, Mosby.

Lipa LA, Mesina CF: Virtual simulation in conjunction with 3-D conformal therapy, *Radiat Therapist* 2:99, 1995.

Marks JE, Armbruster JS: Accreditation of radiation oncology in the US, *Int J Radiat Oncol Biol Phys* 24:863, 1992.

Mell LK et al: A survey of intensity-modulated radiation therapy use in the United States, *Cancer* 98:204, 2003.

Morgan HM: Quality assurance of computer controlled radiotherapy treatments, *Br J Radiol* 65:409, 1992.

National Association of Proton Therapy, Available at http://www.proton-therapy.org/map.htm.

National Cancer Institute: *Genetic testing for breast cancer risk: it's your choice,* Washington, DC, 1997, National Cancer Institute.

National Cancer Institute: *Radiation therapy for cancer: questions and answers,* Available at: http://www.cancer.gov/cancertopics/factsheet/Therapy/radiation. Accessed July 9, 2009.

Navarria P et al: Volumetric modulated arc therapy with flattening filter free beams for stereotactic body radiation therapy in patients with medically inoperable early stage non-small cell lung cancer, *Radiother Oncol* 107:414, 2013.

Order SE: Training in systemic radiation therapy, *Int J Radiat Oncol Biol Phys* 24:895, 1992.

Otto K: Volumetric modulated arc therapy: IMRT in a single gantry arc, *Med Phys* 35:310, 2008.

Palma D et al: Volumetric modulated arc therapy for delivery of prostate radiotherapy: comparison with intensity-modulated radiotherapy and three-dimensional conformal radiotherapy, *Int J Radiat Oncol Biol Phys* 72:996, 2008.

Palma D et al: New developments in arc radiation therapy: a review, *Cancer Treat Rev* 36:393, 2010.

Perez CA: Quest for excellence: ultimate goal of the radiation oncologist: astro Gold Medal address 1992, *Int J Radiat Oncol Biol Phys* 26:567, 1993.

Prado K, Prado C: Dose distributions. In Washington CM, Leaver DT, editors: *Principles and practices of radiation therapy,* ed 3, St Louis, 2010, Mosby.

Qi XS et al: Assessment of interfraction patient setup for head and neck cancer intensity modulated radiation therapy using multiple computed tomography based image guidance, *Int J Radiat Oncol Biol Phys* 86:432, 2013.

Ramsey CR, et al: A technique for adaptive image-guided helical tomotherapy for lung cancer, *Int J Radiat Oncol Biol Phys* 64:1237, 2006.

Rietzel E et al: Four-dimensional image-based treatment planning: target volume segmentation and dose calculation in the presence of respiratory motion, *Int J Radiat Oncol Biol Phys* 61:1535, 2005.

Roberge SL: Virtual reality: radiation therapy treatment planning of tomorrow, *Radiat Therapist* 2:113, 1996.

Sillanpaa J et al: Integrating respiratory gating into a megavoltage cone-beam CT system, *Int J Radiat Oncol Biol Phys* 60:197, 2004.

Simone CH II et al: Stereotactic body radiation therapy for lung cancer, *Chest* 143:1784, 2013.

TomoTherapy, Available at: www.tomotherapy.com. Accessed June 15, 2009.

Vlachaki MT et al: IMRT versus conventional 3D CRT on prostate and normal tissue dosimetry using an endorectal balloon for prostate localization, *Med Dosim* 30:69, 2005.

Wagner LK: Absorbed dose in imaging: why measure it? *Radiology* 178:622, 1991.

Washington CM, Leaver DT, editors: *Principles and practice of radiation therapy,* ed 3, St Louis, 2010, Mosby.

Weber DC et al: Intensity modulated proton and photon therapy for early stage prostate cancer with or without transperineal injection of a polyethylene glycol spacer: a treatment planning comparison study, *Int J Radiat Oncol Biol Phys* 84:e311, 2012.

Wilkinson B et al: Evaluation of current consensus statement recommendations for accelerated partial breast irradiation: a pooled analysis of William Beaumont Hospital and American Society of Breast Surgeon MammoSite Registry trial data, *Int J Radiat Oncol Biol Phys* 85:1179, 2013.

Yamada Y et al: A review of image-guided intensity modulated radiotherapy for spinal tumors, *Neurosurgery* 61:226. 2007.

Yashar CM et al: Initial clinical experience the (SAVI) Breast Brachytherapy Device for accelerated partial-breast irradiation (APBI): first 100 patients with more than 1 year of follow-up, *Int J Radiat Oncol Biol Phys* 80:765, 2011.

INDEX

A

AAA (abdominal aortic aneurysm), **2:**84t, **3:**41
  three-dimensional CT of, **3:**313f
AAA (abdominal aortic aneurysm) endografts, **3:**65-66, 65f-66f
Abbreviations
  for contrast arthrography, **2:**9b
  for digestive system, **2:**107b
  for general anatomy and radiographic positioning terminology, **1:**98b
  for long bone measurement, **2:**2b
  for lower limb, **1:**239b
  for pelvis and proximal femora, **1:**334b
  for preliminary steps in radiography, **1:**52b
  for shoulder girdle, **1:**181b
  for skull, **2:**284b
  for trauma radiography, **2:**30b
  for upper limb, **1:**109b
  for urinary system, **2:**189b
  for vertebral column, **1:**379b
  in Volume One, **1:**521t
  in Volume Two, **2:**475t
ABC (aneurysmal bone cyst), **3:**149, 149f
Abdomen, **2:**81-94
  abbreviations used for, **2:**85b
  anatomy of, **2:**83, 83f, 84b
  AP projection of
    in left lateral decubitus position, **2:**91, 91f-92f
      mobile, **3:**198-199, 198f-199f
      for trauma, **2:**40, 40f
    mobile, **3:**196, 196f-197f
      in left lateral decubitus position, **3:**198-199, 198f-199f
    in neonate, **3:**208-210
      evaluation criteria for, **3:**210b, 210f
      position of part for, **3:**208f-209f, 209
      position of patient for, **3:**208, 208f
      structures shown on, **3:**210, 210f
    in supine position (KUB), **2:**87, 89-90, 89f-90f
    for trauma, **2:**38-39, 38f-39f
      in left lateral decubitus position, **2:**40, 40f
    in upright position, **2:**89-90, 89f-90f
  in children, **3:**112-115
    image assessment for, **3:**123t
    with intussusception, **3:**114, 114f
    with pneumoperitoneum, **3:**115, 115f
    positioning and immobilization for, **3:**112f-113f, 113
  CT of, **3:**336f-338f
  divisions of, **1:**70, 70f

Page numbers followed by "f" indicate figures, "t" indicate tables, and "b" indicate boxes.

Abdomen *(Continued)*
  exposure technique for, **2:**86, 86f
  flat and upright images of, **2:**87
  immobilization for, **2:**86, 87f
  lateral projection of
    in neonate, **3:**211-212, 211f-212f
    in R or L dorsal decubitus position, **2:**94, 94f
    in R or L position, **2:**93, 93f
  mobile radiography of, **3:**196-199
    AP or PA projection in left lateral decubitus position for, **3:**198-199, 198f-199f
    AP projection for, **3:**196, 196f-197f
  MRI of, **3:**360, 360f-361f
  of neonate, **3:**208-212
    AP projection for, **3:**208-210
      evaluation criteria for, **3:**210b, 210f
      position of part for, **3:**208f-209f, 209
      position of patient for, **3:**208, 208f
      structures shown on, **3:**210, 210f
    lateral projection for, **3:**211-212, 211f-212f
  PA projection of, **2:**91, 91f
    in left lateral decubitus position (mobile), **3:**198-199, 198f-199f
  positioning protocols for, **2:**87
  sample exposure technique chart essential projections for, **2:**85t
  scout or survey image of, **2:**87
  sequencing of projections for, **2:**87-94, 87f-88f
  summary of pathology of, **2:**84t
  summary of projections of, **2:**82, 87
  three-way imaging of (acute abdomen series), **2:**87
  trauma radiography of, AP projection in, **2:**38-39, 38f-39f
    in left lateral decubitus position, **2:**40, 40f
  ultrasonography of, **3:**376-383, 376f-377f
Abdominal aorta
  MR angiography of, **3:**364f
  sectional anatomy of, **3:**282f, 284
    in axial (transverse) plane
      at Level A, **3:**285, 285f
      at Level B, **3:**285, 286f
      at Level C, **3:**287f
      at Level D, **3:**288, 288f
      at Level E, **3:**289, 289f
      at Level F, **3:**290, 290f
      at Level G, **3:**291, 291f
    in coronal plane, **3:**298-299, 298f-299f
    in sagittal plane, **3:**297f
Abdominal aortic aneurysm (AAA), **2:**84t, **3:**41
  three-dimensional CT of, **3:**313f
Abdominal aortic aneurysm (AAA) endografts, **3:**65-66, 65f-66f
Abdominal aortography, **3:**41, 41f
Abdominal cavity, **1:**68-69, 69f, **2:**83

Abdominal circumference, fetal ultrasound for, **3:**390, 390f
Abdominal duplex examinations, **3:**392
Abdominal fistulae and sinuses, **2:**180, 180f
Abdominal viscera, **2:**83f
Abdominal wall, ultrasonography of, **3:**383
Abdominopelvic cavity, **1:**68, 69f, **2:**83, 83f
Abdominopelvic region sectional anatomy, **3:**282-299
  on axial (transverse) plane, **3:**284f, 285
    at level A, **3:**285, 285f
    at level B, **3:**285, 286f
    at level C, **3:**287, 287f
    at level D, **3:**288, 288f
    at level E, **3:**289, 289f
    at level F, **3:**290, 290f
    at level G, **3:**291, 291f
    at level H, **3:**292, 292f
    at level I, **3:**293, 293f
    at level J, **3:**294, 294f
    at level K, **3:**295, 295f-296f
  on cadaveric image, **3:**282, 282f
  on coronal plane, **3:**298f-299f, 299
  on sagittal plane, **3:**296, 297f
Abduct/abduction, **1:**96, 96f
ABI (ankle/brachial index), **3:**393, 397
Abscess
  breast, **2:**395
  of epididymis, **2:**253f
Absorbed dose
  in nuclear medicine, **3:**408, 437
  in radiation oncology, **3:**506-507
AC articulation. *See* Acromioclavicular (AC) articulation.
Acanthion, **2:**272, 272f-273f, 285f
Acanthioparietal projection
  for cranial trauma, **2:**46, 46f
  of facial bones, **2:**327, 327f-328f
    for trauma, **2:**328, 328f
Accelerated partial-breast irradiation (APBI), **3:**504
Accelerators, particle, **3:**404, 425, 438, 506
Accessory glands of digestive system, **2:**97, 97f
Accessory process, **1:**374, 374f
Accountability in code of ethics, **1:**3
Acetabulum
  anatomy of, **1:**327, 327f, 329f-330f
  AP oblique projection of (Judet and modified Judet methods), **1:**356-357, 356f-357f
  comminuted fracture of, **3:**201f
  PA axial oblique projection of (Teufel method), **1:**354-355, 354f-355f
  sectional anatomy of, **3:**295-296, 299
Achalasia, **2:**109t
Acinus of breast, **2:**380
Acoustic impedance, **3:**371, 372f, 397-398
Acoustic neuroma, **2:**282t, **3:**357f

Acoustic window in transabdominal ultrasonography, **3:**387, 397
Acromial extremity of clavicle, **1:**175, 175f
Acromioclavicular (AC) articulation
    Alexander method for AP axial projection of, **1:**211-212, 211f-212f
    anatomy of, **1:**178t, 179f, 181, 181f
    Pearson method for bilateral AP projection of, **1:**209, 209f-210f
    sectional anatomy of, **3:**270, 272, 272f
Acromion, **3:**272, 273f
Acromion process, **3:**272f, 273
Acute abdomen series, **2:**87
AD. *See* Alzheimer disease (AD).
AD (architectural distortion) of breast, **2:**393, 393f, 394t-395t
Adam's apple, **2:**72
Adduct/adduction, **1:**96, 96f
Adductor tubercle of femur, **1:**232f, 233
Adenocarcinomas, **3:**483
Adenoids, **2:**71f, 72
Adenomatous polyposis coli *(APC)* gene, **3:**483
ADH (atypical ductal hyperplasia), **2:**395
Adhesion, **2:**245t
Adipose capsule, **2:**184
Adjacent structures, **1:**5
Adolescent development, **3:**104
Adrenal glands
    anatomy of, **2:**183, 183f
    sectional anatomy of, **3:**283, 288-289, 288f-289f
    ultrasonography of, **3:**376f
Adrenaline, **2:**226t
Advanced clinical practice, **1:**14
Adventitia of arterial wall, **3:**65
AEC. *See* Automatic exposure control (AEC).
Afferent arteriole of kidney, **2:**185, 185f
Afferent lymph vessels, **3:**26, 96-97
Age-based development, **3:**102-104
    of adolescents, **3:**104
    of infants, **3:**102
    of neonates, **3:**102
    of premature infants, **3:**102
    of preschoolers, **3:**103, 103f
    of school age children, **3:**104
    of toddlers, **3:**103
Age-related competencies in elderly, **3:**176
Age-specific competencies, **1:**23, 24b, 24t
Aging. *See also* Elderly.
    concept of, **3:**164, 164f
    demographics and social effects of, **3:**162f-164f, 164b, 175
    physical, cognitive, and psychosocial effects of, **3:**166-168, 167b, 167f
    physiology of, **3:**168-173
        endocrine system disorders in, **3:**173
        gastrointestinal system disorders in, **3:**171, 171f
        genitourinary system disorders in, **3:**173
        hematologic system disorders in, **3:**173
        immune system decline in, **3:**172
        integumentary system disorders in, **3:**168
        musculoskeletal system disorders in, **3:**170, 170f-171f
        nervous system disorders in, **3:**168-169
        respiratory system disorders in, **3:**172, 172f
        sensory system disorders in, **3:**169
        summary of, **3:**173
Air calibration for CT, **3:**329, 339-340
Air-contrast study of large intestine, **2:**144
Airway foreign body, **2:**62t
    in children, **3:**139, 139f
Ala of sacrum, **1:**376, 376f
ALARA. *See* As low as reasonably achievable (ALARA).

Alert value (AV) for CT, **3:**330
Alexander method for AP axial projection of acromioclavicular articulation, **1:**211-212, 211f-212f
Algorithm in CT, **3:**302, 339
Alimentary canal, **2:**97, 97 *See also* Digestive system.
Alpha particles, **3:**403, 437-439
Alveolar ducts, **1:**480f, 481
Alveolar process
    anatomy of, **2:**272, 273f
    sectional anatomy of, **3:**254
Alveolar sacs, **1:**480f, 481
Alveolar sockets, **2:**275t
Alveolus(i)
    of breast, **2:**381f
    of lung, **1:**480f, 481
Alzheimer disease (AD), **3:**167-168, 174t
    performing radiography with, **3:**176
    PET for, **3:**434
    stages and symptoms of, **3:**177b
American Health Insurance Portability and Accountability Act of 1996 (HIPAA), **3:**460, 476
American Registry of Radiologic Technologists (ARRT), positioning terminology used by, **1:**85-95
American Society of Radiologic Technologists (ASRT) Code of Ethics, **1:**2
Amnion, **2:**241
Amniotic cavity, ultrasonography of, **3:**388, 389f
Amphiarthroses, **1:**81
Ampulla
    of breast, **2:**381f
    of ductus deferens, **2:**242, 243f
    of uterine tube, **2:**239, 239f
Ampulla of Vater
    anatomy of, **2:**100f, 101, 105, 105f
    sectional anatomy of, **3:**283
Amyloid neurologic study, **3:**434
Anabolic steroids for osteoporosis, **3:**448t
Anal canal
    anatomy of, **2:**102f-103f, 103
    defecography of, **2:**172, 172f
    sectional anatomy of, **3:**283
Analogs, radioactive, **3:**401-402, 437
Anaphylactic reaction, **2:**235
Anastomose, **3:**60, 96
Anatomic markers, **1:**25, 25f-26f, 27, 27b
Anatomic neck of humerus, **1:**104-105, 104f
Anatomic position, **1:**8-12, 8f-9f, 66-67, 66f
Anatomic programmers, **1:**40, 40f
Anatomic snuffbox, **1:**102
Anatomically programmed radiography (APR) systems with obese patients, **1:**52
Anatomy
    anatomic relationship terms in, **1:**85, 85f
    of bones, **1:**75-79
        appendicular skeleton in, **1:**75, 75f, 75t
        axial skeleton in, **1:**75, 75f, 75t
        classification of, **1:**79, 79f
        development in, **1:**77-78, 77f-78f
        fractures of, **1:**84, 84f
        general features in, **1:**76, 76f
        markings and features of, **1:**84
        vessels and nerves in, **1:**77, 77f
    defined, **1:**66
    general, **1:**66-74
        of body cavities, **1:**68-69, 69f
        body habitus in, **1:**72-74, 72f, 73b, 74f
        body planes in, **1:**66-67, 66f-68f
        divisions of abdomen in, **1:**70, 70f
        special planes in, **1:**68, 69f
        surface landmarks in, **1:**71, 71f, 71t

Anatomy *(Continued)*
    of joints, **1:**80-82
        cartilaginous, **1:**80t, 81, 81f
        fibrous, **1:**80f, 80t, 81
        functional classification of, **1:**81
        structural classification of, **1:**80t, 81-82
        synovial, **1:**80t, 82, 82f-83f
    sectional. *See* Sectional anatomy.
Andren–von Rosén method for congenital dislocation of hip, **1:**345
Anechoic structure or mass, **3:**374, 375f, 397
Anemia in older adults, **3:**173
Anencephaly, **3:**391f
Anesthesia provider, **3:**216
Aneurysm, **3:**28, 96
    of anterior communicating artery, **3:**34f
    aortic
        abdominal, **2:**84t, **3:**41
            endografts for, **3:**65-66, 65f-66f
            three-dimensional CT of, **3:**313f
        thoracic, **3:**40
    cerebral, **3:**10f
Aneurysmal bone cyst (ABC), **3:**149, 149f
Angina pectoralis, **3:**75, 96
Angiocatheters, **2:**228f, 229
Angiography, **3:**28-39
    aortic arch, for cranial vessels, **3:**55, 55f
    aortic root, **3:**82, 83f
    aortography as, **3:**40-47
        abdominal, **3:**41, 41f
        thoracic, **3:**40, 40f, 55f
    arteriography as. *See* Arteriography.
    catheterization for, **3:**36-38, 37f-38f
    cerebral. *See* Cerebral angiography.
    contrast media for, **3:**29
    coronary, **3:**40f, 75
        for cardiac catheterization, **3:**84, 85f, 85t
        for percutaneous transluminal coronary angioplasty, **3:**88, 88f-89f
        procedures that may accompany, **3:**76, 76t
    CT. *See* Computed tomography angiography (CTA).
    defined, **3:**18, 28, 96
    definition of terms for, **3:**96b-97b
    digital subtraction. *See* Digital subtraction angiography (DSA).
    electron beam, **3:**95
    future of, **3:**39
    guidewires for, **3:**35, 35f
    historical development of, **3:**20-21
    indications for, **3:**28
    injection techniques for, **3:**29
    introducer sheaths for, **3:**36, 36f
    magnetic resonance, **3:**363-364, 363f-364f
    magnification in, **3:**33
    needles for, **3:**35, 35f
    patient care for, **3:**38
    peripheral, **3:**46
        lower limb arteriograms as, **3:**47, 48f
        lower limb venograms as, **3:**47, 48f
        upper limb arteriograms as, **3:**46, 46f
        upper limb venograms as, **3:**46, 46f
    preparation of examining room for, **3:**39
    radiation protection for, **3:**39
    radionuclide, **3:**416
    renal, **2:**190, 191f
    surgical, **3:**74
    team for, **3:**39
    three-dimensional intraarterial, **3:**34, 34f
    venography as. *See* Venography.
Angioplasty, percutaneous transluminal. *See* Percutaneous transluminal angioplasty (PTA).
Angle of incidence, **3:**397
Angular notch of stomach, **2:**98f
Anisotropic spatial resolution, **3:**339

Ankle
 AP oblique projection of
  with knee included, **1:**294-295, 294f-295f
  in lateral rotation, **1:**286, 286f
  in medial rotation, **1:**283, 283f
 AP projection of, **1:**279, 279f
  with knee included, **1:**290-291, 290f-291f
  stress method for, **1:**287, 287f
  weight-bearing method for, **1:**288-289,
   288f-289f
 lateral projection of
  lateromedial, **1:**282, 282f
  mediolateral, **1:**280, 280f-281f
   with knee included, **1:**292-293,
    292f-293f
 mortise joint of
  anatomy of, **1:**230f-231f, 236t, 238
  AP oblique projection in medial rotation of,
   1:284-289, 284f-285f
 MRI of, **3:**363f
 surgical radiography of, **3:**246f-247f
Ankle joint
 anatomy of, **1:**230f-231f, 238
 AP oblique projection in medial rotation of,
  1:284-289, 284f-285f
Ankle mortise
 anatomy of, **1:**230f-231f, 236t, 238
 AP oblique projection in medial rotation of,
  1:284-289, 284f-285f
Ankle/brachial index (ABI), **3:**393, 397
Ankylosing spondylitis, **1:**331t, 380t
Annihilation radiation photons, **3:**421-424, 421f,
 437
Annotation, **1:**25
Annulus fibrosus
 anatomy of, **1:**368
 sectional anatomy of, **3:**269-270
Anode heel effect, **3:**186-187, 186t
Anomaly, **3:**96
Antenna coil in MRI, **3:**354, 354f
Antenna in MRI, **3:**343, 367-368
Anterior, **1:**85
Anterior arches of soft palate, **2:**59, 59f
Anterior cerebral arteries
 CT angiography of, **3:**325f
 MR angiography of, **3:**363f
 sectional anatomy of, **3:**255, 257-258, 257f-259f,
  260-261
Anterior cervical diskectomy, **3:**227, 227f
Anterior clinoid processes
 anatomy of, **2:**258f, 264f-265f, 265
 sectional anatomy of, **3:**260f, 261-262
Anterior communicating artery
 anatomy of, **3:**51
 aneurysm of, **3:**34f
 CT angiography of, **3:**325f
Anterior cranial fossa, **2:**260
Anterior crest of tibia, **1:**230, 230f
Anterior cruciate ligament, **1:**234f
Anterior facial artery and vein, **3:**22f
Anterior fat pad of elbow, **1:**107, 107f
Anterior fontanel, **2:**259-260, 260f
Anterior horn, **3:**4, 4f
Anterior inferior iliac spine, **1:**327f, 328
Anterior nasal spine, **2:**272, 272f-273f, 332f
Anterior superior iliac spine (ASIS)
 anatomy of, **1:**71f, 71t, 327f, 328, 330f
 as bony landmark, **1:**333, 333f
 with obese patients, **1:**47-49
 sectional anatomy of, **3:**293
Anterior tibial artery
 anatomy of, **3:**22f
 arteriography of, **3:**48f
Anterior tubercle of tibia, **1:**231, 231f
Anteroposterior (AP) oblique projection,
 1:88

Anteroposterior (AP) projection, **1:**10-11, 10f, 86,
 87f
 entry and exit points for, **1:**86, 86f
Anthracosis, **1:**486t
Anthropomorphic, **3:**476-477
Antiarrhythmia device implantation, **3:**94,
 94f
Antisepsis, **3:**250
Antiseptics, **1:**16
Anus
 anatomy of, **2:**102f-103f, 103
 sectional anatomy of, **3:**283
 ultrasonography of, **3:**386f
Aorta
 abdominal. *See* Abdominal aorta.
 anatomy of, **3:**22f, 25
 ascending, **3:**22f, 25
  aortography of, **3:**40f
  sectional anatomy of, **3:**270-271, 275-277
   on axial (transverse) section, **3:**276f
   on coronal section, **3:**281f
   on sagittal section, **3:**278-279, 280f
 descending, **3:**25, 25f
  aortography of, **3:**40f
  sectional anatomy of, **3:**270-271, 271f
   on axial (transverse) section, **3:**275-278,
    276f, 278f
   on coronal section, **3:**281, 281f
   on sagittal section, **3:**279-280, 280f
 sectional image of, **2:**107f
 thoracic, sectional anatomy of, **3:**270-271,
  278-280, 278f-279f
 ultrasonography of, **3:**376f, 380f
Aortic aneurysm
 abdominal, **2:**84t, **3:**41
  endografts for, **3:**65-66, 65f-66f
  three-dimensional CT of, **3:**313f
 thoracic, **3:**40
Aortic arch
 anatomy of, **3:**22f, 25, 25f, 49f
 angiography for cranial vessels of, **3:**55, 55f
 MR angiography of, **3:**364f
 sectional anatomy of, **3:**270-271
  on axial (transverse) plane, **3:**275
  on coronal plane, **3:**280-281, 281f
  on sagittal plane, **3:**278-280, 280f
Aortic artery, **3:**280f
Aortic dissection, **3:**40, 96
Aortic root angiography, **3:**82, 83f
Aortic valve
 anatomy of, **3:**25, 25f
 sectional anatomy of, **3:**270
Aortofemoral arteriography, **3:**47, 48f
Aortography, **3:**40-47
 abdominal, **3:**41, 41f
 defined, **3:**96
 thoracic, **3:**40, 40f, 55f
APBI (accelerated partial-breast irradiation),
 3:504
APC (adenomatous polyposis coli) gene, **3:**483
APDs (avalanche photodiodes), **3:**409
Aperture diameter, maximum, **1:**44-45, 45t
Aperture in CT, **3:**310, 339
Appendicitis, **2:**109t
Appendicular skeleton, **1:**75, 75f, 75t
Apple method for AP oblique projection of glenoid
 cavity, **1:**190-191, 190f-191f
APR (anatomically programmed radiography)
 systems with obese patients, **1:**52
Aquaplast mask, **3:**490f
Arachnoid
 anatomy of, **3:**3, 18
 sectional anatomy of, **3:**254
Arachnoid cisterns, **3:**3
Architectural distortion (AD) of breast, **2:**393,
 393f, 394t-395t

Archiving for CT, **3:**309, 339
Arcuate eminence, **2:**269f
Arcuate line, **1:**328
Areal technique, DXA as, **3:**453, 477
Areola, **2:**380, 381f
Arm. *See* Upper limb.
Array-beam techniques, for DXA, **3:**444, 454-457,
 454f, 476
Arrhythmia, **3:**96
Arrhythmogenic, **3:**96
ARRT (American Registry of Radiologic
 Technologists), positioning terminology used
 by, **1:**85-95
Arterialized venous blood in PET, **3:**430, 437
Arteries, **3:**22f, 23
 coronary, **3:**25, 25f
 defined, **3:**96
 pulmonary, **3:**22f, 23
 systemic, **3:**23
Arteriography, **3:**28
 defined, **3:**96
 peripheral
  lower limb, **3:**47, 48f
  upper limb, **3:**46, 46f
 pulmonary, **3:**42, 42f
 visceral, **3:**42-45, 42f
  celiac, **3:**43, 43f
  hepatic, **3:**43, 43f
  inferior mesenteric, **3:**44, 45f
  other, **3:**45
  renal, **2:**190, 191f, **3:**45, 45f
  splenic, **3:**44, 44f
  superior mesenteric, **3:**44, 44f
Arterioles, **3:**23, 96
Arteriosclerotic, **3:**96
Arteriotomy, **3:**96
Arteriovenous malformation, **3:**96
Arthritis, rheumatoid, **1:**109t, 182t
Arthrography, **1:**82
 contrast. *See* Contrast arthrography.
Arthrology, **1:**80-82
 of cartilaginous joints, **1:**80t, 81, 81f
 defined, **1:**80
 of fibrous joints, **1:**80f, 80t, 81
 functional classification of joints in, **1:**81
 structural classification of joints in, **1:**80t,
  81-82
 of synovial joints, **1:**80t, 82, 82f-83f
Arthroplasty, in older adults, **3:**170, 171f
Articular capsule, **1:**82, 82f
Articular cartilage, **1:**76, 76f
 of vertebrae, **1:**368
Articular pillars. *See* Vertebral arch.
Articular processes, of vertebral arch, **1:**368,
 368f
Articular tubercle
 anatomy of, **2:**268, 268f
 axiolateral oblique projection of, **2:**352f
Artifacts
 with children, **3:**110-111, 110f-111f
 in CT, **3:**319, 319f-320f, 339
 on MRI, **3:**356, 367
 in ultrasonography, **3:**374, 375f
As low as reasonably achievable (ALARA), **1:**2
 in DXA, **3:**458, 476
 in nuclear medicine, **3:**407
Asbestosis, **1:**486t
Ascites, **2:**84t
ASDs (autism spectrum disorders), **3:**105-107,
 105t
Asepsis, **1:**15, **3:**250
 in mobile radiography, **3:**191
Aseptic technique, **3:**250
 for minor surgical procedures in radiology
  department, **1:**17, 17f
 in surgical radiography, **3:**220, 220b

Index

ASIS. *See* Anterior superior iliac spine (ASIS).
Aspiration, **1:**486t
Aspiration pneumonia, **1:**486t
ASRT (American Society of Radiologic Technologists) Code of Ethics, **1:**2
Asterion, **2:**258f, 259
Asthenic body habitus, **1:**72-74, 72f, 73b, 74f
 and gallbladder, **2:**106, 106f
 skull radiography with, **2:**289f
 and stomach and duodenum, **2:**99, 99f, 125f
 and thoracic viscera, **1:**479f
Asymmetric jaws of linear accelerators, **3:**488f, 489, 506
AT. *See* Axillary tail (AT).
ATCM (automatic tube current modulation), **3:**331, 331f
Atelectasis, **1:**486t
Atherectomy, **3:**96
Atherectomy devices, **3:**90, 90f-91f
Atheromatous plaque, **3:**75, 96
Atherosclerosis, **3:**28, 96
 echocardiography of, **3:**393
 in older adults, **3:**170-171, 174t
Atherosclerotic stenosis, balloon angioplasty of, **3:**63f, 64-65
Atlantoaxial joint, **1:**378, 379t
Atlantooccipital joint, **1:**369f, 378, 379t, **2:**266f, 275t
Atlas
 anatomy of, **1:**369, 369f
 AP projection (open mouth) of, **1:**384-385, 384f-385f
 AP tomogram of, **1:**385, 385f
 lateral projection of, **1:**386, 386f
 sectional anatomy of, **3:**267-268
Atom
 components of, **3:**403
 defined, **3:**400, 437
Atomic number, **3:**403, 403f
Atrial septal defect, balloon septoplasty for, **3:**93, 93f
Atrioventricular valve, **3:**25f
Atrium(ia)
 anatomy of, **3:**24-25, 25f, 96
 sectional anatomy of, **3:**270, 271f
  on axial (transverse) plane, **3:**278, 278f
  on coronal plane, **3:**280-281, 281f
  on sagittal plane, **3:**278-280, 280f
Atropine sulfate (Atropine), **2:**226t
Attenuation
 in CT, **3:**339
 in MRI vs. conventional radiography, **3:**342, 367
 in radiation oncology, **3:**494, 506
 in ultrasonography, **3:**397
Attenuation coefficients, **3:**402, 437
Attire of patient, **1:**20, 20f
Atypical ductal hyperplasia (ADH), **2:**395
Atypical lobular hyperplasia, **2:**395
Auditory ossicles, **2:**269f-270f, 271
Auditory tube, **2:**270f, 271
Auricle
 cardiac, **3:**24
 of ear
  anatomy of, **2:**270f, 271, 285f
  sectional anatomy of, **3:**260f, 261-262
Auricular surface
 of ilium, **1:**327f, 328
 of sacrum, **1:**376, 376f
Autism spectrum disorders (ASDs), **3:**105-107, 105t
Automatic collimation, **1:**32
Automatic exposure control (AEC), **1:**38, 42
 for mammography, **2:**409
 with obese patients, **1:**52

Automatic tube current modulation (ATCM), **3:**331, 331f
AV (alert value) for CT, **3:**330
Avalanche photodiodes (APDs), **3:**409
Axial image in CT, **3:**302, 339
Axial plane, **1:**66, 66f-67f
 in sectional anatomy, **3:**252
Axial projection, **1:**86-87, 87f
Axial resolution in ultrasonography, **3:**397
Axial skeletal measurements, **3:**469-471, 469f-471f
Axial skeleton, **1:**75, 75f, 75t
Axilla, labeling codes for, **2:**403t-408t
Axillary arteries, **3:**270-271, 273f, 281f
Axillary lymph nodes
 anatomy of, **2:**380, 381f, **3:**27f
 mammographic findings for, **2:**387
Axillary prolongation. *See* Axillary tail (AT).
Axillary tail (AT)
 anatomy of, **2:**380f, 437f
 axillary projection of, **2:**452-453, 452f-453f
 labeling codes for, **2:**403t-408t
 mediolateral oblique projection of, **2:**412f, 432t, 450-451, 450f-451f
Axillary veins, **3:**271, 273f, 280-281
Axiolateral projection, **1:**88
Axis
 anatomy of, **1:**369, 369f
 AP projection (open mouth) of, **1:**384-385, 384f-385f
 AP tomogram of, **1:**385, 385f
 lateral projection of, **1:**386, 386f
 sectional anatomy of, **3:**267-268
Azygos vein, **3:**271, 271f, 278, 279f, 285, 285f

B
Baby box, **3:**119-120, 119f-120f
Backboard in trauma radiography, **2:**23, 23f
Bacterial pneumonia, **1:**486t
Ball and socket joint, **1:**82, 83f
Ball-catcher's position for AP oblique projection in medial rotation of hand, **1:**130-131
 evaluation criteria for, **1:**131b
 position of part for, **1:**130-131, 131f
 position of patient for, **1:**130
 structures shown on, **1:**131, 131f
Balloon angioplasty, **3:**20, 62-63, 63f
Balloon kyphoplasty for osteoporotic fractures, **3:**449, 449f
Balloon septoplasty, **3:**93, 93f
Barium enema (BE)
 double-contrast method for, **2:**144, 144f, 150-153
  single-stage, **2:**144, 150, 150f-151f
  two-stage, **2:**144
  Wellen method for, **2:**152-153, 152f-153f
 insertion of enema tip for, **2:**148
 preparation and care of patient for, **2:**147
 preparation of barium suspensions for, **2:**147
 single-contrast, **2:**144, 144f, 148-149, 148f-149f
 standard apparatus for, **2:**146, 146f-147f
Barium studies
 of esophagus, **1:**483, 483f, 506f
 of heart
  lateral projection for, **1:**503
  PA oblique projection for, **1:**505, 507
  PA projection for, **1:**499
Barium sulfate
 for alimentary canal imaging, **2:**111, 111f
 high-density, **2:**144
Barium sulfate suspension
 for alimentary canal imaging, **2:**111, 111f-112f
 for barium enema, **2:**147

Barrett esophagus, **2:**109t
Basal ganglia, **3:**254-255
Basal nuclei, **3:**254-255, 258-259, 267
Basal skull fracture, **2:**282t
Basilar artery
 CT angiography of, **3:**325f
 MR angiography of, **3:**363f
 sectional anatomy of, **3:**255
  on axial (transverse) plane, **3:**259f-260f, 260-263, 262f
  on sagittal plane, **3:**264-265
Basilar portion of occipital bone, **2:**266-267, 266f-267f
Basilic vein, **3:**22f
 anatomy of, **3:**22f
 venography of, **3:**46f
BAT (B-mode acquisition technology), **3:**497
BE. *See* Barium enema (BE).
Beam collimation in CT, **3:**331-332, 332t-333t
Beam hardening artifact in CT, **3:**319, 319f
Beam hardening with energy-switching systems for DXA, **3:**452
Beam-shaping filters for CT, **3:**329-330, 329f
Béclère method for AP axial projection of intercondylar fossa, **3:**310, 310f
Becquerel (Bq), **3:**405, 437
Benadryl (diphenhydramine hydrochloride), **2:**226t
Benign prostatic hyperplasia (BPH), **2:**188t
 in older adults, **3:**173, 174t
Bennett fracture, **1:**109t
Beta emitters, **3:**422f
Beta particles, **3:**403, 437
Betatron, **3:**506
Bezoar, **2:**109t
BGO (bismuth germanium oxide) as scintillator for PET, **3:**428t, 437
Biceps brachii muscle, **1:**180f
Bicipital groove
 anatomy of, **1:**104f, 105
 Fisk modification for tangential projection of, **1:**207-208, 207f-208f
Bicornuate uterus, **2:**247f
Bicuspid valve, **3:**25f
Bifurcation, **3:**96
Bile, **2:**104
Bile ducts, **2:**97f, 104f-105f, 105
Biliary drainage procedure, **2:**175, 175f
Biliary stenosis, **2:**109t
Biliary tract
 anatomy of, **2:**97f, 104f-106f, 105
 biliary drainage procedure and stone extraction for, **2:**175, 175f
 cholangiography of
  percutaneous transhepatic, **2:**174-175, 174f
  postoperative (T-tube), **2:**176-177, 176f-177f
 endoscopic retrograde cholangiopancreatography of, **2:**178, 178f-179f
 prefixes associated with, **2:**173, 173t
 radiographic techniques for, **2:**173
 ultrasonography of, **3:**373f, 378, 379f
Biochemical markers of bone turnover, **3:**448, 476
Biometric measurements, fetal ultrasound for, **3:**390, 390f
Biopsy, **3:**480, 506
Biparietal diameter (BPD), **3:**390, 390f, 397
Biplane, **3:**96
Bismuth germanium oxide (BGO) as scintillator for PET, **3:**428t, 437
Bisphosphonates for osteoporosis, **3:**448t
Bit, **3:**437
Bit depth in CT, **3:**308
Black lung, **1:**486t
Bladder. *See* Urinary bladder.
Bladder carcinoma, **2:**188t

Bloch, Felix, **3:**342
Blood, handling of, **1:**16, 16b
Blood oxygen level dependent (BOLD) imaging, **3:**366
Blood pool agents for MRI, **3:**355
Blood-brain barrier, **3:**417, 437
Blood-vascular system, **3:**22-26, 22f
  arteries in, **3:**22f, 23
    coronary, **3:**25, 25f
    pulmonary, **3:**22f, 23
    systemic, **3:**23
  arterioles in, **3:**23
  capillaries in, **3:**23-24
  complete circulation of blood through, **3:**24
  defined, **3:**96
  heart in, **3:**23-24, 25f
  main trunk vessels in, **3:**23
  portal system in, **3:**23, 23f
  pulmonary circulation in, **3:**23, 23f
  systemic circulation in, **3:**23, 23f
  veins in, **3:**22f, 23
    coronary, **3:**25, 25f
    pulmonary, **3:**22f, 23
    systemic, **3:**24
  velocity of blood circulation in, **3:**26
  venules in, **3:**23
Blowout fracture, **2:**46f, 282t, 313, 313f
Blunt trauma, **2:**19
BMC (bone mineral content), **3:**442, 476
BMD (bone mineral density), **3:**442, 476
  calculation of, **3:**453
BMI (body mass index), **1:**44
B-mode acquisition technology (BAT), **3:**497
Body cavities, **1:**68-69, 69f
Body composition dual energy x-ray absorptiometry, **3:**442f, 471, 472f, 476
Body fluids, handling of, **1:**16, 16b
Body habitus, **1:**72-74, 72f, 73b, 74f
  and body position for skull radiography
    in horizontal sagittal plane, **2:**289f
    in perpendicular sagittal plane, **2:**290f
  and gallbladder, **2:**106, 106f
  and stomach and duodenum, **2:**99, 99f
    PA projection of, **2:**124, 125f
  and thoracic viscera, **1:**479, 479f
Body mass index (BMI), **1:**44
Body movement, **1:**96-97
  abduct or abduction as, **1:**96, 96f
  adduct or adduction as, **1:**96, 96f
  circumduction as, **1:**97, 97f
  deviation as, **1:**97, 97f
  dorsiflexion as, **1:**97, 97f
  evert/eversion as, **1:**96, 96f
  extension as, **1:**96, 96f
  flexion as, **1:**96, 96f
  hyperextension as, **1:**96, 96f
  hyperflexion as, **1:**96, 96f
  invert/inversion as, **1:**96f
  plantar flexion as, **1:**97, 97f
  pronate/pronation as, **1:**97, 97f
  rotate/rotation as, **1:**97, 97f
  supinate/supination as, **1:**97, 97f
  tilt as, **1:**97, 97f
Body planes, **1:**66-67
  coronal, **1:**66, 66f-67f
  in CT and MRI, **1:**67, 67f
  horizontal (transverse, axial, cross-sectional), **1:**66, 66f-67f
  imaging in several, **1:**67, 68f
  interiliac, **1:**68, 69f
  midcoronal (midaxillary), **1:**66, 66f
  midsagittal, **1:**66, 66f
  oblique, **1:**66f-67f, 67
  occlusal, **1:**68, 69f
  sagittal, **1:**66, 66f-67f
  special, **1:**68, 69f

Body rotation method for PA oblique projection of sternoclavicular articulations, **1:**465, 465f
Bohr atomic number, **3:**403, 403f
BOLD (blood oxygen level dependent) imaging, **3:**366
Bolus chase method for digital subtraction angiography, **3:**30-31
Bolus in CT angiography, **3:**324, 339
Bone(s), **1:**75-79
  appendicular skeleton of, **1:**75, 75f, 75t
  axial skeleton of, **1:**75, 75f, 75t
  biology of, **3:**445-446
  classification of, **1:**79, 79f
  compact (cortical), **1:**76, 76f
    and bone densitometry, **3:**445, 445t
    defined, **3:**476
  development of, **1:**77-78, 77f-78f
  flat, **1:**79, 79f
  fractures of. *See* Fracture(s).
  functions of, **1:**75
  general features of, **1:**76, 76f
  irregular, **1:**79, 79f
  long, **1:**79, 79f
  markings and features of, **1:**84
  sesamoid, **1:**79, 79f
  short, **1:**79, 79f
  spongy, **1:**76, 76f
  trabecular (cancellous)
    and bone densitometry, **3:**445, 445t
    defined, **3:**477
    in osteoporosis, **3:**446f
  vessels and nerves of, **1:**77, 77f
Bone cyst, **1:**109t, 240t
  aneurysmal, **3:**149, 149f
Bone densitometry, **3:**441-478
  bone biology and remodeling and, **3:**445-446, 445f-446f, 445t
  central (or axial) skeletal measurements in, **3:**469-471, 469f-471f
  defined, **3:**442, 476
  definition of terms for, **3:**476b-477b
  dual photon absorptiometry (DPA) for, **3:**444, 476
  DXA for. *See* Dual energy x-ray absorptiometry (DXA).
  fracture risk models in, **3:**475
  history of, **3:**443-444, 444f
  and osteoporosis, **3:**442, 447-450, 448t
    bone health recommendations for, **3:**450, 450t
    defined, **3:**477
    fractures and falls due to, **3:**449, 449f
  pediatric, **3:**473-474, 473f
  peripheral skeletal measurements in, **3:**474-475, 474f-475f
  principles of, **3:**442-443, 442f
  quantitative computed tomography (QCT) for, **3:**444, 469, 469f, 477
  radiogrammetry for, **3:**443, 477
  radiographic absorptiometry for, **3:**443, 477
  single photon absorptiometry (SPA) for, **3:**444, 444f, 477
  vertebral fracture assessment in, **3:**469-470, 470f-471f, 477
Bone formation, **3:**445, 445f
Bone health, recommendations for, **3:**450, 450t
Bone marrow
  red, **1:**76, 76f
  yellow, **1:**76, 76f
Bone marrow dose, **1:**35, 35t
Bone mass
  defined, **3:**476
  low, **3:**447, 457, 476-477
  peak, **3:**446, 477

Bone mineral content (BMC), **3:**442, 476
Bone mineral density (BMD), **3:**442, 476
  calculation of, **3:**453
Bone remodeling, **3:**445-446, 445f, 476
Bone resorption, **3:**445, 445f
Bone scan, **3:**415-416
Bone scintigraphy, **3:**415-416
Bone studies, **3:**416
Bone turnover, biochemical markers of, **3:**448, 476
Bone windows, **3:**11, 11f
Bony labyrinth, **2:**271
Bony thorax, **1:**445-476
  anatomy of, **1:**447-453
    anterior aspect of, **1:**447f
    anterolateral oblique aspect of, **1:**447f
    articulations in, **1:**449-453, 449t, 450f
    lateral aspect of, **1:**448f
    ribs in, **1:**447f-449f, 448
    sternum in, **1:**447-448, 447f
    summary of, **1:**453b
  body position for, **1:**453
  function of, **1:**447
  respiratory movement of, **1:**451, 451f
    diaphragm in, **1:**452, 452f
  ribs in. *See* Ribs.
  sample exposure technique chart essential projections for, **1:**455t
  sternoclavicular articulations of
    anatomy of, **1:**449, 449t
    PA oblique projection of
      body rotation method for, **1:**465, 465f
      central ray angulation method for, **1:**466, 466f-467f
    PA projection of, **1:**464, 464f
  sternum in. *See* Sternum.
  summary of pathology of, **1:**454t
  summary of projections for, **1:**446
  in trauma patients, **1:**453
Boomerang contact filter
  applications of, **1:**60t, 63-64, 63f
  composition of, **1:**57
  example of, **1:**56f
  placement of, **1:**58, 58f
  shape of, **1:**57
Bowel obstruction, **2:**84t
Bowel preparation, **1:**18
Bowing fractures, **3:**130
Bowman capsule, **2:**185, 185f
Bowtie filters for CT, **3:**329-330, 329f
Boxer fracture, **1:**109t
BPD (biparietal diameter), **3:**390, 390f, 397
BPH (benign prostatic hyperplasia), **2:**188t
  in older adults, **3:**173, 174t
Bq (becquerel), **3:**405, 437
Brachial artery
  anatomy of, **3:**22f, 49f
  arteriography of, **3:**46f
Brachiocephalic artery, **3:**96
  anatomy of, **3:**49f, 50
  arteriography of, **3:**40f
  sectional anatomy of, **3:**270-271, 273-275, 274f, 280-281, 281f
Brachiocephalic vein
  sectional anatomy of, **3:**271
    on axial (transverse) plane, **3:**273-275, 273f-274f
    on coronal plane, **3:**280-281, 281f
  venography of, **3:**60f
Brachycephalic skull, **2:**286, 286f
Brachytherapy, **3:**485, 506
Bradyarrhythmia, **3:**96
Bradycardia, **3:**96
Bragg peak, **3:**505

Brain
  anatomy of, **3:**2, 2f
  CT angiography of, **3:**10f, 324-326, 325f
    perfusion study for, **3:**324-326, 326f
  CT of, **3:**10, 10f-11f, 315f
  defined, **3:**18
  magnetic resonance spectroscopy for, **3:**365, 365f
  MRI of, **3:**12, 13f, 357, 357f
  PET of, **3:**432f, 434
  plain radiographic examination of, **3:**5
  sectional anatomy of, **3:**254
  SPECT study of, **3:**411f, 417
  vascular and interventional procedures of, **3:**14-16, 14f-15f
  ventricular system of, **3:**2, 4, 4f
Brain perfusion imaging, **3:**417
Brain stem
  anatomy of, **3:**2, 2f
  sectional anatomy of, **3:**255, 264
Brain tissue scanner, **3:**305
BRCA1 gene, **2:**378-379, **3:**482
BRCA2 gene, **2:**378-379, **3:**482
Breast(s)
  anatomy of, **2:**380, 380f-381f, 394b
  axillary tail of
    anatomy of, **2:**380f, 437f
    axillary projection of, **2:**452-453, 452f-453f
    mediolateral oblique projection of, **2:**412f, 432t, 450-451, 450f-451f
  connective tissue of, **2:**381f, 382
  density of, **2:**383, 383f
  digital breast tomosynthesis (3D imaging) of, **2:**374-375
  ductography of, **2:**459-460, 459f-460f
  fatty tissue of, **2:**381f, 382
  glandular tissue of, **2:**382
  involution of, **2:**380
  localization and biopsy of suspicious lesions of, **2:**461-470
    breast specimen radiography in, **2:**471, 471f
    for dermal calcifications, **2:**464
    material for, **2:**461, 461f
    stereotactic imaging and biopsy procedures for, **2:**465-470
      calculation of *X*, *Y*, and *Z* coordinates in, **2:**465, 465f-466f, 469, 469f
      equipment for, **2:**466, 467f-468f
      images using, **2:**468, 468f-470f
      three-dimensional localization with, **2:**465, 465f
    tangential projection for, **2:**464
  MRI of, **2:**418-419, 472, **3:**358, 359f
  oversized, **2:**400, 401f
  pathology of, **2:**384-393
    architectural distortions as, **2:**393, 393f, 394t-395t
    calcifications as, **2:**389-393, 389f-392f
    masses as, **2:**384-388, 394t-395t
      circumscribed, **2:**384, 385f, 394
      density of, **2:**384, 386f
      indistinct, **2:**384, 394
      interval change in, **2:**387, 387f
      location of, **2:**387
      margins of, **2:**384, 394t-395t
      palpable, **2:**409, 429-430, 443
      radiolucent, **2:**384, 386f
      seen on only one projection, **2:**388, 388f
      shape of, **2:**384
      spiculated, **2:**384, 385f, 394
    summary of, **2:**394t-395t
  during pregnancy and lactation, **2:**382, 382f
  radiography of. *See* Mammography.

Breast(s) (*Continued*)
  in radiography of sternum, **1:**456
  thermography and diaphanography of, **2:**473
  tissue variations in, **2:**382-393, 382f-383f
  ultrasonography of, **2:**418-419, **3:**375f, 383, 384f
  xerography of, **2:**372, 372f
Breast abscess, **2:**395
Breast augmentation
  complications of, **2:**418
  mammography with, **2:**417-419, 418f
    craniocaudal (CC) projection of
      with full implant, **2:**420-421, 421f
      with implant displaced, **2:**422-423, 422f-423f
      with implant displacement (ID), **2:**403t-408t
    mediolateral oblique (MLO) projection of
      with full implant, **2:**424
      with implant displaced, **2:**425
    MRI with, **2:**418-419
    ultrasonography with, **2:**418-419
Breast cancer
  architectural distortion due to, **2:**393f
  calcifications in, **2:**392f
  genetic factors in, **3:**482
  in men, **2:**426
  prophylactic surgery for, **3:**482, 507
  radiation oncology for, **3:**504, 504f
  risk factors for, **2:**378-379
  ultrasonography of, **3:**375f
Breast cancer screening, **2:**377
  vs. diagnostic mammography, **2:**378
  high-risk, **2:**472
  risk vs. benefit of, **2:**377-378, 377f
Breast specimen radiography, **2:**471, 471f
Breastbone. *See* Sternum.
Breathing, **1:**451, 451f
  for chest radiographs, **1:**490, 490f
  diaphragm in, **1:**452, 452f
  in radiography of ribs, **1:**468
  in radiography of sternum, **1:**456, 457f
  for trauma radiography, **2:**30
Breathing technique, **1:**41
Bregma, **2:**258f-259f, 259
Bridge of nose, **2:**272
Bridgeman method for superoinferior axial inlet projection of anterior pelvic bones, **1:**359, 359f
Broad ligaments, **3:**284
Broadband ultrasound attenuation (BUA), **3:**475
Bronchial tree, **1:**480, 480b, 480f
Bronchiectasis, **1:**486t
Bronchioles, **1:**480, 480f
  terminal, **1:**480, 480f
Bronchitis, **1:**486t
  chronic, in older adults, **3:**172
Bronchomediastinal trunk, **3:**26
Bronchopneumonia, **1:**486t
Bronchopulmonary segments, **1:**482
Bronchoscopy, **3:**226
Bronchus(i)
  mainstem, **1:**480f
  primary, **1:**480, 480f
  secondary, **1:**480, 480f
  sectional anatomy of, **3:**270, 275-277, 276f, 279, 280f-281f
  tertiary, **1:**480, 480f
BUA (broadband ultrasound attenuation), **3:**475
Buckle fracture, **1:**109t
Bucky grid with obese patients, **1:**51
Built-in DR flat-panel IR detector position, **1:**28f
Bulbourethral glands, **2:**242
"Bunny" technique
  for gastrointestinal and genitourinary studies, **3:**116f
  for limb radiography, **3:**127, 127f
  for skull radiography, **3:**132, 133f

Burman method for first CMC joint of thumb, **1:**120-121, 120f-121f
Bursae, **1:**82, 82f, 178
  of shoulder, **1:**178, 178f
Bursitis, **1:**109t, 182t
Butterfly sets, **2:**228f, 229
Byte, **3:**437

C
¹¹C (carbon-11) in PET, **3:**425f, 426t
CAD (computer-aided detection) systems for mammography, **2:**376-379, 376f
Cadaveric sections, **3:**252
Calcaneal sulcus, **1:**229, 229f
Calcaneocuboid articulation, **1:**236f-237f, 236t, 238
Calcaneus
  anatomy of, **1:**228f-229f, 229
  axial projection of
    dorsoplantar, **1:**272, 272f-273f
    plantodorsal, **1:**271, 271f
    weight-bearing coalition (Harris-Beath) method for, **1:**273, 273f
  lateromedial oblique projection (weight-bearing) of, **1:**275, 275f
  mediolateral projection of, **1:**274, 274f
Calcifications of breast, **2:**389-393, 389f-392f, 394t-395t
  amorphous or indistinct, **2:**391, 392f, 394
  arterial (vascular), **2:**389f-390f, 395
  coarse heterogeneous, **2:**389f-390f, 391, 394
  fine heterogeneous, **2:**391, 392f, 394
  linear branching, **2:**392f
  male, **2:**427
  milk of calcium as, **2:**391, 391f, 395
  pleomorphic linear, **2:**392f
  popcorn-type, **2:**389f-390f, 395
  rim, **2:**395
  rodlike secretory, **2:**389f-390f
  round or punctate, **2:**389f-390f, 394
  skin (dermal), **2:**395, 464
Calcitonin for osteoporosis, **3:**448t
Calcium and osteoporosis, **3:**447, 450, 450t
Calculus, **2:**62t
  renal, **2:**188t, 190f
Caldwell method
  for PA axial projection of facial bones, **2:**329-330, 329f-330f
  for PA axial projection of frontal and anterior ethmoidal sinuses, **2:**360-361, 360f-361f
    in children, **3:**136, 136f
  for PA axial projection of skull, **2:**296-300
    evaluation criteria for, **2:**299b
    position of part for, **2:**296, 297f
    position of patient for, **2:**296
    structures shown on, **2:**298f, 299
Calvaria, **2:**257
Camp-Coventry method for PA axial projection of intercondylar fossa, **1:**308, 308f-309f
Canadian Association of Medical Radiation Technologists (CAMRT)
  Code of Ethics of, **1:**2-3
  positioning terminology used by, **1:**85-95
Cancellous bone
  and bone densitometry, **3:**445, 445t
  defined, **3:**477
  in osteoporosis, **3:**446f
Cancer, **3:**481-483
  defined, **3:**481, 506
  epidemiology of, **3:**481
  metastasis of, **3:**481, 507
  most common types of, **3:**482, 482t
  PET imaging of, **3:**433, 433f
  radiation oncology for. *See* Radiation oncology.

Cancer (*Continued*)
  recurrence of, **3:**480
  risk factors for, **3:**482-483, 482t
  tissue origins of, **3:**483, 483t
  TNM classification of, **3:**483, 483t
Cancericidal doses, **3:**480, 506
Canthomeatal (CM) line, **3:**437
Capillaries, **3:**23-24, 26
Capitate, **1:**101f-102f, 102
Capitulum, **1:**104, 104f
Carbon dioxide (CO₂) as contrast medium,
  3:29
Carbon-11 (¹¹C) in PET, **3:**425f, 426t
Carcinogens, **3:**482, 482t, 506
Carcinoma, **2:**109t, **3:**483, 506
Cardia of stomach, **2:**98, 98f
Cardiac catheterization, **3:**75-97
  for advanced diagnostic studies
    of conduction system, **3:**86-88, 87f
    of vascular system, **3:**86, 86f-87f
  for basic diagnostic studies of vascular system,
    3:82-86
    in adults, **3:**82-86
    in children, **3:**86
    of coronary arteries, **3:**84, 85f, 85t
    with exercise hemodynamics, **3:**86
    of left side of heart, **3:**82, 83f-84f
    of right side of heart, **3:**84
  catheter introduction in, **3:**82
  contraindications, complications, and associated
    risks of, **3:**77
  defined, **3:**75
  definition of terms for, **3:**96b-97b
  vs. electron beam tomography, **3:**95-97
  equipment for, **3:**78-80
    angiographic, **3:**78-79
      catheters as, **3:**78, 78f
      contrast media as, **3:**78
      pressure injector as, **3:**79, 79f
    imaging, **3:**79-80
    other, **3:**80, 80f, 80t
    physiologic, **3:**79-80, 79f, 82
  historical development of, **3:**20-21
  indications for, **3:**75-76, 75t
  for interventional procedures of conduction
    system, **3:**94, 94f-95f
  for interventional procedures of vascular system,
    3:88-94
    in adults, **3:**88-92
    in children, **3:**92-94, 93f
    intracoronary stent placement as, **3:**88,
      89f
    vs. intravascular ultrasound, **3:**80t, 91,
      91f-92f
    vs. optical coherence tomography, **3:**80t, 92,
      93f
    percutaneous transluminal coronary
      angioplasty as, **3:**88, 88f-89f
    percutaneous transluminal coronary rotational
      atherectomy as, **3:**80t, 90, 90f-91f
    thrombolytic agents prior to, **3:**92
  vs. MRI, **3:**95
  patient care after, **3:**95
  patient care prior to, **3:**81
  patient positioning for, **3:**81, 81f
  procedures that may accompany, **3:**76, 76t
  trends in, **3:**95-97
Cardiac cycle, **3:**24
Cardiac ejection fraction, **3:**410, 411f, 437
Cardiac gating
  for CT angiography, **3:**324-326, 326f
  for MRI, **3:**356, 356f
Cardiac MRI, **3:**358, 359f
Cardiac muscular tissue, motion control of,
  1:18
Cardiac notch, **1:**481-482, 481f, **2:**98, 98f

Cardiac orifice
  anatomy of, **2:**99
  sectional anatomy of, **3:**283
Cardiac output, **3:**96
Cardiac perfusion study, **3:**414, 414f
Cardiac sphincter, **2:**98f, 99
Cardiac studies with barium
  lateral projection for, **1:**503
  PA oblique projection for, **1:**505, 507
  PA projection for, **1:**499
Cardiac viability, PET imaging for, **3:**435
Cardiology imaging
  nuclear medicine for, **3:**416-417
  PET for, **3:**434-435
Cardiomyopathies, **3:**96
  congestive, **3:**393
Cardiovascular and interventional technologist
  (CIT), **3:**96
Cardiovascular studies in nuclear medicine, **3:**417
Cardiovascular system disorders in older adults,
  3:170-171
Carina
  anatomy of, **1:**480, 480f
  sectional anatomy of, **3:**270
C-arm
  dedicated, **2:**20, 20f
  mobile fluoroscopic, **2:**20, 21f
  in surgical radiography, **3:**221, 221f
    of cervical spine (anterior cervical diskectomy
      and fusion), **3:**227, 227f
    of chest (line placement, bronchoscopy),
      3:226, 226f
    of femoral nailing, **3:**234, 234f
    for femoral/tibial arteriogram, **3:**240
    of hip (cannulated hip screws or hip pinning),
      3:230-231, 230f
    of humerus, **3:**238-239, 238f
    of lumbar spine, **3:**228-229, 228f
    operation of, **3:**221, 222f
    for operative (immediate) cholangiography,
      3:224, 224f
    radiation safety with, **3:**223, 223f
    of tibial nailing, **3:**236, 236f
Carotid arteries. *See also* External carotid artery;
  Internal carotid artery.
  duplex sonography of extracranial, **3:**392, 392f
  MR angiography of, **3:**364f
Carotid canal, **2:**268, 269f
Carotid sinus, **3:**270-271
Carotid sulcus, **2:**264-265, 264f
Carpal(s)
  anatomy of, **1:**101-102, 101f
  terminology conversion for, **1:**101b
Carpal boss, **1:**135, 135f
Carpal bridge, tangential projection of, **1:**145
  evaluation criteria for, **1:**145b
  position of part for, **1:**145, 145f
  position of patient for, **1:**145
  structures shown on, **1:**145, 145f
Carpal sulcus, **1:**102, 102f
Carpal tunnel, **1:**102
Carpometacarpal (CMC) joint(s), **1:**118-119
  anatomy of, **1:**106, 106f
  Burman method for AP projection of, **1:**120-121
    evaluation criteria for, **1:**121b
    position of part for, **1:**120, 120f
    position of patient for, **1:**120
    SID for, **1:**120
    structures shown on, **1:**121, 121f
  Robert method for AP projection of, **1:**118-119
    evaluation criteria for, **1:**119b
    Lewis modification of, **1:**119
    Long and Rafert modification of, **1:**119
    position of part for, **1:**118, 118f
    position of patient for, **1:**118, 118f
    structures shown on, **1:**119, 119f

Cartilaginous joints, **1:**80t, 81, 81f
Cassette with film, **1:**3, 4f
CAT (computed axial tomography), **3:**302
Catheter(s) for cardiac catheterization, **3:**78, 78f
Catheterization
  for angiographic studies, **3:**36-38, 37f-38f
  cardiac. *See* Cardiac catheterization.
Cauda equina
  anatomy of, **3:**3, 3f, 18
  sectional anatomy of, **3:**296, 297f
Caudad, **1:**85, 85f
Caudate nucleus, sectional anatomy of,
  3:253f
  on axial (transverse) plane, **3:**257-259,
    257f-258f
  on coronal plane, **3:**267, 267f
  on sagittal plane, **3:**265f
Cavernous sinus, **3:**262, 262f, 267
CCD (charge-coupled device), **1:**3
CDC (Centers for Disease Control and Prevention),
  1:16, 16b, 16f
Cecum
  anatomy of, **2:**100f, 102, 102f
  sectional anatomy of, **3:**283, 292
Celiac arteriogram, **3:**43, 43f
Celiac artery
  anatomy of, **3:**22f
  sectional anatomy of, **3:**284, 289, 298-299
Celiac axis, arteriography of, **3:**41f
Celiac disease, **2:**109t, **3:**476
Celiac sprue, **2:**109t
Celiac trunk. *See* Celiac artery.
Centering
  for digital imaging, **1:**38
  of obese patients, **1:**47-48
Centers for Disease Control and Prevention (CDC),
  1:16, 16b, 16f
Central nervous system (CNS), **3:**1-18
  anatomy of, **3:**2-4
    brain in, **3:**2, 2f
    meninges in, **3:**3
    spinal cord in, **3:**3, 3f
    ventricular system in, **3:**2, 4, 4f
  CT myelography of, **3:**12, 12f
  CT of, **3:**10-12
    brain in, **3:**10, 10f-11f
    spine in, **3:**11, 11f-12f
  definition of terms for, **3:**18b
  interventional pain management of,
    3:16-18
  MRI of, **3:**12-13, 357-358
    of brain, **3:**12, 13f, 357, 357f
    of spine, **3:**13, 358
      lumbar, **1:**415, 416f, **3:**13f, 358f
      thoracic, **3:**358f
  myelography of. *See* Myelography.
  nuclear medicine imaging of, **3:**417
  plain radiographic examination of, **3:**5
  provocative diskography of, **3:**16, 17f
  vascular and interventional procedures for,
    3:14-16, 14f-15f
  vertebroplasty and kyphoplasty of, **3:**16,
    16f-17f
Central nervous system (CNS) disorders in older
  adults, **3:**168-169
Central ray (CR), **1:**31, 85
  for trauma radiography, **2:**30
Central ray (CR) angulation method for PA oblique
  projection of sternoclavicular articulations,
  1:466, 466f-467f
Central skeletal measurements, **3:**469-471,
  469f-471f
Cephalad, **1:**85, 85f
Cephalic vein
  anatomy of, **3:**22f
  venography of, **3:**46f

Cerebellar peduncles, **3:**255, 265, 265f, 268
Cerebellar tonsils, rami of, **3:**264
Cerebellum
 anatomy of, **2:**259f, **3:**2, 2f
 defined, **3:**18
 sectional anatomy of, **3:**255
  on axial (transverse) plane, **3:**258f-260f,
   259-263, 262f-263f
  on coronal plane, **3:**268, 268f
  on sagittal plane, **3:**264, 265f-266f, 266
Cerebral aneurysm, **3:**10f
Cerebral angiography
 of anterior circulation, **3:**56-58
  AP axial oblique (transorbital) projection for,
   3:58, 58f
  AP axial (supraorbital) projection for, **3:**57,
   57f
  lateral projection for, **3:**56, 56f
 of aortic arch (for cranial vessels), **3:**55,
  55f
 cerebral anatomy and, **3:**49-51, 49f-52f
 of cerebral arteries, **3:**15f
 circulation time and imaging program for, **3:**53,
  53f-54f
 defined, **3:**96
 equipment for, **3:**54
 of internal carotid artery, **3:**14f
 position of head for, **3:**54
 of posterior circulation, **3:**58-59
  AP axial projection for, **3:**59, 59f
  lateral projection for, **3:**58-59, 58f
 technique for, **3:**52-54
 of vertebrobasilar circulation, **3:**49-61
Cerebral aqueduct (of Sylvius)
 anatomy of, **3:**4, 4f, 18
 sectional anatomy of, **3:**255
  on axial (transverse) plane, **3:**258-260,
   258f-259f
  on sagittal plane, **3:**264
Cerebral arteries
 CT angiography of, **3:**325f
 digital subtraction angiography of, **3:**15f
 MR angiography of, **3:**363f
 sectional anatomy of, **3:**255, 257-258, 257f,
  259f, 260-261
Cerebral blood flow, PET images of local, **3:**427,
  427f, 438
Cerebral cortex
 anatomy of, **3:**2, 18
 sectional anatomy of, **3:**256-257
Cerebral hemispheres, **3:**256-257, 264
Cerebral lobes, **3:**256-257
Cerebral peduncles, sectional anatomy of,
  3:255
  on axial (transverse) plane, **3:**258-260,
   258f-259f
  on sagittal plane, **3:**264-265, 265f
Cerebral veins, **3:**255, 258-259
Cerebral vertebral arches, **3:**265
Cerebral vertebral bodies, **3:**265
Cerebrospinal fluid (CSF), **3:**3, 18
 sectional anatomy of, **3:**254, 264-266
Cerebrum
 anatomy of, **2:**259f, **3:**2, 2f
  vascular, **3:**49-51, 49f-52f
 defined, **3:**18
 sectional anatomy of, **3:**254-255
Cerrobend blocks, **3:**489, 506
Certified surgical technologist (CST),
  3:215
Cervical cancer, radiation oncology for, **3:**503,
  503f
Cervical curve, **1:**366f, 367
Cervical diskectomy, anterior, **3:**227, 227f
Cervical myelogram, **3:**9f
Cervical nodes, **3:**27f

Cervical vertebrae
 anatomy of, **1:**366f, 369-371
  atlas in, **1:**369, 369f
  axis in, **1:**369, 369f
  intervertebral transverse foramina and
   zygapophyseal joints in, **1:**370-371, 371f,
   371t
  seventh, **1:**370
  typical, **1:**370-371, 370f-371f
 AP axial oblique projection for trauma of, **2:**34,
  35f-36f
 AP axial projection of, **1:**387-388, 387f-388f
  for trauma, **2:**33, 33f
 AP projection of (Ottonello method), **1:**397-398,
  397f-398f
 atlas of
  anatomy of, **1:**369, 369f
  AP projection (open mouth) of, **1:**384-385,
   384f-385f
  AP tomogram of, **1:**385, 385f
  lateral projection of, **1:**386, 386f
 axis of
  AP projection (open mouth) of, **1:**384-385,
   384f-385f
  AP tomogram of, **1:**385, 385f
  lateral projection of, **1:**386, 386f
 CT of, **2:**53-55, **3:**11, 11f-12f, 336f-338f
 dens of
  anatomy of, **1:**369, 369f
  AP projection of (Fuchs method), **1:**383,
   383f
  PA projection of (Judd method), **1:**383
 dislocation of, **2:**33f
 fracture-dislocation of, **2:**31f
 fusion of, **3:**227, 227f
 intervertebral foramina of
  anatomy of, **1:**370f-371f, 371
  AP axial oblique projection of, **1:**393-394,
   393f-394f
   in hyperflexion and hyperextension,
    1:394
  PA axial oblique projection of, **1:**395,
   395f-396f
  positioning rotations needed to show, **1:**371,
   371t
 lateral projection of
  Grandy method for, **1:**389-390, 389f-390f
  in hyperflexion and hyperextension,
   1:391-392, 391f-392f
  mobile, **3:**206-207, 206f-207f
  swimmer's technique for, **1:**402-403,
   402f-403f
  for trauma, **2:**31, 31f
 mobile radiography of, **3:**206-207
  lateral projection for, **3:**206-207, 206f-207f
  in operating room, **3:**242, 242f-243f
 sectional anatomy of, **3:**265f, 267-268
 surgical radiography of, **3:**227, 227f
 transverse foramina of, **1:**370, 370f-371f
 trauma radiography of
  AP axial oblique projection in, **2:**34, 35f-36f
  AP axial projection in, **2:**33, 33f
  lateral projection in, **2:**31, 31f
 vertebral arch (articular pillars) of
  anatomy of, **1:**368, 368f, 370
  AP axial oblique projection of, **1:**401, 401f
  AP axial projection of, **1:**399-400,
   399f-400f
 zygapophyseal joints of
  anatomy of, **1:**371, 371f
  positioning rotations needed to show, **1:**371,
   371t
Cervicothoracic region, lateral projection of
 in dorsal decubitus position for trauma, **2:**32,
  32f
 swimmer's technique for, **1:**402-403, 402f-403f

Cervix
 anatomy of, **2:**240, 240f
 sectional anatomy of, **3:**284, 295, 295f
 ultrasonography of, **3:**388f-389f
CF (cystic fibrosis), **1:**486t, **3:**141, 141f
Channel, **3:**339
Charge-coupled device (CCD), **1:**3
Chassard-Lapiné method for axial projection of
 large intestine, **2:**169, 169f
Chest CT, **3:**336f-338f
Chest MRI, **3:**358, 359f
Chest radiographs
 AP projection in neonate for, **3:**208-210
  evaluation criteria for, **3:**210b, 210f
  position of part for, **3:**208-209f, 209
  position of patient for, **3:**208, 208f
  structures shown on, **3:**210, 210f
 breathing instructions for, **1:**490, 490f
 in children, **3:**118-124
  with cystic fibrosis, **3:**141, 141f
  image evaluation for, **3:**121, 123t
  less than one year old, **3:**119f-120f, 124
  more than one year old, **3:**121, 122f
  Pigg-O-Stat for, **3:**118, 118f
  with pneumonia, **3:**150-151, 151f
  positioning for, **3:**119
  3 to 18 years old, **3:**124, 124f
 general positioning considerations for,
  1:488
  for lateral projections, **1:**488, 489f
  for oblique projections, **1:**488
  for PA projections, **1:**488, 489f
  upright vs. prone, **1:**488, 488f
 of geriatric patients, **3:**177-178, 178f
 grid technique for, **1:**490, 491f
 lateral projection in neonate for, **3:**211-212,
  211f-212f
 of lungs and heart
  AP oblique projection for, **1:**508-509,
   508f-509f
  AP projection for, **1:**510-511, 510f-511f
  lateral projection for, **1:**500-503
   evaluation criteria for, **1:**502b
   foreshortening in, **1:**501, 501f
   forward bending in, **1:**501, 501f
   general positioning considerations for,
    1:488, 489f
   with pleura, **1:**518-519, 518f-519f
   position of part for, **1:**500-501, 500f
   position of patient for, **1:**500
   structures shown on, **1:**502, 502f-503f
  PA oblique projection for, **1:**504-507
   evaluation criteria for, **1:**507b
   LAO position for, **1:**504f, 505, 506f
   position of part for, **1:**504f-505f, 505
   position of patient for, **1:**504
   RAO position for, **1:**505, 505f, 507f
   SID for, **1:**504
   structures shown on, **1:**506-507,
    506f-507f
  PA projection for, **1:**496-499
   breasts in, **1:**497, 497f
   evaluation criteria for, **1:**499b
   general positioning considerations for,
    1:488, 489f
   with pleura, **1:**516-517, 517f
   position of part for, **1:**496-498, 496f
   position of patient for, **1:**496
   respiration in, **1:**498, 498f
   SID for, **1:**496
   structures shown on, **1:**499, 499f
 of lungs and pleurae
  AP or PA projection for, **1:**483-484,
   516f-517f
  lateral projection for, **1:**518-519,
   518f-519f

Index

Chest radiographs (Continued)
  mobile, 3:192
    AP or PA projection in lateral decubitus
      position for, 3:194-195, 194f-195f
    AP projection in upright or supine position
      for, 3:192, 192f-193f
  of neonate, 3:208-212
    AP projection for, 3:208-210
      evaluation criteria for, 3:210b, 210f
      position of part for, 3:208f-209f, 209
      position of patient for, 3:208, 208f
      structures shown on, 3:210, 210f
    lateral projection for, 3:211-212,
      211f-212f
  of pulmonary apices
    AP axial projection for
      in lordotic position (Lindblom method),
        1:512-513, 512f-513f
      in upright or supine position, 1:515,
        515f
    PA axial projection for, 1:514, 514f
  SID for, 1:490, 491f
  surgical, 3:226, 226f
  technical procedure for, 1:490, 491f
Child abuse, 3:143f-145f
  imaging protocol for, 3:124, 146t
Children, 3:99-159
  abdominal radiography in, 3:112-115
    image assessment for, 3:123t
    with intussusception, 3:114, 114f
    with pneumoperitoneum, 3:115, 115f
    positioning and immobilization for, 3:112f-
      113f, 113
  age-based development of, 3:102-104
    for adolescents, 3:104
    for infants, 3:102
    for neonates, 3:102
    for premature infants, 3:102
    for preschoolers, 3:103, 103f
    for school age children, 3:104
    for toddlers, 3:103
  aneurysmal bone cyst in, 3:149, 149f
  approach to imaging of, 3:100
  artifacts with, 3:110-111, 110f-111f
  with autism spectrum disorders, 3:105-107,
    105t
  cardiac catheterization in
    for advanced diagnostic studies of conduction
      system, 3:86-88
    for advanced diagnostic studies of vascular
      system, 3:86
    for basic diagnostic studies, 3:86
    for interventional procedures of conduction
      system, 3:94, 94f-95f
    for interventional procedures of vascular
      system, 3:92-94, 93f
  chest radiography in, 3:118-124
    for children 3 to 18 years old, 3:124, 124f
    for children less than one year old, 3:119f-
      120f, 124
    for children more than one year old, 3:121,
      122f
    image evaluation for, 3:121, 123t
    Pigg-O-Stat for, 3:118, 118f
    with pneumonia, 3:150-151, 151f
    positioning for, 3:119
  communication with, 3:101
  CT of, 3:156, 156f, 336f-338f
  cystic fibrosis in, 3:141, 141f
  developmental dysplasia of hip in, 3:142,
    142f
  EOS system for, 3:153, 155, 155f
  Ewing sarcoma in, 3:150, 150f
  foreign bodies in, 3:139
    airway, 3:139, 139f
    ingested, 3:139, 140f

Children (Continued)
  fractures in, 3:129-130
    due to child abuse, 3:143-145, 144f-145f
    greenstick, 3:130
    growth plate, 3:131
    due to osteogenesis imperfecta, 3:146t, 147
    pathologic, 3:148-150
    plastic or bowing, 3:130
    Salter-Harris, 3:130, 130f
    supracondylar, 3:131, 131f
    toddler's, 3:130-131
    torus, 3:130
  gastrointestinal and genitourinary studies in,
    3:116-118
    indications for, 3:118t
    radiation protection for, 3:116, 116f
    with vesicoureteral reflux, 3:117-118, 117f
  image assessment for, 3:123t
  immobilization techniques for
    for abdominal radiography, 3:112-113,
      112f-113f
    for chest radiography, 3:118, 118f-120f,
      124f
    for gastrointestinal and genitourinary studies,
      3:116f
    holding as, 3:110
    for limb radiography, 3:127-129, 127f-128f
    for pelvis and hip radiography, 3:126, 126f
    for skull radiography, 3:132, 133f, 135f
  interventional radiography in, 3:157-158,
    157f-158f
  limb radiography in, 3:127-131
    with fractures, 3:129-130, 130f-131f
    image evaluation for, 3:123t, 131
    immobilization for, 3:127-129, 127f-129f
    radiation protection for, 3:129, 129f
  MRI of, 3:155-156, 156f
  nonaccidental trauma (child abuse) in,
    3:143-146, 143f-145f
    imaging protocol for, 3:146, 146t
  osteochondroma in, 3:148, 148f
  osteogenesis perfecta in, 3:147, 147f
  osteoid osteoma in, 3:149, 149f
  osteoporosis in, 3:473-474, 473f
  osteosarcoma in, 3:150
  paranasal sinus series in, 3:135-136,
    136f-137f
  pathologic fractures in, 3:148-150
  pelvis and hip imaging in, 3:125-126
    general principles of, 3:125-126, 125f
    image evaluation for, 3:123t, 126
    initial images in, 3:125
    positioning and immobilization for, 3:126,
      126f
    preparation and communication for, 3:126
  pneumonia in, 3:150-151, 151f
  progeria in, 3:152, 152f
  providing adequate care and service for,
    3:101
  radiation protection for, 3:108-111, 108f-109f,
    109t
  respect and dignity for, 3:101
  safety with, 3:101
  scoliosis in, 3:152-154
    Cobb angle in, 3:154
    congenital, 3:153
    estimation of rotation in, 3:154
    idiopathic, 3:152
    image assessment for, 3:123t
    imaging of, 3:153, 153f
    lateral bends with, 3:154
    neuromuscular, 3:153
    patterns of, 3:154
    skeletal maturity with, 3:154
    symptoms of, 3:152, 152f
    treatment options for, 3:154

Children (Continued)
  skull radiography in, 3:132-135
    AP axial Towne projection for, 3:132,
      135t
    AP projection for, 3:132, 134-135, 134f
    with craniosynostosis, 3:132
    with fracture, 3:132
    immobilization for, 3:132, 133f, 135f
    lateral projection for, 3:132, 134-135,
      134f-135f
    summary of projections for, 3:135t
  soft tissue neck (STN) radiography in,
    3:137-138, 137f-138f
  with special needs, 3:105-107
  ultrasound of, 3:156
  waiting room for, 3:100, 100f-101f
Chloral hydrate (Noctec), 2:226t
Cholangiography, 2:173
  operative (immediate), 3:223-225,
    224f-225f
  percutaneous transhepatic, 2:174-175,
    174f
  postoperative (delayed, T-tube), 2:176-177,
    176f-177f
Cholangiopancreatography
  endoscopic retrograde, 2:178, 178f-179f
  magnetic resonance, 3:361f
Cholecystitis, 2:109t
  ultrasonography of, 3:379f
Cholecystography, 2:173
Cholecystokinin, 2:106
Choledochal sphincter, 2:105
Choledocholithiasis, 2:109t
Cholegraphy, 2:173
Cholelithiasis, 2:109t
Chondrosarcoma, 1:109t, 182t, 240t, 335t,
  454t
Chorion, 2:241
Chorion laeve, ultrasonography of, 3:389f
Chorionic cavity, ultrasonography of, 3:389f
Choroid plexuses, 3:255, 257-259, 257f
Chromium-51 (^{51}Cr), 3:406t
Chromosomes and cancer, 3:482, 506
Chronic bronchitis in older adults, 3:172
Chronic obstructive pulmonary disease,
  1:486t
  in older adults, 3:172, 172f, 174t
Chronologic age, age-specific competencies by,
  1:23
Chyme, 2:99
Ci (curie), 3:405, 437
Cigarette smoking and cancer, 3:482, 482t
Cilia of uterine tube, 2:239
Cineangiography, 3:96
Cinefluorography, 3:96
Circle of Willis
  anatomy of, 3:51, 51f
  CT angiography of, 3:325f
  MR angiography of, 3:363f-364f
  sectional anatomy of, 3:255, 259-261
Circulator, 3:216
Circulatory system, 3:22
  blood-vascular system in, 3:22-26, 22f
    arteries in, 3:22f, 23
      coronary, 3:25, 25f
      pulmonary, 3:22f, 23
      systemic, 3:23
    arterioles in, 3:23
    capillaries in, 3:23-24
    complete circulation of blood through,
      3:24
    heart in, 3:23-24, 25f
    main trunk vessels in, 3:23
    portal system in, 3:23, 23f
    pulmonary circulation in, 3:23, 23f
    systemic circulation in, 3:23, 23f

Circulatory system (*Continued*)
veins in, **3:**22f, 23
coronary, **3:**25, 25f
pulmonary, **3:**22f, 23
systemic, **3:**24
velocity of blood circulation in, **3:**26
venules in, **3:**23
lymphatic system in, **3:**22, 26, 27f
Circumduction, **1:**97, 97f
Cisterna chyli, **3:**26
Cisterna magna, **3:**254, 262-263
Cisternography, radionuclide, **3:**417
CIT (cardiovascular and interventional technologist), **3:**96
Claudication, **3:**28, 47, 96
Claustrum, **3:**253f, 258-259, 258f
Clavicle
anatomy of, **1:**175, 175f
AP axial projection of, **1:**214, 214f
AP projection of, **1:**213, 213f
function of, **1:**175
PA axial projection of, **1:**215, 215f
PA projection of, **1:**215, 215f
sectional anatomy of, **3:**269f, 270
on axial (transverse) plane, **3:**272, 272f-273f
on coronal plane, **3:**280-281, 281f
on sagittal plane, **3:**279-280, 280f
Clavicular notch, **1:**447-448, 447f
Clay shoveler's fracture, **1:**380t
Clear leaded plastic (Clear Pb) filter, **1:**56f, 57
Cleaves method
for AP oblique projection of femoral necks, **1:**342-343
bilateral, **1:**342, 342f
evaluation criteria for, **1:**343b
position of part for, **1:**342, 342f
position of patient for, **1:**342
structures shown on, **1:**343, 343f
unilateral, **1:**342-343, 342f
for axiolateral projection of femoral necks, **1:**344-345, 344f-345f
Clements-Nakamaya modification of Danelius-Miller method for axiolateral projection of hip, **1:**352-353, 352f-353f
Clinical history, **1:**13, 13f
Clivus, **2:**258f-259f, 264-265, 265f, 267
Closed fracture, **1:**84
Clubfoot
defined, **1:**240t
deviations in, **1:**267
Kandel method for dorsoplantar axial projection of, **1:**270, 270f
Kite method for AP projection of, **1:**267, 267f, 269f
Kite method for mediolateral projection of, **1:**268-269, 268f-269f
CM (canthomeatal) line, **3:**437
CMC joints. *See* Carpometacarpal (CMC) joint(s).
CNS. *See* Central nervous system (CNS).
CO_2 (carbon dioxide) as contrast medium, **3:**29
Coagulopathy, **3:**96
Coal miner's lung, **1:**486t
Coalition position for axial projection of calcaneus, **1:**273, 273f
Cobalt-57 (^{57}Co), **3:**406t
Cobalt-60 (^{60}Co) units, **3:**486-487, 487f, 506
Cobb angle, **3:**154
Coccygeal cornua, **1:**376-377, 376f
Coccygeal vertebra, **1:**366
Coccyx
anatomy of, **1:**330f, 366f
AP axial projection of, **1:**431-432, 431f-432f
as bony landmark, **1:**71f, 71t, 333f
lateral projections of, **1:**433-434, 433f-434f
sectional anatomy of, **3:**282, 296, 296f-297f

Cochlea, **2:**269f-270f, 271
Cochlear nerve, **2:**270f
"Code lift" process, **1:**46
Cognitive impairment in older adults, **3:**167
Coils in MRI, **3:**346, 354, 354f, 367
Coincidence circuit, **3:**422-424, 424f
Coincidence counts for PET, **3:**429, 429f
Cold spot, **3:**405, 437
Colitis, **2:**109t
ulcerative, **2:**109t
Collateral, **3:**96
Collecting ducts, **2:**185, 185f
Collecting system, duplicate, **2:**188t
Colles fracture, **1:**109t
Collimation
in digital imaging, **1:**38
multileaf, **3:**489, 489f, 507
with obese patients, **1:**50, 50f
for trauma radiography, **2:**30
of x-ray beam, **1:**32-33, 32f-33f
Collimator(s)
of gamma camera, **3:**408f, 409, 437
for linear accelerators, **3:**488f, 489, 506
Collimator-mounted filter
example of, **1:**56f
foot, **1:**60t, 62f, 63
placement of, **1:**58, 58f-59f
shape of, **1:**57
shoulder, **1:**59f, 60-63, 60t, 63f
swimmer's, **1:**60-63, 60t, 62f
Colloidal preparations for large intestine contrast media studies, **2:**144
Colon
anatomy of, **2:**102f, 103
AP axial projection of, **2:**161, 161f
AP oblique projection of
in LPO position, **2:**162, 162f
in RPO position, **2:**163, 163f
in upright position, **2:**168, 168f
AP projection of, **2:**160, 160f
in left lateral decubitus position, **2:**166
in right lateral decubitus position, **2:**165, 165f
in upright position, **2:**168, 168f
ascending
anatomy of, **2:**100f, 102f, 103
sectional anatomy of, **3:**283, 291, 291f, 298, 298f
axial projection of (Chassard-Lapiné method), **2:**169, 169f
colostomy studies of, **2:**170
contrast media studies of, **2:**144-148
contrast media for, **2:**144-145
double-contrast method for, **2:**144, 144f, 150-153
single-stage, **2:**144, 150, 150f-151f
two-stage, **2:**144
Wellen method for, **2:**152-153, 152f-153f
insertion of enema tip for, **2:**148
opacified colon in, **2:**154
preparation and care of patient for, **2:**147
preparation of barium suspension for, **2:**147
preparation of intestinal tract for, **2:**146, 146f
single-contrast method for, **2:**144, 144f, 148-149, 148f-149f
standard barium enema apparatus for, **2:**146, 146f-147f
CT colonography (virtual colonoscopy) for, **2:**144, 145f
decubitus positions for, **2:**164-172
defecography for, **2:**172, 172f

Colon (*Continued*)
descending, **2:**102f, 103
sectional anatomy of, **3:**283
sectional anatomy on axial (transverse) plane of
at Level D, **3:**288, 288f
at Level E, **3:**289, 289f
at Level F, **3:**290, 290f
at Level G, **3:**291, 291f
at Level H, **3:**292, 292f
at Level I, **3:**293f
sectional anatomy on coronal plane of, **3:**298f
diagnostic enema for, **2:**170, 170f-171f
lateral projection of
in R or L position, **2:**159, 159f
in R or L ventral decubitus position, **2:**167, 167f
in upright position, **2:**168
opacified, **2:**154
PA axial projection of, **2:**156, 156f
PA oblique projection of
in LAO position, **2:**158, 158f
in RAO position, **2:**157, 157f
PA projection of, **2:**154, 154f-155f
in left lateral decubitus position, **2:**166, 166f
in right lateral decubitus position, **2:**165
in upright position, **2:**168, 168f
sectional anatomy of, **3:**283
sigmoid, **2:**102f, 103
axial projection of (Chassard-Lapiné method), **2:**169, 169f
sectional anatomy of, **3:**283, 294, 294f
transverse
anatomy of, **2:**102f, 103
sectional anatomy of, **3:**283
sectional anatomy on axial (transverse) plane of
at Level D, **3:**288, 288f
at Level E, **1:**339, **3:**289f
at Level F, **3:**290, 290f
at Level G, **3:**291, 291f
Colon cancer, familial adenomatous polyposis and, **3:**483
Colonography, CT, **2:**144, 145f
Colonoscopy, virtual, **2:**144, 145f, **3:**335, 335f
Colorectal cancer syndrome, hereditary nonpolyposis, **3:**483
Color-flow Doppler, **3:**396-397
Colostomy stoma, diagnostic enema through, **2:**170, 170f-171f
Colostomy studies, **2:**170
Comminuted fracture, **1:**84f
Common bile duct
anatomy of, **2:**100f, 105, 105f
sectional anatomy of, **3:**283
Common carotid artery
anatomy of, **3:**22f, 49, 49f
arteriography of, **3:**40f, 50f, 57f
digital subtraction angiography of, **3:**31f, 55f
sectional anatomy of, **3:**269f, 270-271
on axial (transverse) plane, **3:**272-275, 272f-274f
on coronal plane, **3:**280-281
on sagittal plane, **3:**278-279, 280f
Common femoral artery, **3:**22f, 25
Common femoral vein, **3:**22f
Common hepatic artery, **3:**284, 289, 289f, 298-299, 298f
Common hepatic duct
anatomy of, **2:**100f, 105, 105f
sectional anatomy of, **3:**283
Common iliac arteries
anatomy of, **3:**22f, 25
arteriography of, **3:**41f, 48f

Common iliac arteries *(Continued)*
  percutaneous transluminal angioplasty of,
    3:64f
  sectional anatomy of, **3:**271, 284, 292, 292f,
    298-299
Common iliac nodes, **3:**27f
Common iliac vein
  anatomy of, **3:**22f
  sectional anatomy of, **3:**284, 292-293,
    292f-293f
  venography of, **3:**48f, 60f
Communication
  with children, **3:**101
    with autism spectrum disorders, **3:**106
  with obese patients, **1:**47
  with older adults, **3:**175
Compact bone, **1:**76, 76f
  and bone densitometry, **3:**445, 445t
  defined, **3:**476
Compensating filters, **1:**53-64
  appropriate use of, **1:**57
  Boomerang contact
    applications of, **1:**60t, 63-64, 63f
    composition of, **1:**57
    example of, **1:**56f
    placement of, **1:**58, 58f
    shape of, **1:**57
  clear leaded plastic (Clear Pb), **1:**56f, 57
  composition of, **1:**57
  convex and concave conical-shaped,
    1:64
  in Danelius-Miller method, **1:**60-63, 62f
  defined, **1:**54-55
  examples of, **1:**55, 56f
  Ferlic collimator-mounted
    examples of, **1:**56f
    placement of, **1:**58, 58f-59f
    shape of, **1:**57
  Ferlic foot, **1:**60t, 62f, 63
  Ferlic shoulder, **1:**59f, 60-63, 60t, 63f
  Ferlic swimmer's, **1:**60-63, 60t, 62f
  highly specialized, **1:**64
  history of, **1:**55
  mounting and removal of, **1:**64, 64f
  need for, **1:**54, 54f
  physical principles of, **1:**57-58
  placement of, **1:**58, 58f-59f
    in position, **1:**55f
  scoliosis, **1:**57, 64, 64f
  shape of, **1:**57
  specific applications of, **1:**60-64, 60t
  in this atlas, **1:**64
  trough
    applications of, **1:**60, 60t, 61f
    example of, **1:**56f
    in position, **1:**55f
    shape of, **1:**57
  wedge
    applications of, **1:**60, 60t, 61f
    example of, **1:**56f
    in position, **1:**55f
    shape of, **1:**57
  specialized, **1:**62f, 63
Compensatory curves, **1:**367
Complete reflux examination of small intestine,
  2:141, 141f
Complex projections, **1:**88
Complex structure or mass in ultrasonography,
  3:374, 374f, 397
Compound fracture, **1:**84f
Compression cone for abdominal imaging, **2:**113,
  113f
Compression devices for abdominal imaging,
  2:113, 113f
Compression fracture, **1:**84f, 380t
  in older adults, **3:**170, 170f, 174t

Compression paddle for abdominal imaging, **2:**113,
  113f
Compression plate for breast lesion localization,
  2:462-464, 462f-463f
Computed axial tomography (CAT), **3:**302
Computed radiography (CR), **1:**36, 36f
Computed tomography (CT), **3:**301-340
  of abdomen, **3:**336f-338f
  of abdominal aortic aneurysm, **3:**313f
  algorithm in, **3:**302, 339
  aperture in, **3:**310, 339
  archiving in, **3:**309, 339
  axial image in, **3:**302, 339
  bit depth in, **3:**308
  body planes in, **1:**67, 67f
  of cervical spine, **3:**336f-338f
  of chest, **3:**336f-338f
  of children, **3:**156, 156f, 336f-338f
  of CNS, **3:**10-12
    brain in, **3:**10, 10f-11f
    spine in, **3:**11, 11f-12f
  contrast media for, **3:**316-318, 316f
    power injector for IV administration of, **3:**317,
      317f
  and conventional radiography, **3:**302-303,
    302f-304f
  of coronal sinuses, **3:**336f-338f
  cradle for, **3:**310
  CT numbers (Hounsfield units) in, **3:**308, 308t,
    339
  curved planar reformations in, **3:**313, 313f
  data acquisition system for, **3:**309, 339
  data storage and retrieval for, **3:**309, 340
  defined, **3:**302, 302f, 339
  definition of terms for, **3:**339-340
  detectors in, **3:**305-306, 309, 339
  diagnostic applications of, **3:**313-314,
    313f-316f
  direct coronal image in, **3:**310, 310f, 339
  dual-energy source, **3:**307, 308f
  dynamic scanning with, **3:**321, 339
  factors affecting image quality in, **3:**318-320
    artifacts as, **3:**319, 319f-320f, 339
    contrast resolution as, **3:**303, 318, 339
    noise as, **3:**318-319, 319f, 340
    patient factors as, **3:**319-320, 321f
    scan diameter as, **3:**320, 340
    scan times as, **3:**320, 340
    spatial resolution as, **3:**318, 340
    temporal resolution as, **3:**318, 340
  field of view in, **3:**308, 339
    scan vs. display, **3:**320
  flat-panel, **3:**307
  fundamentals of, **3:**301f, 302
  future of, **3:**333-335, 335f
  generation classification of scanners for,
    3:305-308, 339
    first-generation, **3:**305-306, 305f-306f
    second-generation, **3:**306
    third-generation, **3:**306-307, 306f
    fourth-generation, **3:**307, 307f
    fifth-generation, **3:**307, 307f
    sixth-generation, **3:**307, 308f
  grayscale image in, **3:**311, 339
  of head, **3:**336f-338f
  high-resolution scans in, **3:**319-320, 321f, 339
  historical development of, **3:**305, 305f
  image manipulation in, **3:**303, 304f, 313, 313f
  image misregistration in, **3:**321-323, 339
  indexing in, **3:**310, 339
  for interventional procedures, **3:**314, 314f-316f
  of knee, **3:**336f-338f
  for long bone measurement, **2:**6, 6f
  of lumbar vertebrae, **1:**415, 416f
  matrix in, **3:**302, 308, 308f, 339
  of mediastinum, **1:**484, 485f

Computed tomography (CT) *(Continued)*
  vs. MRI, **3:**333, 334f
  multiplanar reconstruction in, **3:**309, 313, 313f,
    327f, 340
  vs. nuclear medicine, **3:**401t
  of pelvis, **3:**336f-338f
  with PET, **3:**327-329, 329f, 436
  pixels and voxels in, **3:**308, 308f, 340
  postprocessing techniques in, **3:**326, 340
  primary data in, **3:**302, 340
  projections (scan profiles, raw data) in,
    3:308
  protocols for, **3:**303f, 319-320, 336-340
  quality control for, **3:**329
  quantitative
    for bone densitometry, **3:**444, 469, 469f,
      477
    peripheral, **3:**475, 477
  radiation dose in, **3:**329-331
    equipment to reduce, **3:**329-330, 329f
    estimating effective, **3:**331
    factors that affect, **3:**331-332
      automatic tube current modulation (ATCM)
        as, **3:**331, 331f
      beam collimation as, **3:**331-332,
        332t-333t
      patient shielding as, **3:**331
      patient size as, **3:**332
      "selectable" filters as, **3:**331, 332f
    measurement of, **3:**330, 330f
    reporting of, **3:**330, 331f
  for radiation treatment planning, **3:**327, 328f
  sectional anatomy for, **3:**252
  after shoulder arthrography, **2:**11, 11f
  slice in, **3:**302, 340
  slip ring in, **3:**309, 340
  of soft tissue neck, **3:**336f-338f
  SPECT combined with, **3:**401, 403f, 415, 415f,
    436
  spiral or helical
    defined, **3:**339-340
    multislice, **3:**306, 323-324, 323f-324f
    single slice, **3:**306, 321-323, 322f
  system components for, **3:**309-313, 309f
    computer as, **3:**309, 309f
    display monitor as, **3:**311-312, 312f, 312t
    gantry and table as, **3:**309-310, 309f-310f,
      339
    operator's console as, **3:**311, 311f
    workstation for image manipulation and
      multiplanar reconstruction as, **3:**309, 313,
      313f, 340
  technical aspects of, **3:**308, 308f, 308t
  of thoracic vertebrae, **1:**405, 406f
  of thoracic viscera, **1:**484, 485f
  three-dimensional imaging with, **3:**326-327,
    327f
    of abdominal aortic aneurysm, **3:**313f
    future of, **3:**335, 335f
    maximum intensity projection for,
      3:326
    shaded surface display for, **3:**326
    volume rendering for, **3:**306-307, 321, 322f,
      326-327
  for trauma, **2:**20, 29
    of cervical spine, **2:**53-55
    of cranium, **2:**29, 29f, 53-55, 54f
    of pelvis, **2:**53f, 55
    of thorax, **2:**53-55
  of urinary system, **2:**190, 190f
  volume, **3:**326-327
    defined, **3:**306-307
    multislice spiral CT for, **3:**323-324, 323f
    single-slice spiral CT for, **3:**321, 322f
  windowing (gray-level mapping) in, **3:**10, 312,
    312f, 312t, 340

Computed tomography angiography (CTA), **3**:324-326
  advantages of, **3**:324
  bolus in, **3**:324, 339
  of brain, **3**:10f, 324-326, 325f
    perfusion study for, **3**:324-326, 326f
  cardiac, **3**:324-326, 325f-326f
    with cardiac gating, **3**:324-326, 326f
  defined, **3**:324, 339
  scan duration in, **3**:324, 340
  steps in, **3**:324
  table speed in, **3**:324, 340
  uses of, **3**:324-326
Computed tomography (CT) colonography, **2**:144, 145f
Computed tomography dose index (CTDI), **3**:330, 339
Computed tomography dose index$_{100}$ (CTDI$_{100}$), **3**:330, 339
Computed tomography dose index$_{vol}$ (CTDI$_{vol}$), **3**:330, 339
Computed tomography dose index$_w$ (CTDI$_w$), **3**:330, 339
Computed tomography (CT) enteroclysis, **2**:141, 142f
Computed tomography myelography (CTM), **3**:12, 12f
Computed tomography (CT) simulator for radiation oncology, **3**:489, 490f, 507
Computer(s)
  for CT, **3**:309, 309f
  for DXA, **3**:460
  in gamma ray cameras, **3**:409-410, 410f-411f
Computer-aided detection (CAD) systems for mammography, **2**:376-379, 376f
Computerized planimetry for evaluation of ventricle functions, **3**:82-84, 84f
Concha, **2**:270f
Condylar canals, **2**:266f, 267
Condylar process, **2**:264f, 274, 274f
Condyle, **1**:84
Condyloid joint, **1**:82, 83f
Condyloid process, **3**:254
Cones, **2**:315
Confluence of sinuses, **3**:261-262, 261f
Conformal radiotherapy (CRT), **3**:494, 506
Congenital aganglionic megacolon, **2**:109t
Congenital heart defects, cardiac catheterization for, **3**:92-94, 93f
Congestive heart failure in older adults, **3**:171, 174t
Conjunctiva, **2**:314, 314f-315f
Connective tissue, cancer arising from, **3**:483t
Console for MRI, **3**:345, 345f
Construction in three-dimensional imaging, **3**:326
Contact filter
  applications of, **1**:60t, 63-64, 63f
  composition of, **1**:57
  example of, **1**:56f
  placement of, **1**:58, 58f
  shape of, **1**:57
Contact shield, **1**:33, 33f
Contamination, **3**:250
Contamination control
  CDC recommendations on, **1**:16, 16b, 16f
  chemical substances for, **1**:16
  for minor surgical procedures in radiology department, **1**:17, 17f
  in operating room, **1**:16-17, 16f-17f
  standard precautions for, **1**:15, 15f
Continuous wave transducers for ultrasonography, **3**:372, 397
Contour in radiation oncology, **3**:494, 506
Contractures in older adults, **3**:174t
Contralateral, **1**:85

Contrast, **1**:5, 6f
  in MRI vs. conventional radiography, **3**:342, 367
Contrast arthrography, **2**:7-16
  abbreviations used for, **2**:9b
  defined, **2**:8-9
  double-, **2**:8-9
    of knee, **2**:13, 13f
  of hip, **2**:14
    AP oblique, **2**:14f
    axiolateral "frog", **2**:14f
    with congenital dislocation, **2**:8f, 14, 14f
    prosthetic, **2**:14, 15f
      digital subtraction technique for, **2**:14, 15f
      photographic subtraction technique for, **2**:14, 15f
  of knee, **2**:12
    double-contrast (horizontal ray method), **2**:13, 13f
    vertical ray method for, **2**:12, 12f
  MRI vs., **2**:8, 8f
  of other joints, **2**:16, 16f
  overview of, **2**:8-9
  procedure for, **2**:9, 9f
  of shoulder, **2**:10-11
    CT after, **2**:11, 11f
    double-contrast, **2**:10, 10f-11f
    MRI vs., **2**:8f
    single-contrast, **2**:10, 10f-11f
  summary of pathology found on, **2**:9t
Contrast media
  for alimentary canal, **2**:111-112, 111f-112f
  for angiographic studies, **3**:29
  for cardiac catheterization, **3**:78
  for CT, **3**:316-318, 316f
    power injector for IV administration of, **3**:317, 317f
  for MRI, **3**:355, 355f
  for myelography, **3**:6-7, 6f
  in older adults, **3**:176
  for simulation in radiation oncology, **3**:490, 491f-492f
Contrast media studies
  of esophagus, **2**:115-117, 115f
    barium administration and respiration for, **2**:119, 119f
    barium sulfate mixture for, **2**:115
    double-contrast, **2**:115, 117, 117f
    examination procedures for, **2**:116-117, 116f-117f
    single-contrast, **2**:115, 116f-117f
  of large intestine, **2**:144-148
    contrast media for, **2**:144-145
    double-contrast method for, **2**:144, 144f, 150-153
      single-stage, **2**:144, 150, 150f-151f
      two-stage, **2**:144
      Wellen method for, **2**:152-153, 152f-153f
    insertion of enema tip for, **2**:148
    opacified colon in, **2**:154
    preparation and care of patient for, **2**:147
    preparation of barium suspensions for, **2**:147
    preparation of intestinal tract for, **2**:146, 146f
    single-contrast method for, **2**:144, 144f, 148-149, 148f-149f
    standard barium enema apparatus for, **2**:146, 146f-147f
  of stomach, **2**:121-123
    barium sulfate suspension for, **2**:111, 111f
    biphasic, **2**:123
    in children, **3**:116
    double-contrast, **2**:122, 122f, 124f
    single-contrast, **2**:121, 121f, 124f
    water-soluble, iodinated solution for, **2**:111, 111f

Contrast media studies (*Continued*)
  of urinary system, **2**:190-197
    adverse reactions to iodinated media for, **2**:196
    angiographic, **2**:190, 191f
    antegrade filling for, **2**:191, 191f
    contrast media for, **2**:194, 195f
    CT in, **2**:190, 191f
    equipment for, **2**:198, 198f-199f
    physiologic technique for, **2**:192f, 193
    preparation of intestinal tract for, **2**:196-197, 196f-197f
    preparation of patient for, **2**:197
    retrograde filling for, **2**:192f, 193
    tomography in, **2**:190, 191f
Contrast resolution, **1**:5
  for CT, **3**:303, 318, 339
Contre-coup fracture, **2**:282t
Conus medullaris, **3**:3, 3f, 18
Conus projection, **3**:8
Convolutions, **3**:256-257
Cooper's ligaments, **2**:380, 381f
Coracoid process
  anatomy of, **1**:176, 176f
  AP axial projection of, **1**:222, 222f-223f
  defined, **1**:84
  sectional anatomy of, **3**:270
Coregistration, **3**:402, 402f, 438
Cornea, **2**:314f-315f, 315
Corona radiata, **3**:254-257
Coronal image, direct, in CT, **3**:310, 310f, 339
Coronal image plane in ultrasonography, **3**:397
Coronal plane, **1**:66, 66f-67f
  in sectional anatomy, **3**:252
Coronal sinuses, CT of, **3**:336f-338f
Coronal suture
  anatomy of, **2**:258f, 259, 275t
  lateral projection of, **2**:295f
Coronary angiography, **3**:40f, 75
  for cardiac catheterization, **3**:84, 85f, 85t
  CT, **3**:324-326, 325f-326f
    with cardiac gating, **3**:324-326, 326f
  for percutaneous transluminal coronary angioplasty, **3**:88, 88f-89f
  procedures that may accompany, **3**:76, 76t
Coronary angioplasty, percutaneous transluminal, **3**:66, 88, 88f-89f
  catheter system for, **3**:88, 88f
  with stent placement, **3**:88, 89f
Coronary arteries
  anatomy of, **3**:25, 25f
  sectional anatomy of, **3**:270-271
  stenosis and occlusion of, **3**:75
Coronary arteriography, MRI, **3**:95f
Coronary artery disease, **3**:75
  atherectomy devices for, **3**:90, 90f-91f
  intravascular ultrasound of, **3**:80t, 91, 91f-92f
  tools for diagnosis and treatment of, **3**:80t
Coronary atherectomy devices, **3**:90, 90f-91f
Coronary flow reserve, PET of, **3**:435
Coronary sinus, **3**:25f
Coronary veins, **3**:25, 25f
Coronoid fossa, **1**:104, 104f
Coronoid process
  anatomy of, **1**:103, 103f, **2**:273f-274f, 274
  axiolateral oblique projection of, **2**:344f-345f
  Coyle method for axiolateral projection of, **1**:162-164
    evaluation criteria for, **1**:164
    position of part for, **1**:162, 162f-163f
    position of patient for, **1**:162
    structures shown on, **1**:164, 164f
  defined, **1**:84
  PA axial projection of, **2**:342f
  sectional anatomy of, **3**:254
  submentovertical projection of, **2**:346f

Corpora cavernosa, **3:**297f
Corpora quadrigemina, **3:**255, 259-260, 259f, 264
Corpus callosum
anatomy of, **3:**2, 2f
genu of, **3:**257-258, 257f-258f
sectional anatomy of, **3:**254-255
on axial (transverse) plane, **3:**256-258, 256f-257f
on coronal plane, **3:**266-268, 267f-268f
on sagittal plane, **3:**264, 265f
splenium of, **3:**253f, 257-258, 257f-258f
Cortex of brain, **3:**2, 18
Cortical bone, **1:**76, 76f
and bone densitometry, **3:**445, 445t
defined, **3:**476
Costal cartilage, **1:**447f, 448
Costal facets
of ribs, **1:**447f-448f, 448
of thoracic vertebrae, **1:**372, 372f, 373t
Costal groove, **1:**448, 448f
Costochondral articulations, **1:**449t, 450, 450f
Costophrenic angle
anatomy of, **1:**481-482, 481f-482f
sectional anatomy of, **3:**270
Costosternal articulations, **3:**279-280
Costotransverse joints
in bony thorax, **1:**449f-450f, 449t, 450
sectional anatomy of, **3:**269-270, 272-275, 272f
in thoracic spine, **1:**372f, 378, 378f, 379t
Costovertebral joints
in bony thorax, **1:**449f-450f, 449t, 450
sectional anatomy of, **3:**269-270, 273-275
in thoracic spine, **1:**372f, 378, 378f, 379t
Coyle method for axiolateral projection of radial head and coronoid fossa, **1:**162-164
evaluation criteria for, **1:**164
position of part for, **1:**162, 162f-163f
position of patient for, **1:**162
structures shown on, **1:**164, 164f
CR (central ray). *See* Central ray (CR).
CR (computed radiography), **1:**36, 36f
⁵¹Cr (chromium-51), **3:**406t
Cradle for CT, **3:**310
Cragg, Andrew, **3:**20-21
Cranial bones
anatomy of, **2:**257, 257b
anterior aspect of, **2:**257f
ethmoid bone as
anatomy of, **2:**262, 262f
location of, **2:**259f
frontal bone as
anatomy of, **2:**261, 261f
location of, **2:**257f-259f
function of, **2:**257
lateral aspect of, **2:**258f-259f
in newborn, **2:**259-260, 260f
occipital bone as
anatomy of, **2:**266-267, 266f-267f
location of, **2:**258f-259f, 264f
parietal bones as
anatomy of, **2:**263, 263f
location of, **2:**257f-259f
sectional anatomy of, **3:**253
sphenoid bone as
anatomy of, **2:**264-266, 264f-265f
location of, **2:**257f-258f
temporal bones as
anatomy of, **2:**268, 268f-269f
location of, **2:**257f-259f
Cranial fossae, **2:**258f, 260
Cranial region, sectional anatomy of, **3:**253-268
on axial (transverse) plane, **3:**256, 256f
at level A, **3:**256-257, 256f-257f
at level B, **3:**257-258, 257f

Cranial region, sectional anatomy of (*Continued*)
at level C, **3:**258, 258f
at level D, **3:**259-260, 259f
at level E, **3:**260f-261f, 261-262
at level F, **3:**262, 262f
at level G, **3:**263, 263f
on cadaveric image, **3:**253, 253f
on coronal plane, **3:**266-267, 266f
at level A, **3:**266-267, 267f
at level B, **3:**267-268, 267f
at level C, **3:**268, 268f
on sagittal plane, **3:**256f, 264, 264f
at level A, **3:**264, 265f
at level B, **3:**265, 265f
at level C, **3:**266, 266f
Cranial suture synostosis, premature, **3:**132
Craniosynostosis, **3:**132
Cranium. *See also* Skull.
average or normal, **2:**260
deviations from, **2:**260
Crest, **1:**84
Cribriform plate
anatomy of, **2:**258f, 262, 262f
sectional anatomy of, **3:**253, 261-263
Crista galli
anatomy of, **2:**258f-259f, 262, 262f
PA axial projection of, **2:**298f, 330f
sectional anatomy of, **3:**253, 263, 263f
Crohn disease, **2:**109t
Cross-calibration of DXA machines, **3:**457, 476
The Crosser, **3:**80t
Crossover with K-edge filtration systems for DXA, **3:**452
Cross-sectional plane, **1:**66, 66f-67f
Cross-table projections with obese patient, **1:**49
Crosswise position, **1:**28, 28f
CRT (conformal radiotherapy), **3:**494, 506
Cruciate ligaments, double-contrast arthrography of, **2:**13
Cryogenic magnets for MRI, **3:**346, 367
Cryptorchidism, **2:**245t
Crystalline lens, **2:**314f-315f
CSF (cerebrospinal fluid)
anatomy of, **3:**3, 18
sectional anatomy of, **3:**254, 264-266
C-spine filter for scoliosis imaging, **3:**153
CST (certified surgical technologist), **3:**215
CT. *See* Computed tomography (CT).
CT numbers, **3:**308, 308t, 339
CTA. *See* Computed tomography angiography (CTA).
CTDI. *See* Computed tomography dose index (CTDI).
CTM (computed tomography myelography), **3:**12, 12f
Cuboid bone, **1:**228f, 229
Cuboidonavicular articulation, **1:**236t, 237f, 238
Cuneiforms, **1:**228f, 229
Cuneocuboid articulation, **1:**236t, 237f, 238
Cure, **3:**480, 506
Curie (Ci), **3:**405, 437
Curved planar reformations in CT, **3:**313, 313f, 339
CyberKnife, **3:**499-501, 501f
Cyclotron, **3:**400, 425, 426f, 437
Cyst
bone, **1:**109t, 240t
aneurysmal, **3:**149, 149f
breast, **2:**395
dermoid, **2:**245t
oil, **2:**386f
ovarian
CT of, **3:**315f
ultrasonography of, **3:**375f, 388
renal, **2:**210f-211f
retroareolar, **2:**385f

Cystic duct
anatomy of, **2:**100f, 105-106, 105f
sectional anatomy of, **3:**283
Cystic fibrosis (CF), **1:**486t, **3:**141, 141f
Cystitis, **2:**188t
Cystography, **2:**192f, 214
AP axial or PA axial projection for, **2:**216-217, 216f-217f
AP oblique projection for, **2:**218, 218f-219f
contrast injection for, **2:**214, 215f
contrast media for, **2:**214
defined, **2:**193
excretory
AP axial projection for, **2:**217f
AP oblique projection for, **2:**219f
indications and contraindications for, **2:**214
injection equipment for, **2:**214
lateral projection for, **2:**220, 220f
preliminary preparations for, **2:**214
retrograde
AP axial projection for, **2:**216f-217f
AP oblique projection for, **2:**218f-219f
AP projection for, **2:**215f
contrast injection technique for, **2:**214, 215f
Cystoureterography, **2:**193, 193f, 214
Cystourethrography, **2:**193, 193f, 214
female, **2:**222-224, 222f
metallic bead chain, **2:**222-224, 223f
male, **2:**221, 221f
voiding, **2:**214, 215f
in children, **3:**117, 117f

D
Damadian, Raymond, **3:**342
Danelius-Miller method
for axiolateral projection of hip, **1:**350-351, 350f-351f, 353f
Clements-Nakamaya modification of, **1:**352-353, 352f-353f
compensating filters in, **1:**60-63, 62f
Data acquisition system (DAS) for CT, **3:**309, 339
Data storage and retrieval for CT, **3:**309, 340
Daughter nuclide, **3:**403-404, 437
DBT (digital breast tomosynthesis), **2:**374-375
DCIS (ductal carcinoma in situ), **2:**395
calcifications in, **2:**392f
DDH (developmental dysplasia of hip), **2:**9t, **3:**142, 142f
Deadtime losses in PET, **3:**430, 432, 437
Decay
atomic, **3:**403, 437
in radiation oncology, **3:**486, 506
of radionuclides, **3:**403, 404f
Decidua capsularis, ultrasonography of, **3:**389f
Decidua parietalis, ultrasonography of, **3:**389f
Decidual basalis, ultrasonography of, **3:**389f
DECT (dual-energy source CT), **3:**307, 308f
Decubitus position, **1:**94, 94f-95f
Decubitus ulcers in older adults, **3:**175
Dedicated radiographic equipment for trauma, **2:**20, 20f
Deep, **1:**85
Deep back muscles, **3:**278, 297f
Deep femoral artery
anatomy of, **3:**22f
arteriography of, **3:**48f
Deep inguinal nodes, **3:**27f
Deep vein thrombosis, **3:**70
ultrasonography of, **3:**393, 394f
Defecography, **2:**172, 172f
Degenerative joint disease, **1:**109t, 182t, 240t, 335t, 380t
in older adults, **3:**170, 170f

Deglutition in positive-contrast pharyngography, **2:**74-75, 74f
Delayed cholangiography, **2:**176-177, 176f-177f
Dementia, **3:**167, 174t
  in Alzheimer disease, **3:**167-168, 174t, 176, 177b
  multi-infarct, **3:**169
Demerol (meperidine hydrochloride), **2:**226t
Demifacets, **1:**372, 372f, 373t
Dens
  anatomy of, **1:**369, 369f, **2:**266f
  AP projection of (Fuchs method), **1:**383, 383f
  PA projection of (Judd method), **1:**383
  sectional anatomy of, **3:**267-268
  submentovertical projection of, **2:**311f
Dental ligament, myelogram of, **3:**9f
Depressed skull fracture, **2:**282t
Depressions in bone, **1:**84
Dermoid cyst, **2:**245t
Detail resolution in ultrasonography, **3:**372, 397
Detector(s)
  for CT, **3:**305-306, 309, 339
  for PET, **3:**400, 437
Detector assembly for CT, **3:**302, 339
Deuterons in radionuclide production, **3:**425, 425f, 437
Development, **3:**102-104
  of adolescents, **3:**104
  of infants, **3:**102
  of neonates, **3:**102
  of premature infants, **3:**102
  of preschoolers, **3:**103, 103f
  of school age children, **3:**104
  of toddlers, **3:**103
Developmental dysplasia of hip (DDH), **2:**9t, **3:**142, 142f
Deviation, **1:**97, 97f
DFOV (display field of view) in CT, **3:**320
Diabetes mellitus in older adults, **3:**173
Diagnosis and radiographer, **1:**14
Diagnostic enema through colostomy stoma, **2:**170, 170f-171f
Diagnostic medical sonographers, **3:**370
  characteristics of, **3:**370, 371f
Diagnostic medical sonography. *See* Ultrasonography.
Diagnostic reference levels (DRLs) for CT, **3:**330
Diagonal position, **1:**28, 28f
Diaper, infant, **1:**20
Diaper rash ointment, **1:**20
Diaphanography of breast, **2:**473
Diaphragm
  anatomy of, **1:**479, 479f
  hiatal hernia of
    AP projection of, **2:**134, 135f
    defined, **2:**109t
    PA oblique projection of (Wolf method), **2:**136-137, 136f-137f
    upright lateral projection of, **2:**135f
  in respiratory movement, **1:**452, 452f
  sectional anatomy of
    in abdominopelvic region, **3:**282
      on axial (transverse) plane, **3:**285, 285f-287f
      on coronal plane, **3:**298f
      on sagittal plane, **3:**298
    in thoracic region, **3:**278-279, 280f
Diaphysis, **1:**77, 77f
Diarthroses, **1:**81
Diastole, **3:**96
Diazepam (Valium), **2:**226t
Differentiation, **3:**484, 506
Diffusion study in MRI, **3:**364-365, 365f, 367

Digestive system, **2:**95-180
  abbreviations used for, **2:**107b
  abdominal fistulae and sinuses in, **2:**180, 180f
  anatomy of, **2:**97-106, 97f
    biliary tract and gallbladder in, **2:**97f, 104-106, 104f-106f
    esophagus in, **2:**97, 97f
    large intestine in, **2:**97f, 102-103, 102f-103f
    liver in, **2:**97f, 104-106, 104f-106f
    pancreas and spleen in, **2:**97f, 106, 107f
    small intestine in, **2:**97f, 100f, 101
    stomach in, **2:**97f-99f, 98-99
    summary of, **2:**108b
  biliary tract and gallbladder in
    anatomy of, **2:**97f, 104-106, 104f-106f
    biliary drainage procedure and stone extraction for, **2:**175, 175f
    endoscopic retrograde cholangiopancreatography of, **2:**178, 178f-179f
    percutaneous transhepatic cholangiography of, **2:**174-175, 174f
    postoperative (T-tube) cholangiography of, **2:**176-177, 176f-177f
    prefixes associated with, **2:**173, 173t
    radiographic techniques for, **2:**173
  contrast media for, **2:**111-112, 111f-112f
  endoscopic retrograde cholangiopancreatography of pancreatic ducts in, **2:**178, 178f-179f
  esophagus in
    anatomy of, **2:**97, 97f
    AP, PA, oblique, and lateral projections of, **2:**118, 118f-119f
    contrast media studies of, **2:**115-117, 115f
      barium sulfate mixture for, **2:**115
      double-contrast, **2:**117, 117f
      examination procedure for, **2:**116-117, 116f-117f
    opaque foreign bodies in, **2:**117, 117f
    PA oblique projection of distal (Wolf method), position of part for, **2:**134, 134f
  examination procedure for, **2:**110-114
  exposure time for, **2:**114
  gastrointestinal transit in, **2:**110
  large intestine in. *See* Large intestine.
  nuclear medicine imaging of, **3:**418-419
  preparation of examining room for, **2:**114
  radiation protection for, **2:**114f, 115
  radiologic apparatus for, **2:**113, 113f
  sample exposure technique chart essential projections for, **2:**108t
  small intestine in. *See* Small intestine.
  stomach in. *See* Stomach.
  summary of pathology of, **2:**109t
  summary of projections for, **2:**96
Digestive system disorders in older adults, **3:**171, 171f
Digit(s)
  anatomy of, **1:**101, 101f
  first. *See* Thumb.
  second through fifth
    anatomy of, **1:**101, 101f
    lateral projection of, **1:**112-113
      evaluation criteria for, **1:**113b
      position of part for, **1:**112, 112f
      position of patient for, **1:**112
      structures shown on, **1:**113, 113f
    PA oblique projection in lateral rotation of, **1:**114
      evaluation criteria for, **1:**114b
      medial rotation of second digit in, **1:**114, 115f
      position of part for, **1:**114, 114f
      position of patient for, **1:**114
      structures shown on, **1:**114, 115f

Digit(s) (*Continued*)
  PA projections of, **1:**110-111
    computed radiography for, **1:**111-114
    evaluation criteria for, **1:**111b
    position of part for, **1:**110, 110f
    position of patient for, **1:**110
    structures shown in, **1:**111, 111f
Digital breast tomosynthesis (DBT), **2:**374-375
Digital disk for digital subtraction angiography, **3:**30
Digital imaging, **1:**36-38, 36f
  grids in, **1:**38
  kilovoltage in, **1:**37, 37f
  part centering for, **1:**38
  split cassettes in, **1:**38
  in this atlas, **1:**38
Digital radiographic absorptiometry, **3:**443, 474, 474f
Digital radiography (DR), **1:**3, 4f, 36-37, 37f
  mobile, **3:**184, 185f
  of cervical spine, **3:**207
  of chest, **3:**193-195
  of femur
    AP projection for, **3:**203-205
    lateral projection for, **3:**205
Digital subtraction angiography (DSA), **3:**30-34
  acquisition rate in, **3:**30
  biplane suite for, **3:**31-32, 31f
  bolus chase or DSA stepping method for, **3:**30-31
  cerebral, **3:**14-16, 14f-15f
  of common carotid artery, **3:**31f
  for hip arthrography, **2:**14, 15f
  historical development of, **3:**21
  magnification in, **3:**33
  misregistration in, **3:**31
  postprocessing in, **3:**31
  procedure for, **3:**30-34
  single-plane suite for, **3:**32, 32f
  three-dimensional intraarterial, **3:**34, 34f
Digitally reconstructed radiograph (DRR) in radiation oncology, **3:**491, 493f
Dignity
  in code of ethics, **1:**2-3
  of parents and children, **3:**101
DIP (distal interphalangeal) joints
  of lower limb, **1:**236
  of upper limb, **1:**105, 105f-106f
Diphenhydramine hydrochloride (Benadryl), **2:**226t
Diploë, **1:**79, **2:**258f-259f, 259
Direct coronal image in CT, **3:**310, 310f, 339
Direct effects of radiation, **3:**484, 506
Discordance in DXA, **3:**457, 476
Disinfectants, **1:**16
Disintegration. *See* Decay.
Diskography, provocative, **3:**16, 17f
Dislocation, **1:**109t, 182t, 240t, 335t, **2:**9t
Displaced fracture, **1:**84
Display field of view (DFOV) in CT, **3:**320
Display monitor, **1:**8
  for CT, **3:**311-312, 312f, 312t
Distal, **1:**85, 85f
Distal convoluted tubule, **2:**185, 185f
Distal humerus
  AP projection of
    in acute flexion, **1:**158, 158f
    in partial flexion, **1:**156, 156f
  PA axial projection of, **1:**165, 165f
Distal interphalangeal (DIP) joints
  of lower limb, **1:**236
  of upper limb, **1:**105, 105f-106f
Distal phalanges, **1:**228, 228f
Distal tibiofibular joint, **1:**236t, 238
Distance measurements in CT, **3:**304f

Distortion, **1:**7, 7f
Diverticulitis, **2:**109t
Diverticulosis, **2:**109t
  in older adults, **3:**171
Diverticulum, **2:**109t
  Meckel, **2:**109t
  Zenker, **2:**109t
DLP (dose length product), **3:**330, 339
Documentation
  of medication administration, **2:**235
  for trauma radiography, **2:**30
Dolichocephalic skull, **2:**286, 286f
Dopamine hydrochloride, **2:**226t
Dopamine transporter study, **3:**417
Doppler effect, **3:**397
Doppler ultrasound, **3:**397
Dorsal, **1:**85
Dorsal decubitus position, **1:**94, 94f
Dorsal recumbent position, **1:**90, 90f
Dorsal surface of foot, **1:**228-230
Dorsiflexion, **1:**97, 97f
Dorsum, **1:**85
Dorsum sellae
  anatomy of, **2:**258f, 264-265, 264f-265f
  AP axial projection of
    Haas method for, **2:**309f
    Towne method for, **2:**305f
  PA axial projection of, **2:**298f
  sectional anatomy of, **3:**253-254, 261-262
Dose for nuclear medicine, **3:**405, 437
Dose inhomogeneity in radiation oncology,
    3:495
Dose length product (DLP), **3:**330, 339
DoseRight, **3:**331f
Dosimetry devices, **3:**407
Dosimetry for radiation oncology, **3:**480, 494-496,
    494f-495f, 494t, 506
Dotter, Charles, **3:**20-21
Dotter method for percutaneous transluminal
    angioplasty, **3:**62
Double-contrast arthrography, **2:**8-9
  of knee, **2:**13, 13f
  of shoulder, **2:**10, 10f-11f
DPA (dual photon absorptiometry), **3:**444, 476
DR. *See* Digital radiography (DR).
Dressings, surgical, **1:**20
DRLs (diagnostic reference levels) for CT, **3:**330
DRR (digitally reconstructed radiograph) in
    radiation oncology, **3:**491, 493f
DSA. *See* Digital subtraction angiography (DSA).
DSCT (dual-source CT), **3:**307, 308f
Dual energy vertebral assessment (DVA),
    3:469-470, 470f-471f, 477
Dual energy x-ray absorptiometry (DXA), **3:**442
  accuracy and precision of, **3:**442, 455-457,
    455f-456f
  anatomy, positioning, and analysis for,
    3:463-469
  array-beam (fan-beam) techniques for, **3:**444,
    454-457, 454f, 476
  compare feature (or copy) in, **3:**463, 463f,
    476
  computer competency for, **3:**460
  vs. conventional radiography, **3:**443
  cross-calibration of machines for, **3:**457, 476
  defined, **3:**476
  discordance in, **3:**457, 476
  of forearm, **3:**468-469, 468f
  least significant change (LSC) in, **3:**456, 476
  longitudinal quality control for, **3:**461-462,
    461f-462f, 476
  mean in, **3:**455, 455f-456f, 476
  patient care and education for, **3:**459
  patient history for, **3:**459
  pencil-beam techniques for, **3:**444, 454-457,
    454f, 477

Dual energy x-ray absorptiometry (DXA)
  (*Continued*)
  percent coefficient of variation (%CV) in, **3:**455,
    455f-456f, 477
  peripheral, **3:**475, 475f, 477
  phantom scans for, **3:**461, 462f
  physical and mathematic principles of,
    3:451-453
    in energy-switching systems (Hologic),
      3:451f-452f, 452
      beam hardening in, **3:**452
    in K-edge filtration systems (rare-earth filters,
      GE Lunar and Norland), **3:**451,
      451f-452f
      crossover in, **3:**452
      scintillating detector pileup in, **3:**452
    physics problems with, **3:**452
    soft tissue compensation in, **3:**452, 453f
    volumetric density estimation in, **3:**453, 453f,
      477
  as projectional (areal) technique, **3:**453, 477
  of proximal femur, **3:**466-467, 466f-467f
  radiation protection with, **3:**458, 458t
  reference population in, **3:**457, 477
  regions of interest in, **3:**443, 477
  reporting, confidentiality, record keeping, and
    scan storage for, **3:**460
  scanners for, **3:**442f, 443
  serial scans in, **3:**463-464, 463f, 477
  spine scan in
    equipment for, **3:**442f
    of lateral lumbar spine, **3:**469
    of posteroanterior lumbar spine, **3:**464-466,
      464f-465f
  standard deviation (SD) in, **3:**455, 455f-456f,
    477
  standardized hip reference database for, **3:**457
  as subtraction technique, **3:**443, 477
  T scores in, **3:**457, 458t, 477
  whole-body and body composition, **3:**442f, 471,
    472f
  Z scores in, **3:**457, 477
Dual photon absorptiometry (DPA), **3:**444, 476
Dual-energy source CT (DECT), **3:**307, 308f
Dual-source CT (DSCT), **3:**307, 308f
Ductal carcinoma in situ (DCIS), **2:**395
  calcifications in, **2:**392f
Ductal ectasia, **2:**395
Ductography, **2:**459-460, 459f-460f
Ductus deferens
  anatomy of, **2:**242, 242f-243f
  sectional anatomy of, **3:**284
Duodenal bulb
  anatomy of, **2:**98f, 100f, 101
  sectional anatomy of, **3:**289, 298f
Duodenography, hypotonic, **2:**123, 123f
Duodenojejunal flexure, **2:**100f, 101
Duodenum
  anatomy of, **2:**97f-98f, 100f, 101
  AP oblique projection of, **2:**130-131,
    130f-131f
  AP projection of, **2:**134
    evaluation criteria for, **2:**134b
    position of part for, **2:**134, 134f
    position of patient for, **2:**134, 134f
    structures shown on, **2:**134, 135f
  hypotonic duodenography of, **2:**123, 123f
  lateral projection of, **2:**132-133, 132f-133f
  PA axial projection of, **2:**126-127, 126f-127f
  PA oblique projection of, **2:**128-129,
    128f-129f
  PA projection of, **2:**124-125
    body habitus and, **2:**124-125, 125f
    central ray for, **2:**124
    double-contrast, **2:**124f
    evaluation criteria for, **2:**125b

Duodenum (*Continued*)
    position of part for, **2:**124, 124f
    position of patient for, **2:**124
    single-contrast, **2:**124f
    structures shown on, **2:**124-125, 125f
  sectional anatomy of, **3:**282f, 283
    on axial (transverse) plane, **3:**289-290,
      289f-290f
    on coronal plane, **3:**298
  sectional image of, **2:**107f
Duplex sonography, **3:**392, 392f, 397
Dura mater
  anatomy of, **3:**3, 18
  sectional anatomy of, **3:**254, 256-257
Dural sac, **3:**3, 3f
Dural sinuses, **3:**254
Dural venous sinuses, **3:**255
DVA (dual energy vertebral assessment),
    3:469-470, 470f-471f, 477
DXA. *See* Dual energy x-ray absorptiometry
    (DXA).
Dynamic imaging in nuclear medicine,
    3:412
Dynamic rectal examination, **2:**172, 172f
Dynamic renal scan, **3:**419
Dynamic scanning with CT, **3:**321, 339
Dyspnea, **3:**96

E
EAM. *See* External acoustic meatus (EAM).
Ear, **2:**270f, 271
  external
    anatomy of, **2:**270f, 271
    sectional anatomy of, **3:**267-268
  internal, **2:**269f-270f, 271
  middle, **2:**270f, 271
EBA (electron beam angiography), **3:**95
EBT (electron beam tomography), **3:**95-97
Echo planar imaging, **3:**352-353, 367
Echocardiography, **3:**393-396
  of congenital heart lesions, **3:**396
  history of, **3:**371
  indications for, **3:**393
  pathology in, **3:**393-396, 396f
  procedure for, **3:**393, 395f
Echogenic structure or mass, **3:**374, 374f,
    397
ED (emergency department), **2:**18
Effective dose for CT, **3:**331
Efferent arteriole of kidney, **2:**185, 185f
Efferent lymph vessels, **3:**26, 96
Ejaculatory ducts, **2:**242, 243f
Ejection fraction, **3:**96, 410, 411f, 437
Eklund method or maneuver for mammography,
    2:403t-408t
  with craniocaudal (CC) projection, **2:**422-423,
    422f-423f
  with mediolateral oblique (MLO) projection,
    2:425
Elbow, **1:**151
  AP oblique projection of
    with lateral rotation, **1:**155, 155f
    with medial rotation, **1:**154, 154f
  AP projection of, **1:**151, 151f
    with distal humerus
      in acute flexion, **1:**158, 158f
      in partial flexion, **1:**156, 156f
    with proximal forearm in partial flexion,
      1:157, 157f
  articulations of, **1:**107, 107f
  Coyle method for axiolateral projection of radial
    head and coronoid fossa of, **1:**162-164
    evaluation criteria for, **1:**164
    position of part for, **1:**162, 162f-163f
    position of patient for, **1:**162
    structures shown on, **1:**164, 164f

Elbow (Continued)
  fat pads of, **1:**107, 107f
  lateromedial projection of, **1:**152-153
    evaluation criteria for, **1:**153b
    in partial flexion for soft tissue image, **1:**153, 153f
    position of part for, **1:**152, 152f-153f
    position of patient for, **1:**152
    for radial head, **1:**160-161
      evaluation criteria for, **1:**161b
      four-position series for, **1:**160
      position of part for, **1:**160, 160f
      position of patient for, **1:**160
      structures shown on, **1:**161, 161f
    structures shown on, **1:**152-153, 152f-153f
  PA axial projection of
    with distal humerus, **1:**165, 165f
    with olecranon process, **1:**166, 166f
  PA projection with proximal forearm in acute flexion of, **1:**159, 159f
Elder abuse, **3:**165, 165b
Elderly. See also Aging.
  age-related competencies, **3:**176
  attitudes toward, **3:**165-166
  chronic conditions of, **3:**164, 164b
  contrast agent administration in, **3:**176
  demographics of, **3:**162-166, 162f
  economic status of, **3:**163, 163f
  exercise for, **3:**167
  health care budget for, **3:**163
  health complaints in, **3:**166-167, 167b
  patient care for, **3:**162-166, 175b
    communication in, **3:**175
    patient and family education in, **3:**175
    skin care in, **3:**175
    transportation and lifting in, **3:**175
  radiographer's role with, **3:**176-177, 177b
  radiographic positioning of, **3:**177-181
    for chest, **3:**177-178, 178f
    for lower extremity, **3:**181, 181f
    for pelvis and hip, **3:**179, 179f
    for spine, **3:**178-179, 178f-179f
    technical factors in, **3:**181
    for upper extremity, **3:**180, 180f
  summary of pathology in, **3:**174t
  tips for working with, **3:**175b
Electron(s), **3:**403, 403f, 438
Electron beam angiography (EBA), **3:**95
Electron beam tomography (EBT), **3:**95-97
Electron capture, **3:**403, 438
Electronic portal imaging devices (EPIDs), **3:**497
Electrophysiology studies, cardiac catheterization for, **3:**86, 87f
Ellipsoid joint, **1:**82, 83f
Embolic agents, **3:**66-67, 67b, 67t
Embolization, transcatheter. See Transcatheter embolization.
Embolus, **3:**96
  pulmonary, **3:**70
Embryo, **2:**241
  defined, **3:**397
  ultrasonography of, **3:**388, 389f-390f
Emergency department (ED), **2:**18
Emphysema, **1:**486t
  in older adults, **3:**172, 172f, 174t
Enchondral ossification, **1:**77
Enchondroma, **1:**109t, 240t
Endocarditis, echocardiography of sub-bacterial, **3:**393
Endocardium, **3:**24, 96
Endocavity coil in MRI, **3:**354, 354f
Endocrine system, nuclear medicine imaging of, **3:**417-418
Endocrine system disorders in older adults, **3:**173

Endografts for abdominal aortic aneurysm, **3:**65-66, 65f-66f
Endometrial cancer, phosphorus-32 for, **3:**420
Endometrial polyp, **2:**245t
Endometrium
  anatomy of, **2:**240
  defined, **3:**397
  endovaginal ultrasonography of, **3:**388, 389f
Endomyocardial biopsy, **3:**86, 86f-87f
Endorectal transducer, **3:**396-397
Endoscopic retrograde cholangiopancreatography (ERCP), **2:**178, 178f-179f
Endosteum, **1:**76, 76f
Endovaginal transducers, **3:**375f, 388, 388f, 396-397
Enema
  barium. See Barium enema (BE).
  diagnostic through colostomy stoma, **2:**170, 170f-171f
Energy-switching systems for dual energy x-ray absorptiometry, **3:**451f-452f, 452
  beam hardening in, **3:**452
English/metric conversion, **1:**30
Enteritis, regional, **2:**109t
Enteroclysis procedure, **2:**141
  air-contrast, **2:**141, 141f
  barium in, **2:**141, 141f
  CT, **2:**141, 142f
  iodinated contrast medium for, **2:**141, 142f
Enterovaginal fistula, **2:**250, 250f-251f
EOS system, **3:**153, 155, 155f
Epicardium, **3:**24, 96
Epicondyle, **1:**84
EPID(s) (electronic portal imaging devices), **3:**497
Epididymis, **2:**242, 242f-243f
  abscess of, **2:**253f
Epididymitis, **2:**245t
Epididymography, **2:**253, 253f
Epididymovesiculography, **2:**253
Epidural space, **3:**3, 18
Epigastrium, **1:**70f
Epiglottis, **2:**71f, 72, 73f
Epiglottitis, **1:**486t, **3:**137, 137f
Epilation due to radiation, **3:**481
Epinephrine, **2:**226f
Epiphyseal artery, **1:**77, 77f
Epiphyseal line, **1:**77f-78f, 78
Epiphyseal plate, **1:**77f-78f, 78
Epiphysis, **1:**77f-78f, 78
  slipped, **1:**335t
Epithelial tissues, cancer arising from, **3:**483, 483t, 506
Equipment room for MRI, **3:**345
ERCP (endoscopic retrograde cholangiopancreatography), **2:**178, 178f-179f
Ergometer, **3:**96
Erythema due to radiation, **3:**481
Esophageal stricture, **2:**119, 119f
Esophageal varices, **2:**109t, 119, 119f
Esophagogastric junction, **3:**283
Esophagus
  anatomy of, **1:**483, 483f, **2:**97, 97f
  AP oblique projection of, **2:**118, 118f
  AP projection of, **2:**116f, 118, 119f
  Barrett, **2:**109t
  contrast media studies of, **2:**115-117, 115f
    barium administration and respiration for, **2:**119, 119f
    barium sulfate mixture for, **2:**115
    double-contrast, **2:**115, 117, 117f
    examination procedures for, **2:**116-117, 116f-117f
    single-contrast, **2:**115, 116f-117f

Esophagus (Continued)
  distal
    AP projection of, **2:**119f
    PA oblique projection of (Wolf method), **2:**117f, 136-137, 136f
  exposure time for, **2:**114
  lateral projection of, **2:**116f, 118-119
  oblique projections of, **2:**118-119, 118f
  opaque foreign bodies in, **2:**117, 117f
  PA projection of, **2:**118, 118f-119f
  sectional anatomy in abdominopelvic region of, **3:**283, 285
  sectional anatomy in thoracic region of, **3:**269f, 270, 271f
    on axial (transverse) plane
      at Level A, **3:**272, 272f
      at Level B, **3:**273
      at Level C, **3:**274-275, 274f
      at Level E, **3:**275-277, 276f
      at Level F, **3:**278, 278f
      at Level G, **3:**279f
    on coronal plane, **3:**281, 281f
    on sagittal plane, **3:**279, 280f
Estrogen for osteoporosis, **3:**448t
Ethics, **1:**2-3
Ethmoid bone
  anatomy of, **2:**262, 262f
  location of, **2:**259f, 272f
  in orbit, **2:**275, 275f, 312f
  sectional anatomy of, **3:**253
Ethmoidal air cells. See Ethmoidal sinuses.
Ethmoidal notch, **2:**261, 261f
Ethmoidal sinuses
  anatomy of, **2:**276f-278f, 279
  CT of, **2:**262f
  lateral projection of, **2:**359f
  location of, **2:**261f-262f, 262
  PA axial projection of, **2:**360-361, 360f-361f
    in facial bone radiography, **2:**330f
    in skull radiography, **2:**298f
  parietoacanthial projection of, **2:**363f
  sectional anatomy of, **3:**253, 261-262, 261f, 265f
  submentovertical projection of, **2:**311f, 366-367, 366f-367f
Etiology, **3:**506
EU. See Excretory urography (EU).
Eustachian tube, **2:**270f, 271
Evacuation proctography, **2:**172, 172f
Evert/eversion, **1:**96, 96f
Ewing sarcoma, **1:**109t, 240t
  in children, **3:**150, 150f
ExacTrac/Novalis Body system, **3:**498-499
Excretory cystography
  AP axial projection for, **2:**217f
  AP oblique projection for, **2:**219f
Excretory system, **2:**183
Excretory urography (EU), **2:**201-203
  contraindications to, **2:**201
  contrast media for, **2:**194, 195f
  defined, **2:**191, 191f
  equipment for, **2:**198
  indications for, **2:**201
  patient positioning for, **2:**202, 202f
  postvoiding, **2:**203, 203f
  prevoiding, **2:**203, 203f
  radiation protection for, **2:**201
  radiographic procedure for, **2:**202-203
  time intervals for, **2:**202f-203f, 203
  ureteral compression for, **2:**200, 200f
Exercise
  for older adults, **3:**167
  weight-bearing, and osteoporosis, **3:**450
Exostosis, **1:**240t
Expiration, **1:**41
Explosive trauma, **2:**19

Exposure factors
    for obese patients, **1:**50-52
    for trauma radiography, **2:**23, 23f
Exposure techniques
    adaptation to patients of, **1:**40-41, 41f
    with anatomic programmers, **1:**40, 40f
    chart of, **1:**38, 39f
    factors to take into account in, **1:**40
    foundation, **1:**38-40, 39f
    measuring caliper in, **1:**38, 39f
Exposure time, **1:**42
    for gastrointestinal radiography, **2:**114
Extension, **1:**96, 96f
External, **1:**85
External acoustic meatus (EAM)
    anatomy of, **2:**271, 273f
        in lateral aspect of cranium, **2:**258f
        with sphenoid bone, **2:**264-265
        with temporal bones, **2:**268, 268f-270f
    axiolateral oblique projection of, **2:**352f
    as lateral landmark, **2:**285f
    lateral projection of, **2:**293f, 322f
        in decubitus position, **2:**295f
    sectional anatomy of, **3:**267-268, 267f
External auditory canal, **3:**262-263, 263f, 267-268
External carotid artery
    anatomy of, **3:**49f, 50
    sectional anatomy of, **3:**267
External ear
    anatomy of, **2:**270f, 271
    sectional anatomy of, **3:**267-268
External iliac artery
    anatomy of, **3:**25
    arteriography of, **3:**48f
    sectional anatomy of, **3:**284, 293-294, 293f-294f
External iliac vein
    sectional anatomy of, **3:**284, 293-294, 294f
    venography of, **3:**48f
External oblique muscle, sectional anatomy on
        axial (transverse) plane of
    at Level B, **3:**285, 286f
    at Level C, **3:**287f
    at Level D, **3:**288f
    at Level E, **3:**290
    at Level G, **3:**291
    at Level I, **3:**293, 293f
External occipital protuberance
    anatomy of, **2:**258f, 266, 266f-267f
    sectional anatomy of, **3:**253
External radiation detectors, **3:**400-401, 438
External-beam therapy, **3:**485, 506
Extravasation, **2:**235, **3:**36, 96
Extremity MRI scanner, **3:**347, 347f
Eye
    anatomy of, **2:**314-316, 314f-315f
    lateral projection of, **2:**317, 317f
    localization of foreign bodies within, **2:**316, 316f
    PA axial projection of, **2:**318, 318f
    parietoacanthial projection of (modified Waters
        method), **2:**319, 319f
    preliminary examination of, **2:**316
Eyeball, **2:**314, 315f

F
[18]F. *See* Fluorine-18 (^{18}F).
Fabella of femur, **1:**233
Facet(s), **1:**84, 368, 368f
Facet joints. *See* Zygapophyseal joints.
Facial bones
    acanthioparietal projection of (reverse Waters
        method), **2:**327, 327f-328f
        for trauma, **2:**328, 328f
    anatomy of, **2:**257, 257b, 259f
    function of, **2:**257
    hyoid bone as, **2:**257, 275, 275f
    inferior nasal conchae as, **2:**272f, 273

Facial bones *(Continued)*
    lacrimal bones as, **2:**272, 272f-273f
    lateral projection of, **2:**320-321, 320f, 322f
    mandible as
        anatomy of, **2:**274, 274f
        axiolateral oblique projection of, **2:**343-345,
            343f-345f
        axiolateral projection of, **2:**343-345, 343f
        PA axial projection of body of, **2:**342, 342f
        PA axial projection of rami of, **2:**340, 340f
        PA projection of body of, **2:**341, 341f
        PA projection of rami of, **2:**339, 339f
        panoramic tomography of, **2:**353-354,
            353f-354f
        submentovertical projection of, **2:**346, 346f
    maxillary bones as, **2:**259f, 272, 272f-273f
    modified parietoacanthial projection of (modified
        Waters method), **2:**304, 325f-326f
    nasal bones as
        anatomy of, **2:**259f, 272
        lateral projection of, **2:**331-332, 331f-332f
    orbits as
        anatomy of, **2:**275, 275f
        lateral projection of, **2:**317, 317f
        localization of foreign bodies within, **2:**316,
            316f
        PA axial projection of, **2:**318, 318f
        parietoacanthial projection of (modified
            Waters method), **2:**319, 319f
        preliminary examination of, **2:**316
        radiography of, **2:**312-313, 312f-313f
        PA axial projection of (Caldwell method),
            2:329-330, 329f-330f
    palatine bones as, **2:**259f, 273
    parietoacanthial projection of (Waters method),
        2:323, 323f-324f
    sectional anatomy of, **3:**254
    vomer as, **2:**259f, 272f, 273
    zygomatic bones as, **2:**272f-273f, 273
Facial trauma, acanthioparietal projection (reverse
        Waters method) for, **2:**46, 46f
Fairness in code of ethics, **1:**3
Falciform ligament
    anatomy of, **2:**104, 105f
    sectional anatomy of, **3:**283, 288
Fall(s) due to osteoporosis, **3:**449
Fallopian tubes
    anatomy of, **2:**239, 239f-240f
    hydrosalpinx of, **2:**246f
    hysterosalpingography of, **2:**246-247,
        246f-247f
    sectional anatomy of, **3:**284
Falx cerebri
    anatomy of, **3:**3, 18
    sectional anatomy of, **3:**254
        on axial (transverse) plane, **3:**256-258,
            256f-257f
        on coronal plane, **3:**267, 267f
Familial adenomatous polyposis and colon cancer,
        3:483
Familial cancer research, **3:**483
Family education for older adults, **3:**175
Fan-beam techniques for dual energy x-ray
        absorptiometry, **3:**444, 454-457, 454f, 476
Faraday's law of induction, **3:**343
FAST (focused abdominal sonography in trauma),
        2:55
Fat necrosis, **2:**395
Fat pads of elbow, **1:**107, 107f
Fat-suppressed images, **3:**367
FB. *See* Foreign body (FB).
FDCT (flat-detector CT), **3:**307
Feet. *See* Foot (feet).
Female contraceptive devices, **2:**248, 248f-249f
Female cystourethrography, **2:**222-224, 222f
    metallic bead chain, **2:**222-224, 223f

Female pelvis, **1:**332, 332f, 332t
    PA projection of, **1:**338f
    transabdominal ultrasonography of, **3:**387-388,
        387f
Female reproductive system
    anatomy of, **2:**239-241
        fetal development in, **2:**241, 241f
        ovaries in, **2:**239, 239f
        summary of, **2:**244b
        uterine tubes in, **2:**239, 239f
        uterus in, **2:**240, 240f
        vagina in, **2:**240
    radiography of, **2:**246
        for imaging of female contraceptive devices,
            2:248, 248f-249f
        in nonpregnant patient, **2:**246-251
            appointment date and care of patient for,
                2:246
            contrast media for, **2:**246
            hysterosalpingography for, **2:**246-247,
                246f-247f
            pelvic pneumography for, **2:**246, 250,
                250f
            preparation of intestinal tract for, **2:**246
            radiation protection for, **2:**246
            vaginography for, **2:**246, 250-251,
                250f-251f
        in pregnant patient, **2:**252
            fetography for, **2:**252, 252f
            pelvimetry for, **2:**252
            placentography for, **2:**252
            radiation protection for, **2:**252
    sectional anatomy of, **3:**284
Femoral arteries, **3:**284, 295, 295f
Femoral arteriogram, **3:**240-241, 240f-241f
Femoral head
    accurate localization of, **1:**333, 333f
    anatomy of, **1:**328f-329f, 329
    sectional anatomy of, **3:**295-296, 295f-296f,
        299
Femoral nailing, surgical radiography of,
        3:233-235, 233f
    antegrade, **3:**233
    evaluation criteria for, **3:**235b
    method for, **3:**234, 234f-235f
    retrograde, **3:**234, 234f
    structures shown on, **3:**235, 235f
Femoral neck(s)
    accurate localization of, **1:**333, 333f
    anatomy of, **1:**328f-329f, 329
    angulation of, **1:**330, 330f
    AP oblique projection of (modified Cleaves
        method), **1:**342-343
        bilateral, **1:**342, 342f
        evaluation criteria for, **1:**343b
        position of part for, **1:**342, 342f
        position of patient for, **1:**342
        structures shown on, **1:**343, 343f
        unilateral, **1:**342-343, 342f
    AP projection of, **1:**337-339, 337f
    axiolateral projection of (original Cleaves
        method), **1:**344-345, 344f-345f
Femoral veins
    sectional anatomy of, **3:**284, 295,
        295f-296f
    venography of, **3:**48f
Femorotibial joint. *See* Knee joint.
Femur
    anatomy of, **1:**232-233, 232f-233f
    AP projection of, **1:**318-319, 318f-319f
        mobile, **3:**202-203, 202f-203f
    lateromedial projection of (mobile), **3:**204-205,
        204f-205f
    mediolateral projection of, **1:**320-321,
        320f-321f
        mobile, **3:**204-205, 204f-205f

Index

Femur (Continued)
  mobile radiography of, **3:**202-203
    AP projection for, **3:**202-203, 202f-203f
    lateral projection for, **3:**204-205, 204f-205f
  proximal, **1:**325-360
    anatomy of, **1:**328f-330f, 329-330, 334b
    AP projection of, **1:**337-339, 337f-338f
    DXA of, **3:**466-467, 466f-467f
    lateral projection of, **1:**340-341, 340f-341f
    sample exposure technique chart essential
      projections for, **1:**335t
    summary of pathology of, **1:**335t
    summary of projections for, **1:**326
Femur length, fetal ultrasound for, **3:**390, 390f
Ferguson method
  for AP axial projection of lumbosacral junction
      and sacroiliac joints, **1:**425-426, 425f
  for PA projection of scoliosis, **1:**439-440
    evaluation criteria for, **1:**439b-440b
    first radiograph in, **1:**439, 439f
    position of part for, **1:**439, 439f-440f
    position of patient for, **1:**439, 439f
    second radiograph in, **1:**439, 440f
    structures shown on, **1:**439-440,
      439f-440f
Ferlic collimator-mounted filter
  examples of, **1:**56f
  placement of, **1:**58, 58f-59f
  shape of, **1:**57
Ferlic foot filter, **1:**60t, 62f, 63
Ferlic shoulder filter, **1:**59f, 60-63, 60t, 63f
Ferlic swimmer's filter, **1:**60-63, 60t, 62f
Ferlic wedge filter, **1:**61f
Fetal development, **2:**241, 241f
Fetography, **2:**252, 252f
Fetus, **2:**241, 241f
  defined, **3:**397
  ultrasonography of, **3:**388, 390f-391f
FFDM. See Full-field digital mammography
  (FFDM).
Fibrillation, **3:**96
Fibroadenoma, **2:**385f, 395, 431f
  ultrasonography of, **3:**384f
Fibroid, **2:**245t, 247f
  MRI of, **3:**361f
  transcatheter embolization for, **3:**68, 69f
Fibrous capsule, **1:**82, 82f
Fibrous joints, **1:**80f, 80t, 81
Fibula
  anatomy of, **1:**230f-231f, 231
  AP oblique projections of, **1:**294-295,
    294f-295f
  AP projection of, **1:**290-291, 290f-291f
  lateral projection of, **1:**292-293, 292f-293f
Fibular collateral ligament, **1:**234f
Fibular notch, **1:**230f-231f, 231
Field light size with obese patients, **1:**50, 51f
Field of view (FOV)
  in CT, **3:**308, 339
    scan vs. display, **3:**320
  for PET, **3:**428-429, 428f, 431
Fifth lobe. See Insula.
Film badges, **3:**407
Film size, **1:**30, 30t
Filters, compensating. See Compensating filters.
Filum terminale, **3:**3, 18
Fimbriae
  anatomy of, **2:**239, 239f
  sectional anatomy of, **3:**284
Fine-needle aspiration biopsy (FNAB) of breast,
  2:461
Finger radiographs, display orientation of, **1:**11,
  11f
Fisk modification for tangential projection of
  intertubercular (bicipital) groove, **1:**207-208,
  207f-208f

Fission, **3:**404, 438
Fissure, **1:**84
Fistula
  abdominal, **2:**180, 180f
  defined, **2:**62t
  of reproductive tract, **2:**245t, 250, 250f-251f
  in urinary system, **2:**188t
FLAIR (fluid attenuated inversion recovery),
  3:352-353, 353f
Flat bones, **1:**79, 79f
Flat-detector CT (FDCT), **3:**307
Flat-panel CT (FPCT), **3:**307
Flexion, **1:**96, 96f
  plantar, **1:**97, 97f
Flexor retinaculum, **1:**102, 102f
Flexor tendons, **1:**102
Flocculation-resistant preparations
  for alimentary canal imaging, **2:**111, 111f
  for large intestine contrast media studies,
    2:144
Flow in MRI, **3:**344, 344f
"Flow" study, **3:**412
Fluid attenuated inversion recovery (FLAIR),
  3:352-353, 353f
Fluoride for osteoporosis, **3:**448t
Fluorine-18 (^{18}F), **3:**406t
  decay scheme for, **3:**425f
  in PET, **3:**424, 426t
Fluorine-18 (^{18}F)-2-fluoro-2-deoxy-D-glucose
  (^{18}F-FDG), **3:**427, 427f, 430f, 438
Fluorine-18 (^{18}F)-2-fluoro-2-deoxy-D-glucose
  (^{18}F-FDG) neurologic study, **3:**434
Fluorine-18 (^{18}F)-2-fluoro-2-deoxy-D-glucose
  (^{18}F-FDG) oncologic study, **3:**433-434
Fluorine-18 (^{18}F)-Florbetapir, **3:**434
Fluoroscopic C-arm, mobile, **2:**20, 21f
Fluoroscopic equipment
  for alimentary canal, **2:**110, 113, 113f
  for positive-contrast pharyngography, **2:**75
Fluoroscopic image receptor, **1:**3, 4f
Fluoroscopic surgical procedures, **3:**223-241
  of cervical spine (anterior cervical diskectomy
    and fusion), **3:**227, 227f
  of chest (line placement, bronchoscopy), **3:**226,
    226f
  femoral nailing as, **3:**233-235, 233f
    antegrade, **3:**233
    evaluation criteria for, **3:**235b
    method for, **3:**234, 234f-235f
    retrograde, **3:**234, 234f
    structures shown on, **3:**235, 235f
  femoral/tibial arteriogram as, **3:**240-241,
    240f-241f
  of hip (cannulated hip screws or hip pinning),
    3:230-232, 230f-232f
  of humerus, **3:**238-239, 238f-239f
  of lumbar spine, **3:**228-229, 228f-229f
  operative (immediate) cholangiography as,
    3:223-225, 224f-225f
  tibial nailing as, **3:**236-237
    evaluation criteria for, **3:**237b
    position of C-arm for, **3:**236, 236f
    position of patient for, **3:**236
    structures shown on, **3:**237, 237f
fMRI (functional magnetic resonance imaging),
  3:366
FNAB (fine-needle aspiration biopsy) of breast,
  2:461
Focal spot with obese patients, **1:**51
Focused abdominal sonography in trauma (FAST),
  2:55
Folia
  anatomy of, **3:**2
  sectional anatomy of, **3:**255
Folio method for first MCP joint of thumb, **1:**122,
  122f-123f

Follicular cyst, ultrasonography of, **3:**388, 397
Fontanels, **2:**259-260, 260f
Foot (feet)
  anatomy of, **1:**228-230, 228f-229f
  AP oblique projection of
    in lateral rotation, **1:**258-259, 258f-259f
    in medial rotation, **1:**256, 256f-257f
  AP or AP axial projection of, **1:**252-253
    central ray for, **1:**252f-253f, 253
    compensating filter for, **1:**254-255
    evaluation criteria for, **1:**255b
    position of part for, **1:**252f-253f, 253
    position of patient for, **1:**252
    structures shown on, **1:**254-255,
      254f-255f
  weight-bearing method for
    for both feet, **1:**264, 264f
    composite, **1:**265-266, 265f-266f
  calcaneus of
    anatomy of, **1:**228f-229f, 229
    axial projection of
      dorsoplantar, **1:**272, 272f-273f
      plantodorsal, **1:**271, 271f
      weight-bearing coalition (Harris-Beath)
        method for, **1:**273, 273f
    mediolateral projection of, **1:**274, 274f
    weight-bearing method for lateromedial
      oblique projection of, **1:**275, 275f
  congenital club-
    defined, **1:**240t
    Kandel method for dorsoplantar axial
      projection of, **1:**270, 270f
    Kite method for AP projection of, **1:**267, 267f,
      269f
    Kite method for mediolateral projection of,
      1:268-269, 268f-269f
  dorsum (dorsal surface) of, **1:**228-230
  fore-, **1:**228-230
  hind-, **1:**228-230
  lateromedial weight-bearing projection of, **1:**262,
    262f-263f
  longitudinal arch of
    anatomy of, **1:**228-230, 228f
    weight-bearing method for lateromedial
      projection of, **1:**262, 262f-263f
  mediolateral projection of, **1:**260, 260f-261f
  metatarsals of, **1:**228f, 229
  mid-, **1:**228-230
  phalanges of, **1:**228, 228f
  plantar surface of, **1:**228-230
  sesamoids of
    anatomy of, **1:**228f, 230
    tangential projection of
      Holly method for, **1:**251, 251f
      Lewis method for, **1:**250-251, 250f
  subtalar joint of
    anatomy of, **1:**236t, 237f, 238
    Isherwood method for AP axial oblique
      projection of
      with lateral rotation ankle, **1:**278,
        278f
      with medial rotation ankle, **1:**277,
        277f
    Isherwood method for lateromedial oblique
      projection with medial rotation foot of,
      1:276, 276f
  summary of pathology of, **1:**240t
  summary of projections for, **1:**226
  tarsals of, **1:**228f-229f, 229
  toes of. See Toes.
  transverse arch of, **1:**228-230
  trauma radiography of, **2:**52f
Foot radiographs, display orientation of,
  1:11
Foramen(mina), **1:**77, 84
Foramen lacerum, **2:**258f, 268

Index

Foramen magnum
    anatomy of, **2:**258f, 266, 266f-267f
    AP axial projection of
        Haas method for, **2:**309f
        Towne method for, **2:**305f-307f
    myelogram of, **3:**9f
    sectional anatomy of, **3:**253
Foramen of Luschka, **3:**4
Foramen of Magendie, **3:**4
Foramen of Monro, **3:**4
Foramen ovale, **2:**258f, 264f, 265
Foramen rotundum, **2:**264f, 265
Foramen spinosum
    anatomy of, **2:**258f, 264f, 265
    submentovertical projection of, **2:**311f
Forearm, **1:**148-149
    anatomy of, **1:**102-103, 103f
    AP projection of, **1:**148-149
        CT for, **1:**149-150
        evaluation criteria for, **1:**149b
        position of part for, **1:**148, 148f
        position of patient for, **1:**148
        structures shown on, **1:**149-150, 149f
        for trauma, **2:**47f-48f
    cross-table lateral projection for trauma of,
        2:47f-48f
    DXA of, **3:**468-469, 468f
    lateromedial projection of, **1:**150, 150f
    proximal
        AP projection in partial flexion of, **1:**157,
            157f
        PA projection in acute flexion of, **1:**159,
            159f
    trauma radiography of, **2:**47, 47f-48f
Forearm fracture, surgical radiography of, **3:**247f
Forebrain, **3:**2
Forefoot, **1:**228-230
Foreign body (FB)
    in airway, **2:**62t
        in children, **3:**139, 139f
    aspiration of, **1:**486t
    in children
        airway, **3:**139, 139f
        ingested, **3:**139, 140f
    interventional radiology for removal of, **3:**72
    in orbit or eye, **2:**316, 316f
        lateral projection for, **2:**317, 317f
        PA axial projection for, **2:**318, 318f
        parietoacanthial projection for (modified
            Waters method), **2:**319, 319f
        preliminary examination for, **2:**316
Forward planning in radiation oncology, **3:**495
Fossa, **1:**84
Four-dimensional imaging, ultrasonography for,
    3:372-373
Fourth ventricle
    anatomy of, **3:**4, 4f
    sectional anatomy of, **3:**255
        on axial (transverse) plane, **1:**332f, **3:**259-263,
            260f
        on coronal plane, **3:**268, 268f
        on sagittal plane, **3:**264, 266, 266f
FOV. *See* Field of view (FOV).
Fovea capitis, **1:**328f, 329
Fowler position, **1:**90, 91f
FPCT (flat-panel CT), **3:**307
Fractionation, **3:**480, 506
Fracture(s), **1:**84
    of bony thorax, **1:**454t
    in children, **3:**129-130
        due to child abuse, **3:**143-145, 144f-145f
        greenstick, **1:**84f, **3:**130
        growth plate, **3:**131
        due to osteogenesis imperfecta, **3:**146t, 147
        pathologic, **3:**148-150
        plastic or bowing, **3:**130

Fracture(s) *(Continued)*
    Salter-Harris, **3:**130, 130f
    supracondylar, **3:**131, 131f
    toddler's, **3:**130-131
    torus, **1:**109t, **3:**130
    classification of, **1:**84, 84f
    compression, **1:**84f, 380t
        in older adults, **3:**170, 170f, 174t
    defined, **1:**84
    fragility, **3:**447, 449, 449f, 476
        overall risk of, **3:**474, 477
    general terms for, **1:**84
    greenstick, **1:**84f, **3:**130
    growth plate, **3:**131
    of lower limb, **1:**240t
    mobile radiography with, **3:**191
    pathologic, **3:**148-150
        of pelvis and proximal femora, **1:**335t
    plastic or bow, **3:**130
    Salter-Harris, **3:**130, 130f
    of shoulder girdle, **1:**182t
    of skull, **2:**282t
    supracondylar, **3:**131, 131f
    toddler's, **3:**130-131
    torus, **1:**109t, **3:**130
    of upper limb, **1:**109t
    of vertebral column, **1:**380t
Fracture risk models, **3:**475
Fragility fractures, **3:**447, 449, 449f, 476
    overall risk of, **3:**474, 477
Frank et al. method for PA and lateral projections
    of scoliosis, **1:**437-438, 437f-438f
FRAX tool, **3:**475-476
French size, **3:**96
Frenulum of tongue, **2:**59, 59f
Frequency
    in MRI, **3:**343, 367
    in ultrasonography, **3:**397
Fringe field in MRI, **3:**346, 367
Frog leg position. *See* Cleaves method, for AP
    oblique projection of femoral necks.
Frontal angle of parietal bone, **2:**263f
Frontal bone
    anatomy of, **2:**261, 261f
    location of, **2:**257f-259f
    in orbit, **2:**275, 275f, 312f
    PA axial projection of, **2:**298f
    sectional anatomy of, **3:**253, 256f-257f,
        257-260
Frontal eminence, **2:**261, 261f
Frontal lobe, sectional anatomy of, **3:**254-255, 256f
    on axial (transverse) plane
        at level B, **3:**257-258
        at level C, **3:**258, 258f
        at level D, **3:**259-260, 259f
        at level E, **3:**262f, 263
        at Level E, **3:**260f, 261-262
    on sagittal plane, **3:**264, 265f-266f, 266
Frontal sinuses
    anatomy of, **2:**276f-278f, 279
    lateral projection of, **2:**322f, 359f
    location of, **2:**259f, 261, 261f
    PA axial projection of (Caldwell method),
        2:330f, 360-361, 360f-361f
    parietoacanthial projection of, **2:**363f
    sectional anatomy of, **3:**253
        on axial (transverse) plane, **3:**259-260,
            262-263, 262f-263f
        on sagittal plane, **3:**265f
Frontal squama, **2:**261, 261f
Fuchs method for AP projection of dens, **1:**383,
    383f
Full-field digital mammography (FFDM),
    2:374-375
    labeling for, **2:**409
    technique chart for, **2:**394t

Functional age, age-specific competencies by,
    1:23
Functional image, **3:**421, 438
Functional magnetic resonance imaging (fMRI),
    3:366
Fundus
    of stomach, **2:**98, 98f
    of uterus, **2:**240, 240f
Fungal disease of lung, **1:**486t

G
G (gauss) in MRI, **3:**346, 367
^{67}Ga (gallium-67), **3:**406t
Gadolinium, **3:**18
Gadolinium oxyorthosilicate (GSO) as scintillator
    for PET, **3:**428t
Gadolinium-based contrast agents (GBCAs) for
    MRI, **3:**355, 355f
Galactocele, **2:**395
Gallbladder
    anatomy of, **2:**97f, 100f, 104f-106f, 106
    biliary drainage procedure and stone extraction
        for, **2:**175, 175f
    and body habitus, **2:**106, 106f
    cholangiography of
        percutaneous transhepatic, **2:**174-175, 174f
        postoperative (T-tube), **2:**176-177,
            176f-177f
    endoscopic retrograde cholangiopancreatography
        of, **2:**178, 178f-179f
    MRI of, **3:**361f
    prefixes associated with, **2:**173, 173t
    radiographic techniques for, **2:**173
    sectional anatomy of, **3:**287, 288f
        on axial (transverse) plane, **3:**287, 288f-289f,
            289
        on coronal plane, **3:**298-299, 298f
    ultrasonography of, **3:**373f, 378, 379f
Gallium-67 (^{67}Ga), **3:**406t
Gallstone(s)
    extraction of, **2:**175, 175f
    ultrasonography of, **3:**379f
Gamma camera
    defined, **3:**400, 438
    historical development of, **3:**400
    modern, **3:**408-409, 408f
    multi-crystal, **3:**409
    multihead, **3:**409
Gamma Knife, **3:**486-487, 487f
Gamma ray(s), **3:**403, 438
Gamma ray source for radiation oncology, **3:**485,
    506
Gamma well counter, **3:**430
Gantry for CT, **3:**309-310, 309f, 339
Garth method for AP axial oblique projection of
    glenoid cavity, **1:**205-206, 205f-206f
Gas bubble, **2:**98
Gastric antrum, ultrasonography of, **3:**377f
Gastric artery
    arteriography of, **3:**42f
    sectional anatomy of, **3:**284
Gastritis, **2:**109t
Gastroduodenal artery, arteriography of,
    3:42f
Gastroesophageal reflux, **2:**109t
Gastrografin (meglumine diatrizoate) for simulation
    in radiation oncology, **3:**490
Gastrointestinal (GI) intubation, **2:**143, 143f
Gastrointestinal (GI) series, **2:**120, 120f
    barium sulfate suspension for, **2:**120
    biphasic, **2:**123
    components of, **2:**120
    double-contrast, **2:**122, 122f
    for nonambulatory patients, **2:**120
    preparation of patient for, **2:**120
    single-contrast, **2:**121, 121f

Gastrointestinal (GI) studies in children, **3:**116-118
  indications for, **3:**118t
  radiation protection for, **3:**116, 116f
Gastrointestinal (GI) system. *See* Digestive system.
Gastrointestinal (GI) transit, **2:**110
Gastroschisis, fetal ultrasound of, **3:**391f
Gastroview (meglumine diatrizoate) for simulation
    in radiation oncology, **3:**490
Gating
  cardiac
      for CT angiography, **3:**324-326, 326f
      for MRI, **3:**356, 356f
    for MRI, **3:**356, 356f, 367
    respiratory, for radiation oncology, **3:**498,
        499f
Gauss (G) in MRI, **3:**346, 367
Gaynor-Hart method for tangential projections of
    wrist, **1:**146
  evaluation criteria for, **1:**147b
  inferosuperior, **1:**146, 146f-147f
  superoinferior, **1:**147, 147f
GBCAs (gadolinium-based contrast agents) for
    MRI, **3:**355, 355f
Genant grading system, **3:**470, 470f
Genetic mutations and cancer, **3:**482
Genitourinary nuclear medicine, **3:**419
Genitourinary studies in children, **3:**116-118
  indications for, **3:**118t
  radiation protection for, **3:**116, 116f
  with vesicoureteral reflux, **3:**117-118, 117f
Genitourinary system disorders in older adults,
    3:173
Geriatrics, **3:**161-182
  age-related competencies in, **3:**176
  and attitudes toward older adult, **3:**165-166
  contrast agent administration in, **3:**176
  defined, **3:**161-162, 174t
  demographics and social effects of aging in,
      3:162f-164f, 164b, 175
  and elder abuse, **3:**165, 165b
  Joint Commission criteria for, **3:**176
  patient care in, **3:**162-166, 175b
    communication in, **3:**175
    patient and family education in, **3:**175
    skin care in, **3:**175
    transportation and lifting in, **3:**175
  physical, cognitive, and psychosocial effects of
      aging in, **3:**166-168, 167b, 167f
  physiology of aging in, **3:**168-173
    endocrine system disorders in, **3:**173
    gastrointestinal system disorders in, **3:**171,
        171f
    genitourinary system disorders in, **3:**173
    hematologic system disorders in, **3:**173
    immune system decline in, **3:**172
    integumentary system disorders in, **3:**168
    musculoskeletal system disorders in, **3:**170,
        170f-171f
    nervous system disorders in, **3:**168-169
    respiratory system disorders in, **3:**172, 172f
    sensory system disorders in, **3:**169
    summary of, **3:**173
  radiographer's role in, **3:**176-177, 177b
  radiographic positioning in, **3:**177-181
    for chest, **3:**177-178, 178f
    for lower extremity, **3:**181, 181f
    for pelvis and hip, **3:**179, 179f
    for spine, **3:**178-179, 178f-179f
    technical factors in, **3:**181
    for upper extremity, **3:**180, 180f
  summary of pathology in, **3:**174t
Germicides, **1:**16
Gerontology, **3:**161-162, 174t
Gestational age, **3:**371, 390, 397
Gestational sac, ultrasonography of, **3:**388, 390f,
    397

Gestational weeks, **3:**388
GI. *See* Gastrointestinal (GI).
Giant cell tumor, **1:**240t
Gianturco, Cesare, **3:**20-21
Ginglymus joint, **1:**82, 83f
Glabella
  in anterior aspect of cranium, **2:**257f
  with frontal bone, **2:**261f
  in lateral aspect of cranium, **2:**258f
  in skull topography, **2:**285f
Glabelloalveolar line, **2:**285f
Glenohumeral joint, **1:**178-180, 178t, 179f-181f
Glenoid, **3:**273f
Glenoid cavity
  anatomy of, **1:**176f, 177
  AP axial oblique projection (Garth method) of,
      1:205-206, 205f-206f
  AP oblique projection of
      Apple method for, **1:**190-191, 190f-191f
      Grashey method for, **1:**188-189, 188f-189f
Glenoid process, **1:**179f
Gliding joint, **1:**82, 83f
Globes, **3:**261-262, 266, 266f
Glomerular capsule, **2:**185, 185f
Glomerulonephritis, **2:**188t
Glomerulus, **2:**185, 185f
Glottis, **2:**73
Gloves, **1:**15
Glucagon, **2:**106, 226t
Glucose, local metabolic rate of, **3:**427, 427f
Glucose metabolism, PET image of, **3:**430
Gluteus maximus muscle, **3:**293-294, 293f-296f
Gluteus medius muscle, **3:**293-294, 293f-294f
Gluteus minimus muscle, **3:**293-294, 294f
Gomphosis, **1:**80f, 81
Gonad(s), **2:**242
Gonad dose, **1:**35, 35t
Gonad shielding, **1:**33-35, 33f-34f
  for children, **3:**108, 108f-109f
  for upper limb, **1:**110, 110f
Gonion, **2:**274, 274f
  in lateral aspect of skull, **2:**273f
  as surface landmark, **1:**71f, 71t, **2:**285f
Gout, **1:**109t, 240t
Gowns
  for patients, **1:**20, 20f
  for personnel, **1:**15
Graafian follicle, **2:**239, 239f
Gradient echo pulse sequence, **3:**352-353, 367
Grandy method for lateral projection of cervical
    vertebrae, **1:**389-390, 389f-390f
Granulomatous disease of lung, **1:**486t
Grashey method for AP oblique projection of
    glenoid cavity, **1:**188-189, 188f-189f
Graves disease, radioiodine for, **3:**420
Gray matter, **3:**2
Gray (Gy) units in radiation oncology, **3:**494,
    506
Gray-level mapping in CT, **3:**10, 312, 312f,
    312t
Grayscale image
  in CT, **3:**311, 339
  in ultrasonography, **3:**372, 397
Great cardiac vein, **3:**25f
Great saphenous vein, ultrasonography of,
    3:394f
Great vessels, **3:**23, 25f
  origins of
      anomalous, **3:**50
      digital subtraction angiography of, **3:**55f
  transposition of, **3:**97
Greater curvature of stomach
  anatomy of, **2:**98, 98f
  sectional anatomy of, **3:**283
Greater duodenal papilla, **2:**101
Greater omentum, **3:**283, 285, 286f-287f

Greater sciatic notch
  anatomy of, **1:**327f, 328, 330f
  sectional anatomy of, **3:**282
Greater trochanter
  anatomy of, **1:**232f, 328f-330f, 329
  with obese patients, **1:**49
  sectional anatomy of, **3:**295-296, 295f-296f
  as surface landmark, **1:**71f, 71t, 333, 333f
Greater tubercle
  anatomy of, **1:**104f, 105
  defined, **1:**76f
Greater wings of sphenoid
  anatomy of, **2:**258f, 259, 264f-265f, 265
  sectional anatomy on axial (transverse) plane of,
      3:263
      at Level C, **3:**258
      at Level E, **3:**260f, 261-262
      at Level F, **3:**262-263, 262f
Greenstick fracture, **1:**84f, **3:**130
Grenz rays, **3:**506
Grids
  in digital imaging, **1:**38
  for mammography, **2:**374
  in mobile radiography, **3:**185-186, 185f-186f
  in trauma radiography, **2:**20
Groove, **1:**84
Ground state, **3:**403, 438
Growth hormone for osteoporosis, **3:**448t
Growth plate fractures, **3:**131
Gruntzig, Andreas, **3:**20
GSO (gadolinium oxyorthosilicate) as scintillator
    for PET, **3:**428t
Guidewires for angiographic studies, **3:**35, 35f,
    96
"Gull-wing" sign, **1:**340
Gunson method for positive-contrast
    pharyngography, **2:**75, 75f
Gy (gray) units in radiation oncology, **3:**494, 506
Gynecography, **2:**246, 250, 250f
Gynecologic applications of ultrasonography,
    3:386-388
  anatomic features and, **3:**386, 386f
  endovaginal transducers for, **3:**375f, 388, 388f,
      397
  indications for, **3:**387
  of ovaries, **3:**373f, 375f, 388, 389f
  transabdominal, **3:**387-388, 387f
  of uterus, **3:**387f-389f, 388
Gynecomastia, **2:**426
Gyrus(i), **3:**254-257, 256f

H
Haas method for PA axial projection of skull,
    2:308-309
  central ray for, **2:**308, 308f
  evaluation criteria for, **2:**309b
  position of part for, **2:**308, 308f
  position of patient for, **2:**308
  structures shown on, **2:**309, 309f
Half-life (T ½), **3:**403-404, 404f, 438
  in brachytherapy, **3:**485, 506
Half-value layer, **3:**506
Hamartoma, **2:**386f, 395
Hamate, **1:**101f, 102
Hamulus, **1:**84
Hand, **1:**124
  anatomy of, **1:**99f, 101-102
  articulations of, **1:**105-107, 105f-106f
  bone densitometry of, **3:**474f
  digits of. *See* Digit(s).
  display orientation of, **1:**11, 11f
  fan lateral projection of, **1:**128-129
    evaluation criteria for, **1:**129b
    position of part for, **1:**128, 128f
    position of patient for, **1:**128
    structures shown on, **1:**129, 129f

Hand *(Continued)*
lateromedial projection in flexion of, **1:**130, 130f
mediolateral or lateromedial projection in
extension of, **1:**128-129
evaluation criteria for, **1:**129b
position of part for, **1:**128, 128f
position of patient for, **1:**128
with posterior rotation, **1:**129
structures shown on, **1:**129, 129f
Norgaard method for AP oblique projection in
medial rotation (ball-catcher's position) of,
1:130-131
evaluation criteria for, **1:**131b
position of part for, **1:**130-131, 131f
position of patient for, **1:**130
structures shown on, **1:**131, 131f
PA oblique projection in lateral rotation of,
1:126-127
evaluation criteria for, **1:**127b
position of part for, **1:**126
to show joint spaces, **1:**126, 126f
to show metacarpals, **1:**126, 126f
position of patient for, **1:**126
structures shown on, **1:**127, 127f
PA projection of, **1:**124
computed radiography for, **1:**124-131
evaluation criteria for, **1:**124b
position of part for, **1:**124, 124f
position of patient for, **1:**124
special techniques for, **1:**124
structures shown on, **1:**124, 125f
reverse oblique projection of, **1:**127
tangential oblique projection of, **1:**127
Handwashing, **1:**15, 15f
Hangman's fracture, **1:**380t
Hard palate, **2:**59, 59f, 71f
Hardware, **3:**460
Harris-Beath method for axial projection of
calcaneus, **1:**273, 273f
Haustra, **2:**102, 102f
Haustral folds, **3:**294
HBV (hepatitis B virus) and cancer, **3:**482
HDR (high-dose-rate) brachytherapy, **3:**485,
506
Head. *See also* Skull.
of bone, **1:**84
Head and neck cancers, radiation oncology for,
3:503
Head circumference, fetal ultrasound for, **3:**390,
390f
Head trauma
acanthioparietal projection (reverse Waters
method) for, **2:**46, 46f
AP axial projection (Towne method) for,
2:44-45, 44f-45f
CT of, **2:**29, 29f, 53-55, 54f
lateral projection for, **2:**42-43, 42f-43f
Health Insurance Portability and Accountability Act
of 1996 (HIPAA), **3:**460, 476
Hearing impairment in older adults, **3:**169
Heart
anatomy of, **3:**23-24, 25f
AP oblique projection of, **1:**508-509
catheterization of
left side, **3:**82, 83f-84f
right side, **3:**84
CT angiography of, **3:**324-326, 325f-326f
with cardiac gating, **3:**324-326, 326f
echocardiography of, **3:**393-396
for congenital heart lesions, **3:**396
history of, **3:**371
indications for, **3:**393
pathology in, **3:**393-396, 396f
procedure for, **3:**393, 395f
lateral projection with barium of, **1:**503
nuclear cardiology studies of, **3:**416-417

Heart *(Continued)*
PA chest radiographs with barium of, **1:**499
PA oblique projection with barium of, **1:**505,
507
PET of, **3:**434-435
in radiography of ribs, **1:**468
in radiography of sternum, **1:**456, 457f
sectional anatomy of, **3:**270, 278-279, 285f
Heart shadows, **1:**502f-503f
Heat trauma, **2:**19
Heel, bone densitometry of, **3:**475f
Helical CT, **3:**339
multislice, **3:**306, 323-324, 323f-324f
single slice, **3:**306, 321-323, 322f
Helix, **2:**270f, 271
Hemangioma of liver, **3:**360f
Hematologic studies, in vivo and in vitro, **3:**419
Hematologic system disorders in older adults,
3:173
Hematoma, **2:**395
during catheterization, **3:**36, 96
scalp, **3:**10f
Hematopoietic tissue, cancer arising from,
3:483t
Hemidiaphragm, **3:**278, 285
Hemodynamics, **3:**96
Hemopneumothorax, **2:**37f
Hemostasis, **3:**96
Hepatic arteriogram, **3:**41f-43f, 43
Hepatic artery
anatomy of, **2:**104
sectional anatomy of, **3:**283, 288f
ultrasonography of, **3:**377f
Hepatic bile ducts, **3:**283
Hepatic ducts
anatomy of, **2:**105
sectional anatomy of, **3:**283
Hepatic flexure
anatomy of, **2:**102f, 103
sectional anatomy of, **3:**283
on axial plane, **3:**290, 290f
on coronal plane, **3:**298-299, 298f
Hepatic veins
anatomy of, **2:**104, 105f
sectional anatomy of, **3:**284-285, 285f
Hepatic venography, **3:**61, 61f
Hepatitis B virus (HBV) and cancer, **3:**482
Hepatitis C virus and cancer, **3:**482
Hepatopancreatic ampulla
anatomy of, **2:**100f, 101, 105, 106f
sectional anatomy of, **3:**283
Hereditary nonpolyposis colorectal cancer
syndrome, **3:**483
Hernia
hiatal
AP projection of, **2:**134, 135f
defined, **2:**109t
PA oblique projection of (Wolf method),
2:136-137, 136f-137f
upright lateral projection of, **2:**135f
inguinal, **2:**109t
Herniated nucleus pulposus (HNP), **1:**368, 380t,
3:358f
Heterogeneous structure or mass in
ultrasonography, **3:**374, 374f, 397
Hiatal hernia
AP projection of, **2:**134, 135f
defined, **2:**109t
PA oblique projection of (Wolf method),
2:136-137, 136f-137f
upright lateral projection of, **2:**135f
Hickey method for mediolateral projection of hip,
1:348, 349f
Hickman catheter placement, **3:**226f
High-dose-rate (HDR) brachytherapy, **3:**485,
506

Highlighting in CT, **3:**304f
High-osmolality contrast agents (HOCAs) in
children, **3:**116
High-resolution scans, **3:**319-320, 321f, 339
Hill-Sachs defect, **1:**182t
AP axial oblique projection of, **1:**205
AP axial projection of, **1:**204, 204f
inferosuperior axial projection of
Rafert modification of Lawrence method for,
1:194, 194f-195f
West Point method for, **1:**196-197
Hindbrain, **3:**2, 18
Hindfoot, **1:**228-230
Hinge joint, **1:**82, 83f
Hip(s)
AP projection of, **1:**346-347, 346f-347f
axiolateral projection of (Danelius-Miller
method), **1:**350-351, 350f-351f, 353f
Clements-Nakamaya modification of,
1:352-353, 352f-353f
in children, **3:**125-126
developmental dysplasia of, **2:**9t, **3:**142,
142f
general principles for, **3:**125-126, 125f
image evaluation for, **3:**123t, 126
initial images of, **3:**125
positioning and immobilization for, **3:**126,
126f
preparation and communication for, **3:**126
congenital dislocation of
Andren–von Rosén method for, **1:**345
AP projection for, **1:**339, 339f
contrast arthrography of, **2:**8f, 14, 14f
developmental dysplasia of, **2:**9t, **3:**142, 142f
DXA of, **3:**466-467, 466f-467f
in geriatric patients, **3:**179, 179f
mediolateral projection of (Lauenstein and
Hickey methods), **1:**348, 348f-349f
MRI of, **3:**362f
surgical radiography of, **3:**230-232, 230f-232f
Hip arthrography, **2:**14
AP oblique, **2:**14f
axiolateral "frog", **2:**14f
with congenital dislocation, **2:**8f, 14, 14f
of hip prosthesis, **2:**14, 15f
digital subtraction technique for, **2:**14, 15f
photographic subtraction technique for, **2:**14,
15f
Hip bone
anatomy of, **1:**327-328, 327f-328f, 334b
sample exposure technique chart essential
projections for, **1:**335t
sectional anatomy of, **3:**282
summary of pathology of, **1:**335t
Hip dysplasia, congenital, **1:**331t
Hip fractures due to osteoporosis, **3:**449
Hip joint
anatomy of, **1:**331, 331f, 331t
sectional anatomy of, **3:**299, 299f
Hip joint replacement, surgical radiography of,
3:246f
Hip pads, **3:**449
Hip pinning, **3:**230-232, 230f-232f
Hip prosthesis, contrast arthrography of, **2:**14, 15f
digital subtraction technique for, **2:**14, 15f
photographic subtraction technique for, **2:**14,
15f
Hip screws, cannulated, **3:**230-232, 230f-232f
HIPAA (Health Insurance Portability and
Accountability Act of 1996), **3:**460, 476
Hirschsprung disease, **2:**109t
Histogram in CT, **3:**304f
Histoplasmosis, **1:**486t
History for trauma patient, **2:**26
HNP (herniated nucleus pulposus), **1:**368, 380t,
3:358f

HOCAs (high-osmolality contrast agents) in children, **3:**116
Hodgkin lymphoma, radiation oncology for, **3:**503
Holly method for tangential projection of sesamoids, **1:**251, 251f
Holmblad method for PA axial projection of intercondylar fossa, **1:**306-307
  evaluation criteria for, **1:**307b
  position of part for, **1:**307, 307f
  position of patient for, **1:**306, 306f
  structures shown on, **1:**307, 307f
Homeostasis, **3:**402, 438
Homogeneous structure or mass in ultrasonography, **3:**374, 374f, 397
Hook of hamate, **1:**102, 102f
Horizontal fissure of lungs, **1:**481f, 482
Horizontal plane, **1:**66, 66f-67f
Horizontal plate of palatine bones, **2:**273
Horizontal ray method for contrast arthrography of knee, **1:**13, 13f
Horn, **1:**84
Horseshoe kidney, **2:**188t
Host computer for CT, **3:**309, 339
Hot spots in radiation oncology, **3:**495
Hounsfield units, **3:**308, 308t, 339
HPV (human papillomavirus) and cancer, **3:**482
Hughston method for tangential projection of patella and patellofemoral joint, **1:**313, 313f
Human papillomavirus (HPV) and cancer, **3:**482
Humeral condyle, **1:**104, 104f
Humeral head, **3:**273f
Humeroradial joint, **1:**107, 107f
Humeroulnar joint, **1:**107
Humerus
  anatomy of, **1:**104-105, 104f
  AP projection of
    recumbent, **1:**169, 169f
    for trauma, **2:**49, 49f
    upright, **1:**167, 167f
  distal
    AP projection of
      in acute flexion, **1:**158, 158f
      in partial flexion, **1:**156, 156f
    PA axial projection of, **1:**165, 165f
  lateromedial projection of
    recumbent, **1:**170, 170f
    recumbent or lateral recumbent, **1:**171, 171f
    upright, **1:**168, 168f
  mediolateral projection of, **1:**168, 168f
  proximal
    anatomic neck of, **1:**177
    anatomy of, **1:**177-178, 177f
    greater tubercle of, **1:**177, 177f
    head of, **1:**177, 177f
    intertubercular (bicipital) groove of
      anatomy of, **1:**177, 177f
      Fisk modification for tangential projection of, **1:**207-208, 207f-208f
    lesser tubercle of, **1:**177, 177f
    Stryker notch method for AP axial projection of, **1:**204, 204f
    surgical neck of, **1:**177, 177f
  sectional anatomy of, **3:**269f, 272f, 273
  surgical radiography of, **3:**238-239, 238f-239f
Hutchison-Gilford syndrome, **3:**152
Hyaline membrane disease, **1:**486t
Hybrid imaging, nuclear medicine in, **3:**436
Hydrogen, magnetic properties of, **3:**343, 343f
Hydronephrosis, **2:**188t
  ultrasonography of, **3:**382f
    fetal, **3:**391f
Hydrosalpinx, **2:**246f
Hydroxyzine hydrochloride (Vistaril), **2:**226t

Hyoid bone, **2:**257, 275, 275f
  axiolateral oblique projection of, **2:**344f
  larynx and, **2:**72f
  pharynx and, **2:**72
  in sagittal section of face and neck, **2:**71f
  as surface landmark, **1:**71f, 71t
Hyperechoic structure or mass, **3:**397
Hyperextension, **1:**96, 96f
Hyperflexion, **1:**96, 96f
Hyperparathyroidism, **3:**448, 476
Hypersthenic body habitus, **1:**72-74, 72f, 73b, 74f
  and gallbladder, **2:**106, 106f
  skull radiography with, **2:**289f-290f
  and stomach and duodenum, **2:**99, 99f, 125f
  and thoracic viscera, **1:**479f
Hypertension
  portal, **3:**72
  renal, **2:**188t
Hypochondrium, **1:**70f
Hypodermic needles, **2:**228f, 229
Hypoechoic structure or mass, **3:**397
Hypogastric artery, **3:**25
Hypogastrium, **1:**70f
Hypoglossal canals, **2:**258f, 267, 267f
Hypophysis, **3:**2f
Hyposmia, **3:**169
Hyposthenic body habitus, **1:**72-74, 72f, 73b
  and gallbladder, **2:**106, 106f
  skull radiography with, **2:**289f-290f
  and stomach and duodenum, **2:**99, 99f, 125f
  and thoracic viscera, **1:**479f
Hypothalamus, **3:**259-260
Hypotonic duodenography, **2:**123, 123f
Hysterosalpingography (HSG), **2:**246-247, 247f
  of bicornuate uterus, **2:**247f
  of fibroid, **2:**247f
  of hydrosalpinx, **2:**246f
  of IUD, **2:**248f

I
^{123}I (iodine-123), **3:**406t
  for thyroid scan, **3:**417
^{131}I (iodine-131), **3:**406t
  for residual thyroid cancer or thyroid metastases, **3:**420
^{131}I (iodine-131) thyroid uptake measurement, **3:**418, 418f
IAM (internal acoustic meatus), **2:**259f, 268, 268f, 270f, 271
Iatrogenic, **3:**96
ICD (implantable cardioverter defibrillator), cardiac catheterization for, **3:**94, 94f
ID technique. See Implant displacement (ID) technique.
Identification of radiographs, **1:**25, 25f
IGRT (image-guided radiation therapy), **3:**498, 498f, 506
Ileocecal studies, **2:**139, 140f
Ileocecal valve
  anatomy of, **2:**102, 102f
  sectional anatomy of, **3:**283, 291
Ileum
  anatomy of, **2:**100f, 101, 102f
  sectional anatomy of, **3:**283, 291, 292f
Ileus, **2:**84t, 109t
Iliac arteries, MR angiography of, **3:**364f
Iliac bifurcation, MR angiography of, **3:**364f
Iliac crest
  anatomy of, **1:**327f, 328, 330f
  as bony landmark, **1:**71f, 71t, 333, 333f
  with obese patients, **1:**47-49
  sectional anatomy of, **3:**292
Iliac fossa, **1:**327f, 328
Iliac spine
  anatomy of, **1:**327f, 328
  sectional anatomy of, **3:**282

Iliac vessels as sonographic landmark, **3:**373, 373f
Iliac wings, **3:**299
Iliacus muscle, **3:**293, 293f
Ilioischial column, **1:**327, 327f, 356
Iliopectineal line, **3:**386, 397
Iliopsoas muscles, **3:**295, 295f
Iliopubic column, **1:**327, 327f, 356
Ilium
  anatomy of, **1:**327-328, 327f
  AP and PA oblique projections of, **1:**360, 360f-361f
  sectional anatomy of, **3:**282
    on axial (transverse) plane, **3:**292f-294f, 293-294
    on coronal plane, **3:**298f-299f
Illuminator, **1:**8
Image coregistration, **3:**402, 402f, 438
Image enhancement methods for mammography, **2:**427
  magnification technique (M) as, **2:**403t-408t, 428-429, 428f-429f, 432t
  spot compression technique as, **2:**403t-408t, 429-431, 430f-431f, 432t
Image intensification system, **2:**113, 113f
Image magnification in CT, **3:**304f
Image manipulation in CT, **3:**303, 304f, 313, 313f
Image misregistration in CT, **3:**321-323, 339
Image receptor (IR), **1:**3, 4f
  placement and orientation of anatomy on, **1:**28-29, 28f-29f
  size of, **1:**30, 30t
    with obese patients, **1:**50, 50f
    for trauma radiography, **2:**30
Image receptor (IR) holders for trauma radiography, **2:**20
Image receptor (IR) units, over-table, **1:**44-45, 45f
Image-guided radiation therapy (IGRT), **3:**498, 498f, 506
"Imaging plates" (IPs) in digital radiography, **1:**36, 36f
Immobilization devices, **1:**19, 19f
  for simulation in radiation oncology, **3:**490, 490f-491f
  trauma radiography with, **2:**23, 23f, 28, 30
Immobilization techniques
  for abdominal radiography, **2:**86, 87f
    of children, **3:**112-113, 112f-113f
  for children
    for abdominal radiography, **3:**112-113, 112f-113f
    for chest radiography, **3:**118, 118f-120f, 124f
    for gastrointestinal and genitourinary studies, **3:**116f
    holding as, **3:**110
    for limb radiography, **3:**127-129, 127f-128f
    for pelvis and hip radiography, **3:**126, 126f
    for skull radiography, **3:**132, 133f, 135f
Immune system decline in older adults, **3:**172
Impacted fracture, **1:**84f
Implant displacement (ID) technique for mammography, **2:**403t-408t
  with craniocaudal (CC) projection, **2:**422-423, 422f-423f
  with mediolateral oblique (MLO) projection, **2:**425
Implantable cardioverter defibrillator (ICD), cardiac catheterization for, **3:**94, 94f
Implantation, **2:**241
IMRT (intensity modulated radiation therapy), **3:**489, 496, 506
^{111}In (indium-111), **3:**406t
^{111}In (indium-111) pentetreotide (OctreoScan) for tumor imaging, **3:**415f, 420
In vitro hematologic studies, **3:**419, 438
In vivo examination in nuclear medicine, **3:**415, 438

Index

In vivo hematologic studies, **3:**419, 438
Incontinence in older adults, **3:**173, 174t
Incus, **2:**271
Independent jaws of linear accelerators, **3:**488f, 489, 506
Indexing in CT, **3:**310, 339
Indirect effects of radiation, **3:**484, 506
Indium-111 (^{111}In), **3:**406t
Indium-111 (^{111}In) pentetreotide (OctreoScan) for tumor imaging, **3:**415f, 420
Infant development, **3:**102
Infection, nuclear medicine imaging for, **3:**419
Infection control
  for MRI, **3:**348
  for venipuncture, **2:**228
Inferior angle of scapula, **1:**71f, 71t, 85
Inferior articular process, **1:**368, 368f
Inferior costal margin, **1:**71f, 71t
Inferior horn, **3:**4, 4f
Inferior mesenteric arteriogram, **3:**42f, 44, 45f
Inferior mesenteric artery, **3:**284, 298-299
Inferior mesenteric vein
  anatomy of, **2:**105f, **3:**22f
  sectional anatomy of, **3:**284-285
Inferior nasal conchae
  anatomy of, **2:**272f, 273
  sectional anatomy of, **3:**254, 263f, 264, 265f
Inferior orbital fissure, **2:**272f, 312f, 313
Inferior orbital margin
  modified Waters method for parietoacanthial projection of, **2:**326f
  PA axial projection of, **2:**298f
Inferior ramus, **1:**327f-328f, 328
Inferior rectus muscle, **3:**266, 266f
Inferior sagittal sinus, **3:**257-258, 257f, 267
Inferior thoracic aperture, **1:**479, 479f
Inferior vena cava (IVC)
  anatomy of, **2:**105f, **3:**22f, 24, 25f
  sectional anatomy in abdominopelvic region of, **3:**278, 279f
    on axial (transverse) plane, **3:**282f, 284
      at Level A, **3:**285, 285f
      at Level B, **3:**285, 286f
      at Level C, **3:**287f
      at Level D, **3:**288, 288f
      at Level E, **3:**289, 289f
      at Level F, **3:**290f
      at Level G, **3:**291, 291f
      at Level I, **3:**293
    on coronal plane, **3:**298-299, 298f
  sectional anatomy in thoracic region of, **3:**271
  sectional image of, **2:**107f
  ultrasonography of, **3:**376f-377f
Inferior vena cava (IVC) filter placement, **3:**68-71, 70f-71f
Inferior vena cavogram, **3:**60, 60f
Inferior vertebral notch, **1:**368f
Infiltration, **2:**235
Inframammary crease, **2:**381f
Infraorbital foramen, **2:**272, 272f
Infraorbital margin, **2:**285f, 330f
Infraorbitomeatal line (IOML), **2:**44, 320, 346
Infrapatellar bursa, **1:**82f
Infraspinatus muscle
  anatomy of, **1:**180f
  sectional anatomy of, **3:**271, 273-275, 273f-274f
Infundibulum, **2:**239, 239f
Ingested foreign body, **3:**139, 140f
Inguinal hernia, **2:**109t
Inguinal ligament, **3:**295
Inguinal region, **1:**70f
Inion, **2:**258f, 266, 266f
Initial examination, **1:**14
Inner canthus, **2:**285f

Innominate artery, **3:**96
  anatomy of, **3:**50
  digital subtraction angiography of, **3:**55f
Innominate bone. *See* Hip bone.
In-profile view, **1:**89
Inspiration, **1:**41
Instant vertebral analysis (IVA), **3:**469-470, 470f-471f, 477
In-stent restenosis, **3:**96
Insula, **3:**253f, 254-255, 258, 258f, 266-267
Insulin, **2:**106
Integrity in code of ethics, **1:**3
Integumentary system disorders in older adults, **3:**168
IntellBeam adjustable filter, **3:**332f
Intensity modulated radiation therapy (IMRT), **3:**489, 496, 506
Interarticular facet joints. *See* Zygapophyseal joints.
Intercarpal articulations, **1:**106, 106f
Interchondral joints, **1:**449t, 450, 450f
Intercondylar eminence, **1:**230, 230f
Intercondylar fossa
  anatomy of, **1:**232f-233f, 233
  Béclère method for AP axial projection of, **1:**310, 310f
  PA axial (tunnel) projection of
    Camp-Coventry method for, **1:**308, 308f-309f
    Holmblad method for, **1:**306-307
      evaluation criteria for, **1:**307b
      position of part for, **1:**307, 307f
      position of patient for, **1:**306, 306f
      structures shown on, **1:**307, 307f
Intercostal arteries, arteriography of, **3:**40f
Intercostal spaces, **1:**448, 448f
Intercuneiform articulations, **1:**236t, 237f, 238
Interhemispheric fissure, **3:**2
Interiliac plane, **1:**68, 69f
Intermembranous ossification, **1:**77
Intermetatarsal articulations, **1:**236t, 237f, 238
Internal, **1:**85
Internal acoustic meatus (IAM), **2:**259f, 268, 268f, 270f, 271
Internal capsule, **3:**253f, 258-259, 267, 267f
Internal carotid artery
  anatomy of, **3:**49f, 50
  arteriography of, **3:**50f, 53f-54f
    AP axial oblique projection for, **3:**58f
    AP projection for, **3:**52f
    lateral projection for, **3:**52f-53f, 56f
  digital subtraction angiography of, **3:**31f
  MR angiography of, **3:**363f
  sectional anatomy of, **3:**255
    on axial (transverse) plane
      at Level D, **3:**259f, 260-261
      at Level E, **3:**261-262, 261f
      at Level F, **3:**262-263, 262f
      at Level G, **3:**263f, 264
    on coronal plane, **3:**267
    on sagittal plane, **3:**265, 265f
  stenosis of, **3:**14f
  three-dimensional reconstruction of, **3:**34f
Internal carotid venogram, **3:**52f
Internal iliac artery
  anatomy of, **3:**25
  sectional anatomy of, **3:**284, 293, 293f
Internal iliac vein, **3:**284, 293
Internal jugular vein
  anatomy of, **3:**22f
  sectional anatomy of, **3:**255, 262-264, 262f, 269f, 271
    on axial (transverse) plane, **3:**272-273, 272f-273f
    on coronal plane, **3:**280-281
Internal mammary lymph nodes, **2:**380, 381f

Internal oblique muscle, **3:**288f, 290-291, 293, 293f
Internal occipital protuberance
  anatomy of, **2:**266, 267f
  sectional anatomy of, **3:**253, 259-260, 259f
Interpeduncular cistern, **3:**254, 259-260, 259f
Interphalangeal (IP) joints
  of lower limb, **1:**236, 236t, 237f
  of upper limb, **1:**105, 105f-106f
Interpupillary line, **2:**285f
Intersinus septum, **2:**276f, 279
Interstitial implant technique for brachytherapy, **3:**485
Interstitial pneumonitis, **1:**486t
Intertarsal articulations, **1:**236t, 238
Intertrochanteric crest, **1:**328f, 329
Intertrochanteric line, **1:**328f, 329
Intertubercular groove
  anatomy of, **1:**104f, 105
  Fisk modification for tangential projection of, **1:**207-208, 207f-208f
Intervention, **3:**96
Interventional, **3:**96
Interventional pain management, **3:**16-18
Interventional procedures, CT for, **3:**314, 314f-316f
Interventional radiology (IR), **3:**62-74
  for abdominal aortic aneurysm endografts, **3:**65-66, 65f-66f
  for cardiac catheterization. *See* Cardiac catheterization.
  for children, **3:**157-158, 157f-158f
  of CNS, **3:**15
  defined, **3:**18
  definition of terms for, **3:**96b-97b
  historical development of, **3:**20-21
  for inferior vena cava filter placement, **3:**68-71, 70f-71f
  other procedures in, **3:**72
  percutaneous transluminal angioplasty as, **3:**62-65
    balloon in, **3:**62-63, 63f
    of common iliac artery, **3:**64f
    Dotter method for, **3:**62
    for placement of intravascular stents, **3:**65, 65f
    of renal artery, **3:**64f
  present and future of, **3:**74, 74f
  transcatheter embolization as, **3:**66-68
    in cerebral vasculature, **3:**68, 69f
    embolic agents for, **3:**66-67, 67b, 67t
    of hypervascular uterine fibroid, **3:**68, 69f
    lesions amenable to, **3:**66-67, 67b
    stainless steel occluding coils for, **3:**68, 68f
    vascular plug for, **3:**68, 68f
  for transjugular intrahepatic portosystemic shunt, **3:**72, 72f-73f
Interventricular foramen, **3:**4, 4f
Interventricular septal integrity, **3:**96
Interventricular septum, **3:**270, 278, 278f-279f
Intervertebral disks, **1:**368
Intervertebral foramina
  anatomy of, **1:**368
  sectional anatomy of, **3:**269-270, 278-279, 280f
Intervertebral joints, **1:**378, 379t
Intervertebral transverse foramina, **1:**371, 371f, 371t
Intestinal intubation, **2:**143, 143f
Intestinal tract preparation
  for contrast media studies
    of colon, **2:**146, 146f
    of urinary system, **2:**196-197, 196f-197f
  for female reproductive system radiography, **2:**246
Intima
  anatomy of, **3:**65
  ultrasonography of, **3:**383, 397

Intracavitary implant technique for brachytherapy, **3:**485
Intracoronary stent, **3:**88, 89f, 96
Intraperitoneal organs, **3:**283
Intrathecal injections, **3:**6, 12, 18
Intrauterine devices (IUDs)
  imaging of, **2:**248, 248f-249f
  ultrasonography of, **3:**389f
Intravascular stent placement
  percutaneous transluminal angioplasty for, **3:**65, 65f
  percutaneous transluminal coronary angioplasty for, **3:**88, 89f
Intravascular ultrasound (IVUS), **3:**80t, 91, 91f-92f
Intravenous (IV) medication administration. *See* Venipuncture.
Intravenous urography (IVU). *See* Excretory urography (EU).
Intraventricular foramina (of Monro), **3:**264
Introducer sheaths for angiographic studies, **3:**36, 36f, 97
Intubation examination procedures for small intestine, **2:**143, 143f
Intussusception, **2:**109t
  in children, **3:**114, 114f
Invasive/infiltrating ductal carcinoma, **2:**395, 449f, 458f
  architectural distortion due to, **2:**393f
Inversion recovery, **3:**352-353, 367
Invert/inversion, **1:**96f
Involuntary muscles, motion control of, **1:**18-19
Involution of breasts, **2:**380
Iodinated contrast media
  for alimentary canal imaging, **2:**111-112, 111f-112f
  for angiographic studies, **3:**29
  for large intestine studies, **2:**145
  for urinary system imaging, adverse reactions to, **2:**196
Iodine-123 (^{123}I), **3:**406t
  for thyroid scan, **3:**417
Iodine-131 (^{131}I), **3:**406t
  for residual thyroid cancer or thyroid metastases, **3:**420
Iodine-131 (^{131}I) thyroid uptake measurement, **3:**418, 418f
IOML (infraorbitomeatal line), **2:**44, 320, 346
Ionization, **3:**484, 506
Ionizing radiation and cancer, **3:**482, 506
IP(s) (imaging plates) in digital radiography, **1:**36, 36f
IP (interphalangeal) joints
  of lower limb, **1:**236, 236t, 237f
  of upper limb, **1:**105, 105f-106f
Ipsilateral, **1:**85
IR. *See* Image receptor (IR); Interventional radiology (IR).
Iris, **2:**314f, 315
Iron oxide mixtures for MRI, **3:**355
Irregular bones, **1:**79, 79f
Ischemia, ultrasonography of, **3:**397
Ischemic, **3:**97
Ischial ramus, **1:**327f, 328
Ischial spine
  anatomy of, **1:**327f, 330f
  sectional anatomy of, **3:**296
Ischial tuberosity
  anatomy of, **1:**327f-328f, 328, 330f
  as bony landmark, **1:**333f
Ischium
  anatomy of, **1:**327-328, 327f
  sectional anatomy of, **3:**282, 294-295, 295f-296f

Isherwood method
  for AP axial oblique projection of subtalar joint
    with lateral rotation ankle, **1:**278, 278f
    with medial rotation ankle, **1:**277, 277f
  for lateromedial oblique projection of subtalar joint, **1:**276, 276f
Ishimore, Shoji, **3:**21
Island of Reil. *See* Insula.
Islet cells, **2:**106
Islets of Langerhans, **2:**106
Isocentric machine, cobalt-60 unit as, **3:**486, 506
Isodose line/curve in radiation oncology, **3:**494, 506
Isoechoic structure or mass, **3:**397
Isolation unit
  mobile radiography in, **3:**189
  standard precautions for patient in, **1:**15, 15f
Isotopes, **3:**403, 438
  in radiation oncology, **3:**486, 506
Isotropic emission, **3:**429, 438
Isotropic spatial resolution, **3:**339
Isthmus
  of uterine tube, **2:**239, 239f
  of uterus, **2:**240, 240f
IUDs (intrauterine devices)
  imaging of, **2:**248, 248f-249f
  ultrasonography of, **3:**389f
IV (intravenous) medication administration. *See* Venipuncture.
IVA (instant vertebral analysis), **3:**469-470, 470f-471f, 477
IVC. *See* Inferior vena cava (IVC).
IVU (intravenous urography). *See* Excretory urography (EU).
IVUS (intravascular ultrasound), **3:**80t, 91, 91f-92f

J
Jefferson fracture, **1:**380t
Jejunum
  anatomy of, **2:**100f, 101
  sectional anatomy of, **3:**283, 289
Jewelry, **1:**20, 21f
Joint(s), **1:**80-82
  cartilaginous, **1:**80t, 81, 81f
  fibrous, **1:**80f, 80t, 81
  functional classification of, **1:**81
  in long bone studies, **1:**28, 29f
  structural classification of, **1:**80t, 81-82
  synovial, **1:**80t, 82, 82f-83f
Joint capsule tear, **2:**9t
Joint effusion, **1:**109t
Joint Review Committee on Education in Radiologic Technology (JRCERT), **1:**23
Jones fracture, **1:**240t
Judd method for PA projection of dens, **1:**383
Judet method for AP oblique projection of acetabulum, **1:**356-357, 356f-357f
Judkins, Melvin, **3:**20
Jugular foramen, **2:**258f, 267
Jugular notch
  anatomy of, **1:**447-448, 447f
  with obese patients, **1:**49, 49f
  sectional anatomy of, **3:**256, 273
  as surface landmark, **1:**71f, 71t
Jugular process, **2:**267f
Jugular veins, **3:**271

K
Kandel method for dorsoplantar axial projection of clubfoot, **1:**270, 270f
K-edge filtration systems for DXA, **3:**451, 451f-452f
  crossover in, **3:**452
  scintillating detector pileup in, **3:**452

Kidney(s), **2:**184-185
  anatomy of, **2:**184-185, 185f
  angiography of, **2:**190, 191f
  CT of, **2:**190, 191f
  function of, **2:**183
  horseshoe, **2:**188t
  location of, **2:**183f-184f, 184
  nephrotomography of, **2:**190, 191f
    AP projection in, **2:**209, 209f
    percutaneous renal puncture for, **2:**210-211, 210f
  pelvic, **2:**188t
  polycystic, **2:**188t
  sectional anatomy of, **3:**282f, 283
    on axial (transverse) plane, **3:**290, 290f-291f
    on coronal plane, **3:**299, 299f
  sectional image of, **2:**107f
  ultrasonography of, **3:**382-383, 382f
  urography of. *See* Urography.
Kidney stone, ultrasonography of, **3:**382f
Kilovoltage (kV) in digital imaging, **1:**37, 37f
Kilovoltage peak (kVp)
  control of, **1:**42
  in digital imaging, **1:**37, 37f
  for obese patients, **1:**50
  in this atlas, **1:**42
Kinetics, **3:**421, 438
Kite method
  for AP projection of clubfoot, **1:**267, 267f, 269f
  for mediolateral projection of clubfoot, **1:**268-269, 268f-269f
Kleinschmidt, Otto, **2:**372
Knee
  contrast arthrography of, **2:**12
    double-contrast (horizontal ray method), **2:**13, 13f
    vertical ray method for, **2:**12, 12f
  CT of, **3:**336f-338f
  MRI of, **3:**347, 347f
Knee joint
  anatomy of, **1:**234-235, 234f-235f, 236t, 238, 238f
  AP oblique projection of
    in lateral rotation, **1:**304, 304f
    in medial rotation, **1:**305, 305f
  AP projection of, **1:**296, 296f-297f
    weight-bearing method for, **1:**302, 302f
  mediolateral projection of, **1:**300-301, 300f-301f
  PA projection of, **1:**298-299, 298f-299f
    Rosenberg weight-bearing method for, **1:**303, 303f
Kneecap. *See* Patella.
Knuckles, **1:**101
KUB projection of abdomen, **2:**87, 89-90, 89f-90f
kV (kilovoltage) in digital imaging, **1:**37, 37f
kVp. *See* Kilovoltage peak (kVp).
Kyphoplasty, **3:**16, 18
  balloon, for osteoporotic fractures, **3:**449, 449f
Kyphosis, **1:**367, 367f, 380t
  adolescent, **1:**380t
  and bone densitometry, **3:**476
  in older adults, **3:**170, 170f, 174t
Kyphotic curves, **1:**366f, 367

L
L5-S1 junction
  AP oblique projection of, **1:**421, 422f
  lateral projection of, **1:**419-420, 419f-420f
Labyrinths
  anatomy of, **2:**262
  sectional anatomy of, **3:**253, 253f
Lacrimal bones
  anatomy of, **2:**272, 272f-273f
  in orbit, **2:**275, 275f, 312f
  sectional anatomy of, **3:**254

Index

Lacrimal foramen, **2:**272
Lacrimal fossae, **2:**272
Lacrimal sac, **2:**314f
Lactation, breasts during, **2:**382, 382f
Lactiferous ductules, **2:**380, 381f
Lambda, **2:**258f, 259
Lambdoidal suture, **2:**258f, 259, 275t
Laminae of vertebral arch, **1:**368, 368f
Landmarks, **1:**71, 71f, 71t
    with obese patients, **1:**47-49, 49f
LAO (left anterior oblique) position, **1:**92, 92f
Laquerrière-Pierquin method for tangential
        projection of scapular spine, **1:**224, 224f
Large intestine. *See* Colon.
Large part area shield, **1:**33, 34f
Large saphenous vein, **3:**22f
Large-core needle biopsy (LCNB) of breast,
    2:461
Larmor frequency in MRI, **3:**343
Laryngeal cancer, radiation oncology for,
    3:504
Laryngeal cavity, **2:**73
Laryngeal vestibule, **2:**73
Laryngopharynx, **2:**71f, 72
Larynx
    anatomy of, **2:**71f-73f, 72-73
    AP projection of, **2:**76-77, 76f-77f
    lateral projection of, **2:**78-79, 78f-79f
    methods of examination of, **2:**74-75
Laser printer for digital subtraction angiography,
    3:31
Lateral, **1:**85
Lateral apertures, **3:**4
Lateral collateral ligament, **1:**236f
Lateral condyle
    of femur, **1:**232f-233f, 233
    of tibia, **1:**230, 230f
Lateral decubitus position, **1:**94, 94f
Lateral epicondyle
    of femur, **1:**232f, 233
    of humerus, **1:**104, 104f
Lateral fissure, **3:**258f, 266-267, 267f
Lateral intercondylar tubercle, **1:**230, 230f
Lateral malleolus, **1:**230f-231f, 231
Lateral mass. *See* Vertebral arch.
Lateral meniscus
    anatomy of, **1:**234f-236f, 235
    double-contrast arthrography of, **2:**13, 13f
Lateral position, **1:**91, 91f
Lateral projection, **1:**11, 12f, 88, 88f
    of obese patients, **1:**49
Lateral pterygoid lamina, **2:**265f, 266
Lateral recess, **3:**4f
Lateral recumbent position, **1:**90, 90f
Lateral resolution in ultrasonography, **3:**397
Lateral rotation, **1:**93, 93f, 97, 97f
Lateral sinus, **3:**255
Lateral sulcus, **3:**2f
Lateral ventricles
    anatomy of, **3:**2, 4, 4f
    anterior horn of, **3:**253f, 258f, 264
    posterior horn of, **3:**253f, 258f
    sectional anatomy of, **3:**255
        on axial (transverse) plane, **3:**257-259, 257f
        on coronal plane, **3:**267, 267f-268f
        on sagittal plane, **3:**265-266, 265f-266f
        temporal horn of, **3:**258f-259f
Lateral vertebral assessment (LVA), **3:**469-470,
    470f-471f, 477
Lateromedial projection, **1:**88, 88f
Latissimus dorsi muscle, sectional anatomy of
    in abdominopelvic region, **3:**285,
        285f-287f
    in thoracic region, **3:**278, 278f-279f
Lauenstein method for mediolateral projection of
    hip, **1:**348, 348f-349f

Lauterbur, Paul, **3:**342
Law method (modified) for axiolateral oblique
        projection of TMJ, **2:**345f, 351-352,
        351f-352f
Lawrence method
    for inferosuperior axial projection of shoulder
        joint, **1:**194, 194f-195f
    for transthoracic lateral projection of shoulder,
        1:192-193, 192f-193f
LCBF (local cerebral blood flow), PET images of,
    3:427, 427f, 438
LCIS (lobular carcinoma in situ), **2:**395
LCNB (large-core needle biopsy) of breast,
    2:461
LDR (low-dose-rate) brachytherapy, **3:**485, 506
Le Fort fracture, **2:**282t
Least significant change (LSC) in DXA, **3:**456,
    476
Left anterior oblique (LAO) position, **1:**92, 92f
Left colic flexure, **2:**102f, 103, 114f
Left lower quadrant (LLQ), **1:**70, 70f
Left posterior oblique (LPO) position, **1:**93, 93f
Left upper quadrant (LUQ), **1:**70, 70f
Left ventricular ejection fracture, computerized
    planimetry for evaluation of, **3:**82-84, 84f
Left ventriculography, **3:**82-84, 83f-84f
Leg. *See* Lower limb.
Legg-Calvé-Perthes disease, **1:**335t
Leiomyoma, **3:**397
Lengthwise position, **1:**28, 28f
Lens
    anatomy of, **2:**314f-315f
    sectional anatomy of, **3:**253f
Lentiform nucleus, **3:**253f, 258-259, 258f, 267f
Lesions, **3:**97, 480, 506
Lesser curvature of stomach
    anatomy of, **2:**98, 98f
    sectional anatomy of, **3:**283
Lesser sciatic notch, **1:**327f, 328
Lesser trochanter, **1:**232f, 328f, 329
Lesser tubercle, **1:**104f, 105
Lesser wings of sphenoid
    anatomy of, **2:**258f, 264f-265f, 265
    sectional anatomy of, **3:**253-254, 262
LET (linear energy transfer), **3:**484, 506
Levator scapulae, **2:**272f
Level I trauma center, **2:**19
Level II trauma center, **2:**19
Level III trauma center, **2:**19
Level IV trauma center, **2:**19
Lewis method for tangential projection of
    sesamoids, **1:**250-251, 250f
Life stage, age-specific competencies by, **1:**23
Lifting of older adults, **3:**175
Ligament of Treitz
    anatomy of, **2:**100f, 101
    sectional anatomy of, **3:**283
Ligament tear, **2:**9t
Ligamentum capitis femoris, **1:**329f
Ligamentum teres, **3:**283, 287
Ligamentum venosum, **3:**283
Light pipe of gamma camera, **3:**408f, 409, 438
Limb(s). *See* Lower limb; Upper limb.
Lindblom method for AP axial projection of
    pulmonary apices, **1:**512-513, 512f-513f
Line, **1:**84
Line placement, chest radiography during, **3:**226,
    226f
Linear accelerators (linacs) for radiation oncology,
    3:485, 487-489, 488f, 506
Linear energy transfer (LET), **3:**484, 506
Linear skull fracture, **2:**282t
Linens, **1:**15
Lingula
    anatomy of, **1:**482
    sectional anatomy of, **3:**270, 278

Lipoma, **2:**386f, 395, 447f
Lithotomy position, **1:**90, 91f
Liver
    anatomy of, **2:**104-106, 104f-105f
    combined SPECT/CT of, **3:**415f
    functions of, **2:**104
    hemangioma of, **3:**360f
    MRI of, **3:**360f
    nuclear medicine imaging of, **3:**418
    sectional anatomy in abdominopelvic region of,
        3:282f, 283
        on axial (transverse) plane, **3:**285, 285f-290f,
            287-290
            at Level A, **3:**285, 285f
            at Level B, **3:**285, 286f
            at Level C, **3:**287, 287f
            at Level D, **3:**288, 288f
            at Level E, **3:**289, 289f
            at Level F, **3:**290, 290f
        on coronal plane, **3:**298-299, 298f
    sectional anatomy in thoracic region of, **3:**278,
        279f-280f
    sectional image of, **2:**107f
    ultrasonography of, **3:**373f-374f, 376f-378f,
        378
LLQ (left lower quadrant), **1:**70, 70f
Lobar pneumonia, **1:**486t
    in children, **3:**151
Lobes of breast, **2:**380
Lobular carcinoma in situ (LCIS), **2:**395
Lobular pneumonia, **1:**486t
Lobules of breast, **2:**380, 381f
LOCA(s) (low-osmolality contrast agents) in
    children, **3:**116
Local cerebral blood flow (LCBF), PET images of,
    3:427, 427f, 438
Local metabolic rate of glucose, **3:**427, 427f
Long bone(s), **1:**79, 79f
    anatomy of, **1:**76
    vessels and nerves of, **1:**77, 77f
Long bone measurement, **2:**1-6
    abbreviations for, **2:**2b
    bilateral, **2:**4-5, 4f
    CT for, **2:**6, 6f
    digital imaging for, **2:**2
    digital postprocessing for, **2:**2
    imaging methods for, **2:**2
    with leg length discrepancy, **2:**4f-5f, 5
    localization of joints in, **2:**2-5
    magnification in, **2:**2-3, 3f
    orthoroentgenogram for, **2:**2-3, 3f
    position of part for, **2:**2
    position of patient for, **2:**2
    radiation protection for, **2:**2
    scanogram for, **2:**2
    teleoroentgenogram for, **2:**2
    unilateral, **2:**4f-5f, 5
    of upper limb, **2:**2, 5, 5f
Long bone studies
    joint in, **1:**28, 29f
    in tall patients, **1:**28
Longitudinal angulation, **1:**87
Longitudinal arch
    anatomy of, **1:**228-230, 228f
    weight-bearing method for lateromedial
        projection of, **1:**262, 262f-263f
Longitudinal cerebral fissure, **3:**256-257
Longitudinal fissure, **3:**254-255, 257-258, 257f
Longitudinal plane in MRI, **3:**343, 367
Longitudinal quality control for DXA, **3:**461-462,
    461f-462f, 476
Longitudinal sulcus, **3:**2
Loop of Henle, **2:**185, 185f
Lordosis, **1:**367, 367f, 380t
Lordotic curves, **1:**366f, 367
Lordotic position, **1:**94, 95f

Low-dose-rate (LDR) brachytherapy, 3:485, 506
Lower limb, 1:225-322
  abbreviations used for, 1:239b
  anatomy of, 1:242
    articulations in, 1:236-238, 236f-238f, 236t
    femur in, 1:232-233, 232f-233f
    fibula in, 1:231, 231f
    foot in, 1:228-230, 228f-229f
    knee joint in, 1:234-235, 234f-235f
    patella in, 1:233, 233f
    summary of, 1:239b
    tibia in, 1:230-231, 230f-231f
  ankle of. See Ankle.
  arteriography of, 3:47, 48f
  calcaneus of
    anatomy of, 1:228f-229f, 229
    axial projection of
      dorsoplantar, 1:272, 272f-273f
      plantodorsal, 1:271, 271f
      weight-bearing coalition (Harris-Beath)
        method for, 1:273, 273f
    mediolateral projection of, 1:274, 274f
    weight-bearing method for lateromedial
      oblique projection of, 1:275, 275f
  in children, 3:127-131
    with fractures, 3:129-130, 130f-131f
    image evaluation for, 3:123t, 131
    immobilization for, 3:127-129, 128f
    radiation protection for, 3:129, 129f
  dislocation-fracture of, 2:51f
  femur of
    anatomy of, 1:232-233, 232f-233f
    AP projection of, 1:318-319, 318f-319f
    mediolateral projection of, 1:320-321,
      320f-321f
  fibula of
    anatomy of, 1:230f-231f, 231
    AP oblique projections of, 1:294-295,
      294f-295f
    AP projection of, 1:290-291, 290f-291f
    lateral projection of, 1:292-293, 292f-293f
  foot (feet) of. See Foot (feet).
  of geriatric patients, 3:181, 181f
  intercondylar fossa of
    anatomy of, 1:232f-233f, 233
    Béclère method for AP axial projection of,
      1:310, 310f
    PA axial (tunnel) projection of
      Camp-Coventry method for, 1:308,
        308f-309f
      Holmblad method for, 1:306-307, 306f-307f
  knee joint of
    anatomy of, 1:234-235, 234f-235f
    AP oblique projection of
      in lateral rotation, 1:304, 304f
      in medial rotation, 1:305, 305f
    AP projection of, 1:296, 296f-297f
      weight-bearing method for, 1:302, 302f
    mediolateral projection of, 1:300-301,
      300f-301f
    PA projection of, 1:298-299, 298f-299f
      Rosenberg weight-bearing method for,
        1:303, 303f
  long bone measurement of. See Long bone
    measurement.
  MRI of, 3:360-362, 362f-363f
  patella of
    anatomy of, 1:233, 233f
    mediolateral projection of, 1:312, 312f
    PA projection of, 1:311, 311f
    tangential projection of
      Hughston method for, 1:313, 313f
      Merchant method for, 1:314-315,
        314f-315f
      Settegast method for, 1:316-317,
        316f-317f

Lower limb (Continued)
  patellofemoral joint of
    anatomy of, 1:238, 238f
    tangential projection of
      Hughston method for, 1:313, 313f
      Merchant method for, 1:314-315, 314f-315f
      Settegast method for, 1:316-317, 316f-317f
  radiation protection for, 1:242
  sample exposure technique chart essential
    projections for, 1:241t
  subtalar joint of
    anatomy of, 1:236t, 237f, 238
    Isherwood method for AP axial oblique
      projection of
      with lateral rotation ankle, 1:278, 278f
      with medial rotation ankle, 1:277, 277f
    Sherwood method for lateromedial oblique
      projection with medial rotation foot of,
      1:276, 276f
  surgical radiography of, 3:246-250, 246f-247f,
    249f
  tibia of
    anatomy of, 1:230-231, 230f-231f
    AP oblique projections of, 1:294-295,
      294f-295f
    AP projection of, 1:290-291, 290f-291f
    lateral projection of, 1:292-293, 292f-293f
  toes of. See Toes.
  trauma radiography of, 2:50-53
    patient position considerations for, 2:22f-23f,
      50
    structures shown on, 2:52-53, 52f
    trauma positioning tips for, 2:50, 50f
  venography of, 3:47, 48f
Lower limb alignment, weight-bearing method
  for AP projection to assess, 1:322,
  322f-323f
Lower limb arteries, duplex sonography of,
  3:393
Lower limb length discrepancies, weight-bearing
  method for AP projection to assess, 1:322,
  322f-323f
Lower limb veins, duplex sonography of, 3:393,
  394f
Low-osmolality contrast agents (LOCAs) in
  children, 3:116
LPO (left posterior oblique) position, 1:93, 93f
LSC (least significant change) in DXA, 3:456,
  476
LSO (lutetium oxyorthosilicate) as scintillator for
  PET, 3:428-429, 428t
Lumbar curve, 1:366f, 367
Lumbar discogram, 3:17f
Lumbar fusion, 3:229f
Lumbar intervertebral disks, PA projection of,
  1:435-436, 435f
Lumbar myelogram, 3:8f
Lumbar nodes, 3:27f
Lumbar vein, ultrasonography of, 3:377f
Lumbar vertebrae
  anatomy of, 1:366f, 374-375, 375f
    accessory process in, 1:374, 374f
    intervertebral foramina in, 1:374
    mamillary process in, 1:374, 374f
    pars interarticularis in, 1:374, 374f
    superior aspect in, 1:374, 374f
    transverse processes in, 1:374, 374f
    zygapophyseal joints in, 1:374, 374f-375f,
      375t
  AP projection of, 1:413-415, 413f-415f
    for trauma, 2:36-37, 36f-37f
  compression fracture of, 3:464, 464f
  CT myelogram of, 3:12f
  CT of, 1:415, 416f
    for needle biopsy of infectious spondylitis of,
      3:314f

Lumbar vertebrae (Continued)
  DXA of
    equipment for, 3:442f
    lateral, 3:469
    PA, 3:464-466, 464f-465f
  fracture-dislocation of, 2:35f
  intervertebral disks of, PA projection of,
    1:435-436, 435f
  intervertebral foramina of
    anatomy of, 1:374
    positioning rotations needed to show, 1:371t
  lateral projection of, 1:417-418, 417f-418f
    for trauma, 2:35, 35f
  MRI of, 1:415, 416f, 3:13f, 358f
  PA projection of, 1:413-415, 413f-414f
  sectional anatomy of, 3:282
    on axial (transverse) plane, 3:290-292
    on coronal plane, 3:299
    on sagittal plane, 3:296, 297f
  spinal fusion of
    AP projection of, 1:441-442, 441f-442f
    lateral projection in hyperflexion and
      hyperextension of, 1:443-444, 443f-444f
  spondylolysis and spondylolisthesis of, 1:375,
    375f
  surgical radiography of, 3:228-229, 228f-229f
    mobile, 3:244, 244f-245f
  trauma radiography of
    AP projection in, 2:36-37, 36f-37f
    lateral projections in, 2:35, 35f
  zygapophyseal joints of
    anatomy of, 1:374, 374f-375f, 375t
    AP oblique projection of, 1:421-422
      position of part for, 1:421, 421f
      position of patient for, 1:421
      positioning rotations needed to show, 1:371t
Lumbosacral angle, 1:367
Lumbosacral junction, AP axial projection of
  (Ferguson method), 1:425-426, 425f
Lumbosacral vertebrae
  AP and PA projections of, 1:413-415, 415f
  AP axial projection of (Ferguson method),
    1:425-426, 425f
  lateral projection of, 1:417-418, 418f
    at L5-S1 junction, 1:419-420, 419f-420f
  PA axial projection of, 1:426, 426f
Lunate, 1:101f, 102
Lung(s)
  anatomy of, 1:481-482, 481f-482f
  AP oblique projection of, 1:508-509,
    508f-509f
  AP projection of, 1:510-511, 510f-511f
    with pleura, 1:516-517, 516f-517f
  coal miner's (black), 1:486t
  general positioning considerations for, 1:488
    for lateral projections, 1:488, 489f
    for oblique projections, 1:488
    for PA projections, 1:488, 489f
    upright vs. prone, 1:488, 488f
  lateral projection of, 1:500-503
    evaluation criteria for, 1:502b
    foreshortening in, 1:501, 501f
    forward bending in, 1:501, 501f
    general positioning considerations for, 1:488,
      489f
    with pleura, 1:518-519, 518f-519f
    position of part for, 1:500-501, 500f
    position of patient for, 1:500
    structures shown on, 1:502, 502f-503f
  lobes of, 1:481f, 482
  nuclear medicine for imaging of, 3:419
  PA oblique projection of, 1:504-507
    evaluation criteria for, 1:507b
    LAO position for, 1:504f, 505, 506f
    position of part for, 1:504f-505f, 505
    position of patient for, 1:504

Index

Lung(s) *(Continued)*
  RAO position for, **1:**505, 505f, 507f
  SID for, **1:**504
  structures shown on, **1:**506-507,
    506f-507f
  PA projection of, **1:**496-499
    breasts in, **1:**497, 497f
    evaluation criteria for, **1:**499b
    general positioning considerations for, **1:**488,
      489f
    with pleura, **1:**516-517, 517f
    position of part for, **1:**496-498, 496f
    position of patient for, **1:**496
    respiration in, **1:**498, 498f
    SID for, **1:**496
    structures shown on, **1:**499, 499f
  PET of, **3:**433f
  primary lobules of, **1:**482
  pulmonary apices of
    AP axial projection of
      in lordotic position (Lindblom method),
        1:512-513, 512f-513f
      in upright or supine position, **1:**515,
        515f
    PA axial projection of, **1:**514, 514f
  sectional anatomy of
    in abdominopelvic region, **3:**285f-286f
    in thoracic region, **3:**269f, 270, 271f
      on axial (transverse) plane, **3:**273f,
        274-275, 278, 278f
      on coronal, **3:**280-281
Lung cancer
  in older adults, **3:**172
  PET of, **3:**433f
  radiation oncology for, **3:**502, 502f
Lung markings in radiography of sternum, **1:**456,
  457f
Lung perfusion scan, Tc-99m MAA, **3:**419
Lung ventilation scan, xenon-133, **3:**419
LUQ (left upper quadrant), **1:**70, 70f
Lutetium oxyorthosilicate (LSO) as scintillator for
  PET, **3:**428-429, 428t
Lutetium yttrium orthosilicate (LYSO) as
  scintillator for PET, **3:**428t
LVA (lateral vertebral assessment), **3:**469-470,
  470f-471f, 477
Lymph, **3:**22, 24, 97
Lymph nodes, **3:**26, 27f
Lymph vessels, **3:**26, 97
Lymphadenography, **3:**97
Lymphangiography, **3:**97
Lymphatic system, **3:**22, 26, 27f
Lymphocytes, **3:**26
Lymphography, **3:**26, 27f, 97
Lymphoma, Hodgkin, radiation oncology for,
  3:503
Lymphoreticular tissue, cancer arising from,
  3:483t
LYSO (lutetium yttrium orthosilicate) as scintillator
  for PET, **3:**428t

M
M (magnification technique) for mammography,
  2:403t-408t, 428-429, 428f-429f, 432t
mA (milliamperage), **1:**42
Macroaggregated albumin (MAA) in
  radiopharmaceuticals, **3:**405, 405f
Magnet(s) for MRI, **3:**346
Magnet room for MRI, **3:**346-347,
  346f-347f
Magnetic field strength for MRI, **3:**346
Magnetic resonance (MR), **3:**367
Magnetic resonance angiography (MRA),
  3:363-364, 363f-364f
Magnetic resonance cholangiopancreatography
  (MRCP), **3:**361f

Magnetic resonance imaging (MRI), **3:**341-368
  of abdomen, **3:**360, 360f-361f
  body planes in, **1:**67, 67f
  of breast, **2:**418-419, 472, **3:**358, 359f
  cardiac, **3:**358, 359f
  of chest, **3:**358, 359f
  of children, **3:**155-156, 156f
  claustrophobia in, **3:**349, 353
  of CNS, **3:**12-13, 357-358
    of brain, **3:**12, 13f, 357, 357f
    of spine, **3:**13, 358
      lumbar, **1:**415, 416f, **3:**13f, 358f
      thoracic, **3:**358f
  coils for, **3:**346, 354, 354f, 367
  contrast media for, **3:**355, 355f
  vs. conventional radiography, **3:**342
  CT vs., **3:**333, 334f
  defined, **3:**342, 438
  definition of terms for, **3:**367b-368b
  diffusion and perfusion techniques for,
    3:364-365, 365f
  equipment for, **3:**345-347
    console as, **3:**345, 345f
    equipment room as, **3:**345
    magnet room as, **3:**346-347, 346f-347f
  extremity scanner for, **3:**347, 347f
  fast-imaging pulse sequences for, **3:**357
  functional, **3:**366
  gating for, **3:**356, 356f, 367
  historical development of, **3:**342
  imaging parameters for, **3:**350f-353f, 351-353
  imaging time in, **3:**352
  infection control for, **3:**348
  of musculoskeletal system, **3:**360-362,
    362f-363f
  vs. nuclear medicine, **3:**401t, 402
  patient monitoring for, **3:**354
  of pelvis, **3:**360, 361f
  PET combined with, **3:**401, 436
  planes in, **3:**350f, 351
  positioning for, **3:**353
  principles of, **3:**342
  pulse sequences in, **3:**344, 352, 352f-353f, 367
  in radiation oncology, **3:**494
  safety of, **3:**348-349, 349f
  sectional anatomy of, **3:**252
  signal production in, **3:**343, 343f
  significance of signal in, **3:**344, 344f
  slice in, **3:**342, 368
  slice thickness in, **3:**351-352
  three-dimensional, **3:**351, 351f
  of vessels, **3:**363-364, 363f-364f
Magnetic resonance imaging (MRI) coronary
  arteriography, **3:**95f
Magnetic resonance (MR) mammography,
  2:418-419, 472, **3:**358, 359f
Magnetic resonance spectroscopy (MRS), **3:**365,
  365f-366f
Magnification, **1:**7, 7f
  in angiography, **3:**33
Magnification radiography, **1:**28-29
Magnification technique (M) for mammography,
  2:403t-408t, 428-429, 428f-429f, 432t
Main lobar fissure as sonographic landmark, **3:**373,
  373f
Main trunk vessels, **3:**23, 25f
Major calyx(ces), **2:**185, 185f
Major duodenal papilla, **2:**100f, 105, 105f
Malabsorption syndrome, **2:**109t
Male(s)
  calcifications of breast in, **2:**427
  cystourethrography in, **2:**221, 221f
  mammography in, **2:**426, 426f-427f
  osteoporosis in, **3:**447
Male pelvis, **1:**332, 332f, 332t
  PA projection of, **1:**338f

Male reproductive system
  anatomy of, **2:**242
    ductus deferens in, **2:**242, 242f-243f
    ejaculatory ducts in, **2:**242, 243f
    prostate in, **2:**242f-243f, 243
    seminal vesicles in, **2:**242, 243f
    summary of, **2:**244b
    testes in, **2:**242, 242f
  radiography of, **2:**253-254
    of prostate, **2:**254
    of seminal ducts, **2:**253
      epididymography for, **2:**253, 253f
      epididymovesiculography for, **2:**253
      grid technique for, **2:**253
      nongrid technique for, **2:**253
      vesiculography for, **2:**253, 254f
  sectional anatomy of, **3:**284
Malignancy, **3:**482, 506
Malleolus, **1:**84
Malleus, **2:**271
Mamillary process, **1:**374, 374f
Mammary fat, **2:**381f
Mammary gland. *See* Breast(s).
Mammillary bodies, **3:**259-260
Mammography, **2:**369-474
  artifacts on, **2:**396, 396f
  of augmented breast, **2:**417-419, 418f
    craniocaudal (CC) projection of
      with full implant, **2:**420-421, 421f
      with implant displaced, **2:**422-423,
        422f-423f
    with implant displacement (ID),
      2:403t-408t
    mediolateral oblique (MLO) projection of
      with full implant, **2:**424
      with implant displaced, **2:**425
  automatic exposure control for, **2:**409
  for breast cancer screening, **2:**377
    vs. diagnostic mammography, **2:**378
    risk vs. benefit of, **2:**377-378, 377f
  comfort measures for, **2:**374, 409, 410f
  compression in, **2:**402
  computer-aided detection (CAD) systems for,
    2:376-379, 376f
  descriptive terminology for lesion location in,
    2:411, 413f
  equipment for, **2:**373-374, 373f
  evolution of systems for, **2:**373, 373f
  findings on, **2:**384-393
    architectural distortions as, **2:**393, 393f
    calcifications as, **2:**389-393, 389f-392f
    masses as, **2:**384-388, 385f-388f
  full-field digital, **2:**374-375
    labeling for, **2:**409
    technique chart for, **2:**394t
  grids for, **2:**374
  historical development of, **2:**371-372,
    371f-372f
  image enhancement methods for, **2:**427
    magnification technique (M) as, **2:**403t-408t,
      428-429, 428f-429f, 432t
    spot compression technique as, **2:**403t-408t,
      429-431, 430f-431f, 432t
  labeling for, **2:**402, 402f, 403t-408t
  during lactation, **2:**382, 382f
  magnetic resonance (MR), **2:**418-419, 472,
    3:358, 359f
  male, **2:**426, 426f-427f
  method of examination for, **2:**396
  mosaic imaging or tiling in, **2:**400, 401f
  of oversized breasts, **2:**400, 401f
  patient preparation for, **2:**396, 396f-399f
  posterior nipple line in, **2:**409, 410f
  principles of, **2:**371-374
  procedures for, **2:**400-409, 401f
  respiration during, **2:**409

Index

Mammography *(Continued)*
routine projections in, **2:**411
craniocaudal (CC), **2:**403t-408t, 411f, 413-414, 413f-414f
mediolateral oblique (MLO), **2:**403t-408t, 411f, 415-416, 415f-416f
screening, **2:**377
diagnostic vs., **2:**378
risk vs. benefit of, **2:**377-378, 377f
standards for, **2:**373, 377
summary of projections in, **2:**370-379, 411, 411t-412t
supplemental projections in, **2:**432-457
90-degree lateromedial (LM), **2:**411f, 435-436
applications of, **2:**403t-408t, 432t
evaluation criteria for, **2:**436b
labeling codes for, **2:**403t-408t
position of part for, **2:**435, 435f
position of patient for, **2:**435
structures shown on, **2:**436, 436f
90-degree mediolateral (ML), **2:**411f, 433-434
applications of, **2:**403t-408t, 432t
evaluation criteria for, **2:**434b, 434f
labeling codes for, **2:**403t-408t
position of part for, **2:**433, 433f
position of patient for, **2:**433
structures shown on, **2:**434
axillary for axillary tail as, **2:**452-453, 452f-453f
captured lesion or coat-hanger (CL), **2:**445, 446f-447f
applications of, **2:**403t-408t, 432t
labeling codes for, **2:**403t-408t
caudocranial (FB), **2:**412f, 448-449
applications of, **2:**403t-408t, 432t
evaluation criteria for, **2:**449b
labeling codes for, **2:**403t-408t
position of part for, **2:**448, 448f
position of patient for, **2:**448
structures shown on, **2:**449, 449f
craniocaudal for cleavage (cleavage view, CV) as, **2:**412f, 439-440
applications of, **2:**403t-408t, 432t
evaluation criteria for, **2:**440b, 440f
labeling codes for, **2:**403t-408t
position of part for, **2:**439, 439f
position of patient for, **2:**439
structures shown on, **2:**440
craniocaudal with roll lateral (rolled lateral, RL), **2:**412f, 441-442
applications of, **2:**403t-408t, 432t
evaluation criteria for, **2:**442b
labeling codes for, **2:**403t-408t
position of part for, **2:**441, 441f
position of patient for, **2:**441
structures shown on, **2:**442, 442f
craniocaudal with roll medial (rolled medial, RM), **2:**412f, 441-442
applications of, **2:**403t-408t, 432t
evaluation criteria for, **2:**442b
labeling codes for, **2:**403t-408t
position of part for, **2:**441, 441f
position of patient for, **2:**441
structures shown on, **2:**442
elevated or pushed-up craniocaudal (ECC), **2:**403t-408t
exaggerated craniocaudal (XCCL), **2:**412f, 437-438
applications of, **2:**403t-408t, 432t
evaluation criteria for, **2:**438b, 438f
labeling codes for, **2:**403t-408t
position of part for, **2:**437, 437f
position of patient for, **2:**437
structures shown on, **2:**438

Mammography *(Continued)*
inferolateral to superomedial oblique (LMO), **2:**403t-408t
inferomedial to superolateral oblique (ISO), **2:**403t-408t
lateromedial oblique (LMO), **2:**412f, 454-455, 454f-455f
mediolateral oblique for axillary tail, **2:**412f, 432t, 450-451, 450f-451f
superolateral to inferomedial oblique (SIO), **2:**412f, 456-457
applications of, **2:**403t-408t, 432t
evaluation criteria for, **2:**457b
labeling codes for, **2:**403t-408t
position of part for, **2:**456, 456f
position of patient for, **2:**456
structures shown on, **2:**457, 458f
tangential (TAN), **2:**412f, 443
applications of, **2:**403t-408t, 432t
evaluation criteria for, **2:**443b
labeling codes for, **2:**403t-408t
position of part for, **2:**443, 443f-444f
position of patient for, **2:**443
structures shown on, **2:**443, 444f
xero-, **2:**372, 372f
Mammography Quality Standards Act (MQSA), **2:**377
MammoSite applicator, **3:**504
Mandible
alveolar portion of, **2:**274, 274f
anatomy of, **2:**272f-274f, 274
axiolateral oblique projection of, **2:**343-345
evaluation criteria for, **2:**345b
position of part for, **2:**343, 343f-344f
position of patient for, **2:**343
structures shown on, **2:**343-345, 344f-345f
axiolateral projection of, **2:**343-345, 343f
body of
anatomy of, **2:**274, 274f
axiolateral oblique projection of, **2:**344f-345f
axiolateral projection of, **2:**343f-344f
PA axial projection of, **2:**340f, 342, 342f
PA projection of, **2:**339f, 341, 341f
submentovertical projection of, **2:**346f
lateral projection of, **2:**322f
modified Waters method for parietoacanthial projection of, **2:**326f
panoramic tomography of, **2:**353-354, 353f-354f
rami of
anatomy of, **2:**274, 274f
AP axial projection of, **2:**348f
axiolateral oblique projection of, **2:**344f-345f, 345
axiolateral projection of, **2:**343f, 345, 345f
lateral projection in decubitus position of, **2:**295f
PA axial projection of, **2:**340, 340f, 342f
PA projection of, **2:**339, 339f, 341f
sectional anatomy of, **3:**263f, 264
submentovertical projection of, **2:**346f
sectional anatomy of, **3:**254
submentovertical projection of, **2:**311f, 346, 346f, 367f
symphysis of
anatomy of, **2:**274, 274f
axiolateral oblique projection of, **2:**345, 345f
axiolateral projection of, **2:**343f-344f, 345
PA axial projection of, **2:**342f
PA projection of, **2:**341f
submentovertical projection of, **2:**346f
Mandibular angle
anatomy of, **2:**274, 274f
axiolateral oblique projection of, **2:**344f-345f
in lateral aspect of skull, **2:**273f

Mandibular angle *(Continued)*
parietoacanthial projection of, **2:**324f
modified, **2:**326f
as surface landmark, **1:**71f, 71t, **2:**285f
Mandibular condyle
anatomy of, **2:**273f-274f, 274
AP axial projection of, **2:**306f, 348f
axiolateral oblique projection of, **2:**345f, 352f
PA axial projection of, **2:**342f
PA projection of, **2:**339f
sectional anatomy of, **3:**262, 262f
submentovertical projection of, **2:**311f, 346f
Mandibular fossa
anatomy of, **2:**268, 268f, 274f
axiolateral oblique projection of, **2:**352f
sectional anatomy of, **3:**253-254
Mandibular notch, **2:**273f-274f, 274
Mandrel, **3:**97
Manifold for cardiac catheterization, **3:**78, 78f
Manubriosternal joint, **1:**447f, 449t, 450
Manubrium
anatomy of, **1:**447-448, 447f
sectional anatomy of, **3:**256
on axial (transverse) plane, **3:**274-275, 274f
on coronal plane, **3:**280, 281f
on sagittal plane, **3:**278-280, 280f
Mapping in maximum intensity projection, **3:**326, 339
Marginal lymph sinus, **3:**26
Markers
anatomic, **1:**25, 25f-26f, 27, 27b
of bone turnover, **3:**448, 476
for trauma radiography, **2:**24, 24f
Mass, Dierk, **3:**20-21
Masseter muscles, **3:**255-256, 264
Mastication, **2:**59
Mastoid air cells
anatomy of, **2:**268, 269f-270f
AP axial projection of, **2:**309f
PA projection of, **2:**339f
parietoacanthial projection of, **2:**363f
sectional anatomy of, **3:**259-263
Mastoid angle of parietal bone, **2:**263f
Mastoid antrum, **2:**269f-270f, 271
Mastoid fontanel, **2:**259-260, 260f
Mastoid process
anatomy of, **2:**258f, 268, 268f-269f
PA axial projection of, **2:**342f
submentovertical projection of, **2:**311f
Mastoid tip, **1:**71f, 71t
Mastoidian cells, **2:**269f
Mastoiditis, **2:**282t
Matrix in CT, **3:**302, 308, 308f, 339
Maxilla. *See* Maxillary bones.
Maxillary bones
anatomy of, **2:**259f, 272, 272f-273f
lateral projection of, **2:**322f
in orbit, **2:**275, 275f, 312f
parietoacanthial projection of, **2:**324f
modified, **2:**326f
sectional anatomy of, **3:**254, 262
Maxillary sinuses
acanthioparietal projection of, **2:**328f
anatomy of, **2:**276, 276f-278f
lateral projection of, **2:**322f, 359f
location of, **2:**272
parietoacanthial projection of, **2:**363f, 365f
Waters method for, **2:**324f, 362-363, 362f-363f
open-mouth, **2:**364-365, 364f-365f
sectional anatomy of, **3:**262, 262f, 264, 266, 266f
submentovertical projection of, **2:**311f, 367f
Maximum aperture diameter, **1:**44-45, 45t

Maximum intensity projection (MIP), **3:**326, 339-340
MCP (metacarpophalangeal) joint(s)
  anatomy of, **1:**105, 105f-106f
  folio method for first, **1:**118-119
MDCT (multidetector CT), **3:**306, 323-324, 323f-324f
Mean glandular dose, **2:**377, 377f
Mean in DXA, **3:**455, 455f-456f, 476
Mean marrow dose (MMD), **1:**35, 35t
Meatus, **1:**84
Meckel diverticulum, **2:**109t
Media of arterial wall, **3:**65
Medial, **1:**85
Medial collateral ligament, **1:**236f
Medial condyle
  of femur, **1:**232f-233f, 233
  of tibia, **1:**230, 230f
Medial epicondyle
  of femur, **1:**232f, 233
  of humerus, **1:**104, 104f
Medial intercondylar tubercle, **1:**230, 230f
Medial malleolus, **1:**230f-231f, 231
Medial meniscus
  anatomy of, **1:**234f-236f, 235
  double-contrast arthrography of, **2:**13, 13f
Medial orbital wall, **2:**262f
Medial pterygoid lamina, **2:**265f, 266
Medial pterygoid muscle, **3:**266, 266f
Medial rotation, **1:**93, 93f, 97, 97f
Median aperture, **3:**4
Median nerve, **1:**102, 102f
Mediastinal structures in radiography of sternum, **1:**456, 457f
Mediastinum
  anatomy of, **1:**483-484, 483f-484f
  CT of, **1:**484, 485f
  defined, **1:**479
  lateral projection of superior, **1:**494-495, 494f-495f
  sectional anatomy of, **3:**270, 280
Medical dosimetrist, **3:**480, 506
Medical physicist, **3:**480, 506
Medical terminology, **1:**98, 98t
Medication administration via venipuncture.
  See Venipuncture.
Mediolateral projection, **1:**88
Medulla oblongata
  anatomy of, **3:**2, 2f-3f
  sectional anatomy of, **3:**255
    on axial (transverse) plane, **3:**262-264, 262f-263f
    on sagittal plane, **3:**265f
Medullary cavity, **1:**76, 76f
Medulloblastoma, radiation oncology for, **3:**504, 505f
Megacolon, congenital aganglionic, **2:**109t
Meglumine diatrizoate (Gastrografin, Gastroview)
  for simulation in radiation oncology, **3:**490
Melanoma, PET of, **3:**433f
Membranous labyrinth, **2:**271
Membranous urethra, **2:**186f, 187
Meninges
  anatomy of, **3:**3, 97
  sectional anatomy of, **3:**254
Meniscus, **1:**82, 82f
Meniscus tear, **2:**9t
Menstrual cycle, **2:**240
Mental foramen, **2:**273f-274f, 274
Mental point, **2:**285f
Mental protuberance, **2:**272f, 274, 274f
Mentomeatal line, **2:**327f-328f
Meperidine hydrochloride (Demerol), **2:**226t
Merchant method for tangential projection of patella and patellofemoral joint, **1:**314-315, 314f-315f

Mesentery
  anatomy of, **2:**83
  sectional anatomy of, **3:**283, 290, 293f
Mesocephalic skull, **2:**286, 286f
Mesovarium, **2:**239
Metabolic neurologic study, PET for, **3:**434
Metacarpals, **1:**101, 101f
Metacarpophalangeal (MCP) joint(s)
  anatomy of, **1:**105, 105f-106f
  folio method for first, **1:**118-119
Metal objects, **1:**20, 21f
Metallic bead chain cystourethrography, **2:**222-224, 223f
Metastable technetium-99 (^{99m}Tc). See Technetium-99m (^{99m}Tc).
Metastasis(es)
  to abdomen, **2:**84t
  to bony thorax, **1:**454t
  to lower limb, **1:**240t
  to pelvis and proximal femora, **1:**335t
  radiation oncology for, **3:**481, 507
  to shoulder girdle, **1:**182t
  to skull, **2:**282t
  to thoracic viscera, **1:**486t
  to upper limb, **1:**109t
  to vertebral column, **1:**380t
Metatarsals
  anatomy of, **1:**228f, 229
  surgical radiography of, **3:**249f
Metatarsophalangeal (MTP) articulations, **1:**236f-237f, 236t, 238
Method, **1:**95
Metric/English conversion, **1:**30
MI (myocardial infarction), **3:**75, 97
  echocardiography after, **3:**393, 396f
Microbial fallout, **3:**250
Micturition, **2:**186
Midaxillary plane, **1:**66, 66f
Midazolam hydrochloride (Versed), **2:**226t
Midbrain
  anatomy of, **3:**2, 2f
  sectional anatomy of, **3:**255, 258-259, 265f
Midcoronal plane, **1:**66, 66f
Middle cerebral arteries
  CT angiography of, **3:**325f
  MR angiography of, **3:**363f
  sectional anatomy of, **3:**255
    on axial (transverse) plane, **3:**257-261, 259f
    on coronal plane, **3:**267
Middle cranial fossa, **2:**260
Middle hepatic vein as sonographic landmark, **3:**373, 373f
Middle nasal concha
  anatomy of, **2:**262, 262f
  sectional anatomy of, **3:**253
Middle phalanges, **1:**228, 228f
Midfoot, **1:**228-230
Midsagittal plane, **1:**66, 66f, **2:**285f
Milk ducts, examination of, **2:**459-460, 459f-460f
Milk of calcium, **2:**391, 391f, 395
Miller-Abbott tube, **2:**143, 143f
Milliamperage (mA), **1:**42
Minor calyx(ces), **2:**185, 185f
MIP (maximum intensity projection), **3:**326, 339-340
Misregistration in digital subtraction angiography, **3:**31, 97
Mitral valve
  anatomy of, **3:**25f
  sectional anatomy of, **3:**270
Mitral valve regurgitation, **3:**82-84, 83f
MLC (multileaf collimation), **3:**489, 489f, 507
MMD (mean marrow dose), **1:**35, 35t
^{99}Mo (molybdenum-99), **3:**404, 404f
Mobile PET units, **3:**436, 436f

Mobile radiography, **3:**183-212
  of abdomen, **3:**196-199
    AP or PA projection in left lateral decubitus position for, **3:**198-199, 198f-199f
    AP projection for, **3:**196, 196f-197f
  of cervical spine, **3:**206-207
    lateral projection for, **3:**206-207, 206f-207f
  of chest, **3:**192
    AP or PA projection in lateral decubitus position for, **3:**194-195, 194f-195f
    AP projection in upright or supine position for, **3:**192, 192f-193f
  of chest and abdomen of neonate, **3:**208-212
    AP projection for, **3:**208-210
      evaluation criteria for, **3:**210b, 210f
      position of part for, **3:**208f-209f, 209
      position of patient for, **3:**208, 208f
      structures shown on, **3:**210, 210f
    lateral projection for, **3:**211-212, 211f-212f
  digital, **3:**184, 185f
    of cervical spine, **3:**207
    of chest, **3:**193-195
    of femur
      AP projection for, **3:**203-205
      lateral projection for, **3:**205
  examination in, **3:**190
  of femur, **3:**202-203
    AP projection for, **3:**202-203, 202f-203f
    lateral projection for, **3:**204-205, 204f-205f
  history of, **3:**184
  initial procedures in, **3:**190, 190b
  isolation considerations with, **3:**189
  machines for, **3:**184, 185f
  for obese patients, **1:**52
  patient considerations with, **3:**190-191
    assessment of patient's condition as, **3:**190
    with fractures, **3:**191
    interfering devices as, **3:**191, 191f
    patient mobility as, **3:**191
    positioning and asepsis as, **3:**191
  of pelvis, **3:**200-201
    AP projection for, **3:**200-201, 200f-201f
  principles of, **3:**184, 184f
  radiation safety with, **3:**188, 188f-189f
  surgical, **3:**242-250
    of cervical spine, **3:**242, 242f-243f
    of extremities
      for ankle fracture, **3:**246f
      of ankle with antibiotic beads, **3:**247f
      for fifth metatarsal nonhealing fracture, **3:**249f
      for forearm fracture, **3:**247f
      for hip joint replacement, **3:**246f
      lower, **3:**246-250
      for tibial plateau fracture, **3:**247f
      for total shoulder arthroplasty, **3:**248f
      for wrist fracture, **3:**249f
    of thoracic or lumbar spine, **3:**244, 244f-245f
  technical considerations for, **3:**184-187
    anode heel effect as, **3:**186-187, 186t
    grid as, **3:**185-186, 185f-186f
    radiographic technique charts as, **3:**187, 187f
    source-to-image receptor distance as, **3:**187
  for trauma patients, **2:**21f, 32
Mobility and mobile radiography, **3:**191
Mold technique for brachytherapy, **3:**485
Molybdenum-99 (^{99}Mo), **3:**404, 404f
Moore method for PA oblique projection of sternum, **1:**460-461, 460f-461f
Morphine sulfate, **2:**226t
Morphometric x-ray absorptiometry (MXA), **3:**469-470, 470f, 476

Mortise joint
    anatomy of, **1:**230f-231f, 236t, 238
    AP oblique projection in medial rotation of,
        1:284-289, 284f-285f
Motion artifact on MRI, **3:**356
Motion control, **1:**18-19, 18f
    of involuntary muscles, **1:**18-19
    with obese patients, **1:**50-51
    for trauma radiography, **2:**23, 23f
    of voluntary muscles, **1:**19, 19f
Mouth, **2:**57-67
    anatomy of, **2:**59, 59f, 61b
    salivary glands of. *See* Salivary glands.
    summary of pathology of, **2:**62t
    summary of projections of, **2:**58-59
Movement terminology. *See* Body movement
    terminology.
MPR (multiplanar reconstruction) in CT, **3:**313,
    313f, 327f, 340
MR (magnetic resonance), **3:**367
MR (magnetic resonance) mammography,
    2:418-419, 472, **3:**358, 359f
MRA (magnetic resonance angiography),
    3:363-364, 363f-364f
MRCP (magnetic resonance
    cholangiopancreatography), **3:**361f
MRI. *See* Magnetic resonance imaging (MRI).
MRI conditional implants, **3:**348-349, 367
MRI safe implants, **3:**348-349, 367
MRS (magnetic resonance spectroscopy), **3:**365,
    365f-366f
MSAD (multiple scan average dose) for CT, **3:**330,
    340
MSHCT (multislice helical CT), **3:**306, 323-324,
    323f-324f
MTP (metatarsophalangeal) articulations,
    1:236f-237f, 236t, 238
Multidetector CT (MDCT), **3:**306, 323-324,
    323f-324f
Multiformat camera for digital subtraction
    angiography, **3:**31
Multi-gated acquisition (MUGA) format, **3:**416
Multi-infarct dementia, **3:**169
Multileaf collimation (MLC), **3:**489, 489f, 507
Multiplanar reconstruction (MPR) in CT, **3:**313,
    313f, 327f, 340
Multiple exposures, **1:**29, 29f
Multiple imaging windows in CT, **3:**304f
Multiple myeloma, **1:**335t, 380t, 454t
    of skull, **2:**282t
Multiple scan average dose (MSAD) for CT, **3:**330,
    340
Multislice helical CT (MSHCT), **3:**306, 323-324,
    323f-324f
Musculoskeletal system
    MRI of, **3:**360-362, 362f-363f
    ultrasonography of, **3:**383, 383f
Musculoskeletal system disorders in older adults,
    3:170, 170f-171f
Mutations and cancer, **3:**482
MXA (morphometric x-ray absorptiometry),
    3:469-470, 470f, 476
Mycoplasma pneumonia, **3:**151
Myelography, **3:**6-8
    cervical, **3:**9f
    contrast media for, **3:**6-7, 6f
    conus projection in, **3:**8
    CT, **3:**12, 12f
    of dentate ligament, **3:**9f
    examination procedure for, **3:**7-8, 7f
    of foramen magnum, **3:**9f
    lumbar, **3:**8
    preparation of examining room for, **3:**7, 7f
    of subarachnoid space, **3:**9f
Myeloma, multiple, **1:**335t, 380t, 454t
    of skull, **2:**282t

Myocardial infarction (MI), **3:**75, 97
    echocardiography after, **3:**393, 396f
Myocardial perfusion study
    technetium-99m sestamibi, **3:**416
    thallium-201, **3:**414, 414f, 416
Myocardium, **3:**24
Myometrium, ultrasonography of, **3:**388, 397

N
¹³N (nitrogen-13), **3:**406t
    in PET, **3:**425f, 426t
NaI (sodium iodide) as scintillator for PET, **3:**428t
NaI (sodium iodide) scintillation crystals of gamma
    camera, **3:**408f, 409
Nasal bones
    anatomy of, **2:**259f, 272, 273f
    lateral projection of, **2:**322f, 331-332, 331f-332f
    sectional anatomy of, **3:**254, 261-262, 261f
Nasal conchae
    anatomy of, **2:**262, 262f
    sectional anatomy of, **3:**253-254
        on axial (transverse) plane, **3:**263f, 264
        on sagittal plane, **3:**265, 265f
Nasal septum
    anatomy of, **2:**71f, 273
    modified Waters method for parietoacanthial
        projection of, **2:**326f
    sectional anatomy of, **3:**262
Nasal spine, **2:**261, 261f
Nasion, **2:**261, 261f, 285f
Nasofrontal suture, **2:**332f
Nasopharynx
    anatomy of, **2:**71f, 72
    sectional anatomy of, **3:**263f, 264, 267
National Trauma Database (NTDB), **2:**18-19,
    18f-19f
Navicular bone, **1:**228f, 229
Naviculocuneiform articulation, **1:**236t, 237f, 238
Neck
    anterior part of, **2:**69-79
        anatomy of, **2:**71, 71f
            larynx in, **2:**71f-73f, 72-73
            parathyroid glands in, **2:**71, 72f
            pharynx in, **2:**71f, 72
            summary of, **2:**73b
            thyroid gland in, **2:**71, 72f
        radiography of, **2:**74-79
            AP projection of pharynx and larynx in,
                2:76-77, 76f-77f
            deglutition in, **2:**74-75, 74f
            fluoroscopic, **2:**75
            Gunson method for, **2:**75, 75f
            lateral projection of soft palate, pharynx,
                and larynx in, **2:**78-79, 78f-79f
            methods of examination for, **2:**74-75
            positive-contrast pharyngography for,
                2:74-75
        summary of projections for, **2:**70
    soft tissue
        in children, **3:**137-138, 137f-138f
        CT of, **3:**336f-338f
Neck brace, trauma radiography with, **2:**23, 23f
Needle(s)
    for angiographic studies, **3:**35, 35f
    disposal of, **1:**16, 16f
    for venipuncture, **2:**228-229, 228f
        anchoring of, **2:**233, 233f
        discarding of, **2:**234, 234f
Needle-wire localization of breast lesion,
    2:461-463
Neer method for tangential projection of
    supraspinatus "outlet", **1:**202-203, 202f
Neointimal hyperplasia, **3:**97
Neonatal development, **3:**102
Neonatal neurosonography, **3:**385, 385f
Neonate, cranial bones in, **2:**259-260, 260f

Neoplasm, **3:**506
Nephron, **2:**185, 185f
Nephron loop, **2:**185, 185f
Nephrotomography, **2:**190, 191f, 202
    AP projection in, **2:**209, 209f
    percutaneous renal puncture for, **2:**210-211,
        210f
Nephrotoxic, **3:**97
Nephrourography, infusion, equipment for, **2:**198
Nerve tissue, cancer arising from, **3:**483t
Nervous system disorders in older adults,
    3:168-169
Networking, **3:**409-410
Neuroangiography, surgical, **3:**74
Neurologic imaging, PET for, **3:**434
Neuroma, acoustic, **2:**282t
Neutron(s), **3:**403, 403f, 438
Neutron-deficient nucleus, **3:**422, 423f
Neutron-to-proton ratio, **3:**403
Newborn. *See* Neonate.
Nipple
    anatomy of, **2:**380, 381f
    ductography of, **2:**459-460, 459f-460f
    in mammography, **2:**402
    Paget disease of, **2:**395
Nitrogen-13 (¹³N), **3:**406t
    in PET, **3:**425f, 426t
NMR (nuclear magnetic resonance) imaging,
    3:342, 367
Noctec (chloral hydrate), **2:**226t
Noise
    in CT, **3:**318-319, 319f, 340
    in MRI, **3:**367
Nonaccidental trauma to children, **3:**143f-145f
    imaging protocol for, **3:**124, 146t
Nondisplaced fracture, **1:**84
Noninvasive technique, ultrasonography as, **3:**370,
    397
Nonocclusive, **3:**97
Nonsterile surgical team members, **3:**215f, 216
Norgaard method for AP oblique projection in
    medial rotation of hand, **1:**130-131
    evaluation criteria for, **1:**131b
    position of part for, **1:**130-131, 131f
    position of patient for, **1:**130
    structures shown on, **1:**131, 131f
Notch, **1:**84
Notification values for CT, **3:**330
NTDB (National Trauma Database), **2:**18-19,
    18f-19f
Nuclear cardiology, **3:**416-417
Nuclear magnetic resonance (NMR) imaging,
    3:342, 367
Nuclear medicine, **3:**399-439
    clinical, **3:**415-420
        bone scintigraphy as, **3:**415-416
        of CNS, **3:**417
        of endocrine system, **3:**417-418, 418f
        of gastrointestinal system, **3:**418-419
        genitourinary, **3:**419
        for infection, **3:**419
        in vitro and in vivo hematologic studies as,
            3:419
        nuclear cardiology as, **3:**416-417
        respiratory, **3:**419
        sentinel node, **3:**420
        special procedures in, **3:**420
        therapeutic, **3:**420
        of tumor, **3:**420
    defined, **3:**400
    definition of terms for, **3:**437b-439b
    future of, **3:**435-436
        hybrid imaging as, **3:**436
        for PET, **3:**436, 436f
        radioimmunotherapy as, **3:**435
    historical development of, **3:**400-401

Nuclear medicine *(Continued)*
  imaging methods for, **3:**410-415
    combined SPECT and CT as, **3:**401, 415, 415f
    dynamic, **3:**412
    SPECT as, **3:**413-414, 413f-414f
    static, **3:**410-411
    whole-body, **3:**412, 412f
  instrumentation in, **3:**408-410
    computers as, **3:**409-410, 410f-411f
      quantitative analysis using, **3:**410, 411f, 438
    modern-day gamma camera as, **3:**408-409, 408f
  vs. other modalities, **3:**401-402, 401t, 402f-403f
  patient preparation for, **3:**415
  physical principles of, **3:**403-405
    basic nuclear physics as, **3:**403-404, 403f-404f
    nuclear pharmacy as, **3:**404-405, 405f, 406t
    positron emission tomography (PET) as. *See* Positron emission tomography (PET).
  principles of, **3:**400
  radiation safety in, **3:**407, 407f
  therapeutic, **3:**420
Nuclear particle accelerators, **3:**404, 425, 438
Nuclear pharmacy, **3:**404-405, 405f, 406t
Nuclear physics, **3:**403-404, 403f-404f
Nuclear reactors, **3:**400, 438
  in radiation oncology, **3:**486, 507
Nucleus
  atomic, **3:**343, 367, 403, 403f
  neutron-deficient (proton-rich), **3:**422, 423f
Nucleus pulposus
  anatomy of, **1:**368
  herniated, **1:**368, 380t, **3:**358f
  sectional anatomy of, **3:**269-270
Nuclide, **3:**403, 438
Nulliparous uterus, **2:**240
Nutrient artery, **1:**77, 77f
Nutrient foramen, **1:**77, 77f

O
¹⁵O. *See* Oxygen-15 (¹⁵O).
Obese patients, **1:**44-52
  automatic exposure control and anatomically programmed radiography systems with, **1:**52
  Bucky grid with, **1:**51
  centering of, **1:**47-48
  communication with, **1:**47
  defined, **1:**44, 44f
  equipment for, **1:**44-45, 45f, 45t
  exposure factors for, **1:**50-52
  field light size with, **1:**50, 51f
  focal spot with, **1:**51
  image receptor sizes and collimation with, **1:**50, 50f
  imaging challenges with, **1:**47-50, 47f-48f
  landmarks with, **1:**47-49, 49f
  mobile radiography of, **1:**52
  oblique and lateral projections with, **1:**49
  radiation dose for, **1:**52
  technical considerations for, **1:**52, 52b
  transportation of, **1:**46, 46f
Object–to–image receptor distance (OID), **1:**7, **3:**33
Oblique fissures of lungs, **1:**481f, 482
Oblique fracture, **1:**84f
Oblique plane, **1:**66f-67f, 67
  pancreas in, **3:**380, 397
Oblique position, **1:**92-93, 92f-93f
Oblique projection, **1:**12, 12f, 88, 89f
  of obese patients, **1:**49
Obstetric ultrasonography, **3:**388-391
  in first trimester, **3:**388, 389f-390f
  history of, **3:**371
  in second trimester, **3:**390, 390f
  in third trimester, **3:**390-391, 391f

Obturator foramen
  anatomy of, **1:**327f, 328
  sectional anatomy of, **3:**282
Obturator internus muscle, **3:**295, 295f
Occipital angle of parietal bone, **2:**263f
Occipital bone
  anatomy of, **2:**266-267, 266f-267f
  AP axial projection of, **2:**305f-306f
  fracture of, **2:**44f
  location of, **2:**258f-259f
  PA axial projection of, **2:**309f
  sectional anatomy of, **3:**253, 258-260, 262-263
  submentovertical projection of, **2:**311f
Occipital condyles, **1:**369f, **2:**266-267, 266f
Occipital lobe, sectional anatomy of, **3:**254-255
  on axial (transverse) plane, **3:**258-260
  on sagittal plane, **3:**264, 265f-266f, 266
Occipitoatlantal joints, **2:**267
Occluding coils, stainless steel, **3:**68, 68f
Occlusal plane, **1:**68, 69f
Occlusion, **3:**28, 97
OCT (optical coherence tomography), **3:**80t, 92, 93f
Octagonal immobilizer, **3:**116f
OctreoScan (indium-111 pentetreotide) for tumor imaging, **3:**415f, 420
OD (optical density), **1:**5, 5f
Odontoid process. *See* Dens.
OI (osteogenesis imperfecta), **3:**147, 147f
OID (object–to–image receptor distance), **1:**7, **3:**33
Oil cyst, **2:**386f
Older adults. *See* Aging; Elderly.
Olecranon fossa
  anatomy of, **1:**104, 104f
  PA axial projection of, **1:**166, 166f
Olecranon process, **1:**103, 103f, 107f
-oma, **3:**506
OMAR (orthopedic metal artifact reduction), **3:**319, 320f
Omentum(a), **2:**83, 83f
OML (orbitomeatal line), **2:**44
Oncologist, **3:**480, 507
  radiation, **3:**480, 507
Oncology, **3:**480, 507
  radiation. *See* Radiation oncology.
Oncology imaging, PET for, **3:**433, 433f
Opaque arthrography, **2:**8-9, 8f
Open fracture, **1:**84, 84f
Open mouth technique for atlas and axis, **1:**384-385, 384f-385f
Open surgical biopsy of breast, **2:**461
Operating room (OR), contamination control in, **1:**16-17, 16f-17f
Operating room (OR) attire, **3:**217, 217f
Operating room (OR) suite, **3:**216f
Operator's console
  for CT, **3:**311, 311f
  for MRI, **3:**345, 345f
Optic canal
  anatomy of, **2:**312f, 314f
  correct and incorrect rotation for, **2:**287, 287f
  in lateral aspect of cranium, **2:**258f
  sectional anatomy of, **3:**253-254
  with sphenoid bone, **2:**264f-265f, 265
Optic chiasm, **3:**259-260, 262, 262f, 264, 267f
Optic foramen
  anatomy of, **2:**312f, 314f
  in anterior aspect of cranium, **2:**257f
  and apex of orbit, **2:**312
  with facial bones, **2:**272f
  in lateral aspect of cranium, **2:**258f
  sectional anatomy of, **3:**262, 262f
  with sphenoid bone, **2:**265, 265f
Optic groove, **2:**258f, 264f, 265

Optic nerve
  anatomy of, **2:**314, 314f-315f
  sectional anatomy of, **3:**261-262, 261f, 266, 266f
Optic tracts, **3:**259-260
Optical coherence tomography (OCT), **3:**80t, 92, 93f
Optical density (OD), **1:**5, 5f
OR. *See* Operating room (OR).
Oral cavity. *See* Mouth.
Oral vestibule, **2:**59
Orbit(s)
  acanthioparietal projection of, **2:**328f
  anatomy of, **2:**275, 275f, 312, 312f
  blowout fracture of, **2:**46f, 282t, 313, 313f
  functions of, **2:**313
  lateral projection of, **2:**317, 317f
  localization of foreign bodies within, **2:**316, 316f
  PA axial projection of, **2:**318, 318f
  parietoacanthial projection of, Waters method for, **2:**324f
    modified, **2:**319, 319f
  preliminary examination of, **2:**316
  radiography of, **2:**312-313, 312f-313f
  sectional anatomy of, **3:**262-263, 262f-263f, 266
Orbital base, **2:**312
Orbital fat, **2:**314f
Orbital floor, blowout fracture of, **2:**46f
Orbital mass, CT for needle biopsy of, **3:**314f
Orbital plates, **2:**258f, 261, 261f
Orbital roof
  lateral projection of, **2:**295f
  sectional anatomy of, **3:**262, 262f
Orbital wall, medial, **2:**262f
Orbitomeatal line (OML), **2:**44
Orientation of anatomy on image receptor, **1:**28-29, 28f-29f
Ornaments, **1:**20, 21f
Oropharynx, **2:**59, 71f, 72
Orthopedic metal artifact reduction (OMAR), **3:**319, 320f
Os coxae. *See* Hip bone.
Osgood-Schlatter disease, **1:**240t
Ossification, **1:**77-78
  enchondral, **1:**77
  intermembranous, **1:**77
  primary, **1:**77, 77f
  secondary, **1:**72-74, 77f-78f
Ossification centers, primary and secondary, **1:**77, 77f-78f
Osteoarthritis
  of lower limb, **1:**240t
    in older adults, **3:**170, 170f, 174t
  of pelvis and proximal femora, **1:**335t
  of shoulder girdle, **1:**182t
  of upper limb, **1:**109t
  of vertebral column, **1:**380t
Osteoblasts, **3:**445, 445f, 476
Osteochondroma, **1:**240t
  in children, **3:**148, 148f
Osteoclast(s), **3:**445, 445f, 476
Osteoclastoma, **1:**240t
Osteogenesis imperfecta (OI), **3:**147, 147f
Osteogenic sarcoma. *See* Osteosarcoma.
Osteoid osteoma, **1:**240t
  in children, **3:**149, 149f
Osteology, **1:**75-79
  appendicular skeleton in, **1:**75, 75f, 75t
  axial skeleton in, **1:**75, 75f, 75t
  bone development in, **1:**77-78, 77f-78f
  bone vessels and nerves in, **1:**77, 77f
  classification of bones in, **1:**79, 79f
  defined, **1:**66
  fractures of, **1:**84, 84f
  general bone features in, **1:**76, 76f
  markings and features of, **1:**84

Osteoma
    osteoid, **1:**240t
        in children, **3:**149, 149f
    of skull, **2:**282t
Osteomalacia, **1:**240t, **3:**448, 476
Osteomyelitis, **1:**109t, 240t, 454t, **2:**282t
Osteopenia, **3:**447, 457, 476-477
Osteopetrosis
    of bony thorax, **1:**454t
    of lower limb, **1:**240t
    of pelvis and proximal femora, **1:**335t
    of shoulder girdle, **1:**182t
    of skull, **2:**282t
    of upper limb, **1:**109t
    of vertebral column, **1:**380t
Osteophytosis, **3:**464, 477
Osteoporosis, **3:**447-450
    biochemical markers for, **3:**448
    bone densitometry for, **3:**442
    bone health recommendations for, **3:**450, 450t
    of bony thorax, **1:**454t
    causes of, **3:**447
    cost of, **3:**447
    defined, **3:**447, 477
    epidemiology of, **3:**447
    fractures and falls due to, **3:**447, 449, 449f
    medications for, **3:**448, 448t
    in men, **3:**447
    in older adults, **3:**170, 174t
    pediatric, **3:**473-474, 473f
    of pelvis and upper femora, **1:**335t
    primary, **3:**448, 477
    risk factors for, **3:**447
    secondary, **3:**448, 477
    of shoulder girdle, **1:**182t
    of skull, **2:**282t
    type I, **3:**448, 477
    type II, **3:**448, 477
    of upper limb, **1:**109t
    of vertebral column, **1:**380t
Osteosarcoma, **1:**109t, 240t
    in children, **3:**150
Ottonello method for AP projection of cervical
        vertebrae, **1:**397-398, 397f-398f
Outer canthus, **2:**285f
Oval window, **2:**270f, 271
Ovarian cancer, phosphorus-32 for, **3:**420
Ovarian cyst
    CT of, **3:**315f
    ultrasonography of, **3:**375f, 388
Ovarian follicles, **2:**239, 239f
Ovarian ligament, **2:**240f
Ovaries
    anatomy of, **2:**239, 239f-240f
    sectional anatomy of, **3:**284
    ultrasonography of, **3:**373f, 375f, 388, 389f
Over-table IR units, **1:**44-45, 45f
Over-the-needle cannula, **2:**228f, 229
Ovulation, **2:**239
Ovum(a), **2:**239
Oximetry, **3:**97
    for cardiac catheterization, **3:**80, 80f, 82
Oxygen saturation, **3:**97
Oxygen-15 (^{15}O)
    decay scheme for, **3:**425, 425f
    in PET, **3:**426t
    production of, **3:**425, 425f
Oxygen-15 (^{15}O)-water, production of, **3:**427

P
^{32}P (phosphorus-32), therapeutic use of, **3:**420
PA. *See* Posteroanterior (PA).
Pacemaker implantation, cardiac catheterization
    for, **3:**94, 94f-95f
PACS. *See* Picture archiving and communication
    system (PACS).

Paget disease
    of bony thorax, **1:**454t
    of lower limbs, **1:**240t
    of nipple, **2:**395
    of pelvis and proximal femora, **1:**335t
    of skull, **2:**282t
    of vertebral column, **1:**380t
Pain management, interventional, **3:**16-18
Palatine bones
    anatomy of, **2:**259f, 273
    in orbit, **2:**275, 275f
    sectional anatomy of, **3:**254
Palatine tonsil, **2:**59, 59f
Palliation, **3:**480, 507
Palmar, **1:**85
Palmaz, Julio, **3:**20-21
Pancreas
    anatomy of, **2:**97f, 100f, 105f, 106, 107f
    endocrine, **2:**106
    exocrine, **2:**106
    functions of, **2:**106
    sectional anatomy of, **3:**282f, 283
        on axial (transverse) plane, **3:**288-290,
            288f-290f
        on coronal plane, **3:**299, 299f
    sectional image of, **2:**107f
    ultrasonography of, **3:**377f, 380, 380f
Pancreatic duct
    anatomy of, **2:**100f, 105f, 106
    sectional anatomy of, **3:**283
Pancreatic juice, **2:**106
Pancreatic pseudocyst, **2:**109t
Pancreatitis, **2:**109t
Pangynecography, **2:**246, 250, 250f
Panoramic tomography of mandible, **2:**353-354,
    353f-354f
Pantomography of mandible, **2:**353-354,
    353f-354f
Papilloma, **2:**395
    with atypia, **2:**395
Paramagnetic contrast agents for MRI, **3:**355,
    367
Parametric image, **3:**421, 438
Paranasal sinuses
    anatomy of, **2:**276-279, 276f-278f
    in children, **3:**135-136, 136f-137f
    ethmoidal
        anatomy of, **2:**276-278f, 279
        CT of, **2:**262f
        location of, **2:**261f-262f, 262
        PA axial projection of anterior (Caldwell
            method), **2:**360-361, 360f-361f
        submentovertical projection of, **2:**366-367,
            366f-367f
    frontal
        anatomy of, **2:**276f-278f, 279
        location of, **2:**259f, 261, 261f
        PA axial projection of (Caldwell method),
            2:360-361, 360f-361f
    lateral projection of, **2:**358, 358f-359f
    maxillary
        anatomy of, **2:**276, 276f-278f
        location of, **2:**272
        parietoacanthial projection of
            open-mouth Waters method for, **2:**364-365,
                364f-365f
            Waters method for, **2:**362-363,
                362f-363f
    sphenoidal
        anatomy of, **2:**276f-278f, 279
        location of, **2:**259f, 264-265, 264f-265f
        parietoacanthial projection of
            (open-mouth Waters method),
            2:364-365, 364f-365f
        submentovertical projection of, **2:**366-367,
            366f-367f

Paranasal sinuses *(Continued)*
    technical considerations for radiography of,
        2:355-357
        body position and central ray angulation as,
            2:356, 356f-357f
        exposure level as, **2:**355, 355f
        exudate as, **2:**356
Parathyroid glands, **2:**71, 72f
Parathyroid hormone for osteoporosis, **3:**448t
Parenchyma, ultrasonography of, **3:**376, 397
Parent nuclide, **3:**403-404, 438
Parietal, **1:**85
Parietal bones
    anatomy of, **2:**263, 263f
    AP axial projection of, **2:**305f
    location of, **2:**257f-259f
    PA axial projection of, **2:**298f
    sectional anatomy of, **3:**253, 256f-257f,
        257-258
Parietal eminence, **2:**263, 263f
Parietal lobe, sectional anatomy of, **3:**254-255,
    256f
    on axial (transverse) plane, **3:**257-258, 257f
    on sagittal plane, **3:**264, 265f-266f, 266
Parietal peritoneum, **2:**83, 83f
Parietal pleura, **1:**482
Parietoacanthial projection
    of facial bones, **2:**323, 323f-324f
        modified, **2:**304, 325f-326f
    of maxillary sinuses
        Waters method for, open-mouth, **2:**364-365,
            364f-365f
        Waters methods for, **2:**362-363, 362f-363f
    of orbit, **2:**319, 319f
    of sphenoidal sinuses, **2:**364-365, 364f-365f
Parotid duct, **2:**60, 60f
Parotid gland
    anatomy of, **2:**60, 60f, 97f
    lateral projection of, **2:**66-67, 67f
    sectional anatomy of, **3:**267-268, 267f
    sialography of, **2:**63f
    tangential projection of, **2:**64-65
        evaluation criteria for, **2:**65b
        position of part for, **2:**64-65, 64f
        position of patient for, **2:**64
            in prone body position, **2:**64f, 65
        structures shown on, **2:**64f-65f, 65
            in supine body position, **2:**64, 64f
Pars interarticularis, **1:**374, 374f
Part centering for digital imaging, **1:**38
Partial volume averaging for CT, **3:**340
Particle accelerators, **3:**404, 425, 438, 506
Patella
    anatomy of, **1:**233, 233f
    mediolateral projection of, **1:**312, 312f
    PA projection of, **1:**311, 311f
    tangential projection of
        Hughston method for, **1:**313, 313f
        Merchant method for, **1:**314-315, 314f-315f
        Settegast method for, **1:**316-317, 316f-317f
Patellar surface of femur, **1:**232f, 233
Patellofemoral joint
    anatomy of, **1:**236t, 238, 238f
    tangential projection of
        Hughston method for, **1:**313, 313f
        Merchant method for, **1:**314-315,
            314f-315f
        Settegast method for, **1:**316-317,
            316f-317f
Patency, **3:**97
Patent ductus arteriosus, cardiac catheterization for,
    3:93
Patent foramen ovale, **3:**97
Pathogen contamination control, **1:**16
Pathologic fractures in children, **3:**148-150
Pathologist, **3:**480, 507

Patient(s)
  attire, ornaments, and surgical dressings on, **1:**20, 20f-21f
  ill or injured, **1:**22-23, 22f
  interacting with, **1:**21-23
  preexposure instructions to, **1:**41
Patient care for trauma patient, **2:**26, 27t
Patient care for older adults, **3:**175
Patient moving device, **1:**46, 46f
Patient positioning for trauma radiography, **2:**24, 24f, 28
Patient-centered care in code of ethics, **1:**3
PBL (positive beam limitation), **1:**32
PC (phase contrast) imaging, **3:**363
pDXA (peripheral dual energy x-ray absorptiometry), **3:**475, 475f, 477
Peak bone mass, **3:**446, 477
Pearson method for bilateral AP projection of acromioclavicular articulation, **1:**209, 209f-210f
Pectoralis major muscle
  anatomy of, **2:**380, 380f-381f
  sectional anatomy of, **3:**271, 273-275, 273f-274f, 276f
Pectoralis minor muscle
  anatomy of, **2:**380f
  sectional anatomy of, **3:**271, 273-275, 273f-274f, 276f
Pediatric patients. *See* Children.
Pedicles of vertebral arch, **1:**368, 368f
Pelvic cavity, **1:**68-69, 69f, 332, 332f, **2:**83
Pelvic curve, **1:**366f, 367
Pelvic girdle, **1:**327
Pelvic kidney, **2:**188t
Pelvic pneumography, **2:**246, 250, 250f
Pelvic sacral foramina, **1:**376, 376f
Pelvicaliceal system, **2:**183
  retrograde urography of, **2:**212-213, 212f-213f
Pelvimetry, **2:**252
Pelvis, **1:**325-360
  anatomy of, **1:**332, 332f, 334b
  anterior bones of
    AP axial outlet projection of (Taylor method), **1:**358, 358f
    superoinferior axial inlet projection of (Bridgeman method), **1:**359, 359f
  AP projection of, **1:**337-339, 337f-338f
    for congenital dislocation of hip, **1:**339, 339f
    mobile, **3:**200-201, 200f-201f
    for trauma, **2:**41, 41f
  articulations of, **1:**331, 331f, 331t, 334b
  bony landmarks of, **1:**333-334, 333f
  brim of, **1:**332, 332f
  in children, **3:**125-126
    general principles for, **3:**125-126, 125f
    image evaluation for, **3:**123t, 126
    initial images of, **3:**125
    positioning and immobilization for, **3:**126, 126f
    preparation and communication for, **3:**126
  components of, **1:**327
  CT of, **2:**55, **3:**336f-338f
  false or greater, **1:**332, 332f, **3:**386, 397
  in geriatric patients, **3:**179, 179f
  inferior aperture or outlet of, **1:**332, 332f
  lateral projection of, **1:**340-341, 340f-341f
  localization planes of, **1:**346f
  male vs. female, **1:**332, 332f, 332t
  PA projection of, **1:**338f
  mobile radiography of, **3:**200-201
    AP projection for, **3:**200-201, 200f-201f
  MRI of, **3:**360, 361f
  radiation protection for, **1:**336, 336f
  sample exposure technique chart essential projections for, **1:**335t

Pelvis *(Continued)*
  summary of pathology of, **1:**335t
  summary of projections for, **1:**326
  superior aperture or inlet of, **1:**332, 332f
  trauma radiography of, **2:**41, 41f
  true or lesser, **1:**332, 332f, **2:**83, **3:**386
Pencil-beam techniques for DXA, **3:**444, 454-457, 454f, 477
Penetrating trauma, **2:**19
Penis, **2:**242, 243f
Percent coefficient of variation (%CV) in DXA, **3:**455, 455f-456f, 477
Percutaneous, **3:**97
Percutaneous antegrade pyelography, **2:**211, 211f
Percutaneous antegrade urography, **2:**191
Percutaneous renal puncture, **2:**210-211, 210f-211f
Percutaneous transhepatic cholangiography (PTC), **2:**174-175, 174f
Percutaneous transluminal angioplasty (PTA), **3:**62-65
  balloon in, **3:**62-63, 63f
  of common iliac artery, **3:**64f
  defined, **3:**97
  Dotter method for, **3:**62
  historical development of, **3:**20
  for placement of intravascular stents, **3:**65, 65f
  of renal artery, **3:**64f
Percutaneous transluminal coronary angioplasty (PTCA), **3:**66, 88, 88f-89f
  catheter system for, **3:**88, 88f
  defined, **3:**97
  with stent placement, **3:**88, 89f
Percutaneous transluminal coronary rotational atherectomy (PTCRA), **3:**90, 90f-91f, 97
Percutaneous vertebroplasty, **3:**16
Percutaneously, **3:**97
Perfusion lung scan, **3:**405, 405f
Perfusion study
  for CT angiography of brain, **3:**324-326, 326f
  in MRI, **3:**364-365, 367
Pericardial cavity, **1:**69f, 479, **3:**24
Pericardial sac, **3:**24
Pericardium
  anatomy of, **3:**24, 97
  sectional anatomy of, **3:**270
Periosteal arteries, **1:**77, 77f
Periosteum, **1:**76, 76f
Peripheral, **1:**85
Peripheral angiography, **3:**46
  lower limb arteriograms in, **3:**47, 48f
  lower limb venograms in, **3:**47, 48f
  upper limb arteriograms in, **3:**46, 46f
  upper limb venograms in, **3:**46, 46f
Peripheral dual energy x-ray absorptiometry (pDXA), **3:**475, 475f, 477
Peripheral lymph sinus, **3:**26
Peripheral quantitative computed tomography (pQCT), **3:**475, 477
Peripheral skeletal bone density measurements, **3:**474-475, 474f-475f
Peripherally inserted central catheters (PICCs), **3:**157, 157f
Perirenal fat, **2:**283
Peristalsis, **1:**18, **2:**110
Peritoneal cavity, **2:**83, 83f
Peritoneum
  anatomy of, **2:**83, 83f
  sectional anatomy of, **3:**283
Permanent magnets for MRI, **3:**346, 367
Peroneal artery, arteriography of, **3:**48f
Perpendicular plate
  anatomy of, **2:**262, 262f
  CT of, **2:**262f
  sectional anatomy of, **3:**253, 253f, 262
Personal hygiene in surgical radiography, **3:**217
PET. *See* Positron emission tomography (PET).

Petrosa, submentovertical projection of, **2:**311f, 367f
Petrous apex, **2:**268, 269f
Petrous portion of temporal bone, **2:**258f-259f
Petrous pyramids, **2:**268, 286
Petrous ridge
  acanthioparietal projection of, **2:**328f
  anatomy of, **2:**268, 269f
  AP axial projection of
    Haas method for, **2:**309f
    Towne method for, **2:**305f-306f
  PA axial projection of, **2:**298f, 330f
  parietoacanthial projection of, **2:**324f, 363f
  sectional anatomy of, **3:**261-263
  submentovertical projection of, **2:**346f
Phalanges
  of foot, **1:**228, 228f
  of hand, **1:**101, 101f
Phantom scans for DXA, **3:**461, 462f
Pharmaceuticals, **3:**438
  in radiopharmaceuticals, **3:**404-405, 405f
Pharyngeal tonsil, **2:**71f, 72
Pharyngography, positive-contrast, **2:**74-75
  deglutition in, **2:**74-75, 74f
  fluoroscopic, **2:**75
  Gunson method for, **2:**75, 75f
Pharynx
  anatomy of, **2:**71f, 72, 97f
  AP projection of, **2:**76-77, 76f-77f
  lateral projection of, **2:**78-79, 78f-79f
  methods of examination of, **2:**74-75
  positive-contrast pharyngography of, **2:**74-75
    deglutition in, **2:**74-75, 74f
    fluoroscopic, **2:**75
    Gunson method for, **2:**75, 75f
  sectional anatomy of, **3:**265f, 267f
Phase contrast (PC) imaging, **3:**363
Phasic flow, **3:**393, 397
Phenergan (promethazine hydrochloride), **2:**226t
Philips Medical Systems iDose, **3:**319, 320f
Phleboliths, **2:**188t
Phosphorus-32 (^{32}P), therapeutic use of, **3:**420
Photodiodes, **3:**409
Photographic subtraction technique for hip arthrography, **2:**14, 15f
Photomultiplier tube (PMT), **3:**400, 409, 438
Photopenia, **3:**405, 438
Photostimulable storage phosphor image plate (PSP IP), **1:**3, 4f
Physician assistant, **3:**215
Physiologic equipment for cardiac catheterization, **3:**79-80, 79f, 82
Physiology, defined, **1:**66
Pia mater
  anatomy of, **3:**3
  sectional anatomy of, **3:**254
Pica, **3:**139, 140f
PICCs (peripherally inserted central catheters), **3:**157, 157f
Picture archiving and communication system (PACS)
  for digital subtraction angiography, **3:**31
  for DXA, **3:**460, 477
  for nuclear medicine, **3:**410
Picture element (pixel), **3:**308, 308f, 340
  in nuclear medicine, **3:**438
Piezoelectric effect, **3:**372, 397
Pigg-O-Stat
  for abdominal imaging, **3:**112, 112f
  for chest imaging, **3:**118, 118f
Pilot image in radiation oncology, **3:**490-491
Pineal gland, **3:**258-259, 265f
PIP (proximal interphalangeal) joints
  of lower limb, **1:**236
  of upper limb, **1:**105, 105f-106f
Piriform recess, **2:**71f, 72

Pisiform, **1:**101f-102f, 102
Pituitary adenoma, **2:**282t
Pituitary gland
    anatomy of, **2:**264-265, **3:**2
    sectional anatomy of, **3:**261-262, 264, 265f, 267, 267f
Pituitary stalk, **3:**259-260, 259f
Pivot joint, **1:**82, 83f
Pixel (picture element), **3:**308, 308f, 340
    in nuclear medicine, **3:**438
Placement of anatomy on image receptor, **1:**28-29, 28f-29f
Placenta
    anatomy of, **2:**241, 241f
    previa, **2:**241, 241f
    ultrasonography of, **3:**389f
Placentography, **2:**252
Plane(s), body. *See* Body planes.
Plane joint, **1:**82, 83f
Planimetry, **3:**97
Plantar, **1:**85
Plantar flexion, **1:**97, 97f
Plantar surface of foot, **1:**228-230
Plasma radioactivity measurement in PET, **3:**430
Plastic fractures, **3:**130
"Plates" in digital radiography, **1:**36, 36f
Pledget, **3:**97
Pleura(e)
    anatomy of, **1:**480f, 482
    AP or PA projection of, **1:**483-484, 516f-517f
    lateral projection of, **1:**518-519, 518f-519f
Pleural cavity(ies), **1:**69f, 479, 482
Pleural effusion, **1:**486t
    mobile radiograph of, **3:**195f
Pleural space, **1:**480f
Plural endings for medical terms, **1:**98, 98t
Plural word forms, frequently misused, **1:**98, 98t
PMT (photomultiplier tube), **3:**400, 409, 438
Pneumoarthrography, **2:**8-9
Pneumococcal pneumonia, **3:**151
Pneumoconiosis, **1:**486t, 499f
Pneumonia, **1:**486t
    in children, **3:**150-151, 151f
    in older adults, **3:**172, 172f
Pneumonitis, **1:**486t
Pneumoperitoneum, **2:**84t
    in children, **3:**115, 115f
    mobile radiograph of, **3:**199f
Pneumothorax, **1:**486t, 490, 498f, 503f
PNL (posterior nipple line), **2:**409, 410f
Polonium, **3:**400
Polycystic kidney, **2:**188t
Polycythemia, sodium phosphate for, **3:**420
Polyp, **2:**109t
    cranial, **2:**282t
    endometrial, **2:**245t
Pons
    anatomy of, **2:**259f, **3:**2, 2f-3f
    defined, **3:**18
    sectional anatomy of, **3:**255
        on axial (transverse) plane, **3:**259-262, 259f-260f, 262f
        on sagittal plane, **3:**265f
Pontine cistern, **3:**254, 261-262
Popliteal artery
    anatomy of, **3:**22f
    arteriography of, **3:**48f
    ultrasonography of, **3:**394f
Popliteal surface of femur, **1:**232f
Popliteal vein
    anatomy of, **3:**22f
    ultrasonography of, **3:**394f
    venography of, **3:**48f
Port(s) in children, **3:**158, 158f

Porta hepatis
    anatomy of, **2:**104
    sectional anatomy of, **3:**283, 287-288, 298-299
    ultrasonography of, **3:**376f, 378, 397
Portal hypertension, **3:**72
Portal system, **2:**104, 105f, **3:**23, 23f, 72, 97
Portal vein, **3:**22f
    anatomy of, **2:**104, 105f
    sectional anatomy of, **3:**282f, 283-285
        on axial (transverse) plane, **3:**287-289, 287f-289f
        on coronal plane, **3:**298-299, 298f
Portal venography, **3:**61, 61f
Portal venous system, **3:**284-285, 298-299
Portosystemic shunt, transjugular intrahepatic, **3:**72, 72f-73f
Portsman, Werner, **3:**20
Position(s), **1:**86b, 89-95
    decubitus, **1:**94, 94f-95f
    Fowler, **1:**90, 91f
    general body, **1:**89-90
    lateral, **1:**91, 91f
    lithotomy, **1:**90, 91f
    lordotic, **1:**94, 95f
    note to educators, students, and clinicians on, **1:**95
    oblique, **1:**92-93, 92f-93f
    vs. projection, **1:**95
    prone, **1:**90, 90f
    radiographic, **1:**89
    recumbent, **1:**90, 90f
    seated, **1:**90
    Sims, **1:**90, 91f
    supine, **1:**90, 90f
    Trendelenburg, **1:**90, 90f
    upright, **1:**87f, 90
    uses of term, **1:**89
Position sensitive photomultiplier tubes (PSPMTs), **3:**409
Positioning aids for trauma radiography, **2:**20
Positive beam limitation (PBL), **1:**32
Positive-contrast pharyngography, **2:**74-75
    deglutition in, **2:**74-75, 74f
    fluoroscopic, **2:**75
    Gunson method for, **2:**75, 75f
Positron(s), **3:**421-424
    characteristics of, **3:**422, 423t
    decay of, **3:**421-422, 423f, 425, 425f
    defined, **3:**438
    range of, **3:**424, 424t
Positron emission tomography (PET)
    clinical, **3:**432-435, 432f-433f
        for cardiology imaging, **3:**434-435
        for neurologic imaging, **3:**434
        for oncology imaging, **3:**433, 433f
    data acquisition in, **3:**428-430
        coincidence counts in, **3:**429, 429f
        cross-plane information in, **3:**429, 429f
        deadtime losses in, **3:**430, 432, 437
        decay-corrected radioactivity curves in, **3:**430, 430f
        detector arrangement for, **3:**428-429, 428f
        direct-plane information in, **3:**429, 429f
        electronic collimation for, **3:**430
        field of view for, **3:**428-429, 428f
        for glucose metabolism, **3:**429-430
        for plasma radioactivity measurement, **3:**430
        quantitative parametric images in, **3:**430, 438
        for region of interest (ROI) analysis, **3:**430, 438-439
        resolution in, **3:**428-429
        scanner for, **3:**428-429, 428f
        scintillators, **3:**428-429, 428t
        sensitivity of, **3:**429-430
        three-dimensional, **3:**429-430

Positron emission tomography (PET) *(Continued)*
    defined, **3:**421, 438
    detectors for, **3:**400, 437
    future of, **3:**436, 436f
    historical development of, **3:**400
    image reconstruction and image processing for, **3:**400, 431-432, 431f, 438
    of local cerebral blood flow, **3:**427, 427f
    of local metabolic rate of glucose, **3:**427, 427f
    mobile units for, **3:**436, 436f
    vs. other modalities, **3:**401t, 402, 421, 421f
    patient preparation for, **3:**432
    positrons in, **3:**421-424, 422f-424f, 423t-424t
    principles and facilities for, **3:**421-432, 421f
    in radiation oncology, **3:**494
    radionuclide production in, **3:**425, 425f-426f, 426t
    radiopharmaceuticals for
        choice of, **3:**421
        new, **3:**436
        production of, **3:**427-428, 427f
    septa in, **3:**400, 439
    transmission scan in, **3:**402, 439
Positron emission tomography/computed tomography (PET/CT) scanners, **3:**327-329, 329f, 401, 436
Positron emission tomography/magnetic resonance imaging (PET/MRI) system, **3:**401, 436
Positron-emitting radionuclides, **3:**421-422, 422f
Posterior, **1:**85
Posterior acoustic enhancement, **3:**397
Posterior acoustic shadowing, **3:**375f, 397
Posterior arches of soft palate, **2:**59, 59f
Posterior cerebral arteries
    CT angiography of, **3:**325f
    sectional anatomy of, **3:**255, 260-261
Posterior clinoid processes
    anatomy of, **2:**258f, 264-265, 264f-265f
    AP axial projection of
        Haas method for, **2:**309f
        Towne method for, **2:**305f
    sectional anatomy of, **3:**253-254
Posterior communicating artery
    anatomy of, **3:**51
    arteriography of, **3:**51f, 53f, 56f
    CT angiography of, **3:**325f
    sectional anatomy of, **3:**255
Posterior cranial fossa, **2:**260
Posterior cruciate ligament, **1:**234f, 236f
Posterior fat pad of elbow, **1:**107, 107f
Posterior fontanel, **2:**259-260, 260f
Posterior fossa, **3:**261-262
Posterior horn, **3:**4, 4f
Posterior inferior iliac spine, **1:**327f, 328
Posterior interosseous artery, arteriography of, **3:**46f
Posterior nipple line (PNL), **2:**409, 410f
Posterior superior iliac spine, **1:**327f, 328
Posterior tibial artery
    anatomy of, **3:**22f
    arteriography of, **3:**48f
Posteroanterior (PA) axial projection, **1:**88
Posteroanterior (PA) oblique projection, **1:**88
Posteroanterior (PA) projection, **1:**10-11, 10f, 86, 87f
Postoperative cholangiography, **2:**176-177, 176f-177f
Postprocessing, **3:**97
    in CT, **3:**326, 340
    in digital subtraction angiography, **3:**31
Pott fracture, **1:**240t
Pouch of Douglas, **3:**386, 386f, 398
Power injector for IV administration of contrast media for CT, **3:**317, 317f

Power lifts, **1:**46, 46f
Poznauskis, Linda, **3:**119-120
pQCT (peripheral quantitative computed tomography), **3:**475, 477
Precession, **3:**343, 343f, 367
Preexposure instructions, **1:**41
Pregnancy
  breasts during, **2:**382
  radiography of female reproductive system during, **2:**252
    fetography for, **2:**252, 252f
    pelvimetry for, **2:**252
    placentography for, **2:**252
    radiation protection for, **2:**252
Premature infants, development of, **3:**102
Presbycusis, **3:**169
Presbyopia, **3:**169
Preschoolers, development of, **3:**103, 103f
Pressure injector for cardiac catheterization, **3:**79, 79f
Pressure sores in older adults, **3:**175
Pressure transducers for cardiac catheterization, **3:**79-80, 82
Pressure wire for cardiac catheterization, **3:**80t
Primary curves, **1:**367
Primary data in CT, **3:**302, 340
Primary ossification, **1:**77, 77f
Procedure book, **1:**17
Processes, **1:**84
Proctography, evacuation, **2:**172, 172f
Progeria, **3:**152, 152f
Projection(s), **1:**86-89, 86b
  anteroposterior (AP), **1:**10-11, 10f, 86, 87f
    entry and exit points for, **1:**86, 86f
  anteroposterior (AP) oblique, **1:**88
  axial, **1:**86-87, 87f
  axiolateral, **1:**88
  of bone, **1:**84
  complex, **1:**88
  defined, **1:**86
  entrance and exit points of, **1:**86, 86f
  in-profile, **1:**89
  lateral, **1:**11, 12f, 88, 88f
    of obese patients, **1:**49
  lateromedial and mediolateral, **1:**88, 88f
  note to educators, students, and clinicians on, **1:**95
  oblique, **1:**12, 12f, 88, 89f
  other, **1:**12
  vs. position, **1:**95
  posteroanterior (PA), **1:**10-11, 10f, 86, 87f
  posteroanterior (PA) axial, **1:**88
  posteroanterior (PA) oblique, **1:**88
  tangential, **1:**86-87, 87f
  transthoracic, **1:**88
  true, **1:**89
  vs. view, **1:**95
Projectional technique, DXA as, **3:**453, 477
Promethazine hydrochloride (Phenergan), **2:**226t
Pronate/pronation, **1:**97, 97f
Prone position, **1:**90, 90f
Prophylactic surgery for breast cancer, **3:**482, 507
Prophylaxis, **1:**15
Prostate
  anatomy of, **2:**184f, 186f, 187, 242f-243f, 243
  MRI of, **3:**360
  radiologic examination of, **2:**214, 254
  sectional anatomy of, **3:**284, 296, 296f
Prostate cancer, **2:**245t
  in older adults, **3:**173
  radiation oncology for, **3:**497, 502-503
Prostatic hyperplasia, benign, **2:**188t
  in older adults, **3:**173, 174t
Prostatic urethra, **2:**186f, 187

Prostatography, **2:**214, 254
Protocol book, **1:**17
Protocol(s) for CT, **3:**303f, 319-320, 336-340
Proton(s), **3:**403, 403f, 438
  magnetic properties of, **3:**343, 343f
Proton density in MRI, **3:**344, 367
Proton-rich nucleus, **3:**422, 423f
Protuberance, **1:**84
Provocative diskography, **3:**16, 17f
Proximal, **1:**85, 85f
Proximal convoluted tubule, **2:**185, 185f
Proximal femur, **1:**325-360
  anatomy of, **1:**328f-330f, 329-330, 334b
  AP projection of, **1:**337-339, 337f-338f
  lateral projection of, **1:**340-341, 340f-341f
  sample exposure technique chart essential projections for, **1:**335t
  summary of pathology of, **1:**335t
  summary of projections for, **1:**326
Proximal humerus
  anatomic neck of, **1:**177
  anatomy of, **1:**177-178, 177f
  greater tubercle of, **1:**177, 177f
  head of, **1:**177, 177f
  intertubercular (bicipital) groove of
    anatomy of, **1:**177, 177f
    Fisk modification for tangential projection of, **1:**207-208, 207f-208f
  lesser tubercle of, **1:**177, 177f
  Stryker notch method for AP axial projection of, **1:**204, 204f
  surgical neck of, **1:**177, 177f
Proximal interphalangeal (PIP) joints
  of lower limb, **1:**236
  of upper limb, **1:**105, 105f-106f
Proximal phalanges, **1:**228, 228f
Proximal tibiofibular joint, **1:**236t, 238
Pseudocyst, pancreatic, **2:**109t
Psoas muscle, sectional anatomy of, **3:**282f
  on axial (transverse) plane, **3:**291, 291f-293f
  on coronal plane, **3:**298f-299f
PSP IP (photostimulable storage phosphor image plate), **1:**3, 4f
PSPMTs (position sensitive photomultiplier tubes), **3:**409
PTA. See Percutaneous transluminal angioplasty (PTA).
PTC (percutaneous transhepatic cholangiography), **2:**174-175, 174f
PTCA. See Percutaneous transluminal coronary angioplasty (PTCA).
PTCRA (percutaneous transluminal coronary rotational atherectomy), **3:**90, 90f-91f, 97
Pterion, **2:**258f, 259
Pterygoid hamulus, **2:**259f, 265f, 266
Pterygoid laminae, **2:**265f, 266
Pterygoid muscles, **3:**255-256, 264
Pterygoid processes
  anatomy of, **2:**265f, 266
  sectional anatomy of, **3:**253-254
Pubic symphysis
  anatomy of, **1:**331, 331f, 331t
  with obese patients, **1:**49, 49f
  sectional anatomy of, **3:**282, 290, 296, 299
  as surface landmark, **1:**71f, 71t, 333-334, 333f
Pubis
  anatomy of, **1:**327-328, 327f, 330f
  sectional anatomy of, **3:**282, 294, 295f, 297f
Pulmonary apices
  AP axial projection of
    in lordotic position (Lindblom method), **1:**512-513, 512f-513f
    in upright or supine position, **1:**515, 515f
  PA axial projection of, **1:**514, 514f

Pulmonary arteries
  anatomy of, **3:**22f, 23, 25f
  sectional anatomy of, **3:**270-271
    on axial (transverse) plane, **3:**275-277, 276f
    on coronal plane, **3:**280-281, 281f
    on sagittal plane, **3:**278-280, 280f
Pulmonary arteriography, **3:**42, 42f
Pulmonary circulation, **3:**23, 23f, 97
Pulmonary edema, **1:**486t
Pulmonary embolus, **3:**70
Pulmonary trunk, **3:**275-279, 276f
Pulmonary valve
  anatomy of, **3:**25, 25f
  sectional anatomy of, **3:**270, 280f
Pulmonary veins
  anatomy of, **3:**22f, 23, 25f
  sectional anatomy of, **3:**270, 278-281, 278f, 281f
Pulse, **3:**26, 97
Pulse height analyzer, **3:**409, 438
Pulse oximetry, **3:**97
  for cardiac catheterization, **3:**82
Pulse sequences in MRI, **3:**344, 352, 352f-353f, 367
Pulse wave transducers for ultrasonography, **3:**372, 397
Pupil, **2:**314f
Purcell, Edward, **3:**342
Pyelography, **2:**191
  percutaneous antegrade, **2:**211, 211f
Pyelonephritis, **2:**188t
Pyloric antrum
  anatomy of, **2:**98, 98f
  sectional anatomy of, **3:**283, 288
Pyloric canal
  anatomy of, **2:**98, 98f
  sectional anatomy of, **3:**282f, 289, 289f
Pyloric orifice, **2:**98f, 99
Pyloric portion of stomach, **2:**98, 100f
Pyloric sphincter
  anatomy of, **2:**98f, 99
  sectional anatomy of, **3:**283
Pyloric stenosis, **2:**109t
Pylorus, **3:**282f
Pyrogen-free radiopharmaceuticals, **3:**404-405, 438

Q
Quadrants of abdomen, **1:**70, 70f
Quadratus lumborum muscles, **3:**291, 291f-292f
Quadrigeminal cistern, **3:**254
Quantitative analysis in nuclear medicine, **3:**410, 411f, 438
Quantitative computed tomography (QCT)
  for bone densitometry, **3:**444, 469, 469f, 477
  peripheral, **3:**475, 477
Quantitative ultrasound (QUS), **3:**475, 475f, 477
Quantum noise in CT, **3:**318-319, 340
Quench during MRI, **3:**349

R
RA (radiographic absorptiometry), **3:**443, 474, 474f, 477
RA (radiologist assistant), **1:**14
Ra (radium), **3:**400, 507
Radial artery, **3:**22f, 49f
Radial fossa, **1:**104, 104f
Radial head
  Coyle method for axiolateral projection of, **1:**162-164
    evaluation criteria for, **1:**164
    position of part for, **1:**162, 162f-163f
    position of patient for, **1:**162
    structures shown on, **1:**164, 164f

Radial head *(Continued)*
  lateromedial projection of, **1:**160-161
    evaluation criteria for, **1:**161b
    four-position series for, **1:**160
    position of part for, **1:**160, 160f
    position of patient for, **1:**160
    structures shown on, **1:**161, 161f
Radial notch, **1:**103, 103f
Radial scar, **2:**395
Radial styloid process, **1:**103, 103f
Radial tuberosity, **1:**103, 103f
Radiation, **3:**403, 438
  tolerance doses to, **3:**494, 494t
Radiation dose
  for nuclear medicine, **3:**405, 437
  for obese patients, **1:**52
Radiation dose profile for CT, **3:**330, 330f
Radiation exposure considerations in surgical
    radiography, **3:**223, 223f
Radiation fields, **3:**486-487, 506
Radiation oncologist, **3:**480, 507
Radiation oncology, **3:**479-508
  and cancer, **3:**481-483
    most common types of, **3:**482, 482t
    risk factors for, **3:**482-483, 482t
    tissue origins of, **3:**483, 483t
  clinical applications of, **3:**502-504
    for breast cancer, **3:**504, 504f
    for cervical cancer, **3:**503, 503f
    for head and neck cancers, **3:**503
    for Hodgkin lymphoma, **3:**503
    for laryngeal cancer, **3:**504
    for lung cancer, **3:**502, 502f
    for medulloblastoma, **3:**504, 505f
    for prostate cancer, **3:**497, 502-503
    for skin cancer, **3:**504
  CT for treatment planning in, **3:**327, 328f
  for cure, **3:**480, 506
  defined, **3:**480, 507
  definition of terms for, **3:**506b-507b
  dose depositions in, **3:**485, 485f
  equipment for, **3:**485-489
    cobalt-60 units as, **3:**486-487, 487f, 506
    linear accelerators (linacs) as, **3:**485, 487-489,
      488f, 506
    multileaf collimation system as, **3:**489,
      489f
  external-beam therapy and brachytherapy in,
    3:485
  fractionation in, **3:**480, 506
  future trends in, **3:**505
  historical development of, **3:**481, 481t
  for palliation, **3:**480, 507
  principles of, **3:**480
  skin-sparing effect of, **3:**486, 486f, 507
  steps in, **3:**489-501
    contrast administration as, **3:**490, 491f-492f
    creation of treatment fields as, **3:**491,
      492f-493f
    CyberKnife as, **3:**499-501, 501f
    dosimetry as, **3:**480, 494-496, 494f-495f,
      494t, 506
    immobilization devices as, **3:**490,
      490f-491f
    reference isocenter as, **3:**490-491
    simulation as, **3:**489-491, 490f
    TomoTherapy as, **3:**499, 500f
    treatment as, **3:**496-501, 497f-499f
  theory of, **3:**484, 484t
Radiation protection
  for angiographic studies, **3:**39
  for children, **3:**108-111, 108f-109f, 109t
    for gastrointestinal and genitourinary studies,
      3:116
    for limb radiography, **3:**129, 129f
  with DXA, **3:**458, 458t

Radiation protection *(Continued)*
  for female reproductive system radiography,
    2:246
    during pregnancy, **2:**252
  for gastrointestinal radiography, **2:**114f, 115
  for long bone measurement, **2:**2
  for lower limb, **1:**242
  for pelvis, **1:**336, 336f
  for shoulder girdle, **1:**183
  for skull, **2:**288
  for sternum, **1:**456-462
  for thoracic viscera, **1:**492-493
  for trauma radiography, **2:**25
  for urinary system, **2:**201
Radiation safety
  for children, **3:**101
  with mobile radiography, **3:**188, 188f-189f
  with MRI, **3:**348-349, 349f
  in nuclear medicine, **3:**407, 407f
Radiation therapist, **3:**480, 507
Radiation therapy. *See also* Radiation oncology.
  defined, **3:**480, 507
  image-guided, **3:**498, 498f, 506
  intensity modulated, **3:**489, 496, 506
  stereotactic, **3:**499, 507
Radioactive, **3:**400, 438
Radioactive analogs, **3:**401-402, 437
Radioactive decay, **3:**403, 404f
Radioactive source in radiation oncology, **3:**485,
  507
Radioactivity, **3:**400, 403, 438
Radioactivity concentration in PET, **3:**421
Radiocarpal articulations, **1:**106, 106f
Radiocurable, **3:**507
Radiofrequency (RF) ablation, cardiac
    catheterization for, **3:**94
Radiofrequency (RF) antennas in MRI, **3:**346
Radiofrequency (RF) pulse in MRI, **3:**343, 367
Radiogrammetry, **3:**443, 477
Radiograph(s), **1:**5-12
  adjacent structures on, **1:**5
  anatomic position in, **1:**8-12, 8f-9f
  AP, **1:**10-11, 10f
  contrast on, **1:**5, 6f
  defined, **1:**5
  display of, **1:**8
  of foot and toe, **1:**11
  of hand, fingers, and wrist, **1:**11, 11f
  identification of, **1:**25, 25f
  lateral, **1:**11, 12f
  magnification of, **1:**7, 7f
  oblique, **1:**12, 12f
  optical density (OD) on, **1:**5, 5f
  other, **1:**12
  PA, **1:**10-11, 10f
  shape distortion on, **1:**7, 7f
  spatial resolution of, **1:**5, 6f
  superimposition on, **1:**5
Radiographer, **1:**2
Radiographic absorptiometry (RA), **3:**443, 474,
  474f, 477
Radiographic positioning terminology, **1:**85-95
  for method, **1:**95
  for positions, **1:**86b, 89-95
    decubitus, **1:**94, 94f-95f
    Fowler, **1:**90, 91f
    general body, **1:**90
    lateral, **1:**91, 91f
    lithotomy, **1:**90, 91f
    lordotic, **1:**94, 95f
    note to educators, students, and clinicians on,
      1:95
    oblique, **1:**92-93, 92f-93f
    prone, **1:**90, 90f
    recumbent, **1:**90, 90f
    seated, **1:**90

Radiographic positioning terminology *(Continued)*
    Sims, **1:**90, 91f
    supine, **1:**90, 90f
    Trendelenburg, **1:**90, 90f
    upright, **1:**87f, 90
  for projections, **1:**86-89, 86b, 86f
    AP, **1:**86, 87f
    axial, **1:**87, 87f
    complex, **1:**88
    lateral, **1:**88, 88f
    note to educators, students, and clinicians on,
      1:95
    oblique, **1:**88, 89f
    PA, **1:**86, 87f
    in profile, **1:**89
    tangential, **1:**87, 87f
    true, **1:**89
  for view, **1:**95
Radiographic room, care of, **1:**14, 14f
Radiographic technique charts for mobile
    radiography, **3:**187, 187f
Radiography, defined, **1:**85
Radioimmunotherapy, **3:**435
Radioindicator, **3:**400
Radioiodine for Graves disease, **3:**420
Radioisotope, **3:**438
Radiologic technology, defined, **1:**2
Radiologic vertebral assessment (RVA), **3:**469-470,
  470f-471f, 477
Radiologist assistant (RA), **1:**14
Radiology practitioner assistant (RPA), **1:**14
Radionuclide(s)
  for conventional nuclear medicine, **3:**401-402,
    404-405, 405f, 406t
  decay of, **3:**403, 404f
  defined, **3:**438
  for PET, **3:**425, 425f-426f, 426t
  positron-emitting, **3:**421-422, 422f
  in radiopharmaceuticals, **3:**404-405, 405f
Radionuclide angiography (RNA), **3:**416
Radionuclide cisternography, **3:**417
Radiopaque markers for trauma radiography, **2:**24,
  24f
Radiopaque objects, **1:**20, 21f
Radiopharmaceuticals, **3:**404-405
  commonly used radionuclides in, **3:**404-405,
    406t
  components of, **3:**404-405, 405f
  defined, **3:**400, 438
  dose of, **3:**405
  formation of, **3:**404, 404f
  for perfusion lung scan, **3:**405, 405f
  for PET
    choice of, **3:**421
    new, **3:**436
    production of, **3:**427-428, 427f
  qualities of, **3:**404-405
Radiosensitivity, **3:**484, 507
Radiotracers, **3:**400, 402, 438
Radioulnar joints, **1:**107, 107f
Radium (Ra), **3:**400, 507
Radius(ii)
  of arm, **1:**101f, 102-103, 103f
  defined, **3:**403
Radon, **3:**400
Rafert et al. modification of Lawrence method for
    inferosuperior axial projection of shoulder
    joint, **1:**194, 194f
Rafert-Long method for scaphoid series, **1:**142,
  142f-143f
RANKL inhibitor for osteoporosis, **3:**448t
RAO (right anterior oblique) position, **1:**92,
  92f
Rapid acquisition recalled echo, **3:**367
Rapid film changers, **3:**21
Rapid serial radiographic imaging, **3:**32

Index

Rare-earth filtration systems for DXA, **3:**451, 451f-452f
  crossover in, **3:**452
  scintillating detector pileup in, **3:**452
Raw data in MRI, **3:**345, 367-368
Ray, **3:**438
^{82}Rb (rubidium-82), **3:**406t
RBE (relative biologic effectiveness), **3:**484, 484t, 507
RDCSs (registered diagnostic cardiac sonographers), **3:**370
RDMSs (registered diagnostic medical sonographers), **3:**370
  characteristics of, **3:**370, 371f
Real time, **3:**327, 340
Real-time ultrasonography, **3:**387, 397
Receiving coil in MRI, **3:**343
Recombinant tissue plasminogen activators, **3:**20-21
Reconstruction
  for CT, **3:**309, 340
    multiplanar, **3:**313, 313f, 340
  for PET, **3:**400, 438
Recorded detail, **1:**5, 6f
Rectal ampulla, **2:**103, 103f
Rectal examination, dynamic, **2:**172, 172f
Rectilinear scanner, **3:**408, 438
Rectosigmoid junction, axial projection of (Chassard-Lapiné method), **2:**169, 169f
Rectouterine pouch, ultrasonography of, **3:**386, 386f, 398
Rectouterine recess, ultrasonography of, **3:**388f
Rectovaginal fistula, **2:**251f
Rectum
  anatomy of, **2:**97f, 102f-103f, 103
  axial projection of (Chassard-Lapiné method), **2:**169, 169f
  defecography of, **2:**172, 172f
  sectional anatomy of, **3:**283
    on axial (transverse) plane, **3:**294-296, 294f-296f
    on sagittal plane, **3:**296, 297f
  ultrasonography of, **3:**386f
Rectus abdominis muscle, sectional anatomy of, **3:**285
  on axial (transverse) plane
    at Level B, **3:**286f
    at Level C, **3:**287f
    at Level D, **3:**288f
    at Level E, **3:**290
    at Level G, **3:**291
    at Level I, **3:**293
    at Level J, **3:**294, 294f
  on sagittal plane, **3:**296, 297f
Rectus muscles, **3:**261-262
Recumbent position, **1:**90, 90f
Red marrow, **1:**76, 76f
Reference isocenter in simulation in radiation oncology, **3:**490-491
Reference population in DXA, **3:**457, 477
Reflection in ultrasonography, **3:**372f, 397
Refraction in ultrasonography, **3:**372f, 397
Region(s) of abdomen, **1:**70, 70f
Region(s) of interest (ROI)
  in CT, **3:**340
  in DXA, **3:**443, 477
Region of interest (ROI) analysis in PET, **3:**430, 438-439
Regional enteritis, **2:**109t
Registered diagnostic cardiac sonographers (RDCSs), **3:**370
Registered diagnostic medical sonographers (RDMSs), **3:**370
  characteristics of, **3:**370, 371f
Registered vascular technologists (RVTs), **3:**370
Regurgitation, cardiac valvular, **3:**370, 393, 397

Relative biologic effectiveness (RBE), **3:**484, 484t, 507
Relaxation in MRI, **3:**344, 368
Relaxation times in MRI, **3:**342, 344, 368
Renal angiography, **2:**190, 191f
  CT, **3:**324-326, 325f
Renal arteriography, **2:**190, 191f, **3:**41f-42f, 45, 45f
Renal artery(ies)
  anatomy of, **3:**22f
  MR angiography of, **3:**364f
  percutaneous transluminal angioplasty of, **3:**64f
  sectional anatomy of, **3:**284, 298-299, 299f
  ultrasonography of, **3:**377f
Renal calculus, **2:**188t, 190f
Renal calyx(ces)
  anatomy of, **2:**183, 185, 185f
  sectional anatomy of, **3:**283
Renal capsule, **2:**184, 185f
Renal cell carcinoma, **2:**188t
Renal columns, **2:**185, 185f
Renal corpuscle, **2:**185
Renal cortex, **2:**185, 185f
Renal cyst, **2:**210f-211f
Renal failure in older adults, **3:**174t
Renal fascia
  anatomy of, **2:**184
  sectional anatomy of, **3:**283
Renal hilum, **2:**184, 185f
Renal hypertension, **2:**188t
Renal medulla, **2:**185, 185f
Renal obstruction, **2:**188t
Renal papilla, **2:**185, 185f
Renal parenchyma, nephrotomography of, **2:**209, 209f
Renal pelvis
  anatomy of, **2:**183, 185, 185f
  sectional anatomy of, **3:**283
Renal puncture, percutaneous, **2:**210-211, 210f-211f
Renal pyramids, **2:**185, 185f
Renal scan, dynamic, **3:**419
Renal sinus, **2:**184, 185f
Renal study, nuclear medicine for, **3:**409, 410f
Renal transplant, ultrasonography of, **3:**383
Renal tubule, **2:**185
Renal vein
  anatomy of, **3:**22f
  sectional anatomy of, **3:**284, 290, 290f
Renal venography, **3:**61, 61f
Rendering in three-dimensional imaging, **3:**326, 340
Reperfusion, **3:**97
Reproductive system, **2:**237-254
  abbreviations used for, **2:**245b
  female. *See* Female reproductive system.
  male. *See* Male reproductive system.
  summary of pathology of, **2:**245t
  summary of projections for, **2:**238
Resistive magnets for MRI, **3:**346, 368
Resolution
  of collimator, **3:**409, 439
  in ultrasonography, **3:**371, 397
Resonance in MRI, **3:**343, 368
Respect
  in code of ethics, **1:**2-3
  for parents and children, **3:**101
Respiratory distress syndrome, **1:**486t
Respiratory gating for radiation oncology, **3:**498, 499f
Respiratory movement, **1:**451, 451f
  diaphragm in, **1:**452, 452f
  in radiography of ribs, **1:**468
  in radiography of sternum, **1:**456, 457f
Respiratory syncytial virus (RSV), **3:**150

Respiratory system
  anatomy of, **1:**479-482
    alveoli in, **1:**480f, 481
    bronchial tree in, **1:**480, 480b, 480f
    lungs in, **1:**481-482, 481f-482f
    trachea in, **1:**480, 480b, 480f
  lungs in. *See* Lung(s).
  pleura in
    AP or PA projection of, **1:**516-517, 516f-517f
    lateral projection of, **1:**518-519, 518f-519f
  trachea in
    anatomy of, **1:**480, 480b, 480f
    AP projection of, **1:**492-493, 492f-493f
    lateral projection of, **1:**494, 494f-495f
    radiation protection for, **1:**492-493
Respiratory system disorders in older adults, **3:**172, 172f
Restenosis, **3:**97
Restricted area, **3:**250
Retina, **2:**314f, 315
Retroareolar cyst, **2:**385f
Retrograde cystography
  AP axial projection for, **2:**216f-217f
  AP oblique projection for, **2:**218f-219f
  AP projection for, **2:**215f
  contrast injection technique for, **2:**214, 215f
Retrograde urography, **2:**192f, 193
  AP projection for, **2:**212-213, 212f-213f
  contrast media for, **2:**194, 195f
  defined, **2:**193
  preparation of patient for, **2:**197
Retromammary fat, **2:**381f
Retroperitoneal cavity, ultrasonography of, **3:**380, 382, 397
Retroperitoneal fat, ultrasonography of, **3:**377f
Retroperitoneum
  anatomy of, **2:**83, 83f
  sectional anatomy of, **3:**283
  sectional image of, **2:**107f
  ultrasonography of, **3:**376-383, 376f-377f
Reverse Waters method
  for cranial trauma, **2:**46, 46f
  for facial bones, **2:**327, 327f-328f
  with trauma, **2:**328, 328f
RF. *See* Radiofrequency (RF).
Rheolytic thrombectomy, **3:**80t
Rheumatoid arthritis, **1:**109t, 182t
Rhomboid major muscle, **3:**271, 274-275, 274f
Rhomboid minor muscle, **3:**271, 274-275, 274f
Ribs
  anatomy of, **1:**447f-449f, 448
  anterior, **1:**468
    PA projection of upper, **1:**469-470, 469f-470f
  axillary portion of, **1:**468
    AP oblique projection for, **1:**473-474, 473f-474f
    PA oblique projection for, **1:**475-476, 475f-476f
  cervical, **1:**448
  components of, **1:**448, 448f-449f
  false, **1:**447f, 448
  floating, **1:**447f, 448
  and heart, **1:**468
  localization of lesion of, **1:**468
  lumbar, **1:**448
  positioning for, **1:**453, 468
  posterior, **1:**468
    AP projection of, **1:**471-472, 471f-472f
    in radiography of sternum, **1:**456, 457f
  radiography of, **1:**468
  respiratory movement of, **1:**451, 451f, 468
    diaphragm in, **1:**452, 452f

Ribs (Continued)
  sectional anatomy of
    in abdominopelvic region, 3:298-299
    in thoracic region, 3:269f
      on axial (transverse) plane, 3:273f-274f, 278
      on coronal plane, 3:280-281, 281f
      on sagittal plane, 3:279-280, 280f
    trauma to, 1:453, 468
    true, 1:447f, 448
Rickets, 1:240t
Right anterior oblique (RAO) position, 1:92, 92f
Right colic flexure, 2:102f, 103
Right jugular trunk, 3:26
Right lower quadrant (RLQ), 1:70, 70f
Right lymphatic duct, 3:26
Right posterior oblique (RPO) position, 1:88, 93, 93f
Right upper quadrant (RUQ), 1:70, 70f
Rima glottidis, 2:71f, 73, 73f
RLQ (right lower quadrant), 1:70, 70f
RNA (radionuclide angiography), 3:416
Robert method for first CMC joint of thumb, 1:118-119
  central ray for, 1:119, 119f
  evaluation criteria for, 1:119b
  Lewis modification of, 1:119
  Long and Rafert modification of, 1:119
  position of part for, 1:118, 118f
  position of patient for, 1:118, 118f
  structures shown on, 1:119, 119f
Rods, 2:315
ROI. See Region(s) of interest (ROI).
Rosenberg method for weight-bearing PA projection of knee, 1:303, 303f
Rotablator, 3:90, 90f-91f
Rotate/rotation, 1:97, 97f
  medial and lateral, 1:93, 93f, 97, 97f
Rotational burr atherectomy, 3:97
Rotational tomography of mandible, 2:353-354, 353f-354f
Rotator cuff, sectional anatomy of, 3:271, 274-275
Rotator cuff tear, 2:9t
  contrast arthrography of, 2:10, 10f
Round ligament
  anatomy of, 2:239f-240f
  ultrasonography of, 3:376f
Round window, 2:270f, 271
RPA (radiology practitioner assistant), 1:14
RPO (right posterior oblique) position, 1:88, 93, 93f
RSV (respiratory syncytial virus), 3:150
Rubidium-82 (^{82}Rb), 3:406t
Rugae
  of stomach, 2:98, 98f, 3:283
  of urinary bladder, 2:186
RUQ (right upper quadrant), 1:70, 70f
RVA (radiologic vertebral assessment), 3:469-470, 470f-471f, 477
RVTs (registered vascular technologists), 3:370

S
Sacral canal, 1:376, 377f
Sacral cornua, 1:376, 376f-377f
Sacral hiatus, 1:377f
Sacral promontory, 1:332f, 376, 376f
Sacral teratoma, fetal ultrasound of, 3:391f
Sacral vertebrae, 1:366
Sacroiliac (SI) joints
  anatomy of, 1:331, 331f, 331t, 376f-377f
  AP axial oblique projection of, 1:428, 428f
  AP axial projection of (Ferguson method), 1:425-426, 425f
  AP oblique projection of, 1:427-428, 427f-428f
  PA axial oblique projection of, 1:430, 430f

Sacroiliac (SI) joints (Continued)
  PA axial projection of, 1:426, 426f
  PA oblique projection of, 1:429-430, 429f-430f
  sectional anatomy of, 3:282, 293, 293f
Sacrum
  anatomy of, 1:330f, 366f
  AP axial projection of, 1:431-432, 431f
  lateral projections of, 1:433-434, 433f-434f
  PA axial projection of, 1:431-432, 432f
  sectional anatomy of, 3:282
    on axial (transverse) plane, 3:293f-294f, 294
    on sagittal plane, 3:296, 297f
Saddle joint, 1:82, 83f
Safety. See Radiation safety.
Sagittal plane, 1:66, 66f-67f
  kidneys in, 3:382, 398
  in sectional anatomy, 3:252
Sagittal suture, 2:259, 275t
Salivary duct, 2:62t
Salivary glands
  anatomy of, 2:60-62, 60f-61f, 61b, 97f
  lateral projection of parotid and submandibular glands for, 2:66-67, 66f-67f
  sialography of, 2:62-63, 62f-63f
  summary of pathology of, 2:62t
  summary of projections of, 2:58-59
  tangential projection of parotid gland for, 2:64-65
    evaluation criteria for, 2:65b
    position of part for, 2:64-65, 64f
    position of patient for, 2:64
    in prone body position, 2:64f, 65
    structures shown on, 2:64f-65f, 65
    in supine body position, 2:64, 64f
Salter-Harris fractures, 3:130, 130f
Sarcoidosis, 1:486t
Sarcoma
  of breast, 2:395
  Ewing, 1:109t, 240t
    in children, 3:150, 150f
  osteogenic. See Osteosarcoma.
SAVI (strut adjusted volume implant applicator), 3:504
SBRT (stereotactic body radiation therapy), 3:499
SC articulations. See Sternoclavicular (SC) articulations.
Scan diameter in CT, 3:320, 340
Scan duration in CT angiography, 3:324, 340
Scan field of view (SFOV) in CT, 3:320
Scan in CT, 3:340
Scan times in CT, 3:320, 340
Scaphoid, 1:140-141
  anatomy of, 1:101f, 102
  Rafert-Long method for scaphoid series (PA and PA axial projections with ulnar deviation) of, 1:142, 142f-143f
  Stecher method for PA axial projection of, 1:140-141
    evaluation criteria for, 1:140b
    position of part for, 1:140, 140f
    position of patient for, 1:140
    structures shown on, 1:140, 140f
    variations of, 1:141, 141f
Scaphoid series, 1:142, 142f-143f
Scapula(e)
  acromion of, 1:176, 176f
  anatomy of, 1:176-177, 176f
  AP oblique projection of, 1:220, 220f-221f
  AP projection of, 1:216-217, 216f-217f
  coracoid process of
    anatomy of, 1:176, 176f
    AP axial projection of, 1:222, 222f-223f
  costal (anterior) surface of, 1:176, 176f
  dorsal (posterior) surface of, 1:176, 176f
  function of, 1:175

Scapula(e) (Continued)
  glenoid surface of, 1:176f
  inferior angle of, 1:71f, 71t, 176f, 177
  infraspinous fossa of, 1:176, 176f
  lateral angle of, 1:176f, 177
  lateral border of, 1:176, 176f
  lateral projection of, 1:218, 218f-219f
  medial border of, 1:176, 176f
  neck of, 1:176f, 177
  sectional anatomy of, 3:269f, 270, 273-275, 274f, 278f
  superior angle of, 1:176f, 177
  superior border of, 1:176, 176f
  supraspinous fossa of, 1:176, 176f
Scapular notch, 1:176, 176f
Scapular spine
  anatomy of, 1:176, 176f
  crest of, 1:176, 176f
  Laquerrière-Pierquin method for tangential projection of, 1:224, 224f
  sectional anatomy of, 3:269f, 273f
Scapular Y, PA oblique projection of, 1:199-201
  central ray for, 1:201, 201t
  compensating filter for, 1:199-201
  evaluation criteria for, 1:201b
  position of part for, 1:199, 199f
  position of patient for, 1:199
  structures shown on, 1:200f, 201
Scapulohumeral articulation, 1:178-180, 178t, 179f-181f
Scatter radiation in CT, 3:318-319, 319f
Scattering in ultrasonography, 3:398
Schatzki ring, 2:119f
Scheuermann disease, 1:380t
School age children, development of, 3:104
Schüller method
  for axiolateral projection of TMJ, 2:349-350
    evaluation criteria for, 2:350b
    position of part in, 2:349, 349f-350f
    position of patient in, 2:349
    structures shown on, 2:350, 350f
  for submentovertical projection of cranial base, 2:310-311
    central ray for, 2:310f, 311
    evaluation criteria for, 2:311b
    position of part for, 2:310-311, 310f
    position of patient for, 2:310
    structures shown on, 2:311, 311f
Sciatic nerve, 3:294, 294f-296f
Scintillate, 3:408
Scintillating detector pileup with K-edge filtration systems for DXA, 3:452
Scintillation camera, 3:400, 439
Scintillation counter, 3:444, 477
Scintillation crystals of gamma camera, 3:408f, 409
Scintillation detector, 3:408, 439
Scintillators, 3:400, 438
  for PET, 3:401t, 428-429
Sclera, 2:315
Scoliosis, 3:152-154
  Cobb angle in, 3:154
  congenital, 3:153
  C-spine filter for, 3:153
  defined, 1:380t, 437, 3:152
  DXA with, 3:464, 465f
  estimation of rotation in, 3:154
  idiopathic, 3:152
  image assessment for, 3:123t
  imaging of, 3:153, 153f
  lateral bends with, 3:154
  neuromuscular, 3:153
  PA and lateral projections of (Frank et al. method), 1:437-438, 437f-438f

Index

Scoliosis (Continued)
 PA projection of (Ferguson method), **1:**439-440
  evaluation criteria for, **1:**439b-440b
  first radiograph in, **1:**439, 439f
  position of part for, **1:**439, 439f-440f
  position of patient for, **1:**439, 439f
  second radiograph in, **1:**439, 440f
  structures shown on, **1:**439-440, 439f-440f
 patterns of, **3:**154
 skeletal maturity with, **3:**154
 symptoms of, **3:**152, 152f
 treatment options for, **3:**154
Scoliosis filters, **1:**57, 64, 64f, 367, 367f
Scottie dog
 in AP oblique projection, **1:**421-422,
  421f-422f
 in PA oblique projection, **1:**423, 423f-424f
Scout image
 of abdomen, **2:**87
 in radiation oncology, **3:**490-491
Scrotum, **2:**242
Scrub nurse, **3:**215
SD (standard deviation) in DXA, **3:**455, 455f-456f,
 477
Seated position, **1:**90
Secondary curves, **1:**367
Secondary ossification, **1:**72-74, 77f-78f
Sectional anatomy, **3:**251-300
 of abdominopelvic region, **3:**282-299
  on axial (transverse) plane, **3:**284f, 285
   at level A, **3:**285, 285f
   at level B, **3:**285, 286f
   at level C, **3:**287, 287f
   at level D, **3:**288, 288f
   at level E, **3:**289, 289f
   at level F, **3:**290, 290f
   at level G, **3:**291, 291f
   at level H, **3:**292, 292f
   at level I, **3:**293, 293f
   at level J, **3:**294, 294f
   at level K, **3:**295, 295f-296f
  on cadaveric image, **3:**282, 282f
  on coronal plane, **3:**298f-299f, 299
  on sagittal plane, **3:**296, 297f
 axial (transverse) planes in, **3:**252
 of cadaveric sections, **3:**252
 coronal planes in, **3:**252
 of cranial region, **3:**253-268
  on axial (transverse) plane, **3:**256, 256f
   at level A, **3:**256-257, 256f-257f
   at level B, **3:**257-258, 257f
   at level C, **3:**258, 258f
   at level D, **3:**259-260, 259f
   at level E, **3:**260f-261f, 261-262
   at level F, **3:**262, 262f
   at level G, **3:**263, 263f
  on cadaveric image, **3:**253, 253f
  on coronal plane, **3:**266-267, 266f
   at level A, **3:**266-267, 267f
   at level B, **3:**267-268, 267f
   at level C, **3:**268, 268f
  on sagittal plane, **3:**256f, 264, 264f
   at level A, **3:**264-265, 265f
   at level B, **3:**265, 265f
   at level C, **3:**266, 266f
 of CT, **3:**252
 of MRI, **3:**252
 oblique planes in, **3:**252
 overview of, **3:**252
 sagittal planes in, **3:**252
 of thoracic region, **3:**269-281
  on axial (transverse) plane, **3:**272, 272f
   at level A, **3:**272, 272f
   at level B, **3:**273, 273f
   at level C, **3:**274-275, 274f
   at level D, **3:**275, 275f

Sectional anatomy (Continued)
   at level E, **3:**275-277, 276f-277f
   at level F, **3:**278, 278f
   at level G, **3:**278, 279f
  on cadaveric image, **3:**269, 269f, 271f
  on coronal plane, **3:**280, 281f
   at level A, **3:**280, 281f
   at level B, **3:**280-281, 281f
   at level C, **3:**281, 281f
  on sagittal plane, **3:**278-279, 279f
   at level A, **3:**278-279, 280f
   at level B, **3:**279, 280f
   at level C, **3:**279-280, 280f
Segmentation in three-dimensional imaging, **3:**326,
 340
Segmented regions, **3:**402
Seldinger technique, **3:**20, 36, 37f
Selective estrogen receptor modulators (SERMs)
 for osteoporosis, **3:**448t
Self-efficacy, **3:**166
Sella turcica
 anatomy of, **2:**258f, 264-265, 264f-265f
 lateral projection of, **2:**293f, 322f, 359f
  in decubitus position, **2:**295f
 sectional anatomy of, **3:**253-254, 260f, 261-262
Sellar joint, **1:**82, 83f
Semicircular canals, **2:**269f-270f, 271
Seminal duct radiography, **2:**253
 epididymography for, **2:**253, 253f
 epididymovesiculography for, **2:**253
 grid technique for, **2:**253
 nongrid technique for, **2:**253
 vesiculography for, **2:**253, 254f
Seminal vesicles
 anatomy of, **2:**242, 243f
 sectional anatomy of, **3:**284, 296, 296f
 tuberculous, **2:**254f
Seminoma, **2:**245t
Semirestricted area, **3:**250
Sensitivity of collimator, **3:**409
Sensory system disorders in older adults, **3:**169
Sentinel node imaging, nuclear medicine for, **3:**420
Septum(a)
 pellucidum, **3:**257-258, 257f, 266-267, 267f
 in PET, **3:**400, 439
Serial imaging, **3:**21, 97
Serial scans in DXA, **3:**463-464, 463f, 477
SERMs (selective estrogen receptor modulators)
 for osteoporosis, **3:**448t
Serratus anterior muscle
 anatomy of, **2:**380, 380f
 sectional anatomy of
  in abdominopelvic region, **3:**285, 285f
  in thoracic region, **3:**271, 278, 278f-279f
Sesamoid bones, **1:**79, 79f
 of foot
  anatomy of, **1:**228f, 230
  tangential projection of
   Holly method for, **1:**251, 251f
   Lewis method for, **1:**250-251, 250f
 of hand, **1:**101, 101f
Settegast method for tangential projection of
 patella and patellofemoral joint, **1:**316-317
 evaluation criteria for, **1:**317b
 position of part for, **1:**316-317
 position of patient for, **1:**316
  lateral, **1:**316f
  seated, **1:**316, 316f
  supine or prone, **1:**316, 316f
 structures shown on, **1:**317, 317f
SFOV (scan field of view) in CT, **3:**320
Shaded surface display (SSD), **3:**326, 340
Shading in three-dimensional imaging, **3:**326, 340
Shadow shield, **1:**33, 34f
Shape distortion, **1:**7, 7f
Sheets, **1:**15

Shewhart Control Chart rules, **3:**461, 477
Shielding
 for CT, **3:**331
 gonad, **1:**33-35, 33f-34f
  for children, **3:**108, 108f-109f
Short bones, **1:**79, 79f
Short tau inversion recovery (STIR),
 3:352-353
Shoulder
 AP oblique projection for trauma of, **2:**48,
  48f-49f
 AP projection for, **1:**183-188
  compensating filter for, **1:**185-188, 187f
  evaluation criteria for, **1:**186b-188b
  with humerus in external rotation
   evaluation criteria for, **1:**186
   position of part for, **1:**184f-185f, 185
   structures shown on, **1:**186, 186f
  with humerus in internal rotation
   evaluation criteria for, **1:**186-188
   position of part for, **1:**184f, 185
   structures shown on, **1:**186, 187f
  with humerus in neutral rotation
   evaluation criteria for, **1:**186
   position of part for, **1:**184f, 185
   structures shown on, **1:**186, 186f
  position of part for, **1:**183-185
  position of patient for, **1:**183
  structures shown on, **1:**186-188, 186f
 Lawrence method for transthoracic lateral
  projection of, **1:**192-193, 192f-193f
 surgical radiography of, **3:**238-239,
  238f-239f
 trauma radiography of, **2:**48, 48f-49f
Shoulder arthrography, **2:**10-11
 CT after, **2:**11, 11f
 double-contrast, **2:**10, 10f-11f
 MRI vs., **2:**8f
 single-contrast, **2:**10, 10f-11f
Shoulder girdle, **1:**173-224
 acromioclavicular articulation of
  Alexander method for AP axial projection of,
   1:211-212, 211f-212f
  anatomy of, **1:**178t, 179f, 181, 181f
  Pearson method for bilateral AP projection of,
   1:209, 209f-210f
 anatomy of, **1:**175, 175f
  acromioclavicular articulation in, **1:**178t, 179f,
   181, 181f
  bursae in, **1:**178, 178f
  clavicle in, **1:**175, 175f
  proximal humerus in, **1:**177-178, 177f
  scapula in, **1:**176-177, 176f
  scapulohumeral articulation in, **1:**178-180,
   178t, 179f-181f
  sternoclavicular articulation in, **1:**178t, 179f,
   181-182, 181f
  summary of, **1:**181b
 AP projection of, **1:**183-188
  compensating filter for, **1:**185-188, 187f
  evaluation criteria for, **1:**186b-188b
  with humerus in external rotation
   evaluation criteria for, **1:**186
   position of part for, **1:**184f-185f, 185
   structures shown on, **1:**186, 186f
  with humerus in internal rotation
   evaluation criteria for, **1:**186-188
   position of part for, **1:**184f, 185
   structures shown on, **1:**186, 187f
  with humerus in neutral rotation
   evaluation criteria for, **1:**186
   position of part for, **1:**184f, 185
   structures shown on, **1:**186, 186f
  position of part for, **1:**183-185
  position of patient for, **1:**183
  structures shown on, **1:**186-188, 186f

Index

Shoulder girdle *(Continued)*
  clavicle of
    anatomy of, **1:**175, 175f
    AP axial projection of, **1:**214, 214f
    AP projection of, **1:**213, 213f
    PA axial projection of, **1:**215, 215f
    PA projection of, **1:**215, 215f
  defined, **1:**175
  glenoid cavity of
    Apple method for AP oblique projection of,
      1:190-191, 190f-191f
    Garth method for AP axial oblique projection
      of, **1:**205-206, 205f-206f
    Grashey method for AP oblique projection of,
      1:188-189, 188f-189f
      central ray for, **1:**189
  inferosuperior axial projection of
    Lawrence method and Rafert et al.
      modification of, **1:**194, 194f-195f
    West Point method for, **1:**196-197,
      196f-197f
  Lawrence method for transthoracic lateral
    projection of, **1:**192-193, 192f-193f
  proximal humerus of
    anatomy of, **1:**177-178, 177f
    intertubercular (bicipital) groove of
      anatomy of, **1:**177, 177f
      Fisk modification for tangential projection
        of, **1:**207-208, 207f-208f
    Stryker notch method for AP axial projection
      of, **1:**204, 204f
  radiation protection for, **1:**183
  sample exposure technique chart essential
    projections for, **1:**182t
  scapula of
    anatomy of, **1:**176-177, 176f
    AP axial projection of coracoid process of,
      1:222, 222f-223f
    AP oblique projection of, **1:**220, 220f-221f
    AP projection of, **1:**216-217, 216f-217f
    Laquerrière-Pierquin method for tangential
      projection of spine of, **1:**224, 224f
    lateral projection of, **1:**218, 218f-219f
    scapular Y of, PA oblique projection of,
      1:199-201
      central ray for, **1:**201, 201t
      compensating filter for, **1:**199-201
      evaluation criteria for, **1:**201b
      position of part for, **1:**199, 199f
      position of patient for, **1:**199
      structures shown on, **1:**200f, 201
  summary of pathology of, **1:**182t
  summary of projections for, **1:**174
  superoinferior axial projection of, **1:**198,
    198f
  supraspinatus "outlet" of
    AP axial projection of, **1:**203, 203f
    Neer method for tangential projection of,
      1:202-203, 202f
Shoulder joint
  glenoid cavity of
    Apple method for AP oblique projection of,
      1:190-191, 190f-191f
    Garth method for AP axial oblique projection
      of, **1:**205-206, 205f-206f
    Grashey method for AP oblique projection of,
      1:188-189, 188f-189f
  inferosuperior axial projection of
    Lawrence method and Rafert et al.
      modification of, **1:**194, 194f-195f
    West Point method for, **1:**196-197, 196f-197f
  PA oblique projection of scapular Y of,
    1:199-201
    central ray for, **1:**201, 201t
    compensating filter for, **1:**199-201
    evaluation criteria for, **1:**201b

Shoulder joint *(Continued)*
  position of part for, **1:**199, 199f
  position of patient for, **1:**199
  structures shown on, **1:**200f, 201
  Stryker notch method for AP axial projection of
    proximal humerus of, **1:**204, 204f
  superoinferior axial projection of, **1:**198, 198f
  supraspinatus "outlet" of
    AP axial projection of, **1:**203, 203f
    Neer method for tangential projection of,
      1:202-203, 202f
SI joints. *See* Sacroiliac (SI) joints.
Sialography, **2:**62-63, 62f-63f
SID (source–to–image receptor distance), **1:**7,
  31-32, 31f, **3:**33
  in mobile radiography, **3:**187
Sieverts (Sv), **3:**458, 477
Sigmoid sinuses, **3:**255, 262-263, 262f
Signal in MRI
  defined, **3:**368
  production of, **3:**343, 343f
  significance of, **3:**344, 344f
Silicosis, **1:**486t
Simple fracture, **1:**84f
Sims position, **1:**90, 91f
Simulation in radiation oncology, **3:**489-491
  contrast materials for, **3:**490, 491f-492f
  creation of treatment fields in, **3:**491, 492f-493f,
    507
  CT simulator for, **3:**489, 490f, 507
  immobilization devices for, **3:**490,
    490f-491f
  reference isocenter in, **3:**490-491
Simulator, CT, for radiation oncology, **3:**489, 490f,
  507
Single energy x-ray absorptiometry (SXA), **3:**470,
  475, 477
Single photon absorptiometry (SPA), **3:**444, 444f,
  477
Single photon emission computed tomography
  (SPECT), **3:**413-414
  of brain, **3:**411f, 417
  combined with CT, **3:**401, 403f, 415, 415f,
    436
  common uses of, **3:**414, 414f
  computers for, **3:**409, 411f
  defined, **3:**439
  dual-detector, **3:**413-414, 413f
  historical development of, **3:**400-401
  vs. other modalities, **3:**401t, 402
  reconstruction technique for, **3:**413
Single slice helical CT (SSHCT), **3:**306, 321-323,
  322f
Singular endings for medical terms, **1:**98, 98t
Singular word forms, frequently misused, **1:**98,
  98t
Sinogram data in PET, **3:**431, 439
Sinus(es)
  abdominal, **2:**180, 180f
  defined, **1:**84
  paranasal. *See* Paranasal sinuses.
Sinusitis, **2:**282t
Skeletal metastases, strontium-99 for, **3:**420
Skeletal studies, **3:**416
Skeleton
  appendicular, **1:**75, 75f, 75t
  axial, **1:**75, 75f, 75t
Skin cancer, radiation oncology for, **3:**504
Skin care for older adults, **3:**175
Skin disorders in older adults, **3:**168
Skin-sparing effect in radiation oncology, **3:**486,
  486f, 507
Skull, **2:**255-367
  abbreviations used for, **2:**284b
  anatomy of, **2:**257-260, 257b, 257f-260f
    summary of, **2:**280b-281b

Skull *(Continued)*
  AP axial projection of, **2:**299-300, 301f
    Towne method for, **2:**302-306
      central ray for, **2:**303f, 304
      in children, **3:**132, 135t
      evaluation criteria for, **2:**304b
      for pathologic condition or trauma, **2:**306,
        306f-307f
      position of part for, **2:**302, 303f
      position of patient for, **2:**302
      structures shown on, **2:**304, 305f
      variations of, **2:**302
  articulations of, **2:**275, 275t
    temporomandibular. *See* Temporomandibular
      joint (TMJ).
  asymmetry of, **2:**286
  brachycephalic, **2:**286, 286f
  in children, **3:**132-135
    AP axial Towne projection of, **3:**132, 135t
    AP projection of, **3:**132, 134-135, 134f
    with craniosynostosis, **3:**132
    with fracture, **3:**132
    immobilization of, **3:**132, 133f, 135f
    lateral projection of, **3:**132, 134-135,
      134f-135f
    summary of projections of, **3:**135t
  cleanliness in imaging of, **2:**288
  correct and incorrect rotation of, **2:**287, 287f
  cranial bones of. *See* Cranial bones.
  CT of, **3:**336f-338f
  dolichocephalic, **2:**286, 286f
  ear in, **2:**270f, 271
  eye in
    anatomy of, **2:**314-316, 314f-315f
    lateral projection of, **2:**317, 317f
    localization of foreign bodies within, **2:**316,
      316f
    PA axial projection of, **2:**318, 318f
    parietoacanthial projection of (modified
      Waters method), **2:**319, 319f
    preliminary examination of, **2:**316
  facial bones of. *See* Facial bones.
  general body position for, **2:**288
    adjusting OML to vertical position in, **2:**290f
    adjusting sagittal planes to horizontal position
      in, **2:**289f
  lateral decubitus position of
    for pathologic conditions, trauma, or
      deformity, **2:**306
    for stretcher and bedside examinations,
      2:299-300, 299f
  lateral projection of
    in children, **3:**132, 134-135, 134f-135f
    in dorsal decubitus or supine lateral position,
      2:294-300, 295f
    in R or L position, **2:**291, 292f-293f
  mesocephalic, **2:**286, 286f
  morphology of, **2:**286-287, 286f-287f
  PA axial projection of
    Caldwell method for, **2:**296-300
      evaluation criteria for, **2:**299b
      position of part for, **2:**296, 297f
      position of patient for, **2:**296
      structures shown on, **2:**298f, 299
    Haas method for, **2:**308-309
      central ray for, **2:**308, 308f
      evaluation criteria for, **2:**309b
      position of part for, **2:**308, 308f
      position of patient for, **2:**308
      structures shown on, **2:**309, 309f
  radiation protection for, **2:**288
  sample exposure technique chart essential
    projections for, **2:**283t-284t
  sinuses of. *See* Paranasal sinuses.
  summary of pathology of, **2:**282t
  summary of projections of, **2:**256

Skull (Continued)
technical considerations for radiography of, **2:**288
topography of, **2:**285, 285f
trauma to
acanthioparietal projection (reverse Waters method) for, **2:**46, 46f
AP axial projection (Towne method) for, **2:**44-45, 44f-45f
CT of, **2:**29, 29f, 53-55, 54f
lateral projection for, **2:**42-43, 42f-43f
Skull base, submentovertical projection of (Schüller method), **2:**310-311
central ray for, **2:**310f, 311
evaluation criteria for, **2:**311b
position of part for, **2:**310-311, 310f
position of patient for, **2:**310
structures shown on, **2:**311, 311f
Skull fracture, **2:**43f
in children, **3:**132
Slice, **3:**18
in CT, **3:**302, 340
in MRI, **3:**342, 368
Slice thickness in CT, **3:**331-332, 332t-333t
Slip ring in CT, **3:**309, 340
Slipped disk, **1:**368
Slipped epiphysis, **1:**335t
SMA. See Superior mesenteric artery (SMA).
Small bowel series, **2:**138
Small intestine
anatomy of, **2:**97f, 100f, 101
complete reflux examination of, **2:**141, 141f
duodenum of. See Duodenum.
enteroclysis procedure for, **2:**141
air-contrast, **2:**141, 141f
barium in, **2:**141, 141f
CT, **2:**141, 142f
iodinated contrast medium for, **2:**141, 142f
exposure time for, **2:**114
intubation examination procedures for, **2:**143, 143f
PA or AP projection of, **2:**139
evaluation criteria for, **2:**139b
ileocecal studies in, **2:**139, 140f
position of part for, **2:**139, 139f
position of patient for, **2:**139
structures shown on, **2:**139, 139f-140f
radiologic examination of, **2:**138
oral method for, **2:**138
preparation for, **2:**138
sectional anatomy of, **3:**283
on axial (transverse) plane
at Level E, **3:**289, 289f
at Level G, **3:**291, 291f
at Level H, **3:**292, 292f
at Level I, **3:**293, 293f
at Level J, **3:**294f
on coronal plane, **3:**298-299, 298f
on sagittal plane, **3:**296
SmartShape wedges for CT, **3:**329-330, 329f
Smith fracture, **1:**109t
Smooth muscles, motion control of, **1:**18
SMV projection. See Submentovertical (SMV) projection.
SOD (source-to-object distance), **3:**33
Sodium iodide (NaI) as scintillator for PET, **3:**428t
Sodium iodide (NaI) scintillation crystals of gamma camera, **3:**408f, 409
Sodium phosphate for polycythemia, **3:**420
Soft palate
anatomy of, **2:**59, 59f, 71f
lateral projection of, **2:**78-79, 78f-79f
methods of examination of, **2:**74-75
Soft tissue(s), ultrasonography of, **3:**383
Soft tissue compensation in DXA, **3:**452, 453f

Soft tissue neck (STN)
in children, **3:**137-138, 137f-138f
CT of, **3:**336f-338f
Software, **3:**460
Solid-state digital detectors, **1:**3, 4f
Soloman, Albert, **2:**372
Sonar, **3:**371, 398
Sonography. See Ultrasonography.
SOS (speed of sound), **3:**475
Sound, velocity of, **3:**372, 398
Sound waves
defined, **3:**372, 398
properties of, **3:**372, 372f
Source–to–image receptor distance (SID), **1:**7, 31-32, 31f, **3:**33
in mobile radiography, **3:**187
Source-to-object distance (SOD), **3:**33
Source–to–skin distance (SSD), **1:**31f, 32
SPA (single photon absorptiometry), **3:**444, 444f, 477
Spatial resolution, **1:**5, 6f
for CT, **3:**318, 340
Special needs, children with, **3:**105-107
Special planes, **1:**68, 69f
SPECT. See Single photon emission computed tomography (SPECT).
Spectral analysis, **3:**392
Spectroscopy, **3:**368
magnetic resonance, **3:**365, 365f-366f
Speed of sound (SOS), **3:**475
Spermatic cord, **3:**284, 296, 296f
Sphenoid angle of parietal bone, **2:**263f
Sphenoid bone
anatomy of, **2:**264-266, 264f-265f
greater wings of, **2:**258f, 259, 264f-265f, 265
lesser wings of, **2:**258f, 264f-265f, 265
location of, **2:**257f-258f
in orbit, **2:**275, 275f, 312f
sectional anatomy of, **3:**253-254
Sphenoid sinus effusion, **2:**295f
Sphenoid strut, **2:**265
Sphenoidal fontanel, **2:**259-260, 260f
Sphenoidal sinuses
anatomy of, **2:**276f-278f, 279
AP axial projection of, **2:**309f
lateral projection of, **2:**359f
in decubitus position, **2:**295f
location of, **2:**259f, 264-265, 264f-265f
PA axial projection of, **2:**361f
parietoacanthial projection of, **2:**365f
open-mouth Waters method for, **2:**364-365, 364f-365f
sectional anatomy of, **3:**253-254
on axial (transverse) plane, **3:**261-263, 261f, 263f
on coronal plane, **3:**267, 267f
on sagittal plane, **3:**264, 265f
submentovertical projection of, **2:**311f, 366-367, 366f-367f
Spheroid joint, **1:**82, 83f
Sphincter of Oddi, **2:**105, 105f
Sphincter of the hepatopancreatic ampulla, **2:**105, 105f
Spin echo pulse sequence, **3:**352-353, 368
Spina bifida, **1:**368, 380t
Spinal cord, **2:**259f
anatomy of, **3:**2f-3f, 3
CT myelography of, **3:**12, 12f
CT of, **3:**11, 11f-12f
defined, **3:**18
interventional pain management of, **3:**16-18
MRI of, **3:**12-13, 13f
myelography of, **3:**6-8
cervical, **3:**9f
contrast media for, **3:**6-7, 6f
conus projection in, **3:**8

Spinal cord (Continued)
of dentate ligament, **3:**9f
examination procedure for, **3:**7-8, 7f
of foramen magnum, **3:**9f
lumbar, **3:**8f
preparation of examining room for, **3:**7, 7f
of subarachnoid space, **3:**9f
plain radiographic examination of, **3:**5
provocative diskography of, **3:**16, 17f
sectional anatomy of, **3:**269f, 272f
vertebroplasty and kyphoplasty of, **3:**16, 16f-17f
Spinal fusion
AP projection of, **1:**441-442, 441f-442f
lateral projection in hyperflexion and hyperextension of, **1:**443-444, 443f-444f
Spine examinations for geriatric patients, **3:**178-179, 178f-179f
Spine of bone, **1:**84
Spine scan in DXA
equipment for, **3:**442f
lateral lumbar, **3:**469
PA lumbar, **3:**464-466, 464f-465f
Spin-lattice relaxation, **3:**344, 368
Spinous process, **1:**368, 368f
Spin-spin relaxation, **3:**344, 368
Spiral CT, **3:**340
multislice, **3:**306, 323-324, 323f-324f
single slice, **3:**306, 321-323, 322f
Spiral fracture, **1:**84f
Spleen
anatomy of, **2:**97f, 105f, 106
nuclear medicine imaging of, **3:**418
sectional anatomy of, **3:**282f, 283
on axial (transverse) plane
at Level B, **3:**285, 286f
at Level C, **3:**287, 287f
at Level D, **3:**288, 288f
at Level E, **3:**289, 289f
at Level F, **3:**290, 290f
on coronal plane, **3:**299, 299f
sectional image of, **2:**107f
ultrasonography of, **3:**376f, 381, 381f
Splenic arteriogram, **3:**41f-42f, 44, 44f
Splenic artery
sectional anatomy of, **3:**282f, 284
on axial (transverse) plane, **3:**288-289, 288f-289f
on coronal plane, **3:**298-299, 298f
ultrasonography of, **3:**376f
Splenic flexure
anatomy of, **2:**102f, 103
sectional anatomy of, **3:**283, 287, 287f, 298, 298f
Splenic vein
anatomy of, **2:**105f
sectional anatomy of, **3:**282f, 284-285, 288f, 298-299
ultrasonography of, **3:**380, 380f
Splenomegaly, ultrasonography of, **3:**381f
Split cassettes in digital imaging, **1:**38
Spondylitis, infectious, CT for needle biopsy of, **3:**314f
Spondylolisthesis, **1:**375, 375f, 380t
Spondylolysis, **1:**375, 380t
Spongy bone, **1:**76, 76f
Spongy urethra, **2:**186f, 187
Spot compression technique for mammography, **2:**403t-408t, 429-431, 430f-431f, 432t
Squama of occipital bone, **2:**266, 266f-267f
Squamosal suture. See Squamous suture.
Squamous cell carcinoma, **3:**483
Squamous suture
anatomy of, **2:**258f, 259, 275t
sectional anatomy of, **3:**253-254

⁹⁹Sr (strontium-99) for skeletal metastases, **3:**420
SRS (stereotactic radiosurgery), **3:**486-487, 499, 507
SRT (stereotactic radiation therapy), **3:**499, 507
SSD (shaded surface display), **3:**326, 340
SSD (source–to–skin distance), **1:**31f, 32
SSHCT (single slice helical CT), **3:**306, 321-323, 322f
Stable elements, **3:**422f
Stainless steel occluding coils, **3:**68, 68f
Standard deviation (SD) in DXA, **3:**455, 455f-456f, 477
Standard precautions, **1:**15, 15f
in trauma radiography, **2:**28
Standardized hip reference database for DXA, **3:**457
Stapes, **2:**270f, 271
Starburst artifacts in CT, **3:**319
Starching of gowns, **1:**20
Static imaging in nuclear medicine, **3:**410-411
Statins for osteoporosis, **3:**448t
Statscan, **2:**20, 21f-22f
Stecher method for PA axial projection of scaphoid, **1:**140-141
evaluation criteria for, **1:**140b
position of part for, **1:**140, 140f
position of patient for, **1:**140
structures shown on, **1:**140, 140f
variations of, **1:**141, 141f
Stenosis, **2:**62t, **3:**28, 97
in urinary system, **2:**188t
Stent, **3:**97
Stent graft for abdominal aortic aneurysm, **3:**65-66, 65f-66f
Stereotactic body radiation therapy (SBRT), **3:**499
Stereotactic imaging and biopsy procedures for breast lesions, **2:**465-470
calculation of *X, Y,* and *Z* coordinates in, **2:**465, 465f-466f, 469, 469f
equipment for, **2:**466, 467f-468f
images using, **2:**468, 468f-470f
three-dimensional localization with, **2:**465, 465f
Stereotactic radiation therapy (SRT), **3:**499, 507
Stereotactic radiosurgery (SRS), **3:**486-487, 499, 507
Stereotactic surgery, **3:**18
Stereotaxis. *See* Stereotactic imaging and biopsy procedures.
Sterile, **3:**250
Sterile environment in operating room, **1:**16-17, 16f-17f
Sterile field in surgical radiography
contamination of, **3:**220
image receptor handling in, **3:**219-220, 219f-220f
maintenance of, **3:**218-220, 218f
Sterile surgical team members, **3:**215, 215f
Sternal angle
anatomy of, **1:**447f, 448
sectional anatomy of, **3:**256, 278-279, 280f
as surface marker, **1:**71f, 71t
Sternal extremity, **1:**175, 175f, 447f
Sternal notch, **3:**256
Sternoclavicular (SC) articulations
anatomy of, **1:**178t, 179f, 181-182, 181f, 449, 449t
PA oblique projection of
body rotation method for, **1:**465, 465f
central ray angulation method for, **1:**466, 466f-467f
PA projection of, **1:**464, 464f
sectional anatomy of, **3:**270, 274-275, 274f, 280, 280f
Sternocleidomastoid muscle, **3:**272, 272f

Sternocostal joints
anatomy of, **1:**449t, 450, 450f
sectional anatomy of, **3:**280f
Sternum
anatomy of, **1:**447-448, 447f
and breasts, **1:**456
and heart and other mediastinal structures, **1:**456, 457f
lateral projection of, **1:**462, 462f-463f
PA oblique projection of
in LPO position, **1:**458
in modified prone position (Moore method), **1:**460-461, 460f-461f
in RAO position, **1:**458-459, 458f-459f
and posterior ribs and lung markings, **1:**456, 457f
and pulmonary structures, **1:**456, 457f
radiation protection for, **1:**456-462
radiography of, **1:**456
sectional anatomy of, **3:**269-270, 271f
on axial (transverse) plane, **3:**276f, 278, 278f-279f
on sagittal plane, **3:**280f
and thoracic vertebrae, **1:**456, 456f, 456t
Sthenic body habitus, **1:**72-74, 72f, 73b
and gallbladder, **2:**106, 106f
and stomach and duodenum, **2:**99, 99f, 125f
and thoracic viscera, **1:**479f
STIR (short tau inversion recovery), **3:**352-353
STN (soft tissue neck)
in children, **3:**137-138, 137f-138f
CT of, **3:**336f-338f
Stomach
anatomy of, **2:**97f-99f, 98-99
AP oblique projection of, **2:**130-131, 130f-131f
AP projection of, **2:**134
evaluation criteria for, **2:**134b
position of part for, **2:**134, 134f
position of patient for, **2:**134, 134f
structures shown on, **2:**134, 135f
and body habitus, **2:**99, 99f
contrast studies of, **2:**121-123
barium sulfate suspension for, **2:**111, 111f
biphasic, **2:**123
double-contrast, **2:**122, 122f, 124f
single-contrast, **2:**121, 121f, 124f
water-soluble, iodinated solution for, **2:**111, 111f
exposure time for, **2:**114
functions of, **2:**99
gastrointestinal series for, **2:**120, 120f
lateral projection of, **2:**132-133, 132f-133f
PA axial projection of, **2:**126-127, 126f-127f
PA oblique projection of, **2:**128-129, 128f-129f
Wolf method for, **2:**136-137, 136f-137f
PA projection of, **2:**124-125
body habitus and, **2:**124-125, 125f
double-contrast, **2:**124f
evaluation criteria for, **2:**125b
position of part for, **2:**124, 124f
position of patient for, **2:**124
single-contrast, **2:**124f
structures shown on, **2:**124-125, 125f
sectional anatomy of, **3:**283
on axial (transverse) plane
at Level A, **3:**285f
at Level B, **3:**285, 286f
at Level C, **3:**287, 287f
at Level D, **3:**288f
at Level E, **3:**289, 289f
on coronal plane, **3:**298-299, 298f-299f
sectional image of, **2:**107f
ultrasonography of, **3:**376f
Stopcocks for cardiac catheterization, **3:**78, 78f
Straight sinus, **3:**255, 259f, 260-261, 264-265

Streak artifacts in CT, **3:**319, 319f, 340
Striated muscular tissue, motion control of, **1:**19
Strike-through, **3:**250
Strontium-99 (⁹⁹Sr) for skeletal metastases, **3:**420
Strut adjusted volume implant applicator (SAVI), **3:**504
Stryker notch method for AP axial projection of proximal humerus, **1:**204, 204f
Styloid process
anatomy of, **1:**84, **2:**258f, 268, 268f-269f
sectional anatomy of, **3:**253-254
Subacromial bursa, **1:**178, 178f
Subarachnoid space
anatomy of, **3:**3
myelogram of, **3:**9f
sectional anatomy of, **3:**254
Sub-bacterial endocarditis, echocardiography of, **3:**393
Subclavian arteries
anatomy of, **3:**22f, 49f
arteriography of, **3:**40f, 46f, 55f
sectional anatomy of, **3:**269f, 270-271
on axial (transverse) plane, **3:**273-275, 273f-274f
on coronal plane, **3:**281, 281f
on sagittal plane, **3:**279-280, 280f
Subclavian trunk, **3:**26
Subclavian veins
anatomy of, **3:**22f
sectional anatomy of, **3:**269f, 271, 273, 273f, 280-281
venography of, **3:**46f
Subdural space, **3:**3
Sublingual ducts, **2:**60f, 61-62
Sublingual fold, **2:**59, 59f
Sublingual glands, **2:**60f-61f, 61-62, 97f
Sublingual space, **2:**59, 59f
Subluxation, **1:**380t
Submandibular duct, **2:**60, 60f
Submandibular gland
anatomy of, **2:**60, 60f-61f, 97f
lateral projection of, **2:**66-67, 66f-67f
sialography of, **2:**62f
Submentovertical (SMV) projection
of cranial base, **2:**310-311
central ray for, **2:**310f, 311
evaluation criteria for, **2:**311b
position of part for, **2:**310-311, 310f
position of patient for, **2:**310
structures shown on, **2:**311, 311f
of ethmoidal and sphenoidal sinuses, **2:**366-367, 366f-367f
of mandible, **2:**346, 346f
of zygomatic arch, **2:**333-334, 333f-334f
Subscapular fossa, **1:**176f
Subscapularis muscle
anatomy of, **1:**180f
sectional anatomy of, **3:**271, 273-275, 273f-274f
Subtalar joint
anatomy of, **1:**236t, 237f, 238
Isherwood method for AP axial oblique projection of
with lateral rotation ankle, **1:**278, 278f
with medial rotation ankle, **1:**277, 277f
Isherwood method for lateromedial oblique projection with medial rotation foot of, **1:**276, 276f
Subtraction technique
DXA as, **3:**443, 477
for hip arthrography
digital, **2:**14, 15f
photographic, **2:**14, 15f
Sulci tali, **1:**229
Sulcus(i)
defined, **1:**84
sectional anatomy of, **3:**254-257, 256f

Index

Superciliary arch, **2:**261f
Superconductive magnets for MRI, **3:**346, 368
Superficial, **1:**85
Superficial femoral artery
    anatomy of, **3:**22f
    arteriography of, **3:**48f
Superficial inguinal nodes, **3:**27f
Superficial structures, ultrasonography of, **3:**383, 384f
Superimposition, **1:**5
    of coordinates in CT, **3:**304f
Superior, **1:**85
Superior articular process, **1:**368, 368f
Superior cistern, **3:**254, 258-260, 268, 268f
Superior mesenteric arteriogram, **3:**41f-42f, 44, 44f
Superior mesenteric artery (SMA)
    anatomy of, **3:**22f
    sectional anatomy of, **3:**284, 290, 290f, 298-299, 298f
    ultrasonography of, **3:**376f, 380, 380f
Superior mesenteric vein
    anatomy of, **2:**105f, **3:**22f
    sectional anatomy of, **3:**284-285, 290, 290f, 298-299
    ultrasonography of, **3:**377f
Superior nasal concha
    anatomy of, **2:**262, 262f
    sectional anatomy of, **3:**253
Superior orbital fissures
    anatomy of, **2:**257f, 265, 265f, 272f, 312f, 313
    PA axial projection of, **2:**298f
Superior orbital margin
    lateral projection of, **2:**317f
    PA axial projection of, **2:**298f
Superior ramus, **1:**327f, 328, 329f
Superior sagittal sinus
    anatomy of, **3:**22f
    sectional anatomy of, **3:**255
        on axial (transverse) plane, **3:**256-258, 256f-257f, 260-261
        on coronal plane, **3:**267, 267f
        on sagittal plane, **3:**264-265, 265f
Superior thoracic aperture, **1:**479, 479f
Superior vena cava
    anatomy of, **3:**22f, 24, 25f
    sectional anatomy of, **3:**271
        on axial (transverse) plane, **3:**273, 275-278, 276f
        on coronal plane, **3:**280-281, 281f
Superior vena cavogram, **3:**60, 60f
Superparamagnetic contrast agents for MRI, **3:**355, 368
Supertech trough filter, **1:**61f
Supertech wedge collimator-mounted Clear Pb filter, **1:**56f, 57
Supinate/supination, **1:**97, 97f
Supinator fat pad of elbow, **1:**107, 107f
Supine position, **1:**90, 90f
Supracondylar fracture, **3:**131, 131f
Supraorbital foramen, **2:**257f, 261, 261f
Supraorbital margins
    anatomy of, **2:**261, 261f
    lateral projection of, **2:**293f
Suprapatellar bursa, **1:**82f
Suprarenal glands
    anatomy of, **2:**183, 183f
    sectional anatomy of, **3:**283, 288-289, 288f-289f
    ultrasonography of, **3:**376f
Supraspinatus muscle
    anatomy of, **1:**179f
    sectional anatomy of, **3:**269f, 271, 273, 273f
Supraspinatus "outlet"
    AP axial projection of, **1:**203, 203f
    Neer method for tangential projection of, **1:**202-203, 202f
Surface coils in MRI, **3:**354, 354f

Surface landmarks, **1:**71, 71f, 71t
    with obese patients, **1:**47-49, 49f
Surgeon, **3:**215
Surgical angiography, **3:**74
Surgical assistant, **3:**215
Surgical attire, **3:**216
Surgical bed, **3:**480, 507
Surgical dressings, **1:**20
Surgical neck of humerus, **1:**104-105, 104f
Surgical neuroangiography, **3:**74
Surgical radiography, **3:**213-250
    aseptic techniques in, **3:**220, 220b
    attire for, **3:**217, 217f
    definition of terms for, **3:**250b
    equipment for, **3:**221, 221f-222f
        cleaning of, **3:**222
    fluoroscopic procedures in, **3:**223-241
        of cervical spine (anterior cervical diskectomy and fusion), **3:**227, 227f
        of chest (line placement, bronchoscopy), **3:**226, 226f
        femoral nailing as, **3:**233-235, 233f
            antegrade, **3:**233
            evaluation criteria for, **3:**235b
            method for, **3:**234, 234f-235f
            retrograde, **3:**234, 234f
            structures shown on, **3:**235, 235f
        femoral/tibial arteriogram as, **3:**240-241, 240f-241f
        of hip (cannulated hip screws or hip pinning), **3:**230-232, 230f-232f
        of humerus, **3:**238-239, 238f-239f
        of lumbar spine, **3:**228-229, 228f-229f
        operative (immediate) cholangiography as, **3:**223-225, 224f-225f
        tibial nailing as, **3:**236-237
            evaluation criteria for, **3:**237b
            position of C-arm for, **3:**236, 236f
            position of patient for, **3:**236
            structures shown on, **3:**237, 237f
    mobile, **3:**242-250
        of cervical spine, **3:**242, 242f-243f
        of extremities
            for ankle fracture, **3:**246f
            of ankle with antibiotic beads, **3:**247f
            for fifth metatarsal nonhealing fracture, **3:**249f
            for forearm fracture, **3:**247f
            for hip joint replacement, **3:**246f
            lower, **3:**246-250
            for tibial plateau fracture, **3:**247f
            for total shoulder arthroplasty, **3:**248f
            for wrist fracture, **3:**249f
        of thoracic or lumbar spine, **3:**244, 244f-245f
    personal hygiene in, **3:**217
    radiation exposure considerations in, **3:**223, 223f
    role of radiographer in, **3:**216
    scope of, **3:**214, 214b
    sterile field in
        contamination of, **3:**220
        image receptor handling in, **3:**219-220, 219f-220f
        maintenance of, **3:**218-220, 218f
Surgical suite, **3:**216f
Surgical team, **3:**214-216
    nonsterile members of, **3:**215f, 216
    sterile members of, **3:**215, 215f
Survey image of abdomen, **2:**87
Suspensory muscle of duodenum, **2:**100f, 101
Sustentaculum tali, **1:**229, 229f
Sutures, **1:**80f, 81, **2:**258f, 259, 275t
Sv (sieverts), **3:**458, 477
Swimmer's technique for lateral projection of cervicothoracic region, **1:**402-403, 402f-403f
    mobile, **3:**207

SXA (single energy x-ray absorptiometry), **3:**470, 475, 477
Symphysis, **1:**81, 81f
Symphysis pubis. *See* Pubic symphysis.
Synarthroses, **1:**81
Synchondrosis, **1:**81, 81f
Syndesmosis, **1:**80f, 81
Synostosis, **3:**132
Synovial fluid, **1:**82, 82f
Synovial joints, **1:**80t, 82, 82f-83f
Synovial membrane, **1:**82, 82f
Syringes for venipuncture, **2:**228-229, 228f
    recapping of, **2:**229, 229f
System noise in CT, **3:**340
Systemic arteries, **3:**23
Systemic circulation, **3:**23, 23f, 97
Systemic disease, **3:**480, 506
Systemic veins, **3:**24
Systole, **3:**97

T
T $\frac{1}{2}$ (half-life), **3:**403-404, 404f, 438
    in brachytherapy, **3:**485, 506
T (tesla) in MRI, **3:**343, 346, 368
T scores in DXA, **3:**457, 458t, 477
T1, **3:**344, 368
T1-weighted image, **3:**352, 352f-353f
T2, **3:**344, 368
T2-weighted image, **3:**352, 352f-353f
Table for CT, **3:**309-310, 309f
Table increments in CT, **3:**340
Table pad, **1:**19
Table speed in CT angiography, **3:**324, 340
Tachyarrhythmia, **3:**97
Tachycardia, **3:**97
Taeniae coli, **2:**102, 102f
Talipes equinovarus. *See* Clubfoot.
Tall patients, long bone studies in, **1:**28
Talocalcaneal articulation, **1:**236t, 237f, 238
Talocalcaneonavicular articulation, **1:**236t, 237f, 238
Talofibular joint, **1:**238
Talus, **1:**228f, 229
Tangential projection, **1:**86-87, 87f
Target in nuclear medicine, **3:**439
Targeted lesion, **3:**97
Tarsals
    anatomy of, **1:**228f-229f, 229
    trauma radiography of, **2:**52f
Tarsometatarsal (TMT) articulations, **1:**236f-237f, 236t, 238
Taylor method for AP axial outlet projection of anterior pelvic bones, **1:**358, 358f
TBI (total body iodine-123) scan, **3:**418
TBLH (total body less head) bone densitometry, **3:**477
TEA (top of ear attachment), **2:**268, 270f, 271, 285f
Teamwork, **3:**250
Technetium-99m (^{99m}Tc), **3:**404, 404f-405f, 406t
Technetium-99m (^{99m}Tc) ethylcysteinate dimer (ECD) for brain SPECT study, **3:**417
Technetium-99m (^{99m}Tc) hydroxymethylene diphosphonate (HDP) for bone scan, **3:**415
Technetium-99m (^{99m}Tc)-labeled red blood cells for radionuclide angiography, **3:**416
Technetium-99m (^{99m}Tc) mertiatide (MAG3) for dynamic renal scan, **3:**419
Technetium-99m (^{99m}Tc) microaggregated albumin (MAA) lung perfusion scan, **3:**419
Technetium-99m (^{99m}Tc) pertechnetate for thyroid scan, **3:**417
Technetium-99m (^{99m}Tc) sestamibi myocardial perfusion study, **3:**416

Technetium-99m (^{99m}Tc) sulfur colloid
　for liver and spleen scan, **3:**418
　for sentinel node imaging, **3:**420
Technical factors, **1:**42, 42f-43f
Teeth, **2:**59
Teletherapy, **3:**507
Temporal bones
　anatomy of, **2:**268, 268f-269f
　coronal CT through, **2:**269f
　location of, **2:**257f-259f
　mastoid portion of, **2:**268, 268f-270f
　　sectional anatomy of, **3:**253-254, 259f-260f,
　　　262, 268
　petrous portion of
　　anatomy of, **2:**268, 268f-270f
　　lateral projection of, **2:**293f
　　　in decubitus position, **2:**295f
　　location of, **2:**258f-259f
　　sectional anatomy of, **3:**253-254, 260f, 262,
　　　267-268
　sectional anatomy of, **3:**253-254, 258-260, 267f
　squamous portion of
　　anatomy of, **2:**268, 268f-269f
　　sectional anatomy of, **3:**253-254
　tympanic portion of
　　anatomy of, **2:**268, 268f
　　sectional anatomy of, **3:**253-254
　zygomatic arch of
　　anatomy of, **2:**273
　　AP axial projection of (modified Towne
　　　method), **2:**337, 337f-338f
　　submentovertical projection of, **2:**333-334,
　　　333f-334f
　　tangential projection of, **2:**335-336, 335f-336f
　zygomatic process of
　　anatomy of, **2:**268, 268f
　　sectional anatomy of, **3:**253-254
Temporal lobe, sectional anatomy of, **3:**253f,
　254-255
　on axial (transverse) plane
　　at Level C, **3:**258, 258f
　　at Level D, **3:**259-260
　　at Level E, **3:**260f, 261-262
　　at Level F, **3:**262f
　　at Level G, **3:**263f
　on sagittal plane, **3:**266, 266f
Temporal process of zygomatic bones, **2:**273, 273f
Temporal resolution for CT, **3:**318, 340
Temporalis muscle, sectional anatomy of, **3:**253f,
　255-256
　on axial (transverse) plane, **3:**257-262,
　　257f-259f
Temporomandibular joint (TMJ)
　anatomy of, **2:**268, 275, 275t
　AP axial projection of, **2:**347-348, 347f-348f
　axiolateral oblique projection of, **2:**345f,
　　351-352, 351f-352f
　axiolateral projection of, **2:**349-350
　　evaluation criteria for, **2:**350b
　　position of part for, **2:**349, 349f-350f
　　position of patient for, **2:**349
　　structures shown on, **2:**350f
　lateral projection of, **2:**293f
　panoramic tomography of mandible for,
　　2:353-354, 353f-354f
　sectional anatomy of, **3:**254
Temporomandibular joint (TMJ) syndrome, **2:**282t
Tendinitis, **1:**182t
Tentorium, **3:**3, 18
Tentorium cerebelli, sectional anatomy of, **3:**254
　on axial (transverse) plane, **3:**259-262, 261f
　on coronal plane, **3:**268, 268f
　on sagittal plane, **3:**266
Teres major muscle
　anatomy of, **1:**180f
　sectional anatomy of, **3:**271, 274f

Teres minor muscle
　anatomy of, **1:**180f
　sectional anatomy of, **3:**271, 273-275, 274f
Terminology
　body movement, **1:**96-97
　for positions, **1:**86b, 89-95
　for projections, **1:**86-89, 86b, 86f
Tesla (T) in MRI, **3:**343, 346, 368
Testicles. *See* Testis(es).
Testicular torsion, **2:**245t
Testis(es)
　anatomy of, **2:**242, 242f-243f
　ultrasonography of, **3:**383, 384f
Teufel method for PA axial oblique projection of
　acetabulum, **1:**354-355, 354f-355f
TFT (thin-film transistor), **1:**3
Thalamus, sectional anatomy of, **3:**253f, 258-259,
　264-265, 265f, 267f
Thallium-201 (^{201}Tl), **3:**406t
Thallium-201 (^{201}Tl) myocardial perfusion study,
　3:414, 414f, 416
Therapeutic nuclear medicine, **3:**420
Thermography of breast, **2:**473
Thermoluminescent dosimeters for CT, **3:**330, 330f
Thermoluminescent dosimetry (TLD) rings, **3:**407
Thin-film transistor (TFT), **1:**3
Third ventricle
　anatomy of, **3:**2, 4, 4f, 258
　sectional anatomy of, **3:**255
　　on axial (transverse) plane, **3:**258f
　　on coronal plane, **3:**267-268, 267f
　　on sagittal plane, **1:**331, **3:**267, 267f
Thoracic aortography, **3:**40, 40f, 55f
Thoracic cavity, **1:**68-69, 69f, 479, 479f
Thoracic curve, **1:**366f, 367
Thoracic duct, **3:**26, 27f
Thoracic inlet, **3:**269
Thoracic region, sectional anatomy of, **3:**269-281
　on axial (transverse) plane, **3:**272, 272f
　　at level A, **3:**272, 272f
　　at level B, **3:**273, 273f
　　at level C, **3:**274-275, 274f
　　at level D, **3:**275, 275f
　　at level E, **3:**275-277, 276f-277f
　　at level F, **3:**278, 278f
　　at level G, **3:**278, 279f
　on cadaveric image, **3:**269, 269f, 271f
　on coronal plane, **3:**280, 281f
　　at level A, **3:**280, 281f
　　at level B, **3:**280-281, 281f
　　at level C, **3:**281, 281f
　on sagittal plane, **3:**278-279, 279f
　　at level A, **3:**278-279, 280f
　　at level B, **3:**279, 280f
　　at level C, **3:**279-280, 280f
Thoracic vertebrae
　anatomy of, **1:**366f, 372-373, 373f
　　costal facets and demifacets in, **1:**372, 372f,
　　　373t
　　posterior oblique aspect in, **1:**372, 372f, 373t
　　superior and lateral aspects in, **1:**372, 372f
　　zygapophyseal joints in, **1:**373, 373f
　AP projection of, **1:**404-405, 404f-406f
　　for trauma, **2:**36-37, 36f-37f
　CT of, **1:**405, 406f
　intervertebral foramina of
　　anatomy of, **1:**372f-373f, 373
　　positioning rotations needed to show, **1:**371t
　lateral projection of, **1:**407-409
　　central ray for, **1:**408, 408f
　　evaluation criteria for, **1:**409b
　　improving radiographic quality of, **1:**409
　　position of part for, **1:**407, 407f-408f
　　position of patient for, **1:**407
　　structures shown on, **1:**409, 409f
　　for trauma, **2:**35, 35f

Thoracic vertebrae *(Continued)*
　mobile radiography in operating room of,
　　3:244
　MRI of, **3:**358f
　in radiography of sternum, **1:**456, 456f, 456t
　sectional anatomy of, **3:**269-270, 274-275,
　　278-280
　trauma radiography of
　　AP projection in, **2:**36-37, 36f-37f
　　lateral projections in, **2:**35, 35f
　upper
　　lateral projection of, swimmer's technique for,
　　　1:402-403, 402f-403f
　vertebral arch (pillars of)
　　AP axial oblique projection of, **1:**401,
　　　401f
　　AP axial projection of, **1:**399-400,
　　　399f-400f
　zygapophyseal joints of
　　anatomy of, **1:**372f-373f, 373
　　AP or PA oblique projection of, **1:**410-412
　　　in recumbent position, **1:**411-412,
　　　　411f-412f
　　　in upright position, **1:**410, 410f, 412f
　　　positioning rotations needed to show, **1:**371t
Thoracic viscera, **1:**477-519
　anatomy of, **1:**479-484
　　body habitus and, **1:**479, 479f
　　mediastinum in, **1:**483-484, 483f-484f
　　respiratory system in, **1:**479-482
　　　alveoli of, **1:**480f, 481
　　　bronchial tree of, **1:**480, 480b, 480f
　　　lungs of, **1:**481-482, 481f-482f
　　　trachea of, **1:**480, 480b, 480f
　　　summary of, **1:**484b
　　thoracic cavity in, **1:**479, 479f
　breathing instructions for, **1:**490, 490f
　CT of, **1:**484, 485f, **2:**55
　general positioning considerations for, **1:**488
　　for lateral projections, **1:**488, 489f
　　for oblique projections, **1:**488
　　for PA projections, **1:**488, 489f
　　for upright vs. prone position, **1:**488, 488f
　grid technique for, **1:**490, 491f
　heart as
　　AP oblique projection of, **1:**508-509
　　lateral projection with barium of, **1:**503
　　PA chest radiographs with barium of, **1:**499
　　PA oblique projection with barium of, **1:**507
　lungs as. *See* Lung(s).
　mediastinum as
　　anatomy of, **1:**483-484, 483f-484f
　　CT of, **1:**484, 485f
　　lateral projection of superior, **1:**494-495,
　　　494f-495f
　pleura as
　　AP or PA projection of, **1:**516-517,
　　　516f-517f
　　lateral projection of, **1:**518-519, 518f-519f
　sample exposure technique chart essential
　　projections for, **1:**487t
　SID for, **1:**490, 491f
　summary of pathology of, **1:**486t
　summary of projections for, **1:**478
　technical procedure for, **1:**490, 491f
　trachea as
　　anatomy of, **1:**480, 480b, 480f
　　AP projection of, **1:**492-493, 492f-493f
　　lateral projection of, **1:**494, 494f-495f
　　radiation protection for, **1:**492-493
Thoracolumbar spine, scoliosis of
　PA and lateral projections of (Frank et al.
　　method), **1:**437-438, 437f-438f
　PA projection of (Ferguson method), **1:**439-440
　　evaluation criteria for, **1:**439b-440b
　　first radiograph in, **1:**439, 439f

Thoracolumbar spine, scoliosis of (Continued)
  position of part for, **1:**439, 439f-440f
  position of patient for, **1:**439, 439f
  second radiograph in, **1:**439, 440f
  structures shown on, **1:**439-440,
    439f-440f
Thorax, bony. See Bony thorax.
Three-dimensional conformal radiotherapy (CRT),
  3:494, 506
Three-dimensional imaging
  of breast, **2:**374-375
  CT for, **3:**326-327, 327f
  ultrasonography for, **3:**372-373
Three-dimensional intraarterial angiography, **3:**34,
  34f
Three-dimensional MRI, **3:**351, 351f
Threshold values in shaded surface display, **3:**326,
  340
Thrombectomy, rheolytic, **3:**80t
Thrombogenesis, **3:**97
Thrombolytic, **3:**97
Thrombolytic therapy
  prior to cardiac catheterization, **3:**92
  interventional radiology for, **3:**72
Thrombosis, **3:**97
Thrombus, **3:**97
Through-transmission techniques for
  ultrasonography, **3:**371
Thumb
  anatomy of, **1:**101, 101f
  AP projection of, **1:**116
    evaluation criteria for, **1:**117
    position of part for, **1:**116, 116f
    position of patient for, **1:**116
    structures shown on, **1:**117, 117f
  first CMC joint of, **1:**118-119
    Burman method for AP projection of,
      1:120-121, 120f-121f
    Robert method for AP projection of,
      1:118-119
      evaluation criteria for, **1:**119b
      Lewis modification of, **1:**119
      Long and Rafert modification of,
        1:119
      position of part for, **1:**118, 118f
      position of patient for, **1:**118, 118f
      structures shown on, **1:**119, 119f
  folio method for PA projection of first
    MCP joint of, **1:**122, 122f-123f
  lateral projection of, **1:**116
    evaluation criteria for, **1:**117
    position of part for, **1:**116, 116f
    position of patient for, **1:**116
    structures shown on, **1:**117, 117f
  PA oblique projection of, **1:**117
    evaluation criteria for, **1:**117
    position of part for, **1:**117, 117f
    position of patient for, **1:**117
    structures shown on, **1:**117, 117f
  PA projection of, **1:**116
    evaluation criteria for, **1:**117
    position of part for, **1:**116f
    position of patient for, **1:**116
    structures shown on, **1:**117, 117f
Thymus gland, **1:**484, 484f
Thyroid cancer, iodine-131 for, **3:**420
Thyroid cartilage
  anatomy of, **2:**71-72, 71f-72f
  as surface landmark, **1:**71f, 71t
Thyroid gland
  anatomy of, **2:**71, 72f
  nuclear medicine imaging of,
    3:417-418
  sectional anatomy of, **3:**272, 272f
  ultrasonography of, **3:**375f, 383, 384f
Thyroid scan, **3:**417

Tibia
  anatomy of, **1:**230-231, 230f-231f
  AP oblique projections of, **1:**294-295,
    294f-295f
  AP projection of, **1:**290-291, 290f-291f
  lateral projection of, **1:**292-293, 292f-293f
Tibial arteriogram, **3:**240-241, 241f
Tibial collateral ligament, **1:**234f
Tibial nailing, surgical radiography of, **3:**236-237
  evaluation criteria for, **3:**237b
  position of C-arm for, **3:**236, 236f
  position of patient for, **3:**236
  structures shown on, **3:**237, 237f
Tibial plafond, **1:**231f
Tibial plateau(s), **1:**230, 230f
Tibial plateau fracture, surgical radiography of,
  3:247f
Tibial tuberosity, **1:**230, 230f
Tibiofibular joints, **1:**238
Tilt, **1:**97, 97f
Time of flight (TOF) imaging, **3:**363
TIPS (transjugular intrahepatic portosystemic
  shunt), **3:**72, 72f-73f
²⁰¹Tl (thallium-201), **3:**406t
²⁰¹Tl (thallium-201) myocardial perfusion study,
  3:414, 414f, 416
TLD (thermoluminescent dosimetry) rings,
  3:407
TMJ. See Temporomandibular joint (TMJ).
TMT (tarsometatarsal) articulations, **1:**236f-237f,
  236t, 238
TNM classification, **3:**483, 483t
Toddlers, development of, **3:**103
Toddler's fracture, **3:**130-131
Toes
  anatomy of, **1:**228-230, 228f
  AP axial projection of, **1:**242-249, 243f
  AP oblique projection of, **1:**245, 245f
  AP projection of, **1:**242-249, 243f
  display orientation of, **1:**11
  lateral projections of, **1:**246-249
    evaluation criteria for, **1:**249b
    for fifth toe, **1:**247, 247f, 249f
    for fourth toe, **1:**247, 247f, 249f
    for great toe, **1:**246f, 247, 248f
    position of part for, **1:**247
    position of patient for, **1:**246
    for second toe, **1:**246f, 247, 248f
    structures shown on, **1:**248-249
    for third toe, **1:**246f, 247, 249f
  PA projection of, **1:**244, 244f
  trauma radiography of, **2:**52f
TOF (time of flight) imaging, **3:**363
Tolerance doses to radiation, **3:**494, 494t
TomoTherapy, **3:**499, 500f
Tongue
  anatomy of, **2:**59, 59f, 97f
  sectional anatomy of, **3:**265, 265f
Tonsil
  palatine, **2:**59, 59f
  pharyngeal, **2:**71f, 72
Top of ear attachment (TEA), **2:**268, 270f, 271,
  285f
Torus fracture, **1:**109t, **3:**130
Total body iodine-123 (¹²³I) (TBI) scan, **3:**418
Total body less head (TBLH) bone densitometry,
  3:477
Total joint replacement in older adults, **3:**170,
  171f
Total shoulder arthroplasty, surgical radiography of,
  3:248f
Total-body dual energy x-ray absorptiometry,
  3:442f, 471, 472f
Tourniquet for venipuncture
  application of, **2:**232f, 233
  release of, **2:**233f

Towne method
  for AP axial projection of skull, **2:**44-45,
    44f-45f, 302-306
    central ray for, **2:**303f, 304
    in children, **3:**132, 135t
    evaluation criteria for, **2:**304b
    for pathologic condition or trauma, **2:**306,
      306f-307f
    position of part for, **2:**302, 303f
    position of patient for, **2:**302
    structures shown on, **2:**304, 305f
    variations of, **2:**302
  modified for AP axial projection of zygomatic
    arches, **2:**337, 337f-338f
Trabeculae, **1:**76, 76f
Trabecular bone
  and bone densitometry, **3:**445, 445t
  defined, **3:**477
  in osteoporosis, **3:**446f
Tracer, **3:**400, 405f, 439
Tracer principle, **3:**400
Trachea
  anatomy of, **1:**480, 480b, 480f, **2:**71f-72f
  AP projection of, **1:**492-493, 492f-493f
  lateral projection of, **1:**494, 494f-495f
  sectional anatomy of, **3:**269f, 270
    on axial (transverse) plane, **3:**272-275,
      272f-274f
    on coronal plane, **3:**280-281, 281f
    on sagittal plane, **3:**278-279, 280f
Tragus, **2:**270f, 271
Transabdominal ultrasonography of female pelvis,
  3:387-388, 387f
Transcatheter embolization, **3:**66-68
  in cerebral vasculature, **3:**68, 69f
  embolic agents for, **3:**66-67, 67b, 67t
  of hypervascular uterine fibroid, **3:**68, 69f
  lesions amenable to, **3:**66-67, 67b
  stainless steel occluding coils for, **3:**68, 68f
  vascular plug for, **3:**68, 68f
Transducer, **3:**97
  for ultrasonography, **3:**372, 372f, 398
Transesophageal transducer, **3:**396
Transfer
  of ill patients, **1:**15f, 22
  of obese patients, **1:**46, 46f
Transjugular intrahepatic portosystemic shunt
  (TIPS), **3:**72, 72f-73f
Transmission scan, **3:**402, 439
Transportation
  of obese patients, **1:**46, 46f
  of older adults, **3:**175
Transposition of the great arteries, **3:**97
Transthoracic projection, **1:**88
Transverse abdominal muscles, **3:**290-291, 293,
  293f
Transverse arch of foot, **1:**228-230, 228f
Transverse fracture, **1:**84f
Transverse plane, **1:**66, 66f-67f
  in MRI, **3:**343, 368
  pancreas in, **3:**380, 398
  in sectional anatomy, **3:**252
Transverse processes, **1:**368, 368f
Transverse sinus
  anatomy of, **3:**22f
  sectional anatomy of, **3:**255, 261-262, 268f
Transverse venous sinuses, **3:**262-263, 268
Trapezium
  anatomy of, **1:**101f-102f, 102
  Clements-Nakayama method for PA axial
    oblique projection of, **1:**144, 144f
Trapezius muscle, sectional anatomy of, **3:**269f,
  271
  on axial (transverse) plane, **3:**272-275, 272f,
    274f, 278
Trapezoid, **1:**101f-102f, 102

Trauma
  blunt, **2:**19
  defined, **2:**18
  explosive, **2:**19
  heat, **2:**19
  other imaging procedures for, **2:**53-55
    CT as, **2:**20, 29
      of cervical spine, **2:**53-55
      of cranium, **2:**29, 29f, 53-55, 54f
      of pelvis, **2:**53f, 55
      of thorax, **2:**53-55
    sonography as, **2:**55
  penetrating, **2:**19
  radiography of. *See* Trauma radiography.
  statistics on, **2:**18-19, 18f-19f
Trauma center, **2:**19
Trauma patients, handling of, **1:**22-23, 22f
Trauma radiography, **2:**17-56
  abbreviations used in, **2:**30b
  of abdomen, AP projection in, **2:**38-39, 38f-39f
    in left lateral decubitus position, **2:**40, 40f
  best practices in, **2:**28
  breathing instructions for, **2:**30
    with immobilization devices, **2:**30
  central ray, part, and image receptor alignment
    in, **2:**30
  of cervical spine
    AP axial oblique projection in, **2:**34,
      35f-36f
    AP axial projection in, **2:**33, 33f
    lateral projection in, **2:**31, 31f
  of cervicothoracic region, lateral projection in
    dorsal decubitus position in, **2:**32, 32f
  common projections in, **2:**29-30
  of cranium
    acanthioparietal projection (reverse Waters
      method) in, **2:**46, 46f
    AP axial projection (Towne method) in,
      2:44-45, 44f-45f
    and CT scan, **2:**29, 29f
    lateral projection in, **2:**42-43, 42f-43f
  documentation of, **2:**30
  exposure factors for, **2:**23, 23f
  grids and IR holders for, **2:**20
  image evaluation in, **2:**30
  image receptor size and collimated field for,
    2:30
  with immobilization devices, **2:**23, 23f, 28, 30
  of lower limb, **2:**50-53
    patient position considerations for, **2:**22f-23f,
      50
    structures shown on, **2:**52-53, 52f
    trauma positioning tips for, **2:**50, 50f
  overview of, **2:**18
  patient care in, **2:**26, 27t
  patient preparation for, **2:**29
  of pelvis, AP projection in, **2:**41, 41f
  positioning aids for, **2:**20
  positioning of patient for, **2:**24, 24f, 28
  radiation protection for, **2:**25
  specialized equipment for, **2:**20
    dedicated C-arm–type trauma radiographic
      room as, **2:**20f
    mobile fluoroscopic C-arm as, **2:**20, 21f
    Statscan as, **2:**20, 21f-22f
  standard precautions in, **2:**28
  of thoracic and lumbar spine
    AP projection in, **2:**36-37, 36f-37f
    lateral projections in, **2:**35, 35f
  of upper limb, **2:**47-49
    patient position considerations for, **2:**47-48
      for forearm, **2:**47, 47f-48f
      for humerus, **2:**49, 49f
      for shoulder, **2:**48, 48f-49f
    structures shown on, **2:**49, 49f
    trauma positioning tips for, **2:**47

Trauma team, radiographer's role as part of,
  2:25-26
Treatment fields in radiation oncology, **3:**491,
  492f-493f, 507
Trendelenburg position, **1:**90, 90f
Triceps muscle, **1:**180f
Tricuspid valve
  anatomy of, **3:**25f
  sectional anatomy of, **3:**270
Trigone, **2:**186, 186f
Tripod fracture, **2:**282t
Triquetrum, **1:**101f-102f, 102
Trochanter(s)
  AP projection of, **1:**337-339, 337f
  defined, **1:**84
Trochlea, **1:**229, 229f
Trochlear groove of femur, **1:**233, 233f
Trochlear notch, **1:**103, 103f-104f
Trochlear surface, **1:**228f, 229
Trochoid joint, **1:**82, 83f
Trough filter
  applications of, **1:**60, 60t, 61f
  example of, **1:**56f
  in position, **1:**55f
  shape of, **1:**57
True projections, **1:**89
T-tube cholangiography, **2:**176-177, 176f-177f
Tubercles, **1:**76, 84
Tuberculosis, **1:**486t
Tuberculum sellae
  anatomy of, **2:**258f, 264-265, 264f
  sectional anatomy of, **3:**253-254
Tuberosities, **1:**76, 84
Tumor(s), **3:**480
Tumor imaging, nuclear medicine for, **3:**420
Tumor/target volume, **3:**494, 507
Tunneled catheters in children, **3:**158, 158f
Twining method for mobile radiography of cervical
  spine, **3:**207
Tympanic cavity, **2:**270f, 271
Tympanic membrane, **2:**270f, 271

U
UGI (upper gastrointestinal) series. *See*
  Gastrointestinal (GI) series.
Ulcer, **2:**109t
  decubitus, in older adults, **3:**175
Ulcerative colitis, **2:**109t
Ulna, **1:**101f, 102-103, 103f
Ulnar artery
  anatomy of, **3:**22f, 49f
  arteriography of, **3:**46f
Ulnar styloid process, **1:**103, 103f
Ultrasonography, **3:**369-398
  of abdomen and retroperitoneum, **3:**376-383,
    376f-377f
  anatomic relationships and landmarks for, **3:**373,
    373f
  artifacts in, **3:**374, 375f
  of breast, **2:**418-419, **3:**375f, 383, 384f
  cardiologic applications of, **3:**393-396
    cardiac pathology in, **3:**393-396, 396f
    for congenital heart lesions, **3:**396
    procedure for echocardiography in, **3:**393,
      395f
  characteristics of image in, **3:**374, 374f-375f
  of children, **3:**156
  defined, **3:**370
  definition of terms for, **3:**397b-398b
  of gallbladder and biliary tree, **3:**373f, 378,
    379f
  gynecologic applications of, **3:**386-388
    anatomic features and, **3:**386, 386f
    endovaginal transducers for, **3:**375f, 388,
      388f, 397
  indications for, **3:**387

Ultrasonography (*Continued*)
  of ovaries, **3:**373f, 375f, 388, 389f
  transabdominal, **3:**387-388, 387f
  of uterus, **3:**387f-389f, 388
  historical development of, **3:**371
  intravascular, **3:**80t, 91, 91f-92f
  of kidneys and bladder, **3:**382-383, 382f
  of liver, **3:**373f-374f, 376f-378f, 378
  of musculoskeletal structures, **3:**383, 383f
  for neonatal neurosonography, **3:**385, 385f
  obstetric applications of, **3:**388-391
    in first trimester, **3:**388, 389f-390f
    history of, **3:**371
    in second trimester, **3:**390, 390f
    in third trimester, **3:**390-391, 391f
  of pancreas, **3:**377f, 380, 380f
  personnel for, **3:**370, 371f
  principles of, **3:**370-371
  properties of sound waves in, **3:**372, 372f
  quantitative, **3:**475, 475f, 477
  resource organizations for, **3:**371
  of spleen, **3:**376f, 381, 381f
  of superficial structures, **3:**383, 384f
  through-transmission techniques for, **3:**371
  transducer selection for, **3:**372, 372f
  of trauma, **2:**55
  vascular applications of, **3:**392-393, 392f,
    394f
  volume scanning and three-dimensional and
    four-dimensional imaging in, **3:**372-373
Ultrasound, defined, **3:**372, 398
Umbilical region, **1:**70f
Umbrella, **3:**97
Undifferentiation, **3:**484, 507
Unrestricted area, **3:**250
UPJ (ureteropelvic junction), **2:**185
Upper gastrointestinal (UGI) series.
  See Gastrointestinal (GI) series.
Upper limb, **1:**99-171
  abbreviations used for, **1:**109b
  anatomy of, **1:**101
    arm in, **1:**104-105, 104f
    articulations in, **1:**105-107, 105f-107f, 105t
    fat pads in, **1:**107, 107f
    forearm in, **1:**102-103, 103f
    hand in, **1:**101-102, 101f
    summary of, **1:**108b
    wrist in, **1:**101b, 102, 102f
  arteriography of, **3:**46, 46f
  in children, **3:**127-131
    with fractures, **3:**129-130, 130f-131f
    image evaluation for, **3:**123t, 131
    immobilization for, **3:**127-129, 127f, 129f
    radiation protection for, **3:**129, 129f
  elbow in
    articulations of, **1:**107, 107f
    fat pads of, **1:**107, 107f
    radiography of, **1:**151
  first digit (thumb) in
    anatomy of, **1:**101, 101f
    radiography of, **1:**116-122
  forearm in
    anatomy of, **1:**102-103, 103f
    radiography of, **1:**148-149
  general procedures for, **1:**110
  of geriatric patients, **3:**180, 180f
  hand in
    anatomy of, **1:**101-102, 101f
    articulations of, **1:**105-107, 105f-106f
    radiography of, **1:**124
  humerus in
    anatomy of, **1:**104-105, 104f
    distal
      anatomy of, **1:**104-105, 104f
      radiography of, **1:**165
    radiography of, **1:**167-171

Upper limb (*Continued*)
  long bone measurement of, **2:**2, 5, 5f
  MRI of, **3:**360-362, 362f
  olecranon process in
    anatomy of, **1:**103, 103f, 107f
    radiography of, **1:**166
  sample exposure technique chart essential
      projections for, **1:**108t
  second through fifth digits in
    anatomy of, **1:**101, 101f
    radiography of, **1:**110-111
  shielding gonads for, **1:**110, 110f
  summary of pathology of, **1:**109t
  summary of projections for, **1:**100
  surgical radiography of, **3:**246-250, 247f-249f
  trauma radiography of, **2:**47-49
    for humerus, **2:**49, 49f
    patient position considerations for, **2:**47-48
      for forearm, **2:**47, 47f-48f
      for shoulder, **2:**48, 48f-49f
    structures shown on, **2:**49, 49f
    trauma positioning tips for, **2:**47
  venography of, **3:**46, 46f
  wrist in
    anatomy in, **1:**101b, 102, 102f
    articulations of, **1:**105-107, 106f
    radiography of, **1:**132
Upper limb arteries, duplex sonography of,
    3:393
Upper limb veins, duplex sonography of, **3:**393
Upright position, **1:**87f, 90
Ureter(s)
  anatomy of, **2:**183f-184f, 186, 186f
  defined, **2:**183
  radiologic examination of, **2:**214
  retrograde urography of, **2:**212-213, 212f-213f
  sectional anatomy of, **3:**283, 292, 292f, 294,
    294f
Ureteral compression for excretory urography,
    2:200, 200f
Ureterocele, **2:**188t
Ureteropelvic junction (UPJ), **2:**185
Ureterovesical junction (UVJ), **2:**186
Urethra
  anatomy of, **2:**186f, 187
  defined, **2:**183
  radiologic examination of, **2:**214
  sectional anatomy of, **3:**283, 296, 296f-297f
Urethral orifice, **2:**240, 240f
Urethral stricture, **2:**192f
Urinary bladder
  anatomy of, **2:**186, 186f
  AP axial or PA axial projection of, **2:**216-217,
    216f-217f
  AP oblique projection of, **2:**218, 218f-219f
  cystography of. *See* Cystography.
  cystourethrography of
    female, **2:**222-224, 222f-223f
    male, **2:**221, 221f
    serial voiding, **2:**214, 215f
  defined, **2:**183, 186
  location of, **2:**183f-184f, 186
  MRI of, **3:**360
  sectional anatomy of, **3:**283
    on axial (transverse) plane, **3:**295, 295f
    on coronal plane, **3:**298, 298f-299f
    on sagittal plane, **3:**296, 297f
  ultrasonography of, **3:**382-383, 386f
Urinary incontinence in older adults, **3:**173, 174t
Urinary system, **2:**181-235
  abbreviations used for, **2:**189b
  anatomy of, **2:**183-187, 183f-184f
    kidneys in, **2:**183f-185f, 184-185
    prostate in, **2:**184f, 186f, 187
    summary of, **2:**187b
    suprarenal glands in, **2:**183, 183f

Urinary system (*Continued*)
    ureters in, **2:**183f-184f, 186, 186f
    urethra in, **2:**186f, 187
    urinary bladder in, **2:**183f-184f, 186, 186f
  angiography of, **2:**190, 191f
  AP oblique projection of, **2:**206, 206f
  AP projection of, **2:**204
    evaluation criteria for, **2:**205b
    position of part for, **2:**204
    position of patient for, **2:**204, 204f
    in prone position, **2:**204
    in semi-upright position, **2:**204, 205f
    structures shown on, **2:**204, 205f
    in supine position, **2:**204, 204f-205f
    in Trendelenburg position, **2:**204, 205f
  contrast studies of, **2:**190-197
    adverse reactions to iodinated media for,
      2:196
    angiographic, **2:**190, 191f
    antegrade filling for, **2:**191, 191f
    contrast media for, **2:**194, 195f
    CT in, **2:**190, 191f
    equipment for, **2:**198, 198f-199f
    physiologic technique for, **2:**192f, 193
    preparation of intestinal tract for, **2:**196-197,
      196f-197f
    preparation of patient for, **2:**197
    retrograde filling for, **2:**192f, 193
    tomography in, **2:**190, 191f
  CT of, **2:**190, 190f
  cystography of. *See* Cystography.
  cystoureterography of, **2:**193, 193f, 214
  cystourethrography of, **2:**193, 193f, 214
    female, **2:**222-224, 222f
      metallic bead chain, **2:**222-224, 223f
    male, **2:**221, 221f
    serial voiding, **2:**214, 215f
  image quality and exposure techniques for,
    2:199, 199f
  lateral projection of
    in dorsal decubitus position, **2:**208, 208f
    in R or L position, **2:**207, 207f
  motion control for, **2:**199
  nephrotomography of, **2:**190, 191f
    AP projection in, **2:**209, 209f
    percutaneous renal puncture for, **2:**210-211,
      210f
  overview of radiography of, **2:**190-201
  pelvicaliceal system in, retrograde urography of,
    2:212-213, 212f-213f
  preliminary examination of, **2:**201
  prostate
    anatomy of, **2:**184f, 186f, 187
    radiologic examination of, **2:**214
  pyelography of, **2:**191
    percutaneous antegrade, **2:**211, 211f
  radiation protection for, **2:**201
  renal parenchyma in, nephrotomography of,
    2:209-211
    AP projection for, **2:**209, 209f
    percutaneous renal puncture for, **2:**210-211,
      210f
  respiration for, **2:**200
  sample exposure technique chart essential
      projections for, **2:**189t
  summary of pathology of, **2:**188t
  summary of projections for, **2:**182-183
  ureteral compression for, **2:**200, 200f
  ureters in
    anatomy of, **2:**183f-184f, 186, 186f
    radiologic examination of, **2:**214
    retrograde urography of, **2:**212-213,
      212f-213f
  urethra in
    anatomy of, **2:**186f, 187
    radiologic examination of, **2:**214

Urinary system (*Continued*)
    urinary bladder in
      anatomy of, **2:**183f-184f, 186, 186f
      AP axial or PA axial projection of, **2:**216-217,
        216f-217f
      AP oblique projection of, **2:**218, 218f-219f
      cystourethrography of
        female, **2:**222-224, 222f-223f
        male, **2:**221, 221f
        serial voiding, **2:**214, 215f
      lateral projection of, **2:**220, 220f
      radiologic examination of, **2:**214
    urography of. *See* Urography.
    voiding study of, **2:**192f
Urography
  AP oblique projection for, **2:**206, 206f
  AP projection for, **2:**204
    evaluation criteria for, **2:**205b
    position of part for, **2:**204
    position of patient for, **2:**204, 204f
    in prone position, **2:**204
    in semi-upright position, **2:**204, 205f
    structures shown on, **2:**204, 205f
    in supine position, **2:**204, 204f-205f
    in Trendelenburg position, **2:**204, 205f
    in upright position, **2:**204, 204f
  defined, **2:**190
  equipment for, **2:**198, 198f-199f
  excretory (intravenous). *See* Excretory urography
    (EU).
  image quality and exposure technique for, **2:**199,
    199f
  intestinal tract preparation for, **2:**196-197,
    196f-197f
  lateral projection for
    in dorsal decubitus position, **2:**208, 208f
    in R or L position, **2:**207, 207f
  motion control for, **2:**199
  percutaneous antegrade, **2:**191
  preparation of patient for, **2:**197
  respiration during, **2:**200
  retrograde, **2:**192f, 193
    AP projection for, **2:**212-213, 212f-213f
    contrast media for, **2:**194, 195f
    defined, **2:**193
    preparation of patient for, **2:**197
  ureteral compression for, **2:**200, 200f
Useful patient dose in CT, **3:**340
Uterine fibroid, **2:**245t, 247f
  MRI of, **3:**361f
  transcatheter embolization for, **3:**68, 69f
Uterine ostium, **2:**240, 240f
Uterine tube(s)
  anatomy of, **2:**239, 239f-240f
  hydrosalpinx of, **2:**246f
  hysterosalpingography of, **2:**246-247, 246f-247f
  obstruction of, **2:**245t
  sectional anatomy of, **3:**284
Uterus
  anatomy of, **2:**240, 240f
  bicornuate, **2:**247f
  hysterosalpingography of, **2:**246-247, 246f-247f
  sectional anatomy of, **3:**284, 294, 294f, 296,
    297f
  ultrasonography of, **3:**386f-389f, 388
UVJ (ureterovesical junction), **2:**186
Uvula, **2:**59, 59f, 71f, 72

V
Vacuum bag immobilization device for radiation
    oncology, **3:**491f
Vacuum-assisted core biopsy of breast, **2:**470
Vagina
  anatomy of, **2:**240
  sectional anatomy of, **3:**284
  ultrasonography of, **3:**386f

Index

Vaginal orifice, **2:**240, 240f
Vaginal vestibule, **2:**240
Vaginography, **2:**246, 250-251, 250f-251f
Valium (diazepam), **2:**226t
Valsalva maneuver, **2:**72
Valvular competence, **3:**97
Varices
  defined, **3:**97
  esophageal, **2:**109t, 119, 119f
  venous, **3:**72
Vascular access devices in children, **3:**157, 157f-158f
Vascular access needles for angiographic studies, **3:**35, 35f
Vascular applications of ultrasonography, **3:**392-393, 392f, 394f
Vascular plug, **3:**68, 68f
Vascular procedures of CNS, **3:**14-16, 14f-15f
Vascular stent placement, percutaneous transluminal angioplasty for, **3:**65, 65f
  coronary, **3:**88, 89f
Vascular system. *See* Blood-vascular system.
Vasoconstricting drugs in transcatheter embolization, **3:**67-68
Vasoconstriction, **3:**97
VC (virtual colonoscopy), **2:**144, 145f, **3:**335, 335f
VCT. *See* Volume CT (VCT).
VCUG (voiding cystourethrogram), **2:**214, 215f
  in children, **3:**117, 117f
Veins, **3:**22f, 23
  coronary, **3:**25, 25f
  defined, **3:**97
  pulmonary, **3:**22f, 23
  systemic, **3:**24
Velocity of sound, **3:**372, 398
Venipuncture, **2:**225-235
  discarding needles after, **2:**234, 234f
  documentation of, **2:**235
  infection control during, **2:**228
  medication preparation for, **2:**229-230, 229f
    from bottle or vial, **2:**229, 229f
    identification and expiration date in, **2:**230, 230f
    nonvented tubing in, **2:**230, 230f
    recapping of syringe in, **2:**229, 229f
    tube clamp in, **2:**230, 230f
    vented tubing in, **2:**230, 230f
  medications administered via, **2:**225, 226t
  needles and syringes for, **2:**228-229, 228f
  patient assessment for, **2:**228
  patient education on, **2:**225
  professional and legal considerations for, **2:**225
  reactions to and complications of, **2:**235
  removing IV access after, **2:**234, 234f
  site preparation for, **2:**232, 232f
  site selection for, **2:**230-231, 231f
  technique for, **2:**232-234
    administering medication in, **2:**233-234, 233f
    anchoring needle in, **2:**233, 233f
    applying tourniquet in, **2:**232f, 233
    direct (one-step), **2:**232
    gloves and cleaning of area in, **2:**232f, 233
    indirect (two-step), **2:**232
    local anesthetic in, **2:**233
    releasing tourniquet in, **2:**233f
    stabilizing skin and entering vein in, **2:**233, 233f
    verifying venous access in, **2:**233
Venography, **3:**28, 60
  defined, **3:**97
  inferior venacavogram in, **3:**60, 60f
  peripheral
    lower limb, **3:**47, 48f
    upper limb, **3:**46, 46f
  superior venacavogram in, **3:**60, 60f

Venography *(Continued)*
  visceral, **3:**61
    hepatic, **3:**61, 61f
    portal, **3:**61, 61f
    renal, **3:**61, 61f
Venotomy, **3:**97
Venous insufficiency, ultrasonography of, **3:**393
Venous varices, **3:**72
Ventral, **1:**85
Ventral decubitus position, **1:**94, 95f
Ventral recumbent position, **1:**90, 90f
Ventricles
  cardiac
    anatomy of, **3:**24-25, 25f, 97
    sectional anatomy of, **3:**270, 271f
      on axial (transverse) plane, **3:**278, 278f-279f
      on coronal plane, **3:**280-281, 281f
      on sagittal plane, **3:**278-280, 280f
  cerebral
    anatomy of, **3:**2, 4, 4f
    sectional anatomy of, **3:**255
Ventricular function, echocardiography of, **3:**393
Ventricular system, **3:**2, 4, 4f
Ventriculography, left, **3:**82-84, 83f-84f
Ventriculomegaly, ultrasonography of, **3:**385f
Venules, **3:**23, 97
Vermiform appendix
  anatomy of, **2:**97f, 102, 102f
  sectional anatomy of, **3:**283
Vermis
  anatomy of, **3:**2, 18
  sectional anatomy of, **3:**255
Versed (midazolam hydrochloride), **2:**226t
Vertebra(e)
  defined, **1:**366
  false (fixed), **1:**366
  prominens, **1:**71f, 71t, 370
  true (movable), **1:**366
  typical, **1:**368, 368f
Vertebral arch
  anatomy of, **1:**368, 368f, 370
  AP axial oblique projection of, **1:**401, 401f
  AP axial projection of, **1:**399-400, 399f-400f
  sectional anatomy of, **3:**253, 272
Vertebral arteries
  anatomy of, **3:**49, 49f, 51
  arteriography of, **3:**51f
    AP axial projection for, **3:**59f
    AP projection for, **3:**52f
    lateral projection for, **3:**52f, 58f
  sectional anatomy of, **3:**255, 262-264, 262f-263f
  thoracic aortography of, **3:**55f
  transcatheter embolization of, **3:**68, 69f
Vertebral articulations, **1:**378-382, 378f, 379t
Vertebral canal, **1:**368
Vertebral column, **1:**363-444
  abbreviations used for, **1:**379b
  anatomy of, **1:**366-382, 366f
    cervical vertebrae in, **1:**369-371
    coccyx in, **1:**376f, 377
    lumbar vertebrae in, **1:**374-375, 375f
    sacrum in, **1:**376, 376f-377f
    summary of, **1:**379b
    thoracic vertebrae in, **1:**372-373, 373f
    typical vertebra in, **1:**368, 368f
    vertebral articulations in, **1:**378-382, 378f, 379t
    vertebral curvature in, **1:**367, 367f
  articulations of, **1:**378-382, 378f, 379t
  cervical vertebrae of. *See* Cervical vertebrae.
  coccyx of, **1:**376f, 377
  curvature of, **1:**366f-367f, 367
  defined, **1:**366
  functions of, **1:**366
  lumbar vertebrae in. *See* Lumbar vertebrae.

Vertebral column *(Continued)*
  sacrum of, **1:**376, 376f-377f
  sample exposure technique chart essential projections for, **1:**381t
  summary of pathology of, **1:**380t
  summary of projections for, **1:**364-366
    oblique, **1:**382t
  thoracic vertebrae of. *See* Thoracic vertebrae.
Vertebral curvature, **1:**366f-367f, 367
Vertebral foramen, **1:**368, 368f
Vertebral fracture assessment (VFA), **3:**469-470, 470f-471f, 477
Vertebral fracture(s) due to osteoporosis, **3:**449, 449f
Vertebral notches, **1:**368, 368f
Vertebrobasilar circulation
  AP axial projection for, **3:**59, 59f
  digital subtraction angiography of, **3:**15f
  lateral projection for, **3:**58-59, 58f
Vertebroplasty, **3:**16, 16f-17f, 18
  for osteoporotic fractures, **3:**449
Vertical plate of palatine bones, **2:**273
Vertical ray method for contrast arthrography of knee, **2:**12, 12f
Vesicoureteral reflux, **2:**188t
  in children, **3:**117-118, 117f
Vesicovaginal fistula, **2:**250, 250f
Vesiculography, **2:**253, 254f
Vessels, MRI of, **3:**363-364, 363f-364f
Vestibular folds, **2:**73, 73f
Vestibule of internal ear, **2:**271
VFA (vertebral fracture assessment), **3:**469-470, 470f-471f, 477
View, **1:**95
Viewbox, **1:**8
Villi, **2:**100f, 101
Viral pneumonitis, **1:**486t
Virtual colonoscopy (VC), **2:**144, 145f, **3:**335, 335f
Virtual simulations in radiation oncology, **3:**489, 492f
Visceral, **1:**85
Visceral arteriography, **3:**42-45, 42f
  celiac, **3:**43, 43f
  hepatic, **3:**43, 43f
  inferior mesenteric, **3:**44, 45f
  other, **3:**45
  renal, **2:**190, 191f, **3:**45, 45f
  splenic, **3:**44, 44f
  superior mesenteric, **3:**44, 44f
Visceral pericardium, **3:**24
Visceral peritoneum, **2:**83, 83f
Visceral pleura, **1:**482
Visceral venography, **3:**61
  hepatic, **3:**61, 61f
  portal, **3:**61, 61f
  renal, **3:**61, 61f
Vision in older adults, **3:**169
Vistaril (hydroxyzine hydrochloride), **2:**226t
Vitamin D and osteoporosis, **3:**450
Vitreous body, **2:**314f
VMAT (volumetric modulated arc therapy), **3:**496
Vocal cords, **2:**71f
  false, **2:**73, 73f
  true, **2:**71f, 73, 73f
Vocal folds, **2:**71f, 73, 73f
Voiding cystourethrogram (VCUG), **2:**214, 215f
  in children, **3:**117, 117f
Voiding study, **2:**192f
Volume CT (VCT), **3:**326-327
  defined, **3:**306-307
  multislice spiral CT for, **3:**323-324, 323f
  single-slice spiral CT for, **3:**321, 322f
Volume element (voxel), **3:**308, 308f, 340

Index

Volume rendering (VR), **3:**326-327
  defined, **3:**306-307
  multislice spiral CT for, **3:**323-324, 323f
  single-slice spiral CT for, **3:**321, 322f
Volume scanning, **3:**372-373
Volumetric density in DXA, **3:**453, 453f, 477
Volumetric modulated arc therapy (VMAT), **3:**496
Voluntary muscles, motion control of, **1:**19, 19f
Volvulus, **2:**109t
Vomer
  anatomy of, **2:**259f, 272f, 273
  sectional anatomy of, **3:**254
  submentovertical projection of, **2:**367f
Voxel (volume element), **3:**308, 308f, 340
VR. *See* Volume rendering (VR).

W
Waiting room for children, **3:**100, 100f-101f
Wallsten, Hans, **3:**20-21
Ward triangle, **3:**477
Warren, Stafford, **2:**372
Washout in nuclear medicine, **3:**419, 430f, 439
Waters method
  for facial bones, **2:**323, 323f-324f
    modified, **2:**304, 325f-326f
    reverse, **2:**327, 327f-328f
      with trauma, **2:**328, 328f
  for maxillary sinuses, **2:**362-363, 362f-363f
    in children, **3:**136, 136f
    open-mouth, **2:**364-365, 364f-365f
  modified
    for facial bones, **2:**304, 325f-326f
    for orbits, **2:**319, 319f
    open-mouth, for maxillary and sphenoidal
      sinuses, **2:**364-365, 364f-365f
  reverse
    for cranial trauma, **2:**46, 46f
    for facial bones, **2:**327, 327f-328f
      with trauma, **2:**328, 328f
Water-soluble, iodinated contrast media
  for alimentary canal imaging, **2:**111-112,
    111f-112f
  for large intestine studies, **2:**145
Wedge filter(s)
  applications of, **1:**60, 60t, 61f
  example of, **1:**56f
  in position, **1:**55f
  for radiation oncology, **3:**495, 495f, 507
  shape of, **1:**57
  specialized, **1:**62f, 63
Weight limits, **1:**44-45, 45t
Weight-bearing exercise and osteoporosis, **3:**450
Wellen method for double-contrast barium enema,
  2:152-153, 152f-153f
West Point method for inferosuperior axial
  projection of shoulder joint, **1:**196-197,
    196f-197f

Wheelchairs for obese patients, **1:**46, 46f
White matter
  anatomy of, **3:**2
  sectional anatomy of, **3:**256-257
Whole-body dual energy x-ray absorptiometry,
  3:442f, 471, 472f
Whole-body imaging in nuclear medicine, **3:**412,
  412f
Wilms tumor, **2:**188t
Window level (WL) in CT, **3:**312, 312t, 340
Window width (WW) in CT, **3:**312, 312t, 340
Windowing in CT, **3:**10, 312, 312f, 312t, 340
Wolf method for PA oblique projection of superior
  stomach and distal esophagus, **2:**136-137,
    136f-137f
Wrist, **1:**132
  anatomy of, **1:**102, 102f
  AP oblique projection in medial rotation of,
    1:137, 137f
  AP projection of, **1:**133, 133f
  articulations of, **1:**105-107, 106f
  bone densitometry of, **3:**475f
  display orientation of, **1:**11, 11f
  lateromedial projection of, **1:**134-135
    with carpal boss, **1:**135, 135f
    evaluation criteria for, **1:**135b
    position of part for, **1:**134, 134f
    position of patient for, **1:**134
    structures shown on, **1:**134-135, 134f-135f
  PA oblique projection in lateral rotation of,
    1:136, 136f
  PA projection of, **1:**132, 132f
    with radial deviation, **1:**139, 139f
    with ulnar deviation, **1:**138, 138f
  scaphoid of, **1:**140-141
    anatomy of, **1:**101f, 102
    Rafert-Long method for scaphoid series (PA
      and PA axial projections with ulnar
      deviation) of, **1:**142, 142f-143f
    Stecher method for PA axial projection of,
      1:140-141
  surgical radiography of, **3:**249f
  tangential projections of
    of carpal bridge, **1:**145
    Gaynor-Hart method for, **1:**146
      evaluation criteria for, **1:**147b
      inferosuperior, **1:**146, 146f-147f
      superoinferior, **1:**147, 147f
Wrist arthrogram, **2:**16, 16f
WW (window width) in CT, **3:**312, 312t, 340

X
Xenon-133 (^{133}Xe), **3:**406t
Xenon-133 (^{133}Xe) lung ventilation scan, **3:**419
Xerography of breast, **2:**372-373, 372f
Xeromammography, **2:**372, 372f
Xiphisternal joint, **1:**447f, 449t, 450

Xiphoid process
  anatomy of, **1:**447f, 448
  sectional anatomy of, **3:**256, 285, 285f
  as surface landmark, **1:**71f, 71t
X-ray beam, collimation of, **1:**32-33, 32f-33f

Y
Yellow marrow, **1:**76, 76f
Yolk sac, ultrasonography of, **3:**388,
  389f-390f

Z
Z scores in DXA, **3:**457, 477
Zenker diverticulum, **2:**109t
Zygapophyseal joints, **1:**368, 378, 378f, 379t
  cervical
    anatomy of, **1:**371, 371f, 371t
    positioning rotations needed to show, **1:**371,
      371t
  lumbar
    anatomy of, **1:**374, 374f-375f, 375t
    AP oblique projection of, **1:**421-422
      position of part for, **1:**421, 421f
      position of patient for, **1:**421
      positioning rotations needed to show,
        1:371t
    sectional anatomy of, **3:**269-270, 278-279,
      280f
  thoracic
    anatomy of, **1:**372f-373f, 373
    AP or PA oblique projection of, **1:**410-412
      in recumbent position, **1:**411-412,
        411f-412f
      in upright position, **1:**410, 410f, 412f
      positioning rotations needed to show,
        1:371t
Zygomatic arches
  anatomy of, **2:**273
  AP axial projection of (modified Towne method),
    2:337, 337f-338f
  parietoacanthial projection of, **2:**324f
  sectional anatomy of, **3:**263f, 264
  submentovertical projection of, **2:**333-334,
    333f-334f
  tangential projection of, **2:**335-336,
    335f-336f
Zygomatic bones
  acanthioparietal projection of, **2:**328f
  anatomy of, **2:**272f-273f, 273
  modified Waters method for parietoacanthial
    projection of, **2:**326f
  in orbit, **2:**275, 275f, 312f, 314f
  sectional anatomy of, **3:**254, 262
Zygomatic process
  anatomy of, **2:**268, 268f
  sectional anatomy of, **3:**253-254
Zygote, **2:**241